Fundamentals of EU Regulatory Affairs

Sixth Edition

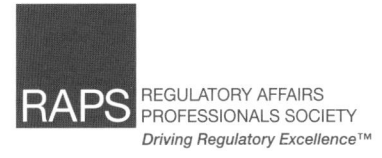
REGULATORY AFFAIRS PROFESSIONALS SOCIETY
Driving Regulatory Excellence™

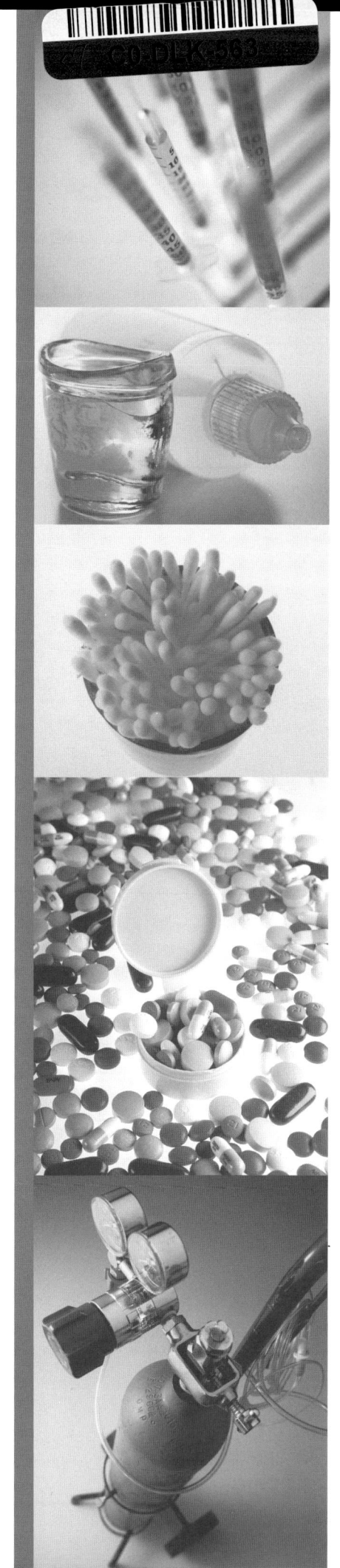

Copyright © 2012 by the Regulatory Affairs Professionals Society.
All rights reserved.

ISBN: 978-0-9829320-1-8

Every precaution is taken to ensure accuracy of content; however, the published cannot accept responsibility for the correctness of the information supplied. At the time of publication, all Internet references (URLs) in this book were valid. However, these references are subject to change without notice.

RAPS Global Headquarters
5635 Fishers Lane
Suite 550
Rockville, MD 20852
USA

RAPS.org

■ NORTH AMERICA ■ EUROPE ■ ASIA

Foreword

The European Union, in accordance with its mandate to eliminate trade barriers between Member States, presents a constantly evolving regulatory environment for healthcare products. Movement toward further harmonisation within the EU and internationally makes it imperative for regulatory professionals to stay current on the latest legislative developments while continously monitoring changes in science and technology that could impact their companies' products.

Fundamentals of EU Regulatory Affairs, Sixth Edition, includes the latest information on EU directives, regulations and guidelines on human and veterinary medicinal products, biologics, medical devices, cosmetics and food supplements, and applicable international standards and guidances.

Several new chapters have been added to this edition that deal with issues of growing importance to EU regulatory professionals. These include reimbursement and the health technology assessments that frequently are the basis for reimbursement decisions. There also is a new chapter on crisis management and one on the special requirements for vaccines. In light of the new legislation in effect in 2012, there also is a chapter devoted to pharmacovigilance.

This edition of *Fundamentals* has been organised into four sections:
- **Section I:** General Information—topics that are applicable across a range of product lines, including a history of EU regulation, crisis management, reimbursement, health technology assessment, paediatric requirements, advertising and promotion, and enforcement and national authorities
- **Section II:** Medical Devices—updated with an eye to the recast of the medical devices directives currently under discussion, covering the legal system, classification, conformity assessments, clinical evaluation, postmarket compliance and varying national regulatory requirements for all device classes
- **Section III:** Medicinal Products—clinical trials, authorisation and registration procedures, quality systems and inspectorate processes, postmarket compliance and pharmacovigilance for prescription, generic and nonprescription products
- **Section IV:** Other Product Classifications—blood and plasma products, tissue products, vaccines, orphan products, combination products, cosmetics, foot supplements and veterinary medicinal products

The text is supplemented by a comparative matrix of directives, regulations and guidelines that spans product lines, a glossary of terms and an extensive index.

Fundamentals is designed to be a reference resource for regulatory professionals at all levels—from those new to the field or preparing for to take the EU RAC exam, to senior management looking for a quick fact or information on a less-familiar product line.

Pamela A. Jones
Senior Editor
Regulatory Affairs Professionals Society

Acknowledgements

The Regulatory Affairs Professionals Society (RAPS) extends its thanks to the following individuals for sharing their expertise in this publication, helping to further the regulatory profession and their colleagues.

Mujadala Abdul-Majid, JD, RAC
Associate, Health Care & Life Sciences
Epstein Becker and Green, PC
Washington, DC, USA

Gordon Bache, PhD, MA, LLB
Associate Consultant, Commercialization
PAREXEL International Consulting
Uxbridge, UK

Nicole Beard. MSc, PhD
Head, Regulatory Affairs International
BiogECHO S.A.R.L.
Carouge, Switzerland

Martha Anna Bianchetto, PharmD, MBA
P & MD Consultants
Venezia, Italy

M. Jason Brooke, MSE, JD
Associate, Health Care & Life Sciences
Epstein Becker & Green, PC
Washington, DC, USA

Jill M.E. Bunyan, PhD, MRPharmS, MTOPRA, MIOS
Regulatory Affairs Consultant
Isle of Man, UK

Gudrun Busch, MSc, PhD, MTOPRA, RAC
Dr. Busch Regulatory Strategy GmbH
Norderstedt/Hamburg, Germany

Rick Clayton, DipM, MTOPRA
Technical Director
International Federation for Animal Health–Europe
Brussels, Belgium

Shailesh S. Dewasthaly
VP, Toxicology
Intercell AG
Vienna, Austria

Martin Gisby, PhD, MRes
Manager, Commercialization
PAREXEL International Consulting
Uxbridge, UK

Claudia Ising, RAC
Head of Regulatory Affairs
Lohmann & Rauscher GmbH & Co. KG
Neuwied, Germany

Gautam Maitra
Head of Regulatory and External Affairs
AC Immune SA
Lausanne, Switzerland

Andrea Martter, RAC
Senior Reguatory Affairs Sepcialist
GOJO Industries
Akron, OH, USA

Salma Michor, PhD, MBA, CMgr, RAC
CEO & Principal Consultant
Michor Consulting e.U.
Vienna, Austria

Tom Padula
VP, Regulatory Compliance
Schiff & Company Inc.
West Caldwell, NJ, USA

Alexander Roussanov
Associate
Hogan Lovells International LLP
Brussels, Belgium

Rodney Ruston, RAC, FRAPS
Director
Priory Analysts Ltd.
Milton Keynes, UK

Robert Schiff, PhD, CQA, RAC, FRAPS
CEO
Schiff & Company Inc.
West Caldwell, NJ, USA

Erik Vollebregt
Partner
Axon Lawyers
Amsterdam, Netherlands

Elisabethann Wright
Partner
Hogan Lovells International LLP
Brussels, Belgium

Isabel Zwart, PhD
Consultant
PAREXEL International Consulting
Uxbridge, UK

Table of Contents

Section I: General Information
Chapter 1   EU Regulatory Affairs—An Historic Perspective 1
Chapter 2   Crisis Management 17
Chapter 3   Reimbursement in the EU 23
Chapter 4   Health Technology Assessment 31
Chapter 5   The Paediatric Regulation 41
Chapter 6   Advertising and Promotion 49
Chapter 7   Enforcement and National Authorities 57

Section II: Medical Devices
Chapter 8   The European Medical Devices Legal System 65
Chapter 9   Classification of Medical Devices 87
Chapter 10   Technical Requirements for Conformity Assessment 93
Chapter 11   Clinical Evaluation of Medical Devices 99
Chapter 12   Conformity Assessment Procedures' Quality System Requirements 107
Chapter 13   In Vitro Diagnostic Medical Devices 119
Chapter 14   Active Implantable Medical Devices 129
Chapter 15   Medical Device Compliance: Postmarket Requirements 133
Chapter 16   Medical Device National Particularities 143

Section III: Medicinal Products
Chapter 17   Overview of Authorisation Procedures for Medicinal Products 151
Chapter 18   Medicinal Product Clinical Trials 169
Chapter 19   Registration Procedures for Medicinal Products 183
Chapter 20   Quality Systems and Inspectorate Process—Medicinal Products 197
Chapter 21   Generic Medicinal Products 205
Chapter 22   Nonprescription Medicinal Products 213
Chapter 23   Marketing Authorisations for Products Derived From Biotechnology 221
Chapter 24   Pharmaceutical Postmarket Requirements and Compliance With the Marketing Authorisation 231
Chapter 25   Pharmacovigilance 241

Section IV: Other Product Classifications
Chapter 26   Products Manufacturers From Human Blood or Plasma 247
Chapter 27   Human Tissue Regulation 255
Chapter 28   Vaccines 269
Chapter 29   Orphan Medicinal Products 283
Chapter 30   Combination Products 293
Chapter 31   Cosmetic Products 301
Chapter 32   Food Supplements, Health Claims and Borderline Issues 311
Chapter 33   Veterinary Medicinal Products 319

Appendices

Comparative Matrix of Regulations, Directives and Guidelines Across Product Lines 343
Glossary of Terms 379
Index 389

Figures

Figure 2-1	Crisis as a Trigger for Change	19
Figure 4-1	Phased Approach to Evaluation of a Health Technology	33
Figure 5-1	Paediatric Investigation Plan (PIP) Approval Process	44
Figure 8-1	EU Legislative Procedure	67
Figure 8-2	Flow Chart for the Conformity Assessment Procedures Provided for in Directive 94/42/EEC on Medical Devices	68
Figure 8-3	Flow Chart for the Conformity Assessment Procedures Provided for in Directive 90/385/EEC on Active Implantable Medical Devices	71
Figure 8-4	Flow Chart for the Conformity Assessment Procedures Provided for in Directive 98/79/EC on In Vitro Diagnostic Medical Devices	72
Figure 8-5	Clinical Evaluation Cycle	79
Figure 11-1	Clinical Evaluation Flow Diagram for all Device Types	101
Figure 11-2	The Clinical Evaluation Process	104
Figure 12-1	CAPS for Active Implantable Medical Devices	109
Figure 12-2	CAP Risk Class I Medical Devices	112
Figure 12-3	CAPs for Risk Class IIa Medical Devices	113
Figure 12-4	CAPs for Risk Class IIb Medical Devices	113
Figure 12-5	CAPs for Rick Class III Medical Devices	114
Figure 12-6	CAP for all In Vitro Medical Devices	115
Figure 12-7	CAPS for Self-testing In Vitro Medical Devices	115
Figure 12-8	CAPS for Annex II List B In Vitro Medical Devices	116
Figure 12-9	CAPS for Annex II List A In Vitro Medical Devices	116
Figure 13-1	Flowchart for the CAPs Provided for in Directive 98/79/EC	123
Figure 18-1	Commencement of a Clinical Trial	172
Figure 18-2	Serious Adverse Event Reporting	175
Figure 28-1	OCABR Decision Flowchart	275
Figure 28-2	Process for Production and Licensing of Seasonal Influenza Vaccines in Europe	278
Figure 29-1	Orphan Designation Criteria	289
Figure 30-1	Consultation Procedure and Timeline	298

Tables

Table 4-1	REA Checklist	37
Table 8-1	European Council Weighted Votes	66
Table 8-2	New Approach Areas	73
Table 8-3	EU Member States and Affiliated Countries Competent Authorities	74
Table 8-4	European Commission Working Groups and Their Activities	76
Table 8-5	European Industrial Trade Associations	78
Table 8-6	MEDDEV Guidance Documents	80
Table 8-7	European Commission Consensus Statements	82
Table 8-8	Interpretive Documents Issues by the European Commission	83
Table 8-9	NBOG Documents	84
Table 10-1	Essential Requirement Checklist: Example (MDD (Directive 93/42/EEC), as amended—Annex I)	95
Table 10-2	Hierarchy of Compliance Document for Technical Documentation	96
Table 11-1	Abbreviations, Definitions and Terms Used in This Chapter	102
Table 12-1	Conformity Assessment Documentation	110
Table 12-2	International Production Control	117
Table 12-3	EC Type-examination	117

Table 12-4	Production Quality Assurance	117
Table 12-5	Product Quality Assurance	117
Table 12-6	Product Verification	117
Table 12-7	Full Quality Assurance System	117
Table 12-8	Authorised Representative in Conformity Assessment	118
Table 13-1	Examples of General Laboratory Use Products and IVD Medical Devices	121
Table 14-1	Comparison of AIMDD and MDD Annexes	130
Table 15-1	Eudamed Data Repository	137
Table 15-2	Comparison of Safeguard Clause and Health Monitoring Measures	140
Table 16-1	Relevant Authorities in Germany	149
Table 17-1	Standard Timetable for Evaluation of a Centralised Appliation	156
Table 17-2	Mutual Recognition Procedure Flowchart	160
Table 17-3	Decentralised Procedure Flowchart	163
Table 18-1	Practical Notes for Clinical Trials	171
Table 19-1	Procedures to Obtain MA	187
Table 19-2	Centralised Procedure	188
Table 19-3	Mutual Recognition Procedure	189
Table 19-4	Decentralised Procedure	190
Table 19-5	A Comparison of the Centralised, Decentralised and Mutual Recognition Procedures	193
Table 22-1	Legal Classification Status of Selected Ingredients in the EU	216
Table 26-1	Medicinal Products Derived From Human Plasma and Their Indications	249
Table 27-1	Donor Testing for Infectious Diseases	259
Table 28-1	Vaccine Guidelines	272
Table 28-2	Adjuvants Licensed in the EU	274
Table 28-3	European Guidelines for Influenza Vaccines	276
Table 28-4	Some Organisations Involved in Vaccine Recommendations in the EU	280
Table 29-1	Comparison of the EU and US Orphan Programmes	286
Table 31-1	Annexes to the Cosmetics Directive and Cosmetic Regulation	305
Table 31-2	Ingredient Nomenclature for Labels	308
Table 32-1	Vitamins and Minerals That May Be Declared and Their Recommended Daily Allowances (RDAs)	313
Table 33-1	Legislative Framework for Registration of Veterinary Medicinal Products Within the EEA	321
Table 33-2	Competent Authorities for the Regulation of Veterinary Medicinal Products in the EEA	330
Table 33-3	Food-producing Species	334
Table 33-4	MUMS Guidelines	337

Chapter 1

EU Regulatory Affairs—An Historic Perspective

Updated by Salma Michor, PhD, MBA, CMgr, RAC

OBJECTIVES

❏ Learn why healthcare regulations for medicinal products and devices were established

❏ Discover the key historical milestones leading to today's healthcare regulations

❏ Understand the major regulations governing medicinal products and medical devices in the European Union (EU)

REGULATIONS AND GUIDELINES COVERED IN THIS CHAPTER

❏ Council Directive 65/65/EEC of 26 January 1965 on the approximation of provisions laid down by law, regulation or administrative action relating to medicinal products, the first European medicinal product directive

❏ Directive 2001/83/EC of the European Parliament and of the Council of 6 November 2001 on the Community code relating to medicinal products for human use

❏ Council Directive 89/432/EEC of 12 June 1989 on the introduction of measures to encourage improvements in the safety and health of workers at work, the first European biologic product directive

❏ Regulation 1394/2007/EC of the European Parliament and of the Council of 13 November 2007 on advanced therapy medicinal products and amending Directive 2001/83/EC and Regulation (EC) No 724/2004

❏ Council Directive 81/851/EEC of 28 September 1981 on the approximation of the laws of the Member States relating to veterinary medicinal products, the first European veterinary product directive

❏ Council Directive 93/42/EEC of 14 June 1993 concerning medical devices

❏ Council Directive 2007/47/EC of the European Parliament and of the Council of 5 September 2007 amending Council Directive 90/385/EEC on the approximation of the laws of the Member States relating to active implantable medical devices, the Council Directive 93/42/EEC concerning medical devices and Directive 98/8/EC concerning the placing of biocidal products on the market

Introduction

Every regulatory system's history provides insight into the circumstances that existed at the time it was established and sheds light on the system's current objectives. Compared to regulation of other industries, regulation of medicinal products in the EU is relatively recent. Medicinal product regulations and regulatory activities were not established until the second half of the 20th century. In common with other regions, the main goal of all European regulatory systems is keeping unsafe products out of the marketplace. Therefore, regulations were established to approve medici-

Regulatory Affairs Professionals Society

nal product Marketing Authorisation Applications (MAAs) and monitor those products in the postauthorisation stage.

A single EU market meets the various interests of healthcare providers, industry and consumers, although the involved parties' viewpoints may differ. Providers and reimbursement bodies focus on minimising healthcare costs, whereas consumers demand easy access to a broad range of safe and effective products and treatments without necessarily considering the cost implications. Industry prefers a regulatory system that enables an "approved once, accepted everywhere" approach to reduce the time and cost of multiple registrations resulting from heterogeneous national requirements; i.e., if a country approves a product on the basis of its regulatory system, then other countries should accept the product without further testing or application review.

This chapter simplifies the complex subject of EU medicinal product regulations. After briefly describing the history of EU healthcare regulations, it summarises those governing today's medicinal product industry.

Historic Factors in the Development of Medicinal Product Regulations

Healthcare regulations have their beginnings in ethics. Their main objective was to protect individuals against unethical and unsafe human trials. The need for ethical standards stemmed from the inhumane practices of infamous Nazi physician Josef Mengele during World War II. However, prior to those experiments, research-oriented physicians had conducted private clinical trials that exceeded the bounds of common ethical standards. For example, the first vaccine trials were performed without any regulatory supervision and the results were never published. Although these first human experiments were subject to internal ethical discussions by healthcare professionals, they were not regulated officially. Press reports about research incidents sensitised the public to the need for healthcare regulations to protect public safety. Therefore, by the early 20th century, the public increasingly viewed medicines and surgery not as treatments for illness but as sources of injury and failure if not used properly.

The first European healthcare regulations concerned the ethical treatment of human subjects and were promulgated midway through the 20th century. The *Helsinki Declaration* in 1964 set forth ethical standards for the first time. Subsequently, laws were passed regulating which products could be placed on the market and the claims manufacturers could make about those products. Today, medicinal product regulations not only target ethical, safety and efficacy concerns but also address economic issues, increased availability of information, continuing technological and product innovations, market structure changes and the groundswell of consumer activism.

Consequences of Unsafe Products

Certain safety incidents have been catalysts for medicinal product regulations. The thalidomide scandal in Europe and Canada was a milestone in the development of pharmaceutical product regulations. In the late 1950s, the German pharmaceutical company Grünenthal launched Contergan, a sedative containing thalidomide that also was used to treat morning sickness. Contergan was advertised by the company as "atoxic," "without danger" and "non-poisonous." Soon after the product was introduced, thousands of babies were born with malformations, particularly to their limbs; the deformities soon were associated with thalidomide. In 1961, the turnover through Contergan reached its sales zenith with 1.3 million deutsche mark per day. In 1961–62, the link to Contergan was officially established; this was the peak of the Contergan scandal. At the time, no premarket reproductive toxicity testing was legally required, so the teratogenic potential of new medicinal products was unknown prior to marketing authorisation (MA).

Awareness of the potential transmission of bovine spongiform encephalopathy (BSE, also known as "mad cow disease") and transmissible spongiform encephalopathy (TSE) to humans during the 1990s led to heightened legislative activity to regulate medicinal products containing bovine-derived materials. In the early 1990s, cases of BSE were reported in the UK, as were a growing number of new forms of Creutzfeldt-Jakob disease (i.e., TSE), the human equivalent of BSE. Suspicions that these cases were associated with consuming BSE-infected beef led to dramatic export restrictions on British beef, resulting in significant economic impact on British farmers. The crisis led to amended medicinal products regulations because many products contain ingredients derived from bovine material (e.g., lactose, gelatine and magnesium stearate). One example of this type of regulation is Directive 2003/32/EC,[1] which is designed to reduce the risks of transmitting TSE to patients under normal conditions via medical devices manufactured with animal tissue.

Economic Issues

Although public health protection is the primary driver of healthcare regulation, economic considerations also began to have an impact in the second half of the 20th century. With the establishment of the first health insurance system, it became obvious that the growing availability and number of healthcare products would lead to increased costs for EU Member States because of higher medicinal product consumption and the subsequent rise in risks of side effects and misuse. The transfer of healthcare costs from individual consumers to private or public insurance systems necessitated product pricing transparency. It quickly became clear that limited economic resources had to be spent prudently. Awareness of healthcare's economic limits continues to build.

Availability of Information

Triggered by the media and supported by such worldwide communication systems as the Internet, medicinal product information is available almost immediately to virtually everyone. This information, both good and bad, can no longer be controlled or presented in an appropriate context by industry. For example, entering the word "Ritalin" into a common search engine may provide numerous hits, including some from anti-Ritalin activist groups fighting the drug's use in children with attention deficit hyperactivity disorder. In view of the extensive and often inaccurate material available to consumers, maintaining public confidence in the healthcare system necessitates timely and appropriate regulations that ensure medicinal product quality, safety and efficacy and clear instructions for use.

Product Innovations

Tremendous technological advances have made many novel therapies available. Such new developments as biologics, blood products and in vitro diagnostics initially entered a market and a regulatory system that were not prepared for them. For example, the introduction of recombinant products led to implementation of the Concertation Procedure in 1987, in which Member States agreed to conduct a common MAA dossier assessment; this enabled Member States to collaborate across borders. This need to share expertise has driven the regulation development process.

Innovative product developers may both benefit from and exploit the existence of a "regulatory vacuum," as some areas still lack adequate regulations. Consequently, manufacturers can become involved in defining the regulatory framework of a new area and influence public and official opinion.

Changes in the Market Structure

Removal of trade barriers within the EU is another factor influencing healthcare regulations. The markets have been opened to products from many sources, and product quality control is an increasing concern. For example, importing single-use products (e.g., injection needles) signalled the need to include medical devices in existing medicinal product laws and regulations. Problems arose with imported products because manufacturers in the exporting countries were not fully governed by the importing country's product regulations. The range of European healthcare regulations—from practically none for certain products in some countries to well-defined frameworks in other countries—had to be brought under the same regulatory umbrella. This need led to a new product regulation approach.

Consumer Advocacy

Regulatory authorities consider safety to be of paramount importance. They ensure that adequate safety data are generated through clinical trials to support authorisation and that these data are monitored throughout the product's postauthorisation lifecycle. They also promptly communicate any safety profile changes to the public when concerns arise—all while ensuring that products are available to patients in a timely manner.

Consumers' perceptions of health and healthcare have changed. The economic prosperity of most European countries has led to expectations of improved quality of life, improved survival rates and longevity, and a growing demand for not only the treatment and prevention of illness, but also improvements in consumers' general well-being. This demand also drives new regulations.

Healthcare professionals who direct the use of healthcare products and the consumers of these products have divergent interests. Providers focus on reimbursement for services, whereas consumers want to protect their health by using products of maximum safety. Healthcare providers are subject to increased oversight by newly empowered consumers. Consumers are increasingly well educated and informed about health and health products and services, and are not afraid to challenge companies and regulatory and enforcement authorities.

Evolution of Current Regulations

Europe is the world's second-largest pharmaceutical market and is highly regulated. Since the adoption of the first pharmaceutical directive in 1965, European pharmaceutical legislation has consistently pursued two objectives: protection of public health and free movement of products among the Member States. The approval criteria and procedures for human medicines, as well as several other important aspects of pharmaceutical legislation, have been extensively harmonised within the EU. European pharmaceutical legislation now covers all industrially manufactured medicines, including vaccines, blood derivatives, biopharmaceuticals and homeopathic medicines.

The following legal framework for medicinal products for both human and veterinary use is available as a series of volumes entitled, *The Rules Governing Medicinal Products in the European Union,* published by the European Commission:[2]

- pharmaceutical legislation (directives, regulations, decisions and other communications of the European Council and the European Commission)
- *Notice To Applicants* describing administrative procedures for MAs and the MAA dossier format including:
  o MA submission procedures
  o dossier presentation and content (including the Common Technical Document (CTD) and electronic Common Technical Document (eCTD))
  o regulatory guidelines

- guidelines on conducting recommended quality, safety and efficacy studies to support an MAA; the subgroups are:
  - quality and biotechnology
  - safety, environment and information
  - efficacy (clinical guidelines)
- detailed Good Manufacturing Practice (GMP) guide
- detailed drug monitoring (pharmacovigilance) guide

The aforementioned legislation consists of directives, which are to be incorporated into each Member State's national laws; regulations that are directly applicable in each Member State; and notes for guidance, which are nonbinding texts to help applicants fulfil regulatory approval obligations to place medicinal products on the market. National regulatory authorities frequently use the notes for guidance and other European nonbinding guidelines to interpret their own national laws.

Medicinal Products for Human and Veterinary Use

The first regulations governing medicinal products for human use came into force in the early 1960s. The Contergan catastrophe was the driving force for the first European medicinal product directive: Council Directive 65/65/EEC[3] (later codified into the unified Directive 2001/83/EC, as amended). For the first time, detailed MA requirements for medicinal products for human use were described and applicable across the European Community. The directive reflects many of the requirements established by the US Food and Drug Administration (FDA). By the 1970s, the directive had been incorporated into the national laws of all Member States. The directive also regulated the registration of medicinal products already marketed in Member States.

Council Directive 75/318/EEC (later codified into the unified Directive 2001/83/EC in Article 8(3)(a)–(i) and Article 10a) defined legal requirements relating to MAA analytical, pharmacotoxicological and clinical documentation. Scientific and technological progress have been reflected in supplemental amendments to the directives, such as the amendment involving requirements for minimising TSE contamination risks, among others.

In 1991, Directive 91/356/EEC[4] described GMP principles, which Member States incorporated into their regulations over the next 10 years. Prescription status (Directive 92/26/EEC, later codified into the unified Directive 2001/83/EC as Articles 70–75), medicinal product labelling and package leaflets (Directive 92/27/EEC, later codified into the unified Directive 2001/83/EC as Articles 54–69) and medicinal product advertising (Directive 92/28/EEC, later codified into the unified Directive 2001/83/EC as Articles 86–100) all were regulated somewhat later, in 1992. The national transition period in some countries was rather long (e.g., package leaflets were not mandatory in the UK and Denmark before 1995).

At the end of 2001, the European Council adopted the *Medicinal Products Directive* (Directive 2001/83/EEC),[5] replacing all previous medicinal product directives. This huge project simplified the existing *Medicinal Products Directive*, unified recommendations that had diverged over time, clarified definitions of terms and enabled the repeal of directives that were no longer necessary. This made the regulatory environment clearer for authorities and industry.

Since then, the *Medicinal Products Directive* has been amended by:

- Directive 2002/98/EC,[6] setting standards of quality and safety for the collection, testing, processing, storage and distribution of human blood and blood components
- Directive 2003/63/EC,[7] establishing the analytical, pharmacotoxicological and clinical standards and protocols for medicinal product testing
- Directive 2004/24/EC,[8] regarding traditional herbal medicinal products
- Directive 2004/27/EC,[9] regarding GMP process requirements for APIs
- Regulation (EC) No 1901/2006,[10] regarding medicinal products for paediatric use and amendments
- Council Regulation (EC) No 1394/2007[11] on advanced therapy medicinal products
- Directive 2008/29/EC,[12] relating to medicinal products for human use, as regards the implementing powers conferred on the Commission
- Directive 2009/53/EC,[13] regarding variations to the terms of MAs for medicinal products
- Directive 2009/120/EC,[14] relating to medicinal products for human use as regards advanced therapy medicinal products
- Directive 2010/84/EU,[15] amending, as regards pharmacovigilance, Directive 2001/83/EC on the Community code relating to medicinal products for human use
- Directive 2011/62/EU,[16] regarding the prevention of the entry into the legal supply chain of falsified medicinal products

Directives 2004/24/EC and 2004/27/EC and a new Regulation (EC) 726/2004[17] regarding the European Agency for the Evaluation of Medicinal Products (EMEA) were the result of a legislatively mandated review of EU pharmaceutical legislation that began in 2000 and was finalised in 2004, improving the EU medicinal product regulatory system. Directive 2004/27/EC introduced changes to labelling and packaging and the MA ("Sunset Clause") and a "compassionate use" regulatory framework. Moreover, pharmacovigilance has been improved by implementing a database and an electronic notification system regarding adverse events.

Also in 2003, Directive 2003/94/EC[18] laid down further GMP principles and guidelines with respect to medicinal products and investigational medicinal products for human use.

Regulation (EC) No 1901/2006 established rules concerning the development of medicinal products for human use in order to meet the specific therapeutic needs of the paediatric population, without subjecting the paediatric population to unnecessary clinical or other trials and in compliance with Directive 2001/20/EC.[19]

In 1995, pursuant to Council Regulation (EEC) No 2309/93,[20] the EU implemented a pan-European registration system known as the "Centralised Procedure" and established the EMEA. In 2004, Council Regulation (EC) No 2309/93 was superseded by Regulation (EC) No 726/2004[21] of the European Parliament and the Council of 31 March 2004. The regulation aimed to improve the authorisation procedure, amending certain administrative aspects. Further, the name of the European Agency for the Evaluation of Medicinal Products was changed to the European Medicines Agency, while retaining the acronym EMEA. This acronym was shortened to EMA in 2010.

This system enabled a single medicinal product MA for the entire EU. The option of submitting an MAA through the Centralised Procedure also is available for biotechnology-derived products and products that are considered highly innovative. Moreover, Regulation (EC) No 726/2004 expanded application of the Centralised Procedure to orphan drugs (established by Regulation (EC) No 141/2000[22]) and products with new active substances dealing with acquired immune deficiency syndrome, cancer, neurodegenerative disorders, diabetes and, from 20 May 2008, autoimmune diseases and other immune dysfunctions and viral diseases.

Starting 30 December 2008, Regulation (EC) No 1394/2007 on advanced therapy medicinal products (ATMPs) expanded the applicability of Regulation (EC) No 726/2004 to advanced therapy medicinal products (such as gene and somatic therapy medicinal products as well as tissue-engineered products). This expansion has strengthened EMA by increasing its responsibilities and influence on the European pharmaceutical market.

EMA is headquartered in London and provides the administrative centre and support for MAA reviews.

One of six scientific committees conducts the technical review of all Centralised Procedure applications on the EU's behalf: the Committee for Medicinal Products for Human Use (CHMP); the Committee for Medicinal Products for Veterinary Use (CVMP); the Committee on Orphan Medicinal Products (COMP); the Committee on Herbal Medicinal Products (HMPC); the Committee for Advanced Therapies (CAT); and the Paediatric Committee (PDCO).

CAT is responsible for reviewing ATMPs qualifying for the Centralised Procedure. COMP's role in reviewing orphan products is defined in Regulation (EC) No 141/2000. HMPC was established by Directive 2004/24/EC on traditional herbal medicine products. This directive also defines its role and duties. The roles of CHMP and CVMP in reviewing medicinal products for humans and animals, respectively, are defined in Regulation (EC) No 726/2004.

These committees are composed of regulatory agency representatives from each Member State. They meet at EMA's offices on a predefined schedule. The centralised medicinal product review procedure and associated timelines are clearly defined in the *Notice to Applicants, Volume 2A*. Further information about this procedure is available from EMA.

Medicinal products that do not meet Centralised Procedure criteria may receive MAs through two mechanisms: national registration and decentralised mutual recognition (commonly referred to as mutual recognition). MA through the National Procedure is possible only for medicinal products that do not qualify for centralised approval and are intended for marketing in only one EU country. If these conditions apply, the requirements, review procedure and timelines are governed by the individual Member State's own process; reference should be made to the specific country's website for further information.

If, however, the intent is to market the product in more than one country, the MAA is reviewed through the Mutual Recognition Procedure. The Decentralised Procedure, a modified form of the Mutual Recognition Procedure, should be used for products for which no MA exists. In essence, the MAA will be evaluated by one Member State (chosen by the company) that will act as the Reference Member State (RMS). If an MA is granted by that state, other Member States (chosen by the company, depending upon where the product will be sold), known as the Concerned Member States (CMS), are asked to "mutually recognise" the RMS approval. If the approval is recognised, a MA will be granted in all the CMS.

Commission Regulation (EC) No 1234/2008 of 24 November 2008 (which is based on Commission Regulations (EC) No 1084/2003[23] and (EC) No 1085/2003 of June 2003) concerning the examination of variations to the terms of MAs for medicinal products for human use and veterinary medicinal products uses a simplified approach to handling variations.

Biologics

In 1989, Council Directive 89/342/EEC[24] defined requirements for immunological medicinal products consisting of vaccines, toxins or sera and allergens; Directive 89/381/EEC covers medicinal products derived from human blood or plasma. Council Directive 2001/18/EEC,[25] which replaced Council Directives 90/219/EEC and 90/220/EEC, regulates the use of genetically modified microorganisms and their deliberate release into the environment. This directive was amended by Regulation (EC) No 1830/2003,[26] establishing a clear EU system for tracing and labelling genetically modified organisms.

Biological medicinal product safety was increased by Directive 2003/63/EC, amending Annex I of Directive 2001/83/EC. Part III of Annex I now includes special biological pharmaceutical requirements. It established a new system that simplified approval and subsequent change procedures for human plasma-derived medicinal products. Moreover, it introduced a Vaccine Antigen Master File (VAMF), which allows the pooling of national expertise and, through EMA coordination, a single evaluation of the concerned vaccine antigen.

The regulations and directives are complemented by various guidance documents that can be found on EMA's website.

Advanced Therapy Products

On 30 December 2007, Regulation (EC) No 1394/2007 on advanced therapy medicinal products (ATMPs) (the *ATMP Regulation*) entered into force. The regulation included a "grandfather clause" with a transition period for products that were legally on the Community market when it came into force. Products new to the market had to comply with the regulation by 30 December 2008. "Grandfathered" products had to be in compliance by 30 December 2011, unless they are tissue-engineered products, in which case they must comply by 30 December 2012.

The regulation's purpose is to facilitate research, development and authorisation of ATMPs and to improve patient access to them. ATMPs covered by the regulation are gene therapy medicinal products as defined in Part IV of Annex I to Directive 2001/83/EC, somatic cell therapy medicinal products as defined in Part IV of Annex I to Directive 2001/83/EC and tissue-engineered products as defined in the regulation itself.

Under this regulation, all ATMPs are required to have an EU-wide MA as defined in Regulation (EC) No 726/2004. Moreover, it created centralised supervision and pharmacovigilance of ATMPs and the CAT within EMA. This provision combines expertise from different Member States to enable ATMP evaluation, and provides advice on the authorisation process, long-term follow-up of patients and risk management strategies for the postauthorisation phase. CAT is in charge of developing evaluation criteria and guidelines for these products.

A further effect of the *ATMP Regulation* was the applicability of the provisions of Directive 2001/83/EC governing GMP- and GCP-compliance, and ATMP advertising, labelling, classification and distribution.

The *ATMP Regulation* has been complemented by:

- Commission Directive 2009/120/EC of 14 September 2009 amending Directive 2001/83/EC of the European Parliament and of the Council on the Community code relating to medicinal products for human use as regards advanced therapy medicinal products
- Commission Regulation (EC) No 668/2009 of 24 July 2009 implementing Regulation (EC) No 1394/2007 of the European Parliament and of the Council with regard to the evaluation and certification of quality and nonclinical data relating to advanced therapy medicinal products developed by micro, small and medium-sized enterprises

The regulations and directives are supported by a number of guidance documents that can be found on EMA's website.

Veterinary Products

The basic regulatory principles applied to human products also govern veterinary medicinal products. EU Directive 81/851/EEC[27] was the first Community directive regulating veterinary medicinal products and the analytical, pharmacotoxicological and clinical standards and protocols related to the testing of those products. A maximum residue limit regulation (Council Regulation (EEC) No 2377/90, now replaced by Regulation (EC) No 470/2009) and the *GMP Directive* (Directive 91/412/EEC) supplemented Directive 81/851/EEC in 1990 and 1991, respectively. Additional directives adopted during the 1990s recently have been codified into the unified Directive 2001/82/EC,[28] the Community code related to veterinary medicinal products.

Directive 2004/28/EC[29] of March 2004 amended Directive 2001/82/EC on veterinary medicinal products. As a result of scientific and technical progress in the animal health field, the definitions and scope of Directive 2001/82/EC needed to be clarified to meet high quality, safety and efficacy standards for veterinary medicinal products. Another aim of Directive 2004/28/EC was to eliminate remaining obstacles to free movement of these products within the European Community.

Directive 2006/130/EC[30] of 11 December 2006, laying down criteria for exempting certain veterinary medicinal products for food-producing animals from the requirement for a veterinary prescription, implements Directive 2001/82/EC.

Commission Directive 2009/9/EC of 10 February 2009 amended Directive 2001/82/EC on the Community code relating to medicinal products for veterinary use. It was introduced mainly to simplify current procedures for the assessment of veterinary vaccines, both for the granting of a first MA and for subsequent changes due to modifications to the manufacturing process and testing of individual antigens involved in combined vaccines. A new system based on the concept of a VAMF should be introduced for vaccines that involve several antigens.[31]

Directive 2009/53/EC of the European Parliament and of the Council of 18 June 2009 amended Directive 2001/82/EC and Directive 2001/83/EC, as regards variations to the terms of MAs for medicinal products.

Regulation (EC) 1950/2006[32] of 13 December 2006 established—in accordance with Directive 2001/82/EC on the Community code relating to veterinary medicinal products—a list of substances essential for the treatment of *equidae*.

Traditional Herbal Medicinal Products

In 2004, Directive 2004/24/EC amended Directive 2001/83/EC on traditional herbal medicinal products. Given the particular characteristics of these medicinal products—especially their long tradition—the European Commission established a special, simplified procedure for them. HMPC is responsible for reviewing registry documents and providing scientific opinions on traditional herbal medicines.

Medical Devices

To remove barriers to the free movement of goods, two innovative regulatory instruments regarding medical devices were developed in the EU: the New Approach to device regulation and the Global Approach to conformity assessment. The medical device regulations are the best-known examples.

New Approach directives describe a fast legislative pathway with a defined content and structure. Their legal basis is Article 95 of the *European Council Treaty*. The New Approach is not limited to healthcare devices; it also applies to toys, electromagnetic compatibility, lifts and radio and telecommunication equipment. Devices that are granted market access using the New Approach can be recognised by the *Conformité Européenne* (CE) Mark. New Approach directives are harmonised across the EU; the Member States must repeal all contradictory national legislation and are not allowed to maintain or introduce more-stringent measures than those in the directives. When Member States incorporate the New Approach requirements, they may include additional provisions considered necessary to apply the requirements more effectively. These harmonised directives limit public intervention and enable industry to meet its obligations in a manner suitable to the specific situation or device without the need for a cumbersome regulatory approval process. About 20 New Approach directives came into force during the mid-1980s. As a result, the reduced regulatory burden for authorities enabled approval processes to advance much more quickly than before. In addition, the changes enabled the creation of a single European market for devices by December 1992—an objective of the *European Council Treaty*.

Council Directive 90/385/EEC[33] (June 1990), relating to active implantable medical devices, was the first application of the New Approach to the field of medical devices. The New Approach has not been applied in sectors where Community legislation was well advanced before 1985 or where provisions for finished products and hazards related to such products cannot be established. For instance, Community legislation on foodstuffs, chemical products and pharmaceutical products does not follow New Approach principles.

The Global Approach supplements the New Approach by defining the basis for Conformity Assessment Procedures (CAPs) within the New Approach directives. The Global Approach does not give conformity assessment details; those are described in the directives themselves. Its broader scope is to facilitate conditions to implement conformity assessment evidence when mutual recognition agreements are signed. Conformity assessments are to be found in regulatory and nonregulatory fields.

The *Guide to the implementation of directives based on the New Approach and the Global Approach*, a detailed description of New Approach and Global Approach directives, is available from the European Commission.[34]

The 1993 *Maastricht Treaty* introduced public health into the EU's areas of competence. The mission of the European Commission and, particularly, its Directorate-General for Health and Consumer Protection, is to ensure a high level of protection of consumers' health, safety and economic interests, as well as public health. Scientific advice for drafting and amending EU regulations is provided by a number of committees, including the Scientific Committee on Medicinal Products and Medical Devices. The Directorate-General for Enterprise promotes innovation, entrepreneurship, e-business, standardisation and New Approach EU regulations, which are of direct concern to the medical technologies and devices sector.

The medical devices definition is similar to the definition of medicinal products in Council Directive 65/65/EEC, and relevant medical device regulation sections were driven by pharmaceutical regulation experience. The difference between product groups is the mode of action. If the product's mode of action is primarily pharmacological, immunological or metabolic, it is classified as a medicinal product. In other cases—mainly, if the product acts by physical means—it is classified as a medical device. The heterogeneity of medical devices and the high degree of innovation in new product development, including software and new technologies such as chromatographic procedures, provide the rationale for establishing specific medical device regulations.

Interestingly, the *Medical Devices Directive* (*MDD*)[35] (Directive 93/42/EEC) regulates only products for human use. Therefore, medical devices for veterinary use, such as special drug delivery systems, are still under the medicinal products regulations. This situation may be a disadvantage for medical device manufacturers if the product is intended for use by both humans and animals. The products follow two different guidelines and must be labelled in two different ways, according to the intended use.

In Europe, medical devices are a €30 billion market. Recognising the growing need for international harmonisation of medical device regulatory control, senior government officials and regulated industry representatives in the EU, US, Australia, Canada and Japan have been working to harmonise regulations through the medical device Global Harmonization Task Force (GHTF). GHTF is phasing out in 2012 and will be replaced by the International Medical Device Regulators Forum (IMDRF). IMDRF has indicated that it will continue to use those GHTF guidance documents that are still relevant and up to date. Others may be revised or updated and some retired. Further details will be forthcoming.

The EU has an open medical device regulatory system that is transparent, based on harmonised standards and spans all EU Member States. Medical devices sold within the EU must meet the health and safety requirements set forth in the EU medical devices directives. These directives, which are listed below, consolidate EU regulatory requirements under one system, meaning that if the device receives CE designation in one Member State, it can be sold in all EU Member States:

- *Active Implantable Medical Devices Directive* (*AIMDD*) (Directive 90/385/EEC) as amended
- *Medical Devices Directive* (*MDD*) (Directive 93/42/EEC) as amended
- Directive 2001/104/EC[36] amending Council Directive 93/42/EEC
- *In Vitro Diagnostic Devices Directive* (*IVDD*) (Directive 98/79/EC)
- *Clinical Trials Directive* (Directive 2001/20/EC)
- *Human Blood and Human Plasma Derivatives Directive* (Directive 2000/70/EC)[37]
- *Personal Protective Equipment Directive* (Directive 89/686/EEC)
- Directive 2003/12/EC on the reclassification of breast implants in the framework of Directive 93/42/EEC concerning medical devices
- Directive 2003/32/EC introducing detailed specifications regarding requirements laid down in Council Directive 93/42/EEC on medical devices manufactured utilising tissues of animal origin
- Directive 2007/47/EC[38] amending Directive 90/385/EEC on the approximation of the laws of the Member States relating to active implantable medical devices, Directive 93/42/EEC concerning medical devices and Directive 98/8/EC concerning the placing of biocidal products on the market

The medical devices directives have been under revision by the European Commission. Directive 2007/47/EC of the European Parliament and of the Council of 5 September 2007 amending Directive 90/385/EEC on the approximation of the laws of the Member States relating to active implantable medical devices (*Active Implantable Medical Devices Directive* (*AIMD*)), Directive 93/42/EEC concerning Medical Devices (*Medical Devices Directive* (*MDD*)) and Directive 98/8/EC concerning the placing of biocidal products on the market, was formally adopted and published on 21 September 2007.[39]

The most significant changes concern, *inter alia*, the expansion of the medical device definition to software products; clarification of the Essential Requirements and Requirements for Design Examinations; provision of a procedure of Scientific Advice on substance quality and safety for borderline products; conformity procedure and review of the validity of existing classifications; and clinical evaluation.

Moreover, in certain cases, additional regulations apply; for example, the statements on devices for special purposes required by Annex VIII of the *MDD* must also conform to regulations governing the field of human blood derivatives. However, the *In Vitro Diagnostic Medical Devices Directive* (*IVDD*) 98/79/EC is not affected by Directive 2007/47/EC.

The new directive's key regulatory environment elements are:

- Legislative harmonisation is limited to Essential Requirements that devices must meet.
- Device technical specifications must meet the Essential Requirements. Harmonised standards can help determine conformance with these requirements. The application of harmonised or other standards remains voluntary, and the manufacturer may always apply other technical specifications to meet the requirements.

Although this directive does not apply to blood products, plasma or blood cells of human origin, or to human tissue-engineered products as such, provision has been made to bring devices with an ancillary human tissue-engineered product within its scope. This completes the *Regulation on Advanced Therapy Medicinal Products*[40] and thereby avoids a regulatory gap.

Member States adopted the laws, regulations and administrative provisions necessary to comply with this directive by 21 December 2008; it was implemented 21 March 2010.

To make the New Approach function reliably, conformity assessment conditions must build confidence through competence and transparency. Member States' obligation to ensure that only devices that do not endanger public safety and health or affect other public interests are placed on the market also entails market surveillance responsibility.

Essential Requirements are set forth in annexes to the directives and include all criteria necessary to achieve a directive's objective. When the manufacturer has not (or has only partially) applied national standards that incorporate harmonised standards, the measures taken and their adequacy must be documented to comply with the Essential Requirements.

Medical devices must fulfil the corresponding directive's Essential Requirements. They should provide patients, users and third parties with a high level of protection and attain the performance levels the manufacturer has ascribed to them. The Essential Requirements and other conditions, including those intended to minimise or reduce risk, must be interpreted and applied to take into account technology and practices in use at the time of design, as well as technical and economic considerations compatible with a high level of health and safety protection.

Before a manufacturer places a device on the Community market, the product must be subjected to the CAP denoted in the applicable directive, with a view to affixing the CE Mark. For some device categories, a third-party CAP is carried out by so-called Notified Bodies (NBs), which have been designated by the Member States as fulfilling directive requirements and being established in their territory. NBs are public institutes or private companies; they are not Competent Authorities.

Devices in compliance with all of the directives' provisions concerning CE marking may bear the CE Mark. The mark is an indication that the products meet the Essential Requirements of applicable directives, have undergone a CAP and, hence, may be placed on the market.

Member States are required to incorporate the directives' provisions into their national legislation. Five-year transition periods are typical. The Member States also must inform the Commission of measures taken. Member States must permit products that comply with regulations in force in their territory to be marketed when a directive is implemented.

For CAPs, medical devices are grouped into four product classes. The classification rules are based on the human body's vulnerability and take into account potential risks associated with the device's technical design and manufacture. Manufacturers can carry out CAPs for Class I devices. However Class I devices that are sold in a sterile condition and devices that have a measuring function require the involvement of an NB. Devices falling into Classes IIa, IIb and III, which have a high risk potential, require design and manufacture inspection by an NB. Class III is set aside for the riskiest devices; explicit prior conformity authorisation is required before Class III devices can be placed on the market. Interestingly, hip, knee and shoulder joint replacements were reclassified as Class III devices by Directive 2005/50/EC. Reclassification by derogation to the classification rules set out in Annex IX to Directive 93/42/EEC is indicated where the shortcomings identified due to a product's specific characteristics will be more properly addressed under the CAPs corresponding to the new category.

Pursuant to Directive 2003/12/EC, breast implants also were reclassified as Class III medical devices.

Medical devices must bear the CE Mark to indicate their conformity with the provisions of the medical devices directives to enable them to move freely within the Community and be put into service in accordance with their intended purpose.

MEDDEV guidance documents are developed by representatives of the national Competent Authorities, European Commission, industry and other partners. The guidelines promote a common approach by the Competent Authorities charged with implementing the medical devices directives, as incorporated into national law. The guidelines are not legally binding. Because interested parties and Competent Authorities' experts participate in the development process, it is anticipated that these guidelines will be followed within the Member States and, therefore, ensure uniform application of relevant directive provisions.

Developments in both FDA's GMP regulations and the EU medical devices directives are part of a movement toward harmonising regulatory processes and requirements in an effort to diminish trade barriers. The EU and FDA have adopted a harmonised international management system standard for design, control and manufacturing (i.e., ISO 13485, which has minor variations in the US and the EU).

Mutual Recognition Agreements (MRAs) between the EU and the US, Canada, Australia, New Zealand and Switzerland provide an improved way for foreign medical device manufacturers to enter the European market. The US/EU MRA began in 1998 with a three-year transition that was viewed as a "confidence-building" period. Its operational phase was postponed in 2002 when FDA and European regulators extended the medical device transition period for another two years to enable both sides to complete verification of conformity assessment bodies (CABs). This agreement recognises that certain CABs in the US can conduct product approval reviews and quality system evaluations that meet European regulatory requirements and are equivalent to those conducted by the EU. Similarly, the agreement recognises that EU CABs can conduct preliminary product approval reviews for listed medical devices and evaluations according to FDA requirements.

Funding of public health and health insurance programs relating directly or indirectly to devices is not subject to the regulations. Interpretation of EU legislation may vary in practice, as may the economic situation in Member States. Moreover, national authorities have an exclusive right to regulate many areas that directly or indirectly affect medical technology and device development—particularly reimbursing medical treatment expenses, encouraging research and development and promoting patient access to new medical breakthroughs.

In 2008, the European Commission held a public consultation concerning the recast of the medical devices directives.[41] In addition, a public consultation regarding the technical aspects of the revision of the *IVDD* was held in 2010. The proposed recast aims to address various issues in the pre- and postmarket phases and to extend the scope of the legislation.

Scope

- transform the current directives into regulations
- extend the scope of device legislation to cover:
  1. products manufactured utilising nonviable tissues and cells of human origin
  2. certain implantable, injectable or otherwise invasive products for aesthetic purposes
- address the issues of genetic tests and "in-house" tests in the EU legislation on IVDs
- address the issue of reprocessing of single-use medical devices
- address the issue of "borderline" cases and diverging determination of the regulatory status of a given product and product type by Member States
- align, where appropriate, to the New Legislative Framework for the Marketing of Products[42]

Premarket Phase

- strengthen and harmonise the oversight of NBs in terms of demonstrating competence, impartiality and transparency
- simplify and streamline CAPs
- ensure uniform high standards and criteria for CAPs by NBs, particularly regarding the assessment of the manufacturer's clinical evaluation and in the field of new technologies
- coordinate Member States' approvals regarding multi-centre clinical investigations
- clarify basic concepts related to clinical investigation and evaluation
- align IVD classification with GHTF guidance
- clarify the concept of clinical evidence in the EU legislation on IVDs[43]

Postmarket Phase

- develop a tool for the central reporting of incidents by manufacturers and improve coordination of authorities in vigilance and market surveillance
- clarify key concepts in postmarket safety
- regulate the distribution and traceability of medical devices to address counterfeiting and device identification (e.g., Unique Device Identifier)
- centralise the EU registration process for manufacturers/Authorised Representatives and medical devices (further develop Eudamed)[44]

System Management

- introduce a legal basis for a Medical Device Expert Group (MDEG) to be composed of experts designated by the Member States and to be established at an EU body (e.g., agency or Commission):
  o to ensure consistent application of the medical device regulatory framework throughout the EU
  o to enhance coordination between national Competent Authorities in postmarket safety and multi-national clinical investigations
- mandate an EU body to provide administrative, technical and scientific support to the MDEG to ensure sustainable management of the regulation regime and:
  o organise and participate in the assessment of NBs
  o manage an expert panel and network of Reference Laboratories
  o develop, maintain and manage the IT infrastructure[45]

Blood Derivatives

In 2000, an amendment to the *MDD* through Directive 2000/70/EC passed the decision-making process. This amendment extended the *MDD*'s scope to include devices that incorporate stable derivatives of human blood or blood products. Later, a mistranscription was found in the wording agreed to by the Council. To avoid confusion in interpreting the provisions, a new directive, 2001/104/EC, amending Council Directive 93/42/EEC, was published in the *Official Journal of the European Union* on 10 January 2002.

In 2003, Directive 2002/98/EC increased the quality and safety requirements for human blood and blood components, also influencing blood derivative manufacturing. The directive set quality and safety standards for the collection, testing, processing, storage and distribution of human blood and blood components. The directive established a system that ensures traceability of blood and blood components through accurate donor, patient and laboratory identification procedures, record maintenance, and an appropriate identification and labelling system. It also introduced surveillance procedures to collect and evaluate information on adverse or unexpected events or reactions resulting from the collection of blood or blood components to prevent similar or equivalent events or reactions.

Directive 2004/33/EC[46] implemented Directive 2002/98/EC regarding certain technical requirements for blood and blood components. Directive 2005/61/EC[47] and Directive 2005/62/EC[48] implemented Directive 2002/98/

EC concerning traceability requirements and notification of serious adverse reactions and events, as well as Community standards and specifications relating to a quality system for blood collection establishments.

Cosmetics

In the early 1970s, Member States decided to harmonise their national cosmetic regulations to enable the free circulation of cosmetic products within the European Community. After numerous discussions among experts from all Member States, Directive 76/768/EEC[49] was adopted in July 1976. The principles set forth in the *Cosmetics Directive* take into account the consumer's needs while encouraging commercial exchange and eliminating barriers to trade. One of the directive's main objectives was to give clear guidance on the requirements a safe cosmetic product must meet in order to freely circulate within the EU without national MA. Cosmetic product safety relates to composition, packaging and information, which are the responsibility of the producer or EU importer, as is marketing liability. There are no cosmetic product premarket controls. Cosmetic product control within the EU, including a simple manufacturing and importing site notification and an in-market surveillance system, is the responsibility of the entity that places the product on the market.

Directive 95/17/EC[50] set forth detailed rules for the application of the basic *Cosmetics Directive* of 1976. The basic directive has already undergone several amendments and adaptations in response to technical progress; e.g., the sixth amendment (Directive 2003/15/EC[51]) provided *inter alia* more-detailed provisions on phasing out animal testing and introduced the "period-after-opening labelling." Moreover, the directive has been subject to numerous adaptations to adjust annex provisions to technical progress, for example, Directive 2005/80/EC.[52] The last amendments for the purpose of adapting Annexes II, III, IV and V to technical progress were the Commission Directives 2006/65/EC,[53] 2006/78/EC,[54] 2007/1/EC,[55] 2007/17/EC,[56] 2007/22/EC,[57] 2007/53/EC[58] and 2007/54/EC.[59]

The *Cosmetics Directive* has been recast into a regulation. On 30 November 2009, the new *Cosmetic Products Regulation*, Regulation (EC) No 1223/2009 of the European Parliament and of the Council of 30 November 2009 on cosmetic products was adopted, replacing the Cosmetics Directive. The aim of the recast was a robust, internationally recognised regime that reinforces product safety, taking into consideration the latest technological developments, including the possible use of nanomaterials. Most of the provisions of this new regulation will be applicable from 11 July 2013.[60]

Food and Dietary Products

On 28 January 2002, the European Parliament and the Council adopted Regulation (EC) No 178/2002 laying down the general principles and requirements of food law.61 Food and dietary supplements are also governed by this regulation.

The European Commission's horizontal legislation initially focused on additives, colours and materials intended to come into contact with foodstuffs. Directive 89/107/EEC[62] addressed the approximation of Member States' laws concerning food additives authorised for use in foodstuffs intended for human consumption.

In 2000, Directive 2000/13/EC[63] combined all previous directives on foodstuff labelling. The directive was amended by Directive 2001/101/EC[64] on the approximation of the laws of the Member States relating to the labelling, presentation and advertising of foodstuffs, by Directive 2003/89/EC[65] as regards indication of the ingredients present in foodstuffs, and by Directives 2006/107/EC[66] and 2006/142/EC.[67]

Two years later, Directive 2002/46/EC,[68] regulating food supplements, was adopted. Annex II to this directive has been amended by Directive 2006/37/EC[69] regarding the inclusion of certain substances.

Annex II of Directive 2002/46/EC is a list of permitted vitamin or mineral preparations that may be added for specific nutritional purposes in food supplements. It has been amended by Commission Directive 2006/37/EC,[70] Commission Regulation (EC) 1170/2009[71] and Commission Regulation (EU) No 1161/2011[72] to include additional substances. The trade of products containing vitamins and minerals not listed in Annex II has been prohibited since 1 August 2005. In addition, Directive 2002/46/EC has been aligned with the Regulatory Procedure with Scrutiny by Regulation (EC) 1137/2008.[73]

In addition, several directives describe specific policies. Foods resulting from technological innovations as well as baby foods, sweeteners and dietary foods are subject to Commission regulations and directives. For example, European Council Directive 89/398/EEC[74] concerns foodstuffs that, owing to their special composition or manufacturing process, are clearly distinguishable from foodstuffs for normal consumption. Such foodstuffs intended for particular nutritional uses are suitable for their claimed nutritional purposes and can be marketed in such a way as to indicate such suitability. These products may be characterised as "dietetic" or "dietary." Foodstuffs for normal consumption may not use the adjectives "dietetic" or "dietary" in labelling, presentation or advertising.

Following a series of food scares in the 1990s, the European Food Safety Agency (EFSA) was established. Provisionally organised in Brussels in 2002, it has been located in Parma, Italy, since 2003. EFSA deals with all matters related to food and feed safety, scientific advice on nutrition in relation to Community legislation and communication with the public.

In July 2003, the EU Council of Ministers formally adopted two European Commission proposals on genetically modified organisms (GMOs). The proposals establish a clear EU system for tracing and labelling GMOs (Regulation 1830/2003/EC[75]) and for regulating the marketing and labelling of food and feed products derived from GMOs (Regulation 1829/2003/EC[76]).

More information can be found at http://ec.europa.eu/food/food/labellingnutrition/supplements/index_en.htm.

Future Issues

Healthcare regulations must balance the interests of patients, manufacturers, authorities, insurance companies and others in a fast-moving and complex environment. In Europe, the mechanisms for healthcare product review and approval must be robust enough to ensure patient safety throughout the Community. Those mechanisms, however, must be efficient and balance safety considerations with the need to make new therapeutics available to the public in a timely manner.

Advances in such novel therapies as cell technologies, tissue engineering and gene therapy led to a new proposal for a regulation by the European Parliament and Council on advanced therapy medicinal products. This proposal was adopted by the European Commission on 16 November 2005. It resolved the regulatory gap involving these innovative technologies by addressing such therapy products within a single, integrated and tailored framework. It covers the harmonisation and facilitation of market access and improves advanced therapy product safety by establishing a premarketing approval requirement.

Product classifications as we know them today (drugs, devices and biologics) are being redefined to include new technologies such as gene replacement therapy and the use of agricultural products as biofactories to produce human proteins.

Third-party inspections and self-certification programs may become more common, and inspection standards will be harmonised globally. MRAs will increasingly allow nations' sovereignty over local industry to eclipse inspection by foreign regulatory authorities as the move toward transparency continues.

Biological research will partially fulfil its promise. The resulting new products, services and information will challenge current regulatory systems and push industry and authorities into new discussions and debates concerning risks. New ethical and moral benchmarks will guide risk management. Oversight must continue to evolve as health and risk management knowledge expands, and as power and influence are redistributed within the global regulatory system.

Medical device regulations were revised by Directive 2007/47/EC. The growing number of medical devices on the market and the expansion of the EU have led to an increased need to coordinate activities of national authorities related to the *MDD* (93/42/EEC), involving a number of Member States and/or third countries. The majority of this directive's amendments are intended to clarify the process of bringing medical devices to market and monitoring them. Additionally, they seek to close certain gaps and update the framework for dealing with new developments, such as the increasing importance of software in medical devices. Moreover, safety is enhanced through the emphasis on clinical evaluation documentation included in the file, which NBs must now evaluate.

References

1. Directive 2003/32/EC of 23 April 2003 introducing detailed specifications as regards the requirements laid down in Council Directive 93/42/EEC with respect to medical devices manufactured utilising tissues of animal origin. EUR-Lex website. http://eur-lex.europa.eu/LexUriServ/LexUriServ.do?uri=OJ:L:2003:105:0018:0023:EN:PDF. Accessed 28 March 2012.
2. European Commission. *EudraLex: The Rules Governing Medicinal Products in the European Union* (European Commission, April 1998). EC website. http://ec.europa.eu/health/documents/eudralex/. Accessed 28 March 2012.
3. Directive 65/65/EEC of 26 January 1965 on the approximation of provisions laid down by law, regulation or administrative action relating to medicinal products. EUR-Lex website. http://eur-lex.europa.eu/LexUriServ/LexUriServ.do?uri=CELEX:31965L0065:EN:HTML. Accessed 28 March 2012.
4. Directive 91/356/EEC of 13 June 1991 laying down the principles and guidelines of good manufacturing practice for medicinal products for human use.
5. Directive 2001/83/EC of the European Parliament and of the Council of 6 November 2001 on the Community code relating to medicinal products for human use. EC website. http://ec.europa.eu/health/files/eudralex/vol-1/dir_2001_83_cons/dir2001_83_cons_20081230_en.pdf. Accessed 28 March 2012.
6. Directive 2002/98/EC of the European Parliament and of the Council of 27 January 2003 setting standards of quality and safety for the collection, testing, processing, storage and distribution of human blood and blood components and amending Directive 2001/83/EC. EUR-Lex website. http://eur-lex.europa.eu/LexUriServ/LexUriServ.do?uri=OJ:L:2003:033:0030:0040:EN:PDF. Accessed 28 March 2012.
7. Directive 2003/63/EC of 25 June 2003 amending Directive 2001/83/EC of the European Parliament and of the Council on the Community code relating to medicinal products for human use (replacing Annex 1). EC website. http://ec.europa.eu/health/files/eudralex/vol-1/dir_2003_63/dir_2003_63_en.pdf. Accessed 28 March 2012.
8. Directive 2004/24/EC of the European Parliament and of the Council of 31 March 2004 amending, as regards traditional herbal medicinal products, Directive 2001/83/EC on the Community code relating to medicinal products for human use. EUR-Lex website. http://eur-lex.europa.eu/LexUriServ/LexUriServ.do?uri=OJ:L:2004:136:0085:0090:en:PDF. Accessed 28 March 2012.
9. Directive 2004/27/EC of the European Parliament and of the Council of 31 March 2004 amending Directive 2001/83/EC on the Community code relating to medicinal products for human use. EC website. http://ec.europa.eu/health/files/eudralex/vol-1/dir_2004_27/dir_2004_27_en.pdf. Accessed 28 March 2012.
10. Regulation (EC) 1901/2006 of the European Parliament and of the Council of 12 December 2006 on medicinal products for paediatric use and amending Regulation (EEC) 1768/92, Directive 2001/20/EC, Directive 2001/83/EC and Regulation (EC) 726/2004. EC website.

http://ec.europa.eu/health/files/eudralex/vol-1/reg_2006_1901/reg_2006_1901_en.pdf. Accessed 28 March 2012.
11. Regulation (EC) 1394/2007 of the European Parliament and of the Council of 13 November 2007 on advanced therapy medicinal products and amending Directive 2001/83/EC and Regulation (EC) 726/2004. EUR-Lex website. http://eur-lex.europa.eu/LexUriServ/LexUriServ.do?uri=OJ:L:2007:324:0121:0137:en:PDF. Accessed 28 March 2012.
12. Directive 2008/29/EC of the European Parliament and of the Council of 11 March 2008 amending Directive 2001/83/EC on the Community code relating to medicinal products for human use, as regards the implementing powers conferred on the Commission. EC website. http://ec.europa.eu/health/files/eudralex/vol-1/dir_2008_29/dir_2008_29_en.pdf. Accessed 28 March 2012.
13. Directive 2009/53/EC of the European Parliament and of the Council of 18 June 2009 amending Directive 2001/82/EC and Directive 2001/83/EC, as regards variations to the terms of marketing authorisations for medicinal products. EC website. http://ec.europa.eu/health/files/eudralex/vol-1/dir_2009_53/dir_2009_53_en.pdf. Accessed 28 March 2012.
14. Commission Directive 2009/120/EC of 14 September 2009 amending Directive 2001/83/EC of the European Parliament and of the Council on the Community code relating to medicinal products for human use as regards advanced therapy medicinal products. EC website. http://ec.europa.eu/health/files/eudralex/vol-1/dir_2009_120/dir_2009_120_en.pdf. Accessed 28 March 2012.
15. Directive 2010/84/EU of the European Parliament and of the Council of 15 December 2010 amending, as regards pharmacovigilance, Directive 2001/83/EC on the Community code relating to medicinal products for human use. EC website. http://ec.europa.eu/health/files/eudralex/vol-1/dir_2010_84/dir_2010_84_en.pdf. Accessed 28 March 2012.
16. Directive 2011/62/EU of the European Parliament and of the Council of 8 June 2011 amending Directive 2001/83/EC on the Community code relating to medicinal products for human use, as regards the prevention of the entry into the legal supply chain of falsified medicinal products. EC website. http://ec.europa.eu/health/files/eudralex/vol-1/dir_2011_62/dir_2011_62_en.pdf. Accessed 28 March 2012.
17. Regulation (EC) 726/2004 of the European Parliament and of the Council of 31 March 2004 laying down Community procedures for the authorisation and supervision of medicinal products for human and veterinary use and establishing a European Medicines Agency. EUR-Lex website. http://eur-lex.europa.eu/LexUriServ/LexUriServ.do?uri=OJ:L:2004:136:0001:0033:en:PDF. Accessed 28 March 2012.
18. Commission Directive 2003/94/EC of 8 October 2003 laying down the principles and guidelines of good manufacturing practice in respect of medicinal products for human use and investigational medicinal products for human use. EC website. http://ec.europa.eu/health/files/eudralex/vol-1/dir_2003_94/dir_2003_94_en.pdf. Accessed 28 March 2012.
19. Directive 2001/20/EC of the European Parliament and of the Council of 4 April 2001 on the approximation of the laws, regulations and administrative provisions of the Member States relating to the implementation of good clinical practice in the conduct of clinical trials on medicinal products for human use. EUR-Lex website. http://eur-lex.europa.eu/LexUriServ/LexUriServ.do?uri=OJ:L:2001:121:0034:0044:EN:PDF. Accessed 28 March 2012.
20. Council Regulation (EEC) 2309/93 of 22 July 1993 laying down Community procedures for the authorisation and supervision of medicinal products for human and veterinary use and establishing a European Agency for the Evaluation of Medicinal Products. EC website. http://ec.europa.eu/health/files/eudralex/vol-1/reg_1993_2309/reg_1993_2309_en.pdf. Accessed 28 March 2012.
21. Regulation (EC) 726/2004 of the European Parliament and of the Council of 31 March 2004 laying down Community procedures for the authorisation and supervision of medicinal products for human and veterinary use and establishing a European Medicines Agency. EUR-Lex website. http://eur-lex.europa.eu/LexUriServ/LexUriServ.do?uri=OJ:L:2004:136:0001:0033:en:PDF. Accessed 28 March 2012.
22. Regulation (EC) 141/2000 of the European Parliament and of the Council of 16 December 1999 on orphan medicinal products. EUR-Lex website. http://eur-lex.europa.eu/LexUriServ/LexUriServ.do?uri=OJ:L:2000:018:0001:0005:en:PDF. Accessed 28 March 2012.
23. Commission Regulation (EC) 1084/2003 of 3 June 2003 concerning the examination of variations to the terms of a marketing authorisation for medicinal products for human use and veterinary medicinal products granted by a competent authority of a Member State. EC website. http://ec.europa.eu/health/files/eudralex/vol-1/reg_2003_1084/reg_2003_1084_en.pdf. Accessed 28 March 2012.
24. Council Directive 89/342/EEC of 3 May 1989 extending the scope of Directives 65/65/EEC and 75/319/EEC and laying down additional provisions for immunological medicinal products consisting of vaccines, toxins or serums and allergens. EUR-Lex website. http://eur-lex.europa.eu/LexUriServ/LexUriServ.do?uri=OJ:L:1989:142:0014:0015:EN:PDF. Accessed 28 March 2012.
25. Directive 2001/18/EC of the European Parliament and of the Council of 12 March 2001 on the deliberate release into the environment of genetically modified organisms and repealing Council Directive 90/220/EEC. EUR-Lex website. http://eur-lex.europa.eu/LexUriServ/LexUriServ.do?uri=OJ:L:2001:106:0001:0038:EN:PDF. Accessed 28 March 2012.
26. Regulation (EC) 1830/2003 of the European Parliament and of the Council of 22 September 2003 concerning the traceability and labelling of genetically modified organisms and the traceability of food and feed products produced from genetically modified organisms and amending Directive 2001/18/EC. EUR-Lex website. http://eur-lex.europa.eu/LexUriServ/LexUriServ.do?uri=OJ:L:2003:268:0024:0028:EN:PDF. Accessed 28 March 2012.
27. Council Directive 81/851/EEC of 28 September 1981 on the approximation of the laws of the Member States relating to veterinary medicinal products. EUR-Lex website. http://eur-lex.europa.eu/LexUriServ/LexUriServ.do?uri=OJ:L:1981:317:0001:0015:EN:PDF. Accessed 28 March 2012.
28. Directive 2001/82/EC of the European Parliament and of the Council of 6 November 2001 on the Community code relating to veterinary medicinal products. EC website. http://ec.europa.eu/health/files/eudralex/vol-5/dir_2001_82/dir_2001_82_en.pdf. Accessed 28 March 2012.
29. Directive 2004/28/EC of the European Parliament and of the Council of 31 March 2004 amending Directive 2001/82/EC on the Community code relating to veterinary medicinal products. EC website. http://ec.europa.eu/health/files/eudralex/vol-1/dir_2004_27/dir_2004_27_en.pdf. Accessed 28 March 2012.
30. Commission Directive 2006/130/EC of 11 December 2006 implementing Directive 2001/82/EC of the European Parliament and of the Council as regards the establishment of criteria for exempting certain veterinary medicinal products for food-producing animals from the requirement of a veterinary prescription. EUR-Lex website. http://eur-lex.europa.eu/LexUriServ/LexUriServ.do?uri=OJ:L:2006:349:0015:0016:EN:PDF. Accessed 28 March 2012.
31. Commission Directive 2009/9/EC of 10 February 2009 amending Directive 2001/82/EC of the European Parliament and of the Council on the Community code relating to medicinal products for veterinary use. EC website. http://ec.europa.eu/health/files/eudralex/vol-5/dir_2009_9/dir_2009_9_en.pdf. Accessed 28 March 2012.
32. Commission Regulation (EC) 1950/2006 of 13 December 2006 establishing, in accordance with Directive 2001/82/EC of the European Parliament and of the Council on the Community code relating to veterinary medicinal products, a list of substances essential for the treatment of equidae. EUR-Lex website. http://eur-lex.europa.eu/LexUriServ/LexUriServ.do?uri=OJ:L:2006:367:0033:0045:EN:PDF. Accessed 28 March 2012.
33. Council Directive 90/385/EEC of 20 June 1990 on the approximation of the laws of the Member States relating to active implantable medical

devices. EUR-Lex website. http://eur-lex.europa.eu/LexUriServ/LexUriServ.do?uri=CELEX:31990L0385:en:HTML. Accessed 28 March 2012.
34. *Guide to the implementation of directives based on the New Approach and the Global Approach.* EC website. http://ec.europa.eu/enterprise/policies/single-market-goods/files/blue-guide/guidepublic_en.pdf. Accessed 29 March 2012.
35. Council Directive 93/42/EEC of 14 June 1993 concerning medical devices. EUR-Lex website. http://eur-lex.europa.eu/LexUriServ/LexUriServ.do?uri=CONSLEG:1993L0042:20071011:en:PDF. Accessed 28 March 2012.
36. Directive 2001/104/EC of the European Parliament and of the Council of 7 December 2001 amending Council Directive 93/42/EEC concerning medical devices. EUR-Lex website. http://eur-lex.europa.eu/LexUriServ/LexUriServ.do?uri=OJ:L:2002:006:0050:0051:EN:PDF. Accessed 28 March 2012.
37. Directive 2000/70/EC of 16 November 2000 amending Council Directive 93/42/EEC as regards medical devices incorporating stable derivates of human blood or human plasma. EUR-Lex website. http://eur-lex.europa.eu/LexUriServ/LexUriServ.do?uri=OJ:L:2000:313:0022:0024:EN:PDF. Accessed 28 March 2012.
38. Directive 2007/47/EC of the European Parliament and of the Council of 5 September 2007 amending Council Directive 90/385/EEC on the approximation of the laws of the Member States relating to active implantable medical devices, Council Directive 93/42/EEC concerning medical devices and Directive 98/8/EC concerning the placing of biocidal products on the market. EUR-Lex website. http://eur-lex.europa.eu/LexUriServ/LexUriServ.do?uri=OJ:L:2007:247:0021:0055:en:PDF. Accessed 28 March 2012.
39. Directive 2007/47/EC of the European Parliament and of the Council of 5 September 2007 amending Council Directive 90/385/EEC on the approximation of the laws of the Member States relating to active implantable medical devices, Council Directive 93/42/EEC concerning medical devices and Directive 98/8/EC concerning the placing of biocidal products on the market. EUR-Lex website. http://eur-lex.europa.eu/LexUriServ/LexUriServ.do?uri=OJ:L:2007:247:0021:0055:en:PDF. Accessed 28 March 2012.
40. Op cit 11.
41. EC Medical Devices Regulatory Framework. EC website. EC website. http://ec.europa.eu/health/medical-devices/regulatory-framework/index_en.htm. Accessed 7 March 2012
42. EC Roadmap for Medical Device Regulation: 1. Proposal for a Regulation of the European Parliament and of the Council concerning medical devices and repealing Directives 90/385/EEC and 93/42/EEC; 2. Proposal for a Regulation of the European Parliament and of the Council concerning in vitro diagnostic medical devices and repealing Directive 98/79/EC; 3. Communication regarding the innovation in medical devices for the benefit of patients, consumers and healthcare professionals (7th Nov 2011). EC website. http://ec.europa.eu/governance/impact/planned_ia/docs/2008_sanco_081_proposal_medical_devices_en.pdf. Accessed 28 March 2012.
43. Ibid.
44. Ibid.
45. Ibid.
46. Commission Directive 2004/33/EC of 22 March 2004 implementing Directive 2002/98/EC of the European Parliament and of the Council as regards certain technical requirements for blood and blood components. EUR-Lex website. http://eur-lex.europa.eu/LexUriServ/LexUriServ.do?uri=OJ:L:2004:091:0025:0039:EN:PDF. Accessed 28 March 2012.
47. Commission Directive 2005/61/EC of 30 September 2005 implementing Directive 2002/98/EC of the European Parliament and of the Council as regards traceability requirements and notification of serious adverse reactions and events. EUR-Lex website. http://eur-lex.europa.eu/LexUriServ/LexUriServ.do?uri=OJ:L:2005:256:0032:0040:EN:PDF. Accessed 28 March 2012.
48. Commission Directive 2005/62/EC of 30 September 2005 implementing Directive 2002/98/EC of the European Parliament and of the Council as regards Community standards and specifications relating to a quality system for blood establishments. EUR-Lex website. http://eur-lex.europa.eu/LexUriServ/LexUriServ.do?uri=OJ:L:2005:256:0041:0048:EN:PDF. Accessed 28 March 2012.
49. Council Directive 76/768/EEC of 27 July 1976 on the approximation of the laws of the Member States relating to cosmetic products. EUR-Lex website. http://eur-lex.europa.eu/LexUriServ/LexUriServ.do?uri=CONSLEG:1976L0768:20080424:en:PDF. Accessed 28 March 2012.
50. Commission Directive 95/17/EC of 19 June 1995 laying down detailed rules for the application of Council Directive 76/768/EEC as regards the non- inclusion of one or more ingredients on the list used for the labelling of cosmetic products. EUR-Lex website. http://eur-lex.europa.eu/LexUriServ/LexUriServ.do?uri=OJ:L:2006:362:0092:0093:EN:PDF. Accessed 28 March 2012.
51. Directive 2003/15/EC of the European Parliament and of the Council of 27 February 2003 amending Council Directive 76/768/EEC on the approximation of the laws of the Member States relating to cosmetic products. EUR-Lex website. http://eur-lex.europa.eu/LexUriServ/LexUriServ.do?uri=OJ:L:2003:066:0026:0035:en:PDF. Accessed 28 March 2012.
52. Commission Directive 2005/80/EC of 21 November 2005 amending Council Directive 76/768/EEC, concerning cosmetic products, for the purposes of adapting Annexes II and III thereto to technical progress. EUR-Lex website. http://eur-lex.europa.eu/LexUriServ/LexUriServ.do?uri=OJ:L:2005:303:0032:0037:en:PDF. Accessed 28 March 2012.
53. Commission Directive 2006/65/EC of 19 July 2006 amending Council Directive 76/768/EEC, concerning cosmetic products, for the purpose of adapting Annexes II and III thereto to technical progress. EUR-Lex website. http://eur-lex.europa.eu/LexUriServ/LexUriServ.do?uri=OJ:L:2006:198:0011:0014:en:PDF. Accessed 28 March 2012.
54. Commission Directive 2006/78/EC of 29 September 2006 amending Council Directive 76/768/EEC, concerning cosmetic products, for the purposes of adapting Annex II thereto to technical progress. EUR-Lex website. http://eur-lex.europa.eu/LexUriServ/LexUriServ.do?uri=OJ:L:2006:271:0056:0057:en:PDF. Accessed 28 March 2012.
55. Commission Directive 2007/1/EC of 29 January 2007 amending Council Directive 76/768/EEC, concerning cosmetic products, for the purposes of adapting Annex II thereof to technical progress. EUR-Lex website. http://eur-lex.europa.eu/LexUriServ/LexUriServ.do?uri=OJ:L:2007:025:0009:0011:en:PDF. Accessed 28 March 2012.
56. Commission Directive 2007/17/EC of 22 March 2007 amending Council Directive 76/768/EEC, concerning cosmetic products, for the purposes of adapting Annexes III and VI thereto to technical progress. EUR-Lex website. http://eur-lex.europa.eu/LexUriServ/LexUriServ.do?uri=OJ:L:2007:082:0027:0030:en:PDF. Accessed 28 March 2012.
57. Commission Directive 2007/22/EC of 17 April 2007 amending Council Directive 76/768/EEC, concerning cosmetic products, for the purposes of adapting Annexes IV and VI thereto to technical progress. EUR-Lex website. http://eur-lex.europa.eu/LexUriServ/LexUriServ.do?uri=OJ:L:2007:101:0011:0013:en:PDF. Accessed 28 March 2012.
58. Commission Directive 2007/53/EC of 29 August 2007 amending Council Directive 76/768/EEC concerning cosmetic products for the purposes of adapting Annex III thereto to technical progress. EUR-Lex website. http://eur-lex.europa.eu/LexUriServ/LexUriServ.do?uri=CONSLEG:2007L0053:20070919:EN:PDF. Accessed 28 March 2012.
59. Commission Directive 2007/54/EC of 29 August 2007 amending Council Directive 76/768/EEC, concerning cosmetic products, for the purpose of adapting Annexes II and III thereto to technical progress. EUR-Lex website. http://eur-lex.europa.eu/LexUriServ/

LexUriServ.do?uri=OJ:L:2007:226:0021:0027:en:PDF. Accessed 28 March 2012.
60. Regulation (EC) No 1223/2009 of the European Parliament and of the Council of 30 November 2009 on cosmetic products (recast). EUR-Lex website. http://eur-lex.europa.eu/LexUriServ/LexUriServ.do?uri=OJ:L:2009:342:0059:0209:EN:PDF. Accessed 28 March 2012.
61. Regulation (EC) No 178/2002 of the European Parliament and of the Council of 28 January 2002 laying down the general principles and requirements of food law, establishing the European Food Safety Authority and laying down procedures in matters of food safety. EUR-Lex website. http://eur-lex.europa.eu/LexUriServ/LexUriServ.do?uri=OJ:L:2002:031:0001:0024:EN:PDF. Accessed 28 March 2012.
62. Council Directive 89/107/EEC of 21 December 1988 on the approximation of the laws of the Member States concerning food additives authorized for use in foodstuffs intended for human consumption. EUR-Lex website. http://eur-lex.europa.eu/LexUriServ/LexUriServ.do?uri=CELEX:31989L0107:EN:HTML. Accessed 29 March 2012.
63. Directive 2000/13/EC of the European Parliament and of the Council of 20 March 2000 on the approximation of the laws of the Member States relating to the labelling, presentation and advertising of foodstuffs. EUR-Lex website. http://eur-lex.europa.eu/LexUriServ/LexUriServ.do?uri=OJ:L:2000:109:0029:0042:EN:PDF. Accessed 28 March 2012.
64. Commission Directive 2001/101/EC of 26 November 2001 amending Directive 2000/13/EC of the European Parliament and of the Council on the approximation of the laws of the Member States relating to the labelling, presentation and advertising of foodstuffs. EUR-Lex website. http://eur-lex.europa.eu/LexUriServ/LexUriServ.do?uri=CELEX:32001L0101:EN:HTML. Accessed 28 March 2012.
65. Directive 2003/89/EC of the European Parliament and of the Council of 10 November 2003 amending Directive 2000/13/EC as regards indication of the ingredients present in foodstuffs. EUR-Lex website. http://eur-lex.europa.eu/LexUriServ/LexUriServ.do?uri=OJ:L:2003:308:0015:0018:EN:PDF. Accessed 28 March 2012.
66. Council Directive 2006/107/EC of 20 November 2006 adapting Directive 89/108/EEC relating to quick-frozen foodstuffs for human consumption and Directive 2000/13/EC of the European Parliament and of the Council relating to the labelling, presentation and advertising of foodstuffs, by reason of the accession of Bulgaria and Romania. EUR-Lex website. http://eur-lex.europa.eu/LexUriServ/LexUriServ.do?uri=OJ:L:2006:363:0411:0413:EN:PDF. Accessed 28 March 2012.
67. Commission Directive 2006/142/EC of 22 December 2006 amending Annex IIIa of Directive 2000/13/EC of the European Parliament and of the Council listing the ingredients which must under all circumstances appear on the labelling of foodstuffs. EUR-Lex website. http://eur-lex.europa.eu/LexUriServ/LexUriServ.do?uri=OJ:L:2006:368:0110:0111:EN:PDF. Accessed 28 March 2012.
68. Directive 2002/46/EC of the European Parliament and of the Council of 10 June 2002 on the approximation of the laws of the Member States relating to food supplements. EUR-Lex website. http://eur-lex.europa.eu/LexUriServ/LexUriServ.do?uri=OJ:L:2002:183:0051:0057:EN:PDF. Accessed 28 March 2012.
69. Commission Directive 2006/37/EC of 30 March 2006 amending Annex II to Directive 2002/46/EC of the European Parliament and of the Council as regards the inclusion of certain substances. EUR-Lex website. http://eur-lex.europa.eu/LexUriServ/LexUriServ.do?uri=OJ:L:2006:094:0032:0033:EN:PDF. Accessed 28 March 2012.
70. Commission Directive 2006/37/EC of 30 March 2006 amending Annex II to Directive 2002/46/EC of the European Parliament and of the Council as regards the inclusion of certain substances. EUR-Lex website. http://eur-lex.europa.eu/LexUriServ/LexUriServ.do?uri=OJ:L:2006:094:0032:0033:EN:PDF. Accessed 29 March 2012.
71. Commission Regulation (EC) No 1170/2009 of 30 November 2009 amending Directive 2002/46/EC of the European Parliament and of Council and Regulation (EC) No 1925/2006 of the European Parliament and of the Council as regards the lists of vitamin and minerals and their forms that can be added to foods, including food supplements. EUR-Lex website. http://eur-lex.europa.eu/LexUriServ/LexUriServ.do?uri=OJ:L:2009:314:0036:0042:EN:PDF. Accessed 29 March 2012.
72. Commission Regulation (EU) No 1161/2011 of 14 November 2011 amending Directive 2002/46/EC of the European Parliament and of the Council, Regulation (EC) No 1925/2006 of the European Parliament and of the Council and Commission Regulation (EC) No 953/2009 as regards the lists of mineral substances that can be added to foods. EUR-Lex website. http://eur-lex.europa.eu/LexUriServ/LexUriServ.do?uri=OJ:L:2011:296:0029:0030:EN:PDF. Accessed 29 March 2012.
73. Food Supplements. EC website. http://ec.europa.eu/food/food/labellingnutrition/supplements/index_en.htm. Accessed 7 March 2012.
74. Council Directive of 3 May 1989 on the approximation of the laws of the Member States relating to foodstuffs intended for particular nutritional uses (89/398/EEC). EC website. http://ec.europa.eu/food/food/labellingnutrition/nutritional/d89-398-ec.pdf. Accessed 29 March 2012.
75. Regulation (EC) No 1830/2003 of the European Parliament and of the Council of 22 September 2003 concerning the traceability and labelling of genetically modified organisms and the traceability of food and feed products produced from genetically modified organisms and amending Directive 2001/18/EC. EUR-Lex website. http://eur-lex.europa.eu/LexUriServ/LexUriServ.do?uri=OJ:L:2003:268:0024:0028:EN:PDF. Accessed 29 March 2012.
76. Regulation (EC) 1829/2003 of the European Parliament and of the Council of 22 September 2003 on genetically modified food and feed. EC website. http://ec.europa.eu/food/food/animalnutrition/labelling/Reg_1829_2003_en.pdf. Accessed 28 March 2012.

Chapter 2

Crisis Management

By Salma Michor, MBA, PhD, CMgr, RAC

OBJECTIVES

- To gain a basic understanding of crisis management
- Learn about types of crises
- Learn the importance of crisis leadership
- Gain a basic understanding of crisis management techniques

Introduction

A crisis can be defined as a time of intense difficulty or danger.[1] In an organisation, a crisis can be any event that threatens to harm the organisation or its stakeholders. Crisis management is a process by which an organisation deals with such a crisis.[2] Common to most crisis situations is an unexpected event(s) that pose a major threat(s) to the organisation and must be dealt with quickly. A crisis situation can be caused by internal or external factors. Internal factors could include crises arising from such internal hazards as production failure, quality issues and batch recalls, to name a few. External factors could include natural disasters, a financial crisis or other serious external situation affecting an organisation. The former are usually situations that could have been avoided, whereas the latter are those events over which the organisation has no control. In all cases, early identification and management of crises and issues are vital for the organisation's survival. As opposed to risk management, which involves assessing potential threats and finding the best ways to avoid them, crisis management generally involves dealing with threats before, during and after their occurrence. This chapter looks at both external and internal crisis situations in the context of the life sciences industry.

Crisis Management

Crisis management comprises various methods to respond to a crisis, establishing metrics to deal with crises including defining what scenarios constitute a crisis and possible response mechanisms. A crisis management plan should include possible worst-case scenarios and solutions in the form of a contingency plan. For example, dealing with a fire in a building requires proper preparation and a rapid response plan. This can be achieved via drills and exercises to ensure a timely response in the event of a fire.

The way an organisation acts in time of crisis can have an effect on its credibility and reputation. Many companies have a so called emergency or business continuity plan for the short term, complemented by a longer-term recovery plan.

Furthermore, a crisis can be sudden such as natural disasters, sabotage, a hostile takeover or a plant explosion; or a smouldering crisis, such as a product defect, workplace safety or whistle blowing.[3]

Internal Crises

Internal crises can take on many forms, including a production breakdown, batch recalls and personnel strikes, among others. For businesses, several types of crises may be relevant:[4]

- technical or technological crises
- confrontation crises
- crisis of malevolence
- organisational misdeeds
- workplace violence
- rumours
- terrorist attacks/man-made disasters

Chapter 2

Technical or Technological Crises

These types of crises arise when, for example, machines fail to produce expected results. Human error also can cause a technological crisis. A good example of this is the recent BP oil spill. This created both a local environmental crisis as well as an internal company crisis for BP. In the pharmaceutical and medical device industries, a technical crisis could arise when there is a production failure resulting in products of unacceptable quality, a production breakdown or any other technical hazard. As in the BP example, human failure sometimes can lead to a hazard and a potential crisis. This can be in the form of a physical hazard such as a chemical leak resulting in an environmental and safety problem, or a technical problem resulting in compromised processes and/or products. Substandard products could cause a potential health risk resulting in a batch recall. This, in itself, could negatively impact the company image, resulting in a crisis situation.

Confrontation Crises

A typical example of a confrontation crisis is a strike by company personnel to win acceptance of their demands and expectations. This could be in the form of boycotts, sit-ins, ultimatums to those in authority, blockades or occupation of buildings and resisting or disobeying police.[5] This type of crisis is not specific to the life sciences industry. It can arise during periods of stress, e.g., after a merger and/or acquisition, during a financial crisis when companies are forced to lay off workers or any other stressful situation. Often, this happens in countries where there are strong workers' unions, supporting such employee actions.

Crises of Malevolence

These are rare in the life sciences industry, but could occur when opponents or miscreant individuals use criminal means or other extreme tactics for the purpose of expressing hostility or anger toward, or seeking gain from, a company.

Organisational Misdeeds

This could occur when stakeholder interests are put at risk by mismanagement, also known as management misconduct. There are several cases in recent years that have caught the media's attention, e.g., the Italian multinational dairy and food corporation Parmalat SpA's collapse in 2003 with a €14 billion ($20 billion (US); £13 billion (UK)) hole in its accounts, in what remains the EU's biggest bankruptcy.[6]

Workplace Violence

In stressful situations, employees could physically attack others in the workplace. In the life sciences industry, such incidents are rare.

Rumours

Rumours can seriously harm an individual's and/or organisation's reputation. In severe cases, these can cause a crisis situation.

Terrorist Attacks/Man-made Disasters

Although not a common occurrence, pharmaceutical and medical device manufacturers are not immune from terrorist attacks.

External Crises

These are natural crises, such as earthquakes, volcanic eruptions, tornadoes, hurricanes, droughts and other natural disasters that normally are not under an organisation's control. Although external in nature, such crisis situations could adversely affect an organisation and its ability to carry out its normal operations. Some of these, for example a hurricane, may be temporary but others, such as a nuclear catastrophe or financial crisis, may have a longer lasting effect.

Crisis Leadership

A deciding factor for companies in time of crisis is leadership. The most damaging thing to a company about a crisis is the loss of its reputation. For example, the cyanide-laced Tylenol scandal that led to numerous deaths in the 1980s was very well managed by of Johnson & Johnson.[7] In contrast, Exxon Corporation badly managed the oil spill off the coast of Alaska, resulting in a negative image even 20 years later. Erika Hayes James[8] groups crises into two classifications: sudden crises and smouldering crises. The former come about quickly and the organisation usually has little control over the situation. As a result, organisations usually are not blamed, and there is little negative publicity; to the contrary, a sudden crisis such as a terrorist attack may engender solidarity.

Smouldering crises, on the other hand, creep up on a company and usually are the result of mismanagement. In this type of situation there is usually a lot of negative publicity and finger pointing that erode public trust in leadership. James[9] identifies five leadership competencies to deal with a crisis.

1. building trust
2. reforming an organisation's mindset
3. identifying the organisation's vulnerabilities
4. making decisions and taking courageous action
5. learning from crisis to effect change

In comparison to other areas, crisis management is a relatively new field of management.[10] Crisis management incorporates elements of risk management, including such proactive activities as forecasting potential crises and planning how to deal with them. Today, crisis management is an important part of managing a business. An effective leader must institutionalise a process of crisis management to anticipate, prepare and mitigate impending crises.[11]

Crisis Management

Management Commitment

Since some crisis situations cannot be anticipated, any crisis management plan, which is the first step in dealing with the situation, should be more generic; any particular known risks can be more specifically addressed. Upper management should show commitment to and support such an initiative by helping to draft and support a crisis management policy, which provides definitions for general terms and identifies different levels of crisis in the organisation.[12] To effectively implement a crisis management plan, a team should be formed.

Core Team

This core team should identify all possible and probable crises the company could face. Such a plan should also allow for unforeseen situations and unexpected crises. The plan should include roles and responsibilities for crisis preparation and mitigation.

Communication

Vital in any crisis situation is effective communication. Any crisis plan should have an efficient and detailed communication strategy. Companies should ensure they have an adequate infrastructure to support rapid communication with both internal and external stakeholders in times of crisis.

For example, in the case of a critical batch recall, a company must have a system to communicate rapidly with the relevant internal departments, as well as with external agencies such as the Competent Authorities. For a batch recall, relevant departments may include: regulatory, vigilance, medical, logistics, marketing and quality assurance. Other departments also may be involved, depending on the company, the criticality and the type of products being recalled. Internal communication is vital for efficient crisis management; however, communication with external agencies is often more critical and could involve political elements requiring a certain amount of diplomacy.

Training

Training is an important part of crisis management. This ensures organisational preparedness for facing the crisis and usually is carried out in the form of mock drills. Many companies have regular fire alarm drills, which while usually a bother, form part of a wider crisis management plan.

Crisis Resolution

As noted previously, a crisis by its nature has an element of surprise, hence a crisis management plan must be generic

Figure 2-1. Crisis as a Trigger for Change

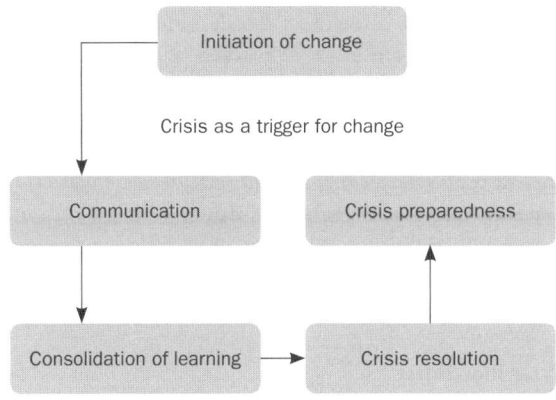

Source: www.alagse.com/leadership/l1.php

enough to cater to unexpected situations. Good leadership in times of crisis ensures a good outcome and a positive perception of the company by stakeholders and the general public.[13] This must be drilled into a company's organisational values to ensure a quick and proper response in times of crisis. An effective response and follow-up could ensure that a company emerges from the crisis with an enhanced image and reputation rather than the opposite.

Crisis as a Trigger for Change

Crisis management demands an adept response based on lessons learned and often leads to change. Hence, change and crisis management often go hand in hand.

Figure 2-1 shows a crisis management cycle that includes: identifying crises, managing crises, extracting learning, communications and initiating a change programme to overcome the organisation's vulnerability.

Case Studies

As noted above, how a company deals with a crisis is vital in determining how the crisis will affect its reputation and public image. Several case studies highlighting good and bad management of crisis situations follow.

Good Crisis Management

Tylenol (Johnson & Johnson)
In the 1980s, someone added cyanide to some Tylenol capsules on store shelves, killing seven people in the US. Johnson & Johnson immediately recalled and destroyed 31 million capsules at a cost of $100 million. The situation was handled very well by Johnson & Johnson, which rapidly introduced tamper-resistant packaging, and Tylenol sales swiftly bounced back to near pre-crisis levels. This crisis had a minimum negative effect due to the way the company responded to the situation.

Chapter 2

Odwalla Foods

In the mid-1990s, the Odwalla company's apple juice was thought to be the cause of an *E. coli* outbreak, causing the company to lose a third of its market value. The company acted swiftly, conferring with the US Food and Drug Administration and Washington state health officials. The company's management organised daily press briefings and sent out press releases that announced a recall. In addition, they expressed remorse and concern and apologised, and took responsibility for anyone harmed by the company's products. The efficient handling of the crisis ensured a minimal negative impact for the company.

Water Pipe Burst

In Los Angeles, during a long drought, a huge water pipe burst right in the middle of one of the city's busiest streets, Ventura Boulevard. This caused the road to split apart, and water flooded the street and sidewalks, closing all the businesses. One of the businesses in the flood area was a hamburger restaurant called Mel's Diner. The manager did not have any customers, so started giving away free hamburgers to the workers repairing the water pipe. Since this incident was covered by the media, the burger restaurant received a lot of media attention by reacting swiftly to an otherwise bad situation.[14]

Bad Crisis Management

Snow Brand Milk Products Co.

For Snow Brand, Japan's premier dairy foods company, a badly handled food poisoning scandal in 2000 damaged the company's reputation so severely that is still impacted today. Large numbers of people (more than 15,000), mostly in western Japan, suddenly came down with food poisoning. This was linked to consuming milk or other dairy products made by Snow Brand. An analysis traced the illnesses to staphylococcus aureus bacteria on the production line in Snow Brand's Osaka factory that processed low-fat milk. Inspections of the factory found that the company's hygiene standards were appalling.

The company initially sought to downplay the incident in an attempt to limit the extent of the product recall. Although requested by the Osaka city public health centre to voluntarily recall other products, the company was reluctant to do so. It tried to hide the request, but the city publicised both the recall and the request.

Media reports on the incident gave the impression that the poisoning was the end-product of a company rife with corporate arrogance, which led to very bad publicity for the company.[15]

Exxon

In the late 1980s, as the Exxon Valdez oil tanker entered Prince William Sound on its way to California, the ship ran aground and began spilling oil. Within a very short period of time, significant quantities of its 1,260,000 barrels had leaked into the waters.[16]

At the time of the collision, the third mate, who was not certified to take the tanker into those waters, was at the helm because the ship's captain and many of the crew had been drinking alcohol in considerable quantities.

Action to contain the spill was very slow and communication was poor. Shortly after the accident took place and international media began extensive coverage of the spill, the Exxon chairman refused to talk with the press. The spill continued to spread and the situation worsened, in part due to bad weather. As the company continued to communicate poorly, the media coverage became hostile.[17]

Eventually, the chairman did give a live interview where it became apparent that he had neglected to read the latest plans for the clean-up, and stated his belief that it was not the chairman's job to read such reports, blaming others for the mishandling of the spill. This made Exxon's catastrophe complete.

Japan's Reactors and the BP Spill

More recently, two major badly managed crises include the earthquake and tsunami damage to Japan's nuclear reactors and the BP spill in the Gulf of Mexico. Both crises involved potentially catastrophic technological problems, incomplete crisis response plans, misleading early information, divided private and public authority and ineffective initial actions.[18]

Conclusions

A crisis usually is associated with a drop in an organisation's stock value. A study carried out in 1996[19] identified organisations that recovered and even exceeded pre-catastrophe stock prices (Recoverers) and those whose stock prices did not recover (Non-recoverers). One of the key conclusions of this study is, "Effective management of the consequences of catastrophes is very significant in determining whether a company can effectively recover from a crisis situation." To achieve this, there needs to be a strong commitment from upper management moving from reacting to a crisis to generating crisis leadership. This calls for the type of leader who can perform well under considerable pressure. Effective communication with the media can affect public opinion and the company's reputation with shareholders, its financial well-being and its survival. Effective leadership during a crisis should address immediate action as well as long-term implications and opportunities for change and improvement.

References
1. "Crisis," Oxford Dictionaries. http://oxforddictionaries.com/definition/crisis. Accessed 26 May 2012.
2. "Crisis Management," Wikipedia. http://en.wikipedia.org/wiki/Crisis_management. Accessed 29 May 2012.
3. James EH. "Crisis Leadership." Social Science Research Network. Available at SSRN: http://ssrn.com/abstract=1281843.

4. Lerbinger, O. *The Crisis Manager: Facing Risk and Responsibility*. 1997; Mahwah, NJ: Lawrence Erlbaum Associates.
5. Op cit 2.
6. "Italian dairy boss gets 10 years." BBC news website. http://news.bbc.co.uk/2/hi/business/7790803.stm. Accessed 8 June 2012.
7. Op cit 3.
8. Ibid.
9. James EH and Wooten LP. "Leadership as (Un)usual: How to Display Competence in Times of Crisis." Erika Hayes James website. http://erikahayesjames.com/2009/04/leadership-as-unusual-how-to-display-competence-in-times-of-crisis/. Accessed 10 June 2012.
10. "All About Crisis Management." Free Management Library website. http://managementhelp.org/crisismanagement/index.htm. Accessed 9 June 2012.
11. "Crisis management—a leadership challenge." www.alagse.com/leadership/l1.php. Alagse website. Accessed 9 June 2012.
12. Ibid.
13. Ibid.
14. "Crisis Management Moments: Making the most of a bad situation." All About Public Relations website. www.aboutpublicrelations.net/aa021701b.htm. Accessed 10 June 2012.
15. "Companies in Crisis—What not to do when it all goes wrong." Mallenbacker.net corporate social responsibility website. www.mallenbaker.net/csr/crisis04.html. Accessed 10 June 2012.
16. Ibid.
17. Ibid.
18. Op cit 2.
19. Knight RF and Pretty D. *The Impact of Catastrophes on Shareholder Value*, 1996. ASSE website. www.asse.org/professionalaffairs-new/bosc/docs/Catastrophesandshareholdervalue.pdf. Accessed 11 June 2012.

Chapter 3

Reimbursement in the EU

By Gordon Bache, PhD, MA, LLB, and Martin Gisby, PhD, MRes

OBJECTIVES

❑ To enable an understanding of the key models of reimbursement utilised by healthcare systems in the EU

❑ To appreciate and clarify the differences and links between reimbursement and the related processes of pricing regulation and health technology assessment

❑ To provide case studies and examples to illustrate the operation of reimbursement and related processes in the EU

DIRECTIVES AND GUIDELINES COVERED IN THIS CHAPTER

❑ Council Directive 89/105/EEC of 21 December 1988 relating to the transparency of measures regulating the prices of medicinal products for human use and their inclusion in the scope of national health insurance systems

❑ European Commission, Proposal for a Directive of the European Parliament and of the Council relating to the transparency of measures regulating the prices of medicinal products for human use and their inclusion in the scope of public health insurance systems

Introduction

In the current environment, institutions that cover the costs of medicines are increasingly utilising cost-containment measures to reduce the burden of their drug bills. As such, if a product is to successfully gain access to a market, it has to negotiate a variety of measures to secure a price and obtain payment from the relevant institution. Moreover, as described in this chapter, these measures vary widely among different EU Member States. Therefore, it is important that regulatory professionals have a basic knowledge of what may be expected from states after they have obtained regulatory approval so they can work with commercial and payer-evidence colleagues to ensure reimbursement. Moreover, when considering study designs, it is important that the payer constituency is considered as well as the regulatory agencies.

Before exploring some of the key concepts involved in the pricing and reimbursement of medicinal products, an important starting point is an appreciation of the complexity of pricing and reimbursement regulation across the EU. Three points represent useful insights for understanding this complexity.

First, a useful concept for understanding the setup of different healthcare systems across the EU is the "financing mix." Medicinal products provided under healthcare systems may be funded by both public (indirect taxation, general taxation, national insurance) and private sources (e.g., out-of-pocket payments, co-payments, private health insurance, employer-provided benefits). EU healthcare systems use different mixes of these sources of finance.

Second, the principal "payer" will differ among countries, and there may be multiple payers in one state based upon a geographical hierarchy (e.g., national, regional, local) or point of delivery (e.g., hospital-based care or community care). The principal payer may be a public body (e.g., the soon-to-be abolished local Primary Care Trusts [PCTs] in the UK), a publically mandated scheme (e.g., Statutory Health Insurance in Germany) or private enterprises (e.g., private health insurance). In France, depending on the product and the level of determined benefit, the state and a private insurer may reimburse different proportions of a single prescription, e.g., 65% and 35% respectively.

Third, the nature of the pricing and reimbursement system may be different based upon the nature of the product concerned. For example, the maximum reimbursed price for generics, innovative medicines or medicines considered to be therapeutically equivalent may be entirely different. In the UK, the Pharmaceutical Price Regulation Scheme (PPRS), which is a voluntary scheme, largely governs the pricing of innovative pharmaceuticals, and Scheme M outlines the voluntarily agreed system for generic medicines.[1]

These three insights alone illustrate the extremely complex environment in the EU for obtaining pricing and reimbursement of medicinal products. As such, the purpose of this chapter is not to provide a comprehensive overview of the area, but to provide some of the basic concepts and processes used within the EU, supported by clear examples.

This chapter first outlines the responsibility (i.e., competence) of Member States and the EU with regard to pricing and reimbursement policy. Second, so far as is possible, it delineates the key differences between pricing, reimbursement and health technology assessment (HTA). Third, the chapter identifies the key pricing processes utilised in the EU. Fourth, there is an exploration of the main reimbursement models and the impact that reimbursement requirements have on evidence-generation plans. Fifth, two different country reimbursement case studies (Spain and Germany) are presented. Finally, a brief summary of some emerging trends in the pricing and reimbursement environment concludes the chapter.

Competence: Responsibility for Pricing and Reimbursement Policy

In the EU, competence for the pricing and reimbursement of medicinal products rests with the 27 individual Member States. The *Treaty on the Functioning of the European Union*, Article 168 states:

> "Union action shall respect the responsibilities of the Member States for the definition of their health policy and for the organisation and delivery of health services and medical care. The responsibilities of the Member States shall include the management of health services and medical care and the allocation of the resources assigned to them."

As such, pricing and reimbursement policy is organised by Member States, and each Member State has a different system that must be negotiated to obtain pricing approval and reimbursement by the relevant healthcare system. There has, however, been some limited intervention at the EU level in the form of the *Transparency Directive*, which was adopted in 1989.[2] Essentially, the *Transparency Directive* puts an upper limit on the duration of the initial pricing and reimbursement process at 180 days,[3] reasons must be supplied for the decision and it must be possible to appeal the decision. Moreover, for Member States using profit controls (e.g., the UK) the methodology used must be published. The justification for EU-level intervention here was that non-transparent measures may represent hidden barriers to the free movement of goods and services in the internal market. At the time of writing, the European Commission has proposed a new directive to replace the existing one, which proposes a shortening of the upper limit to 120 days for innovative medicines and 30 days for generics.[4] Moreover, the proposal aims to strengthen the enforcement of the *Transparency Directive*'s provisions by allocating a responsible body and calling for the imposition of stronger sanctions for noncompliance with timelines. However, besides the requirement for transparency and imposition of specified duration for the pricing and reimbursement process, policy is formed and executed primarily at the Member State level.

The Difference Between Pricing, Reimbursement and Health Technology Assessment

Before exploring the differing policies that have been adopted for the EU, it is important to understand what pricing and reimbursement are in the first place, and how they relate to the concept of health technology assessment (HTA). It can be very easy to confuse the processes of securing a price for a medicinal product, of obtaining reimbursement for a product and negotiating (or being subjected to) a process of HTA. The reason for this is that many systems in different Member States combine two or more steps together into a single process that makes them difficult to separate. For example, in France there is an assessment of medical benefit that informs the reimbursement rate decision and additional medical benefit (a comparative assessment) that feeds into the pricing decision. As such, in distinguishing between the processes of pricing, obtaining reimbursement and negotiating (or being subject to) an HTA, it should be recognised that, in practice, the processes may be tightly mixed together (or a consecutive process). Another complicating factor is the distinction between what is commonly referred to as the ex-factory price and what is often referred to as the "reimbursed price." For example, there may often be two different processes, e.g., free pricing for the former and contractual negotiations for the latter. Thus, there may be more than one price in a market (e.g., ex-factory, wholesale, pharmacy price), which is regulated under a different system. Therefore, it is important to always check the context under which a particular price is applicable and how it has been agreed.

To provide clarity for the purposes of this chapter:
- Obtaining reimbursement can be considered to be the process/system through which an enterprise that markets a medicinal product receives payment from a third-party payer (e.g., social insurance, a national healthcare system [or subcomponent thereof], private insurance, "patient-as-payer"—e.g., out-of-pocket costs). However, the chain of reimbursement may also involve other bodies such as the manufacturer itself, wholesalers and pharmacies.
- Pricing of a medicinal product is considered to be the process through which a maximum price is set, either without government controls (e.g., free pricing) or with such controls (e.g., reference pricing or pricing negotiations).
- HTA is considered in its broadest sense as any form of assessment (using a defined methodology) conducted of a healthcare technology, which is intended to influence decision making. This does not necessarily have to directly inform a formal decision process (for example, HTAs may be independently conducted by universities or other bodies not formally linked to a decision-making institution).

Consideration of HTA is not a focus of this chapter, but it is covered to a limited extent as it is directly or indirectly tied into reimbursement decisions in some countries. (For more information on HTA, see Chapter 4.)

Pricing

An extensive variety of mechanisms is used to regulate the pricing process in the EU. Therefore, the following section aims to outline three key examples of processes that are widely used in the EU. The country-specific case studies considered toward the end of this chapter provide fuller examples, which demonstrate how this array of mechanisms is used in practice.

As mentioned previously, medicinal products may be priced or obtain pricing approval in many different ways, depending on the design of the system in place in a particular Member State. A first approach to pricing is free pricing. Under a free pricing system, the enterprise that is marketing the medicinal product is able to freely set its price when the product launches in the market. The states that have traditionally been regarded as free pricing states are the UK and Germany, but such categorisation can be misleading. An ex-factory price, as used in this chapter, is the price that is generally published in a public instrument (e.g., the *British National Formulary* in the UK) and is the maximum price that the payer is likely to pay, although discounts may be provided against this price. For example,

in Germany there is a mandatory 16% statutory rebate from the price that is published, which means this price largely is relevant only for purposes of external benchmarking in other states. Moreover, securing a free price may be based on the condition of agreeing to mandatory reductions in price at a later date,[5] price freezes, mandatory discounts or controls on profit.[6] As such, this initial free pricing is usually conditional.

A second approach to pricing, broadly speaking, is "pricing control." Such controls can operate either directly or indirectly. For example, prices may be set unilaterally by a legal measure (e.g., Romania), may be agreed through a process of negotiation (e.g., Italy[7]) or may be based on public procurement (e.g., tendering by hospitals). The basis for this statutory process may be "international reference pricing." This method takes the price from other listed countries (the basket), which are normally specified and uses that data as the basis for its own price or to inform pricing negotiations. For example, Romania bases the maximum price on the average of the lowest three prices from 12 reference states: Czech Republic, Bulgaria, Hungary, Poland, Slovakia, Austria, Belgium, Italy, Lithuania, Spain, Greece and Germany.[8] Internal reference pricing is another widely used method. For example, in Germany, products that are deemed therapeutically equivalent can be placed in a reference price group, with each priced at the same level. Again, some states may use a mix of these different approaches.

A third pricing approach with increasing prominence within the policy environment is value-based pricing. Value-based pricing incorporates consideration of a concept of "value" within the process through which price is agreed. The concept of value may differ by country and can include:
- the assessment of additional clinical benefit (Germany)[9]
- additional medical benefit (France)[10]
- level of innovation, burden of illness and wider societal benefit (proposed value-based pricing framework set to be introduced in the UK)[11]

Reimbursement

This section moves from consideration of pricing to an exploration of 1) the models of reimbursement in the EU and 2) the impact the increased role of payers has on evidence-generation requirements.

Models of Reimbursement

Reimbursement is often fundamentally linked to pricing approval. This link is particularly evident in a first example, which is use of selected lists. Often, there will be a "positive list" (usually a formulary), which is a list containing the products that will be reimbursed by a particular healthcare institution. There may be a formal allocation of budget to medicines that are included on this list. For example, in Italy price-volume agreements may be a condition of gaining national approval for reimbursement from the Italian Medicines Agency, *Agenzia Italiana del Farmaco* (AIFA). In addition, AIFA has secured legislation to ensure that where a positive decision is made, regional authorities are required to provide access to these therapies (often through regional formularies). The exact process for inclusion on these lists can be unclear and will be defined to different degrees in different systems.

Pressure for a clear understanding of the rationale behind inclusion (or non-inclusion) on reimbursement formularies has led to the development of more explicit and transparent decision-making methodologies. A second key model of reimbursement that incorporates this is a defined pharmacoeconomic or value-based assessment of a medicinal product. Under such a model, a reimbursement decision may incorporate a defined methodology such as cost-effectiveness analysis (e.g., UK), budget impact analysis (e.g., Spain), other health-economic data (e.g., the Netherlands),[12] a methodology that assesses improvement of medical benefit (e.g., France)[13] or another determination of value. At present, there are distinctly different methodologies being used by Member States, which, from a Marketing Authorisation Holder's (MAH) perspective, complicates the collection of the relevant evidence to address payer requirements.

A third reimbursement model to be aware of, but which is not used extensively in the EU, is the benefit design given to the coverage of a particular medicinal product in a competitive market. For example, in the US, private insurance companies and Medicaid and Medicare programmes may apply a different level of co-payment or deductible, i.e., the part that the patient pays, for different drugs. Where the co-payment required of patients is higher, this can impact prescribing patterns and thus limit reimbursement of particular drugs. In the EU, this method is less relevant, but it is applicable where a decision necessitates out-of-pocket expenses from patients. For example, in Spain, there are different levels of reimbursement status (100%, 90% and 60% covered by the state), and patients have to cover the outstanding cost where the product is not fully reimbursed.

A final phenomenon of which to be aware, which does not necessarily constitute an independent model, is a conditional reimbursement approach. In certain Member States (e.g., the UK and Italy), there has been increasing use of what are known as "risk share schemes" (commonly referred to in the UK as patient access schemes). Under such schemes, the Member State may reimburse a product (which they might not have otherwise) based on its per-patient performance (pay-for-performance), an initial defined period of free stock or an agreed upper limitation of financial exposure. Conditional reimbursement may also be granted for a fixed period of time to enable an MAH to collect additional data, either as part of a standardised process (e.g., the Netherlands), or to address specific information gaps (e.g., real-world effectiveness or compliance rates).

The three reimbursement models outlined above make it clear that demonstrating value to payers is different from demonstrating safety, efficacy and quality to a regulatory agency. As payers are the key to reimbursement, these processes need to be understood by all involved in drug commercialisation.

A point that needs to be noted here is that differences in the reimbursement process may exist in a specific country depending on the setting of treatment. For example:

- Hospitals may purchase medicines directly, frequently at a discount against the ex-factory price, whereas community-dispensed medicine is generally reimbursed at the ex-factory price.
- Reimbursement may be through diagnosis related group (DRG)-based tariff payments for bundles of care in a secondary care setting.
- Some systems only regulate reimbursement in the community, allowing local decision making around purchasing in acute care (e.g., Sweden), or may direct reimbursement through hospitals to take advantage of lower costs (e.g., Spain).

As such, the setting of care is an important consideration in many EU states when planning for commercialisation of a product after obtaining regulatory approval.

Evidence Requirements to Support Reimbursement

In an environment where enterprises have to negotiate these country-specific reimbursement processes after they have secured regulatory approval, there is an increasing need to generate data that are relevant to the "payer" constituency, which can be quite different to that of the regulatory agency assessment.

First, there is pressure for investment in health economics and outcomes research (HEOR) studies. Outcomes research may include such data as clinician-reported outcomes for secondary clinical endpoints (e.g., scoring physical functioning), patient-reported outcomes (PROs) (e.g., quality of life) or healthcare resource utilisation (e.g., number of secondary care visitations). Outcomes research can be conducted either as independent studies or can be added into a traditional clinical trial. Studies that collect data to support health economic modelling, for example cost-effectiveness analyses, are a necessary part of ensuring reimbursement in some Member States (e.g., the UK and the Netherlands).

Second, there is increasing pressure from payers for MAHs to complete clinical trials that demonstrate therapeutic value beyond that required to gain regulatory approval. For example, the concepts of comparative efficacy or effectiveness research and collection of "Real World Evidence" (RWE) are important in states like France (in the ASMR rating, a rating of added clinical value in comparison with existing therapies) and Germany (in the medical benefit-assessment process) which require studies that show additional benefit compared to a relevant clinical comparator. The aim of such studies is to demonstrate the efficacy of medicines as compared to a relevant comparator in clinical trials (with an emphasis on head-to-head trials) and also effectiveness in real-world clinical practice (rather than under randomised controlled trial conditions). An example of where such an approach is being adopted in the EU is Germany, where the law regulating the reimbursement of drugs (AMNOG) requires demonstration of additional benefit against a predefined appropriate comparator.

A useful concept when considering the evidence-generation requirements for a particular state is the "payer archetype" that exists there, i.e., the kind of evidence that is likely to support claims of value in that state. For example, the UK is often considered to be an example where the cost-effectiveness archetype is prominent, and Italy is an example where a budget impact archetype is emphasised. Therefore, when developing evidence for the Italian market, the need for strong budget impact data is paramount; in the UK, the key concern is cost-effectiveness.

This chapter now turns to consideration of two different case studies, which will demonstrate how some of the measures explored in this chapter are used in practice within a single system.

Case Study 1: Germany

In Germany, everyone is insured under the statutory health insurance (*Gesetzliche Krankenversicherung*, GKV) scheme. Approximately 80% of the German population receives the same services to the extent necessary, provided those services are appropriate and cost-efficient. Thus, both the extent and the amount of reimbursement for medicines supplied outside the hospital setting are, for the most part, determined centrally by laws, regulations and collective agreements. Consequently, individual agreements between pharmaceutical companies and individual health insurance funds do not define the content of the services provided, but rather they contain additional price reductions or special reimbursement models for particular medicinal products.

In the German market, all authorised prescription-only medicines are inherently reimbursable by virtue of their marketing authorisation, unless they are prescribed for such "lifestyle disorders," as controlling obesity or treating minor ailments (e.g., common colds), or they have been explicitly excluded from the reimbursement scheme by means of secondary regulations. Nonprescription-only medicines for adults have, since 2004, only been reimbursable to a very minor extent and under strictly defined circumstances. It is the responsibility of the Federal Joint Committee (*Gemeinsamer Bundesausschuss*, G-BA)—the self-regulatory body for health insurance funds, physicians and hospitals—to issue binding directives on drug reimbursement.

The reimbursement of a medicinal product by GKV funds is based on the selling price as determined by the pharmaceutical company itself, though this is not paid in full. Various central control instruments are designed to limit GKV spending on medicines, such as reference prices for particular groups of medicines, whereby GKV will cover the cost up to the amount fixed in each case. This amount is calculated by the Federal Association of Statutory Health Insurance Funds (*GKV-Spitzenverband*, GKV-SV), based on an average of current prices, and is constantly adjusted. Where medicines are not eligible for reference prices, health insurance funds are to receive discounts for each medicine sold, generally amounting to 6% of the manufacturer's selling price, but sometimes rising to 16%. In addition, there are reductions for generics (10%) and occasional price freezes. Furthermore, the individual health insurance funds are able to reach discount agreements for specific medicines with individual pharmaceutical companies in order to generate additional savings.

For reimbursable medicines containing new active substances launched in Germany on or after 1 January 2011, there is a new system of benefit assessment that informs pricing negotiations. Where products are not deemed to provide an additional benefit, they will normally fall into one of the reference price groups, at an amount corresponding to the cost of the appropriate comparator therapy. Medicines with additional benefit move forward to negotiate a reimbursement discount between the pharmaceutical company and GKV-SV, which will then apply to all health insurance funds—including private funds. This applies for 12 months after the medicinal product is first brought onto the market and is granted as a discount on the manufacturer's price. Thus, for 12 months, GKV pays the manufacturer's price minus the statutory discounts for new medicines, and from month 13 onward, the health insurance funds additionally receive the centrally agreed discount.

To obtain an "early benefit assessment," the pharmaceutical company must, at the time of launching the new medicinal product, submit a dossier to G-BA containing evidence of the following:
- approved indications
- medical benefit
- additional medical benefit in relation to the appropriate comparator therapy
- the number of patients and patient subgroups for whom there is a meaningful additional therapeutic benefit
- the costs of the treatment to the statutory health insurance scheme
- the requirement for quality-assured implementation

If no dossier is submitted, the additional benefit is regarded as unproven. The benefit assessment must have been completed within three months of submission. As a rule, it is performed by the Institute for Quality and Efficiency in Health Care (*Institut für Qualität und Wirtschaftlichkeit im Gesundheitswesen*, IQWiG), an independent scientific body established under private law. G-BA reaches a binding decision on the additional benefit within a further three months. Additional benefit is understood to mean qualitative or quantitative greater benefit—as demonstrated by studies supported by high-level evidence (Randomised Controlled Clinical Trials, RCTs)—compared with the relevant standard therapy in terms of endpoints of relevance to the patient, such as morbidity or mortality. Consideration is only given to surrogate endpoints in isolated exceptional cases. There are six levels of benefit, which range from minor benefit through to a considerable additional benefit compared with the comparator therapy. The additional benefit in each case is established for identifiable patient subgroups. G-BA likewise stipulates the standard therapy with which the new medicine is compared according to the international standards of evidence-based medicine. If there are several alternatives, the most cost-efficient treatment is to be chosen. This is chiefly of relevance to medicines without any additional benefit, since their reimbursement is capped at an amount corresponding to the cost of this comparator therapy. For medicines belonging to a specific class of active substance, the same comparator therapy will apply. If the pharmaceutical company, when compiling the dossier, deviates from the comparator therapy selected by G-BA, it must comprehensively justify the change. G-BA decides whether or not to accept this justification. Before commencing the benefit assessment, G-BA provides the pharmaceutical company with advice, for a fee of approximately €10,000, which includes identifying what G-BA considers to be the appropriate comparator therapy. Although the costs of the treatment to GKV also are to be specified in the dossier itself, these only become relevant in connection with the reimbursement agreement between GKV-SV and the pharmaceutical company. Only the direct costs to GKV are considered here. In the negotiations concerning the reimbursement discount, a monetary value is to be placed on the established additional benefit of the drug. Here the parties to the agreement should also take into consideration the annual treatment costs of comparable medicines and the anticipated selling prices in a basket of other European countries, if the drug is marketed there. If the negotiations are not concluded after six months, the reimbursement discount is determined by an arbitration body.

For the first time, the new reimbursement system in Germany for innovative medicines includes the pharmaceutical industry in the complex web of agreements reached by GKV and thus, henceforth, requires cooperation from the pharmaceutical industry, the self-governing body and health insurance funds. For the German healthcare system, in contrast to other EU countries, this is an entirely new situation, which in the first instance confronts all stakeholders with the challenge of creating a platform for objective discussion. This is still necessary in relation to many aspects of the early benefit assessment (such as assessment methods, for example). Whether the negotiations on reimbursement discounts between the health insurance funds' umbrella organisation and the individual pharmaceutical companies will lead to a system of reimbursement for new medicines that suits both sides will not become apparent until the second half of 2012 at the earliest.

Case Study 2: Spain

In Spain, once regulatory approval is granted by *Agencia Española del Medicamento y Productos Sanitarios* (AEMPS),[14] the manufacturer can submit an application for pricing and reimbursement. Pharmaceutical regulation is an exclusive responsibility of the national administration, although the responsibility for pharmaceutical management (including funding) is fully transferred to the regional health systems (Autonomous Communities).[15]

There are three main stakeholders in the process for pricing and reimbursement of pharmaceuticals in Spain. The first stakeholder is the *Comisión interministerial de Precios del medicamento* (CIPM, the Inter-Ministerial Commission on Drug Prices).[16] This body is responsible for defining drug prices, after reviewing the manufacturer's application. Price decisions are based on therapeutic utility of drugs from AEMPS and the drug's average price, if available, in reference EU countries. Price setting will comprise one of two elements: 1) defining a reference price for therapeutic drug groups when generics with the same active ingredient are available[17] or 2) defining limits on the prices of new licensed drugs.

The second key stakeholder is the *Dirección General de Cartera Básica de Servicios del Sistema Nacional de Salud y Farmacia* (General Directorate for Basic Services Portfolio of National Health Service and Pharmacy).[18] This body decides whether to reimburse a new drug in the public health system, for what indications and under what conditions. If the reimbursement status is approved, the pricing decision will be communicated to the manufacturer. If the reimbursement decision is negative, the product will be placed on a "negative list" and the price can be freely determined by the manufacturer. There are three reimbursement categories:[19]

- 100% reimbursement for hospital pharmaceuticals
- 90% reimbursement for pharmaceuticals for the management of chronic illnesses (e.g., diabetes, asthma)
- 60% reimbursement for the majority of prescription-only pharmaceuticals

At a national level, decision criteria for granting reimbursement status to drugs in Spain include:
- severity, duration and consequences of the condition for which they are indicated
- specific needs of some population groups
- the drug's therapeutic and social utility
- rationalisation of public pharmaceutical expenditure
- existence of other drugs or therapies for the same indication(s)
- new drug's degree of innovation

Each company is free to submit as much documentation as is considered necessary to the General Directorate for Basic Services Portfolio of National Health Service and Pharmacy to support a positive decision. Among these documents, only the *Escandallo* (Price application) is compulsory. No HEOR data are formally required for a pricing and reimbursement application. There are no opportunities for presubmission formal advice or use of risk-share or patient access schemes.

The third main group of stakeholders is the *Comunidades Autónomas* (Autonomous Communities). As mentioned previously, pharmaceutical management is fully transferred to the Autonomous Communities in Spain.[20] Each Autonomous Community has a regional health department and health minister responsible for health policy within the geographical region, plus a health service that manages service delivery.

In Spain, central and regional governments are looking to strengthen the mechanisms for selective reimbursement of drugs (factors such as incremental clinical benefit, budget impact and cost-minimisation studies will be considered). There have been calls for formation of a committee for selection of drugs that would operate in a similar way to the UK's National Institute for Health and Clinical Excellence (NICE).[21] However, most recent opinion indicates that rather than opting for the creation of a new evaluating body, central government will rely on the existing network of national and regional HTA agencies. Reports from this network will be used to decide what technologies and procedures are to be incorporated in the common health service portfolio and, most importantly, which are to be excluded from reimbursement. In addition, opinion in early 2012 indicated that autonomous communities could have a voice in the CIPM.[22]

Conclusion

This chapter provides a starting point for regulatory professionals in understanding the complex, but increasingly pivotal, pricing and reimbursement landscape in the EU. After reading this chapter, it should be clear that the placement of responsibility (or competence) for formation of pharmaceutical policy rests primarily with Member States, which have all developed their own individual systems that need to be negotiated after regulatory approval. Three modes of pricing have been outlined that can be used as the basis for considering the mix of mechanisms used in practice; these are free pricing, pricing controls and value-based pricing. The chapter makes it clear that when considering reimbursement models, in most markets, a fundamental link to pricing exists. This chapter presented four different reimbursement approaches (which may often be present as a mix in a specific country): selected lists, pharmacoeconomic or value-based assessment, benefit design and conditional reimbursement. In light of the rapidly changing EU environment for pricing and reimbursement, some implications for evidence-generation plans were highlighted. These include the increased need for health economic analyses (e.g., cost-effectiveness analysis, budget impact analysis) and outcomes research studies (clinician reported outcomes and patient reported outcomes) as well as payer focussed study designs that consider comparative efficacy, effectiveness and real-world evidence. The preexisting trend for payers to request more country-specific data looks set to intensify, both from clinical and economic perspectives. Finally, two case studies for Germany and Spain have provided overview examples of how these different mechanisms can be set up in practice within a country.

References

1. UK Department of Health, "Revised long-term arrangements for reimbursement of generic medicines Scheme M' March 2010 – An agreement reached between the Department of Health and the British Generic Manufacturers Association." UK Department of Health website. www.dh.gov.uk/en/Publicationsandstatistics/Publications/PublicationsPolicyAndGuidance/DH_115260. Accessed 9 April 2012.
2. Council Directive 89/105/EEC of 21 December 1988 relating to the transparency of measures regulating the prices of medicinal products for human use and their inclusion in the scope of national health insurance systems. *Transparency Directive*. EudraLex website. http://eur-lex.europa.eu/LexUriServ/LexUriServ.do?uri=CELEX:31989L0105:en:HTML. Accessed 9 April 2012.
3. *Transparency Directive*. Article 6. The price is to be agreed and communicated to the applicant within 90 days.
4. European Commission, *Proposal for a Directive of the European Parliament and of the Council relating to the transparency of measures regulating the prices of medicinal products for human use and their inclusion in the scope of public health insurance systems* COM(2012) 84 final. EC website. http://ec.europa.eu/governance/impact/ia_carried_out/docs/ia_2012/com_2012_0084_en.pdf. Accessed 9 April 2012.
5. For example in the UK the agreement between the Association of the British Pharmaceutical Industry and the Department of Health periodically (around every five years) agrees a particular price cut from the initial price, which is to be implemented as part of the agreement.
6. In the UK, the PPRS contains a maximum return on investment (ROC) and a maximum margin of tolerance regarding levels of profit. In Italy, it is not profit, but the volume of sales based on a particular price, that is capped. If enterprises sell more than that cap, they are required to pay back additional revenue generated.
7. Although Italy is a mixed system in that the negotiated price is then published in the *Official Gazzette*. See Law n. 326 of November 24, 2003 and *Comitato Interministeriale per la Programmazione Economia* (CIPE, Interministerial Committee for Economic Planning) Resolution of 1 February 2001.

8. Norm no. 220 from 12.03.2010. Romanian law specifying price-setting strategy as the average price of the three lowest prices at which the drug is sold, among the 12 reference European countries (Czech Republic, Bulgaria, Hungary, Poland, Slovakia, Austria, Belgium, Italy, Lithuania, Spain, Greece and Germany).
9. See The Act on the Reform of the Market for Medicinal Products (Gesetz zur Neuordnung des Arzneimittelmarktes - AMNOG) 2011. Bundesministerium für Gesundheit. www.bmg.bund.de/krankenversicherung/arzneimittelversorgung/arzneimittelmarktneuordnungsgesetz-amnog/das-gesetz-zu-neuordnung-des-arzneimittelmarktes-amnog.html. Accessed 9 April 2012.
10. For example, according to research conducted by the International Society for Pharmacoeconomics and Outcomes Research (ISPOR) CEPS will consider improvement of medical benefit level in price negotiations. ISPOR website. www.ispor.org/htaroadmaps/. Accessed 9 April 2012.
11. UK Department of Health. "A new value-based approach to the pricing of branded medicines: A consultation." 16 December 2010 – s4.10. UK Department of Health website. www.dh.gov.uk/en/Consultations/Liveconsultations/DH_122760. Accessed 9 April 2012.
12. *Zorgverzekeringswet* (Netherlands Healthcare Insurance Act 2006, An addition to the Exceptional Medical Expenses Act). Netherlands government website. www.rijksoverheid.nl/onderwerpen/zorgverzekering. Accessed 10 April 2012.
13. *Amélioration du Service Médical Rendu* (ASMR). France Pharmaceuticals. ISPOR website. www.ispor.org/htaroadmaps/france.asp. Accessed 10 April 2012.
14. *Agencia Española del Medicamento y Productos Sanitarios* (Spanish agency for drugs and health products), AEMPS website. www.aemps.gob.es/. Accessed 10 April 2012.
15. *Ley 29/2006, de 26 de julio, de garantías y uso racional de los medicamentos y productos sanitarios* (Law 29/2006 on guarantees and rational use of medicines and health products). Noticias Juridicas website. http://noticias.juridicas.com/base_datos/Admin/l29-2006.t1.html. Accessed 10 April 2012.
16. *Comisión Interministerial de Precios de los Medicamentos.* Spain Pharmaceutical. ISPOR website. www.ispor.org/htaroadmaps/spain.asp. Accessed 10 April 2012.
17. Real Decreto-ley 9/2011, de 19 de agosto, de medidas para la mejora de la calidad y cohesión del sistema nacional de salud, de contribución a la consolidación fiscal, y de elevación del importe máximo de los avales del Estado para 2011 (Royal decree 9/2011, of 19 August, for measures to improve the quality and cohesion of the national health system). Following the adoption of this measure, it is mandatory for healthcare professionals to prescribe by international nonproprietary name. Noticias Juridicas website. http://noticias.juridicas.com/base_datos/Admin/rdl9-2011.html. Accessed 10 April 2012.
18. *Dirección General de Cartera Básica de Servicios del Sistema Nacional de Salud y Farmacia.* Ministerio de Sanidad, Servicios Sociales, e Igualdad website. www.msps.es/en/organizacion/ministerio/organizacion/sgralsanidad/dgcbssnsyfF.htm. Accessed 10 April 2012.
19. There is a cap on the maximum out of pocket expense for the patient.
20. 17 regions plus 2 Autonomous Cities, Ceuta and Melilla.
21. Rodríguez C. "El Interterritorial sienta las bases para establecer acuerdos de mínimos en materia de prestaciones." *El Global.* 2 March 2012. Issuu website. http://issuu.com/el_global/docs/555. (Subscription required.)
22. Ibid.

Acknowledgements
Special thanks to Iván Viejo Viejo (PAREXEL Consulting) and Christine Lietz for contributing information for the Spanish and German case studies respectively. Thanks also to Dieter Russmann (PAREXEL Consulting) for his assistance in the preparation of this chapter.

Chapter 4

Health Technology Assessment

By Mujadala Abdul-Majid, JD, RAC and M. Jason Brooke, MSE, JD

OBJECTIVES

☐ Understand the role of HTA in health product market access

☐ Recognise the importance of HTA locally and globally

☐ Compare and discuss various HTA models

☐ Understand the significance of the Relative Effectiveness Assessment paradigm for pharmaceuticals

REGULATIONS AND GUIDELINES COVERED IN THIS CHAPTER

☐ Directive 2011/24/EU of the European Parliament and the Council of 9 March 2011 on the application of patients' rights in cross-border healthcare

☐ European Commission, Final Conclusions and Recommendations of the High Level Pharmaceutical Forum

☐ European Commission, High Level Pharmaceutical Forum, Core principles on relative effectiveness

Background

History

The concept of a health technology assessment (HTA) emerged in the mid-1960s in the US in recognition of the growing importance of accurate, timely and independent information to enhance and evaluate the impact of technological developments. This led to the establishment of the Office of Technology Assessment (OTA) within the US Congress in 1972.[1] Independent of developments in the US, researchers in Europe were increasingly focusing on policy implications of health technologies.[2] As a result, university-based HTA groups, then national HTA agencies began to emerge. As an example, the first national agency in the EU was the Swedish Council on Technology Assessment in Health Care (*Statensberedning för medicinsk utvardering* (SBU)).[3] By 2007, nine regional and 18 national HTA agencies had been established throughout Europe. Today, HTA organisations maintain a presence across the globe, with the International Network of Agencies for Health Technology Assessment (INAHTA) serving as the international association for national and regional publicly-funded HTA agencies. INAHTA currently represents 59 member agencies from 29 countries spanning from North and Latin America to Europe, Asia and Australia.[4] The INAHTA network serves as a platform for organisations around the world that are engaged in assessments of healthcare technology, to cooperate and share information from different cultures.[5]

In the EU, organisational structuring and activities have overlap as well as variations within the HTA agencies across Member States. For example, operational setting, funding, types and scopes of assessments, and relation to decision making are a few areas in which HTA agencies may diverge or converge.[6] Variations in these areas can create a difficult scheme for stakeholders involved in health technology development across different European markets. In recent years, the EU has expressed recognition of a "clear area of European added-value [in harmonising HTA] to reduce overlap and duplication of efforts in this field and hence promote the effective and efficient use of resources."[7] However, bringing harmonisation and a more collaborative scheme to the forefront has limitations set forth in the *Treaty on the Functioning of the EU*, which does not allow the EU to directly intervene in Member States' healthcare policies. Opponents to EU-wide collaboration on HTA argue that healthcare implementation and reimbursement decisions are driven by distinct Community and national standards and should not adhere to an EU-wide set of principles.[8]

Despite obstacles, there was a growing recognition of the need for formalised collaboration among EU institutions and increased transparency among stakeholders, and in 2006, the European Network for Health Technology Assessment (EUnetHTA) emerged as a pilot programme co-funded by the EC and industry members to collaborate on HTA. Further, in 2008, the EC issued a proposed directive entitled, *A Community framework on the application of patients' rights in cross-border healthcare*, with an aim to improve cooperation between Member States and clarify patients' rights to access safe and good quality treatment across EU borders and be reimbursed accordingly.[9] To that end, HTA was indicated as one of the directive's major provisions and as a field in which collaboration between Member States can yield relevant added value.[10]

Directive 2011/24/EU,[11] which was adopted in 2011, refers to the EUnetHTA Project as a basis for a permanent EU structure of cooperation in the health technology assessment field. Article 15 of the *Cross Border Patients' Rights Directive*, regarding the cooperation of Member States on HTA, states the EUnetHTA's objectives:

- support cooperation between national authorities or bodies
- support Member States in the provision of objective, reliable, timely, transparent, comparable and transferable information on the relative efficacy as well as on the short- and long-term effectiveness, when applicable, of health technologies and to enable an effective exchange of this information between the national authorities or bodies
- support the analysis of the nature and type of information that can be exchanged
- avoid duplication of assessments[12]

Article 15 also specifies its limitations as not to interfere with "Member States' competences in deciding on the implementation of health technology assessment conclusions and shall not harmonise any laws or regulations of the Member States."[13] This language connotes a balance between the reach of mandated collaboration and the limitations set forth under the *Treaty on the Functioning of the EU*. Thus, the directive manages to indirectly increase HTA collaboration and resolve issues affecting the cross-border provision of medical services without impinging on Member States' dominions.

The following sections focus primarily on standards and initiatives established by EUnetHTA. In some cases, definitions and standardised approaches established by INAHTA are also provided.

Conceptualising HTA

The delivery of healthcare in the EU and elsewhere around the world depends in large part on the technologies available to the clinician or caregiver at the point of care. In general, these health technologies can range from drugs and medical devices, to clinical diagnostic and treatment methodologies (e.g., surgical procedures), to disease prevention and rehabilitation methodologies, to the organisational and supportive systems within which care is provided.[14] INAHTA, for example, defines "healthcare technology" as "[a]ny intervention that may be used to promote health, to prevent, diagnose or treat disease or for rehabilitation or long-term care. This includes the pharmaceuticals, devices, procedures and organisational systems used in health care."[15] Despite the expansive range that exists today, health technologies are constantly evolving to improve the quality and delivery of care. Therefore, the systematic evaluation of health technologies can be considered essential to healthcare delivery.

Broadly speaking, the systematic evaluation of a health technology can be broken into a three-phase process: 1) market authorisation, 2) technology assessment (i.e., HTA), and 3) utilisation decision making (see **Figure 4-1**). The first phase involves the evaluation of a given technology's safety and effectiveness to support authorisation for its use. For example, a medical device must undergo a rigorous evaluation process before receiving CE marking, which is required before the device may be legally marketed in the EU (see Chapter 8 for more details). Similarly, new surgical procedures are subject to peer review and broader clinical scrutiny before becoming the standard of care. But simply demonstrating that a given health technology is safe and effective in achieving its desired clinical goal does not ensure that the technology 1) is the optimal means by which to achieve the clinical goal, or 2) will be adopted for use across the EU or at all levels within a national healthcare system. Such utilisation decisions (the third phase in the process) are influenced by numerous factors, including the outcome of HTA (the second phase, often viewed as the bridge between research and decision-making).

In general, HTA is the systematic and multidisciplinary evaluation of health technologies that uses research to support their adoption and utilisation. More specifically, INAHTA defines HTA as "the systematic evaluation of

Figure 4-1. Phased Approach to Evaluation of a Health Technology

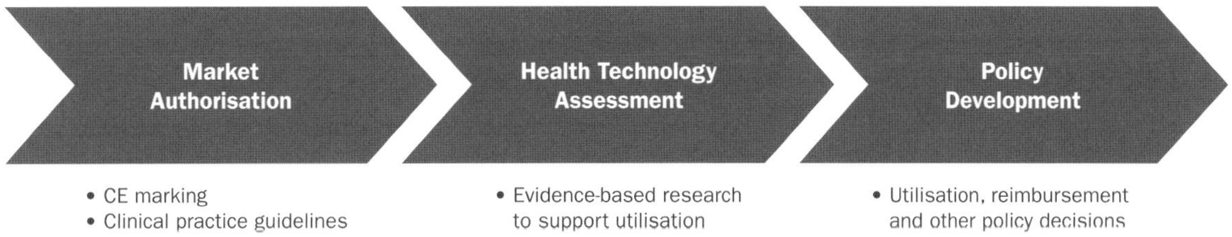

Market Authorisation → Health Technology Assessment → Policy Development

- CE marking
- Clinical practice guidelines

- Evidence-based research to support utilisation

- Utilisation, reimbursement and other policy decisions

properties, effects, and/or impacts of health care technology...conducted by interdisciplinary groups using explicit analytical frameworks drawing from a variety of methods... to inform technology-related policy making in healthcare."[16] The EUnetHTA Project focuses on the process and goals of an assessment, defining HTA as:

"[A] multidisciplinary process that summarises information about the medical, social, economic and ethical issues related to the use of a health technology in a systematic, transparent, unbiased, robust manner. Its aim is to inform the formulation of safe, effective, health policies that are patient focused and seek to achieve best value. Despite its policy goals, HTA must always be firmly rooted in research and the scientific method."[17]

It is important to note that the HTA process includes collaborative input from various stakeholders, including healthcare professionals, decision makers, patients, regulators, payers and industry. Given the broad definition of HTA, it is not surprising that manifestation of HTA varies considerably across national settings.[18] It has been posited that to be most relevant, HTA should be undertaken within the policy context of a particular country, taking into account its national priorities and systems.[19] However, there is a clear distinction between assessment, which is considered a scientific process, and the role of HTA and subsequent appraisal by policy-makers.[20] Therefore, HTA is generally accepted "as a bridge between research and decision making," with a majority of EU Member States using public sector HTA agencies to influence decision and policy making at regional and national levels.[21]

Although HTAs are used to inform policy decisions, including whether to use a particular health technology and to what extent a particular health technology should be reimbursed, this chapter focuses on HTA itself. It summarises the historical development of HTAs and introduces a harmonised core model for performing an objective product assessment, briefly discussing the European Medicines Agency's (EMA) increasingly collaborative role with EUnetHTA and focuses on relative efficacy and effectiveness as a non-contextual evaluation of certain product assessments.

EUnetHTA and the Development of a Core HTA Model

HTA developed as a concept that was variably defined in its practical applications. For example, in some countries, HTA is limited to clinical- and cost-effectiveness. Other countries may extend the assessment more broadly into social and ethical impacts of an assessed technology. Differences in national implementation and organisation present challenges to international use of technology.[22] EUnetHTA brings together national health insurance organisations, academia, government agencies and health ministries, and national and regional health authorities to support an effective collaborative approach that brings added value at the European, national and regional levels.[23] Based on that mission, EUnetHTA undertook a two-year project from 2006 to 2008 with the following strategic objectives:[24]

- Reduce overlap and duplication of effort and hence promote more effective use of resources.
- Increase HTA input to decision making in Member States and the EU and, hence, increase the impact of HTA.
- Strengthen the link between HTA and healthcare policy making in the EU and its Member States.
- Support countries with limited experience with HTA.

Adopting the methods and tools established by the 2006–08 project and incorporating initiatives developed by the Working Group on Relative Effectiveness of the High Level Pharmaceutical Forum, EUnetHTA initiated the "EUnetHTA Joint Action 2010–2012" with the following specific objectives:[25]

- Develop a general strategy and a business model for sustainable European collaboration on HTA.
- Develop HTA tools and methods.
- Field test and apply developed tools and methods.

The following sections focus on the establishment of a core model for HTA methodology and reporting. As an example of the HTA Core Model's application, this chapter will conclude by examining a methodological guidance used to assess the relative effectiveness of pharmaceuticals—a major initiative in the EU as described above in the discussion on EMA collaboration with EUnetHTA.

Methodological Aspects

The HTA Core Model is a tool developed by the EUnetHTA based on the fundamental premise that there are common issues in each HTA and across Member States that can be more efficiently addressed at the EU level. The model attempts to define and standardise HTAs by providing structure for HTA methodology and reporting. At the outset, an important step for a successful HTA process is the selection of relevant and targeted topics that are adequately prioritised. These topics may be identified by recognising the overarching policy questions involved and translating them into relevant research questions to establish a protocol.

Once an overarching policy question is identified, relevant aspects of the problem can be described. Such aspects may range from safety or effectiveness to legal or economic. For each aspect, a specific research plan and relevant methodologies for such research can be developed. The methodologies used in the assessment vary based on the context of the policy issues being addressed.[26] Questions that give rise to contextual aspects of the policy issue include:[27]

- Who initiated/commissioned the assessment?
- Why is the assessment needed right now?
- Which decision is the assessment going to support?
- Who represents the primary target audience for the report?

Contextualising the policy issues allows the researchers to specify aspects that will need to be determined to provide evidence-based solutions. The process of identifying and developing the most critical questions to determine what evidence is needed gives rise to the context necessary to make determinations relevant to overarching policy issues.

Core Concepts and Structure: Domains, Topics, and Issues

The core model is based on nine domains identified in the EUR-ASSESS Project. The EUR-ASSESS Project, started in 1994, is aimed at coordinating HTA activities in Europe to improve the quality and value for money of HTAs undertaken in European countries and improving decision making concerning adoption and use of healthcare technology.[28] The culmination of the project was a document outlining the theory, practice and principles of setting HTA priorities. Based on the EUR-ASSESS outline, a core model was proposed that aimed to construct a clear structure and presentation of information by structuring HTA according to these basic concepts:[29]

- Domain—a wide framework within which the technology is considered to view its use and consequences
- Topic—a specific area of consideration within a domain
- Issue—a more specific area of consideration, more than one of which typically makes up one topic

A domain can be divided into several topics. Likewise, similar topics may be addressed within more than one domain. An issue is usually expressed as a focused question. For example, life expectancy may be a topic in two domains, such as "effectiveness" and "ethical analysis," and an issue under that topic may be expressed as: "What is the direct effect of the technology on patient mortality?"

EUnetHTA identified the following nine domains and their related methodologies, which were put forth in the *HTA Core Model Online Handbook*. Note that some assessments under a given domain may be context-dependent or context-independent. A context-dependent domain will be limited in its application, whereas a context-independent assessment may have broader implications, including those that span domains:[30]

1. Health problem and current use of technology: This domain uses published epidemiological, prognostic and qualitative research as well as statistical data and registries as sources of information. Furthermore, use of websites and databases for horizon scanning and ongoing research is often relevant. Both national and EU information can be valuable.

2. Description and technical characteristics of technology: This domain focuses on a review of articles, textbooks and technical reports from governmental agencies or scientific research groups and manufacturers' websites. A systematic review is not always needed; however, explicit documentation is required for transparency.

3. Safety: The purpose of this domain is to review and predefine safety issues and outcome measures. Harms are not always well-reported in randomised trials. Terms specified for adverse effects have to be defined and added to each search strategy. Information about new, serious, rare or long-term adverse effects typically are found in observational studies.

4. Effectiveness: The core of this domain is the randomised controlled trial (RCT). Because test RCTs are rare, inferences regarding the effectiveness of diagnostic technologies are often made based on linked evidence from studies on accuracy, change-in-management and treatment effectiveness.

5. Cost and economic considerations: The type of analysis and data collected for this domain will depend on the specific research question. Modelling is useful when economic and clinical data are missing. Sensitivity analysis shows the decision maker the robustness of the conclusions of an economic analysis. Ideally the analysis is conducted from the broad

societal perspective instead of for one or two narrow contexts or settings.

6. Ethical analysis: This domain involves an ongoing process that lasts throughout the HTA project performed with content experts. The analysis should never be a philosophical add-on input by ethicists. The method should be tailored to suit the topic under study, local culture and healthcare system, and the HTA organisation itself. The various approaches include:
   - casuistry (i.e., case-based reasoning)
   - coherence analysis
   - interactive, participatory HTA approach
   - principalism
   - social shaping of technology
   - wide reflective equilibrium methodologies

7. Organisational analysis: Both qualitative and quantitative research data are required in this domain. Registries and routinely collected statistics are often useful for this analysis. Comparing results from two or more data collection methods (e.g., interview and observation) may reduce bias. At least two different views on causality and transferability are used in the organisational research: the diffusion model[31] and the translation model.[32] The assessment of the organisational issues is in many cases context-dependent.

8. Social aspects: In this domain, the focus is on relevant social issues associated with organisational and ethical issues. Qualitative studies are highly relevant, along with quantitative studies with various observational designs. If no relevant studies are found, a primary study (e.g., an interview, survey or participant observation) should be considered. A thematic synthesis, a thorough description of relevant themes and sub-themes identified in literature or interviews (thematic mapping), is more important than finding every single study or opinion.

9. Legal Aspects: Compulsory legal sources (e.g., international laws, EU laws and national legislation) form the regulatory framework of any given question in this domain. These sources are often complemented by various "soft law" instruments, agreements, documentation by the technology supplier and legal scientific literature.

The domain will determine the methodology and assessment elements. Elements are the basic unit of the model that will describe the technology or impact of its use. In general, an element will "provide information" so that each domain can be better understood. Some elements may be described as context-independent, which implies that the information may be transferable across another context (e.g., location, system or policy setting) for the same technology. Although HTA may encompass many different elements, the core model adopts those that are both context-independent and/or considered particularly significant for HTA.[33]

HTA Reports

The product of the HTA assessment is the HTA report. HTA reports typically have followed the traditional scientific paper format: abstract, background, methods, results, conclusions and references. In terms of standards for presentation, requirements have been presented with regard to requisite content and, in some cases, how and in what order the content should be presented.[34] This has been useful in circumventing reports based on authors' personal judgments with regard to presentation and content selection. Despite current guidance, there is still great variation in the internal structures of various sections of HTA reports.[35] However, expanded utilisation of the HTA Core Model can serve to alleviate two problems concerning HTA reports: varying content and unrefined structure. It accomplishes this by facilitating a shared understanding of what information should be found in an HTA report and, perhaps, in an ideal comprehensive assessment. The production of Core HTAs and structured output is carried out in five phases:

1. project definition
2. protocol design
3. research
4. entering results
5. reviewing and publishing results

The "project definition phase" is used to identify which HTA models should be used, define the scope of the entire project (i.e., technology, indication and comparison) and identify the project participants and their roles.

The "protocol design phase" can be divided into four steps: 1) selecting applicable issues by going through each element and deciding whether each particular issue is relevant in the context of the technology that is being assessed; 2) formulating research questions by producing a list of practical and answerable questions according to the research tradition of each domain; 3) identifying and mapping the relations between issues to assess overlap and avoid duplication of research efforts; and 4) framing domains to the commonly defined specific project scope.

The "research phase" is the one in which the questions defined by the core protocol are answered for each domain.[36] To ensure that research questions are formulated in a useful way, they should be clearly worded, answerable, limited in number, address meaningful outcomes and address other relevant treatment alternatives.[37]

"Entering results" includes the use of an electronic database where each protocol is associated with a collected "Core HTA" frame that places the assessment element in the proper context. Each Core HTA consists of the following parts:

- general introduction
- domain-specific sections (one for each domain)
  - introduction of domain
  - domain methodology
  - assessment elements within domain; for each element:
    - methods
    - results (answers)
    - comment (optional)
  - discussion of findings within domain
  - references of domain
  - appendices of domain
    - summary of findings for whole Core HTA

The results should be peer-reviewed and the final phase is the "review and publishing" of the Core HTA. The prior phases should produce a report that follows a standardised structure that can be read, used and interpreted across multiple contexts.

The Relative Effectiveness Assessment (REA) Paradigm

On the road to market access in the EU, a new drug is subject to assessment and approval by EMA. Approval is obtained based on assessments of quality, safety and efficacy.[38] Market Authorisation Holders must further seek reimbursement from third-party payers. The payers will require an assessment, sometimes by independent HTA bodies, to determine the new drug's cost-effectiveness for reimbursement purposes.[39]

As discussed above, an HTA is a broad assessment that can encompass elements (e.g., social, ethical and cost aspects of a technology). The EUnetHTA positions relative effectiveness assessment (REA) as a specific element of HTA that focuses on the clinical implications of an intervention.[40] HTA bodies may compare the relative effectiveness of medicines to take their financial cost into account, which may lead to differences in the types of studies carried out to support EMA assessments.

Due to growing concerns over these differences, the European Commission launched a High Level Pharmaceutical Forum (HLPF) that aimed to serve as a platform for the exchange of best practice and examination of efficiency gains.[41] In the context of the pharmaceutical industry and related public health considerations, specific focuses of the forum were competitiveness in the areas of disease and treatment options, REAs and pricing and reimbursement of medicinal products. HLPF adopted a report in October 2008 in which it "[acknowledged] the distinction between scientific assessment of the relative effectiveness of medicinal products and health-economic assessments of their costs and benefits [and endorsed] the aim of relative effectiveness assessment to compare healthcare interventions in daily practice and classifying them according to their added therapeutic value."[42] The report also gave a political mandate for EMA to interact with HTA agencies. Since the 2008 mandate, EMA has been collaborating with HTA bodies at an increasing level and has recognised that, more frequently, decisions by regulators and payers are conducted at nearly the same time and often based on identical data sets for new drugs;[43] therefore, an important emerging issue at the regulator-payer interface is the assessment of relative effectiveness.

The aim of relative effectiveness is to categorically assign therapeutic value to compare healthcare interventions.[44] Thus, the first step in an REA is to identify "relative efficacy." HLPF endorsed the following four definitions differentiating the efficacy-effectiveness spectrum:[45]

- Efficacy—the extent to which an intervention does more good than harm under ideal circumstances
- Effectiveness—the extent to which an intervention does more good than harm when provided under the usual circumstances of healthcare practice
- Relative efficacy—the extent to which an intervention does more good than harm, under ideal circumstances, compared to one or more alternative interventions
- Relative effectiveness—the extent to which an intervention does more good than harm compared to one or more intervention alternatives for achieving the desired results when provided under the usual circumstances of healthcare practice

HLPF also asked its working group to explore different ways of encouraging the production of additional relevant data.[46] In turn, the working group suggested the following principles for HLPF to endorse for nonbinding use, as appropriate, in Member States:[47]

1. Individual Member States may use REAs for different purposes. Decisions on the detailed operation of REAs, including methods and relevant stakeholders, are most appropriately made at a national level.
2. REA processes, selection of products to be assessed, working methodologies and quality assurance processes should be transparent to all parties and should be evidence-based.
3. Relevant stakeholders should be able to contribute to the development of assessment methodologies. The purpose of the REA and the organisation(s) responsible for its conduct should be clearly identified.
4. REA processes should remain separate from product market authorisation procedures (though this does not mean that they are necessarily performed by different organisations).
5. REA processes should be time-framed and should minimise or avoid causing unnecessary procedural delays consistent with any associated *Transparency Directive*[48] requirements, where applicable.

Table 4-1. REA Checklist

Purpose and Responsibilities	
Q1:	Is the purpose of the REA specifically described?
Q2:	Is the organisation responsible for its conduct clearly identified?
Transparency	
Q3:	Is the REA process transparent to all parties?
Q4:	Is the selection of products to be assessed in the REA transparent to all parties?
Q5:	Is the REA working methodology transparent to all parties?
Q6:	Is the REA quality assurance process transparent to all parties?
Evidence Base	
Q7:	Is the REA evidence-based?
Stakeholders	
Q8:	Are the relevant stakeholders able to contribute to the development of REA methodologies?
Q9:	Have the sources of evidence that form the relevant REA inputs been specifically discussed between the key stakeholders?
Q10:	Are the key stakeholders able to submit evidence or arguments for appraisals??
Processes	
Q11:	Are the REA processes separate from product market authorisation procedures?
Q12:	Are the REA processes time-framed?
Q13:	Do the REA processes minimise or avoid causing any unnecessary procedural delays and are they consistent with any associated Transparency Directive requirements (timing, appeals, etc.), where applicable?
Q14:	Has the national assessment body established contacts with other national or international agencies to exchange views, methodologies and information?
Quality of Assessment	
Q15:	Is the REA capable of addressing uncertainty in the evidence base transparently?
Q16:	Is the REA capable of addressing uncertainty in the methodological challenges transparently?
Q17:	Does the REA include a comparison with the most appropriate healthcare interventions built on the results of active controlled clinical trials, where available?
Communication	
Q18:	Are the outcomes of the REA communicated clearly and in good time to all interested parties?
Q19:	Are the outcomes and supporting evaluation of the REA published on a publicly accessible website?
Other Aspects	
Q20:	Is the REA capable of subsequent revision and updating as the evidence base develops?
Q21:	Does the REA identify areas in which the evidence base on an intervention could be most usefully developed in the future?
Q22:	Does the REA include input from other national or international agencies on the same or closely related projects?

6. REA should be capable of transparently addressing uncertainty in the evidence base and the methodological challenge of translating evidence on relative efficacy and other appropriate available data into conclusions on relative effectiveness.
7. The sources of evidence that are to form the relevant relative effectiveness input should be specifically discussed among the identified key stakeholders, who should each be able to submit evidence or argumentation for appraisal.
8. REA should include comparison with the most appropriate healthcare interventions. Such comparison should build on the results of active controlled clinical trials, where available.
9. When concluded, outcomes should be communicated in a clear and timely manner to all interested parties. Communication by means of publishing the supporting evaluation on a publicly accessible website is strongly encouraged.
10. REA should be capable of subsequent revision and updating as the evidence base develops.
11. REA should aim to identify areas in which the evidence base on an intervention could be developed most usefully in the future.

In EMA's draft *Road Map to 2015*,[49] the agency expresses a vision for collaboration with HTA bodies that concentrates on the goal of improving the information available on centrally authorised medicines based on recommendations established by HLPF.[50] HLPF developed a checklist to be used by Member States as a framework for the evaluation of their own REA systems (**Table 4-1**).[51] It was posited that the checklist can be used to improve REAs by simplifying the method of evaluating the strength of the REA system or program in place, collecting views from relevant stakeholders and establishing a basis for cross-national comparisons.[52]

Summary

This chapter reviews a wide range of available information aimed at adding efficiency to the delivery of new healthcare technologies. Recently adopted and proposed directives demonstrate that the EU will continue to encourage collaboration on HTA among Member States. While this chapter does not attempt to capture the full spectrum of HTA's impact, it provides an overview of the emphasis on collaboration and standardisation in the employment of HTA. New developments in the core model, its application and breadth of use are likely to ensue in the coming years as the EU continues its initiative to further strengthen informed decision making by health authorities.

References

1. Velasco Garrido M, Kristensen FB, Nielsen CPP and Busse R. *Health Technology Assessment and Health Policy-Making in Europe— An introduction to objectives, role of evidence, and structure in Europe* [hereinafter European Observatory HTA Policy Report]. 2008: 34. World Health Organization, European Observatory on Health Systems and Policies. WHO website. www.euro.who.int/__data/assets/pdf_file/0003/90426/E91922.pdf. Accessed 16 May 2012.
2. Ibid., p. 80.
3. Ibid., p. 81.
4. Ibid.
5. International Network of Agencies for Health Technology Assessment (INAHTA) website. www.inahta.net/. Accessed 16 May 2012.
6. Op cit 1, p.81. (See also "About INAHTA." INAHTA website. www.inahta.net/. Accessed 16 May 2012.)
7. Op cit 1, p 8.
8. *Policy Brief: Cross Border Health Technology Assessment.* Stockholm Network (2010). Stockholm network website. www.stockholm-network.org/downloads/publications/CBHTA_Polybrief.pdf. Accessed 16 May 2012.
9. Proposal for a Directive of the European Parliament and of the Council on the application of patients' rights in cross-border healthcare (COM(2008) 414 final). Brussels; 2 July 2008. EC website. http://ec.europa.eu/health-eu/doc/com2008414_en.pdf. Accessed 16 May 2012. (See also Europa Press Release (MEMO/11/32), Q&A: Patients' Rights in Cross Border Healthcare. (19 January 2011). Europa website. http://europa.eu/rapid/pressReleasesAction.do?reference=MEMO/11/32&format=HTML&aged=0&language=en&guiLanguage=en. Accessed 16 May 2012.
10. Ibid.
11. Directive 2011/24/EU of the European Parliament and the Council of 9 March 2011 on the application of patients' rights in cross-border healthcare. EUR-Lex website. http://eur-lex.europa.eu/LexUriServ/LexUriServ.do?uri=OJ:L:2011:088:0045:0065:EN:PDF. Accessed 16 May 2012.
12. Ibid.
13. Ibid.
14. HTA definition. EUnetHTA website. "About," http://www.eunethta.eu/Public/About_EUnetHTA/HTA/. Accessed 16 May 2012.
15. "HTA Resources" webpage. INAHTA website. http://inahta.net/. Accessed 16 May 2012.
16. Ibid.
17. Op cit 14.
18. Op cit 1, pp. 31–32.
19. Ibid., p. 6.
20. Ibid., p. 33.
21. Ibid., p. 32.
22. Ibid., p. 40.
23. European network for Health Technology Assessment European network for Health Technology Assessment (EUnetHTA) "Mission." EUnetHTA website. www.eunethta.eu/Public/About_EUnetHTA/EUnetHTA-Mission/. Accessed 16 May 2012.
24. "EUnetHTA Project 2006–08." EUnetHTA website. www.eunethta.eu/Public/Work_Packages/EUnetHTA-Project-2006-08. Accessed 16 May 2012.
25. "EUnetHTA Joint Action 2010–12." EUnetHTA website. www.eunethta.eu/Public/Work_Packages/EUnetHTA-Joint-Action-2010-12. Accessed 16 May 2012.
26. Op cit 1, pp. 49-50.
27. Ibid.
28. "The EUR-Assess Project." WHO Collaborating Center for Knowledge Translation and Health Technology Assessment in Health Equity. www.cgh.uottawa.ca/whocc/projects/nb_toolkit/chp2/t_eur.htm. Accessed 16 May 2012.
29. Op cit 1, p. 43.
30. *HTA Core Model Online Handbook.* EUnetHTA website. https://fio.stakes.fi/htacore/ViewHandbook.aspx. Accessed 16 May 2012.
31. The diffusion model treats the establishment of an organizational practice as evidence of diffusion by assuming that practice is reproduced locally following a prototype.
32. The translation model emphasizes that not all ideas are translated locally and each process requires careful analysis.
33. Op cit 1, p. 42.
34. *HTA Checklist.* INAHTA. http://inahta.episerverhotell.net/upload/HTA_resources/Checklist_instructions_2007.doc. Accessed 16 May 2012.
35. Op cit 1, p. 41.
36. Op cit 30.
37. Busse R et al. "Best practice in undertaking and reporting health technology assessments." *International Journal of Technology Assessment in Health Care.* 18:361–422 (2002).
38. Council Regulation (EEC) No 2309/93 of 22 July 1993 laying down Community procedures for the authorization and supervision of medicinal products for human and veterinary use and establishing a European Agency for the Evaluation of Medicinal Products. EC website. http://ec.europa.eu/health/files/eudralex/vol-1/reg_1993_2309/reg_1993_2309_en.pdf. Accessed 16 May 2012.
39. Eichler HG, Bloechl-Daum B, Abadie E, Barnett D, Konig F and Pearson S. "Relative efficacy of drugs: an issue between regulatory agencies and third-party payors." Nature Reviews: Drug Discovery; 9:277; April 2010. http://www.ncbi.nlm.nih.gov/pubmed/20186141. Accessed 16 May 2012.
40. "JA WP5:Relative Effectiveness Assessment (REA) of Pharmaceuticals," July 2011. EUnetHTA website. www.eunethta.eu/upload/WP5/Link1.pdf. Accessed 16 May 2912.
41. *High Level Group on innovation and provision of medicines recommendations for actions.* EC website. http://ec.europa.eu/enterprise/sectors/healthcare/files/phabiocom/docs/g10-medicines_en.pdf. Accessed 16 May 2012.
42. Ibid.
43. Ibid.
44. *Core Principles on Relative Effectiveness.* HLPF Working Group on Relative Effectiveness. EC website. http://ec.europa.eu/enterprise/sectors/healthcare/files/docs/rea_principles_en.pdf. Accessed 16 May 2012. "Relative effectiveness" can be defined as the extent to which an intervention does more good than harm compared to one or more intervention alternatives for achieving the desired results when provided under the usual circumstances of health care practice.
45. Op cit 41. (The INAHTA offers some similar definitions for these terms.)
46. *Availability of Data to Conduct Relative Effectiveness Assessments.* HLPF Working Group on Relative Effectivness. EC website. http://ec.europa.eu/enterprise/sectors/healthcare/files/docs/rea_data_en.pdf. Accessed 16 May 2012.
47. Op cit 41.
48. Council Directive 89/105/EEC of 21 December 1988 relating to the transparency of measures regulating the prices of medicinal

products for human use and their inclusion in the scope of national health insurance systems. EUR-Lex website. http://eur-lex.europa.eu/LexUriServ/LexUriServ.do?uri=CELEX:31989L0105:en:HTML. Accessed. 16 May 2012.
49. *Roadmap to 2015—The European Medicines Agency's contribution to science, medicines and health.* EMA website. http://www.ema.europa.eu/ema/pages/includes/document/open_document.jsp?webContentId=WC500101373. Accessed 16 May 2012.
50. Op cit 41.
51. Op cit 44.
52. Ibid.

Chapter 5

The Paediatric Regulation

Updated by Nicole Beard, MSc, PhD

OBJECTIVES

❏ Understand key aspects of the *Paediatric Regulation*

❏ Identify the role of the European Medicines Agency's Paediatric Committee (PDCO)

❏ Become aware of other guidances applicable to European paediatric drug development

REGULATIONS AND GUIDELINES COVERED IN THIS CHAPTER

❏ Regulation (EC) 1901/2006, as amended, of the European Parliament and of the Council of 12 December 2006 on medicinal products for paediatric use and amending Regulation (EEC) 1768/92, Directive 2001/20/EC, Directive 2001/83/EC and Regulation (EC) 726/2004

❏ Regulation (EC) 1902/2006 of the European Parliament and of the Council of 20 December 2006 amending Regulation 1901/2006 on medicinal products for paediatric use

❏ Communication from the Commission 2008/C 243/01 - Guideline on the format and content of applications for agreement or modification of a paediatric investigation plan and requests for waivers or deferrals and concerning the operation of the compliance check and on criteria for assessing significant studies

Background and Scope

In October 2004, when the European Commission issued a proposal for a regulation on medicines for paediatric use, the potential advantages and risks of dedicated European legislation in this field had been under intense debate for several years. A focal point for the discussion was how to strike the right balance between new requirements for the pharmaceutical industry and possible incentives and rewards. Second, if companies were to be rewarded in some way for paediatric research, how would these rewards be delivered and how much would they be? Understandable ethical concerns voiced about conducting clinical trials in children had to be balanced against equally valid concerns about the potential harmful effects of the continued practice of unlicenced and off-licence prescribing of adult medicines for children. After a public consultation and an unusually quick review by the European institutions, a regulation was approved by the European Parliament and the Council of Ministers in 2006 and entered into force on 26 January 2007.

The stated overall policy objective of the *Paediatric Regulation* (Regulation (EC) No 1901/2006),[1] as amended by Regulation (EC) No 1902/2006,[2] is "to improve the health of the children in Europe." This goal is to be achieved by:

- increasing the development of medicines for use in children
- ensuring that medicines used to treat children are subject to high-quality research and are appropriately authorised for use in children
- improving the information available on the use of medicines in children
- achieving the above objectives without subjecting children to unnecessary or duplicative trials and in full compliance with the EU Clinical Trials Directive[3]

Patient Population(s)

In fact, the *Paediatric Regulation* text does not employ the term "children" but instead uses "the paediatric population," here defined as the population aged between birth and 18 years of age. A Commission guideline clarifies that this should be understood as "up to but not including 18 years."[4] As for the different subsets of paediatric patients, the ICH E11 guideline[5] definitions apply, i.e., preterm neonates, term neonates (0–27 days), infants (1–23 months), children (2–11 years) and adolescents (12–16 to 18 years, depending on the geographic region). However, different age subsets may be acceptable for a given condition if they can be justified.

Which Products are Concerned?

The regulation's scope includes medicinal products for human use within the meaning of Directive 2001/83/EC, as amended by Directive 2004/27/EC.[6] In other words, the legislation, in principle, applies to all human medicines (but not to medical devices) regardless of registration pathway (Centralised, Mutual Recognition or Decentralised Procedure or purely National Procedures) or prescription status. The medicines are subdivided in three categories:

1. products in development (unauthorised in the Community)
2. authorised products still covered by patents or Supplementary Protection Certificates (SPCs)
3. authorised products no longer covered by patents or SPCs ("generics")

A combination of incentives, obligations and rewards aims to increase pharmacological research and enhance paediatric labelling information for all three product categories.

Paediatric Investigation Plan (PIP)

A Paediatric Investigation Plan (PIP) is a development plan aimed at ensuring the necessary data are obtained through studies in children, when it is safe to do so, to support the authorisation of a medicine for children.

A PIP prepared by the applicant or Marketing Authorisation Holder (MAH) and approved by the European Medicines Agency (EMA), is expected to address the entire disease or condition that encompasses each of the adult indications authorised or under development and should propose measures to assess the medicine's quality, safety and efficacy in all subsets of the paediatric population (unless justified). The PIP also should include a time schedule for these measures. The PIP may be required to describe a strategy to make the formulation more acceptable, easier, safer or more effective for the paediatric population. Detailed instructions for the preparation of PIPs are provided in the Commission guideline.[7] For instance, the PIP documentation should describe similarities and differences in the disease or condition and the anticipated effect of the product among different age groups (adult and paediatric, paediatric subsets); paediatric prevalence and incidence (including the earliest age of onset); current methods of diagnosis, prevention or treatment; and whether the product might provide a significant therapeutic benefit or fulfil a paediatric therapeutic need (comparing the product with current standard of care).

Paediatric Committee (PDCO)

A key element of the regulation is a European committee with combined expertise covering multiple aspects of the research, development, authorisation and use of medicines for children. The Paediatric Committee (PDCO) is attached to the EMA organisational structure and can rely on administrative and scientific support from the agency. The chair is elected from the committee members, all of whom are appointed to three-year, renewable terms:

- five Committee for Medicinal Products for Human Use (CHMP) members with their alternates, appointed by CHMP
- one member and one alternate appointed by each Member State (except Member States already represented through the members appointed by CHMP)
- three members and alternates representing healthcare professionals
- three members and alternates representing patients' associations

PDCO's main tasks are to:

- assess the content of PIPs and adopt opinions on them
- evaluate full or partial waiver and deferral requests
- check PIP compliance (in all cases for Centralised Procedure products)
- adopt opinions on the quality, safety and efficacy of a medicine for use in the paediatric population, at the request of the CHMP or a national health authority

The committee also:

- prepares an inventory of paediatric uses, therapeutic needs and priorities for research; the inventory is intended as an information source for physicians and patients and to help companies identify business development opportunities
- provides support and advice to a European paediatric investigator network

It is important to emphasize that PDCO does not provide opinions on Marketing Authorisation Applications (MAAs). This remains the formal responsibility of CHMP. On the other hand, CHMP (or a national Competent Authority) may, as mentioned above, ask PDCO to make recommendations on quality, safety and efficacy data generated in accordance with an approved PIP.

Waivers

Many medicines are, of course, irrelevant, unnecessary or simply unsuitable for children. Waivers from the requirements will, in such situations, be issued by PDCO. The regulation defines three alternative criteria for granting either product-specific or class waivers:
- the product is likely to be ineffective or unsafe in part or all of the paediatric population
- the disease or condition occurs only in adult populations
- the product does not represent a significant therapeutic benefit over existing treatments for paediatric patients

In such instances, a waiver can be issued for:
- any or all of the paediatric subpopulations
- one or more therapeutic indication(s)
- a combination of the above

A list of class waivers is maintained on the EMA website and is updated regularly. Currently listed are diseases clearly irrelevant to children, including Alzheimer's disease; age-related macular degeneration; and breast, endometrial and prostate carcinomas.

Applicants or MAHs can only request product-specific waivers, which normally should be granted (or rejected) within 60 days. PDCO may revisit a granted waiver at any time. However, if a product-specific waiver or a class waiver is revoked, the mandatory requirements for paediatric data (or an approved deferral) will only start to apply 36 months from the date of removal from the list.

It is worth noting that the *Paediatric Regulation* does not explicitly provide for granting waivers on the basis of small patient numbers and/or geographic dispersion, because studies are impractical or because formulation efforts have failed. However, inclusion of a robust, evidence-based explanation for the infeasibility of conducting paediatric clinical studies on a product in a given condition in certain cases may be accepted. The justification should include actual feasibility data reflecting low prevalence of the condition or ethical or cultural issues.

Deferrals

At the time of PIP submission, the MAH or applicant can request a deferral of the initiation or completion of some (or all) of the measures it sets forth. A deferral may be granted on scientific or technical grounds or related to public health. In any event, deferrals can (and should) be granted whenever it is more appropriate to conduct studies in adults before initiating studies in children, and when studies in children will take longer than those in adults. The deferral must nevertheless forecast a deadline for the initiation and/or completion of the PIP. A report on progress with deferred paediatric measures is due to EMA annually, based on the date of marketing authorisation (MA).

When, then, is it appropriate and ethically defensible to initiate clinical trials in children? The relevant reference for Europe is the ICH E11 guideline,[8] which describes a number of factors to be weighed when deciding on the best timing. These factors include, for instance, the condition's prevalence and seriousness, availability of alternative treatments, whether the product is novel or belongs to a known class of medicines, whether there are unique paediatric subsets and the need to develop paediatric-specific endpoints.

Application Procedure

Initial Submission

At what stage should the PIP be submitted? Importantly, the intention of the *Paediatric Regulation* is clearly that a PIP (or a waiver application) should be submitted early in clinical development, "…except in duly justified cases, not later than upon completion of the human pharmacokinetic studies in adults." This requirement is intended to "ensure an early dialogue" between the applicant and PDCO. However, the "completion of human PK studies" is somewhat ambiguous. It has been observed that while healthy volunteer PK studies are indeed conducted early in product development, this is not necessarily true for other types of adult PK studies (e.g., special populations, drug-drug interactions, population PK). By contrast, the US Food and Drug Administration (FDA) encourages sponsors to submit their paediatric development plans no later than the End-of-Phase 2 meeting, and for products intended to treat life-threatening or severely debilitating illnesses, by the End of Phase 1.

At best, the proposed PIP can be formally approved in 140 days. However, EMA may suspend the validation phase for an unspecified period (if the dossier is deemed incomplete), and PDCO can extend the evaluation by another 60 days if modifications to the PIP are judged necessary (see **Figure 5-1**). Preliminary experience indicates that the majority of applications have to pass two 60-day cycles plus company response time ("clock-stop period"), which can vary, but is usually up to three months. A teleconference during the clock-stop period between the applicant or MAH and the assigned rapporteur and peer reviewer at PDCO may be valuable for clarifying the requested modifications to the PIP prior to submission of responses.

The applicant or MAH has the right to appeal a PDCO decision. In such a case, a request for a "re-examination" must be filed within 30 days after receiving the original opinion. If EMA has not received a re-examination request at the end of the 30-day period, the PDCO opinion becomes definitive.

Figure 5-1. Paediatric Investigation Plan (PIP) Approval Process

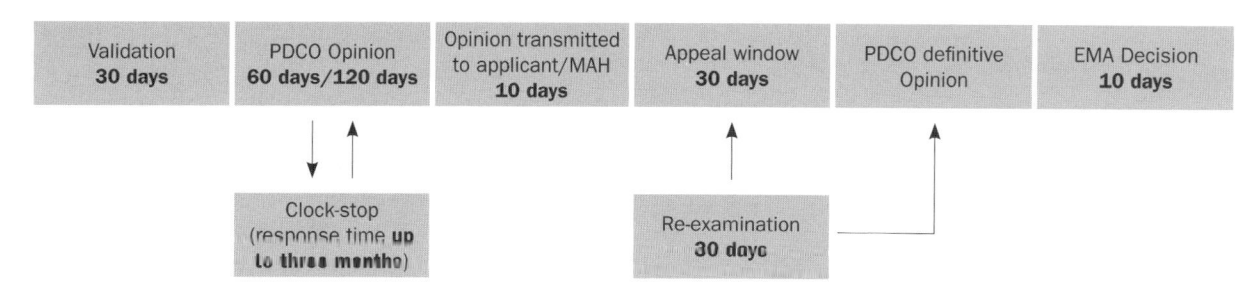

| Validation 30 days | PDCO Opinion 60 days/120 days | Opinion transmitted to applicant/MAH 10 days | Appeal window 30 days | PDCO definitive Opinion | EMA Decision 10 days |

Clock-stop (response time up to three months)

Re-examination 30 days

EMA decisions are published on the agency's website after removal of any commercially sensitive information.

Changes to a PIP

Product development is a dynamic process with frequent changes. Therefore, provision has been made for modifications to the PIP. If the PIP is no longer appropriate or if difficulties encountered make the plan unworkable, the applicant or MAH can propose changes or request a deferral or a waiver based on detailed grounds. A procedure similar to the submission of the initial application for a PIP or waiver applies. The request should be reviewed within 60 days. However, it is important to remember that changes to an agreed PIP have to be fully justified and should be prospectively approved by EMA.

Rewards for Paediatric Research

Extended Intellectual Property Protection Period

The *Paediatric Regulation* stipulates that paediatric research shall be rewarded by granting a six-month extension of the SPC subject to meeting all the following conditions:[9]
- compliance with all measures included in the approved PIP
- protection of the product by an SPC (or by a patent qualifying for an SPC)
- authorisation of the product in all EU Member States
- inclusion of relevant information on results in the product information (by means of a variation)

Since the patent restoration reward is for conducting clinical studies and not for demonstrating that the product is safe and effective in the paediatric population, it will be granted even if the results are negative and no paediatric indication is achieved.

The extension application had to be submitted no later than six months before the SPC expiry for the first five years after the regulation's entry into force. Since this interim period ended 26 January 2012, the extension application must be submitted no later than two years before SPC expiry.

Alternatively, the MAH can apply for a one-year extension of data protection on the grounds that a new paediatric indication "brings significant clinical benefit in comparison with existing therapies" in accordance with the EU Regulation (EC) No 726/2004[10] or Directive 2001/83/EC,[11] as amended. However, it will not be possible to combine one year of extra data protection and a six-month SPC extension for the same product.

A Different Reward for Orphan Medicinal Products

Under EU orphan legislation, products that have been designated orphan medicinal products gain 10 years of market exclusivity upon the granting of a MA for the orphan indication. Frequently, these products no longer benefit from intellectual property protection. The *Paediatric Regulation*, therefore, in return for compliance with an approved PIP, provides a two-year extension of the orphan market exclusivity. This extension applies whether or not the orphan product is subject to intellectual property protection. An alternative six-month SPC extension is not possible.

In comparison, the US offers no corresponding special incentive for conducting paediatric studies with orphan products.

Marketing Authorisation Requirements

For products not approved within the Community, the MAA must contain one (or a combination) of the following:
- results of paediatric studies and details of all information collected in compliance with an approved PIP
- an EMA decision granting a product-specific waiver
- an EMA decision granting a class-specific waiver
- an EMA decision granting a deferral

The above must cover all subsets of the paediatric population.

For products authorised in the Community and protected by an SPC (or a patent qualifying for an SPC), any application for a new indication, new pharmaceutical form or new route of administration must contain:

- results of paediatric studies and details of all information collected in compliance with an agreed PIP
- an EMA decision granting a product-specific waiver
- an EMA decision granting a class-specific waiver
- an EMA decision granting a deferral letter

The above must cover both the new and previously authorised indications in adults, pharmaceutical forms and routes of administration included in the Summary of Product Characteristics (SmPC).

Regarding these requirements, EMA has established a procedure for a paediatric validation check of MAAs and applications for a new indication, pharmaceutical form or route of administration, conducted by the agency, and compliance checks conducted by PDCO.[12] The validity of a proposed application cannot be decided until compliance with the PIP has been demonstrated. When paediatric development is still ongoing at the time of the submission of the application, the compliance check will concern only the measures related to the applied condition, and only those that should have been completed by the time of submission of the application, as reflected in the PIP.

Paediatric Use Marketing Authorisation (PUMA)

To provide an incentive for off-patent medicines, the regulation creates a new type of MA, the Paediatric Use Marketing Authorisation (PUMA) for products developed exclusively for use in children. Interestingly, a PUMA medicine can utilise an existing brand name (of the corresponding product approved for adult use) and it benefits from 10 years of data protection. However, this protection is limited to the paediatric indication(s) and paediatric formulation, where relevant. For the first time, this makes it possible to combine new data of direct relevance to the paediatric population with an otherwise generic application. Cross-references can be made to data contained in a dossier for a product that is (or has been) authorised in the Community (according to Article 14(11) of Regulation (EC) No 726/2004 and Article 10 of Directive 2001/83/EC, as amended).

Obligation to Market

When an agreed PIP has led to the authorisation of a paediatric indication for a product already available for other (adult) indications, the MAH is obliged to implement labelling changes and market the product accordingly in all EU Member States within two years. The applicant must also describe measures to follow up on efficacy and possible adverse reactions linked to the paediatric use. The obligation to market within two years does not apply to products with a PUMA. If an MAH that has benefited from a paediatric SPC extension decides to discontinue commercialisation, the MA will be transferred or a third party will be allowed to use the pharmaceutical, preclinical and clinical documentation contained in the file.

Enforcement Tools

By way of a cross-reference to an infringement provision in the EMA regulation,[13] the European Commission may, if requested by EMA, impose financial penalties for infringement of the *Paediatric Regulation*'s provisions or implementing measures. In such instances, the company name and reasons for the financial penalties imposed will be made public. Infringement procedures are detailed in separate Community legislation.[14]

Other Measures

The *Paediatric Regulation* also contains other measures, which cannot be covered in detail in this chapter. For instance:

- MAHs are obligated to submit any existing data from paediatric trials that were completed by the date the regulation entered into force within one year of study completion, and from any other MAH-sponsored studies within six months of study completion.
- Free EMA Scientific Advice is available on the design and conduct of tests and studies necessary to demonstrate quality, safety or efficacy, or the design of pharmacovigilance or risk management systems for medicines in the paediatric population. The free Scientific Advice is not limited to Centralised Procedure products.
- The EMA-managed EudraCT database for clinical trials will be expanded to non-EU trials included in PIPs.[15] Selected data fields concerning paediatric protocols stored in the EudraCT database will be made accessible to the public. In a second implementation step, the agency will publish trial results; results of MAH-sponsored studies conducted with an authorised product in the paediatric population should be submitted to EMA for entry into EudraCT no later than six months after their completion.
- Article 32 of the regulation stipulates that products with an authorised paediatric indication must display a dedicated paediatric use symbol on the package label to facilitate identification. However, in December 2007, PDCO announced it would not recommend any symbol because it considered the risks identified (including potentially fatal medication errors) outweighed the benefits. As a consequence, the European Commission publicly announced in January 2008 that Article 32 could not be implemented.

Other Development Guidances

Expanded clinical testing in children and adolescents offers a range of new challenges. The *Paediatric Regulation* cross-references the ICH E11 guideline, which addresses several important ethical considerations. Ethical and GCP aspects are further developed in a Commission guideline[16] that, for instance, discusses the issue of "informed consent" (from a parent or a legal guardian) vs. "informed assent" (from a child). Other issues of relevance to the paediatric population, e.g., juvenile toxicology studies, organ maturity and pharmacokinetics, trials in small patient populations[17–23] and issues specific to paediatric pharmacovigilance,[24] are addressed in a series of dedicated EMA guidelines. A sometimes overlooked aspect is the potential necessity to develop age-specific formulation(s). While solid tablets may be a preferred dosage form for adolescents, they are (as any parent surely has observed) of little or no use for very young children. Conversely, intravenous solutions may be convenient for administration to newborns but may not be the preferred form for older children.[25] Refer to the EMA and DG Enterprise and Industry websites for an exhaustive compilation of guidelines of particular relevance to the development of paediatric medicines in Europe.

Summary

In 2007, the EU became the second major pharmaceutical market with a regulatory framework dedicated to the improvement of paediatric labelling information. In the US, the *Best Pharmaceuticals for Children Act* and *Pediatric Research Equity Act* were re-authorised in October 2007 for an additional five years (sunset 1 October 2012). In contrast, the EU *Paediatric Regulation* does not require a re-authorisation. The more recent EU regulation is largely inspired by two main components of the US legislation, i.e., the voluntary "paediatric incentive" (for both off- and on-patent products) and the obligatory "paediatric rule" for new and on-patent drugs. However, the EU legislation is arguably more constraining for MAHs and sponsors of new drugs in development since the potential paediatric utility has to be considered not only for every investigational medicinal product but also for all licensed, on-patent products whenever a lifecycle submission is planned.

Potential paediatric needs must further be examined for all adult indications and for all paediatric subsets (i.e., premature neonates, term neonates, infants, children and adolescents) unless the condition or disease falls into one of the blanket (class) waivers published by EMA. An approved EU PIP includes timelines for the completion of the various elements and is considered an agreement between the company and the agency. Companies failing to comply with the agreed plan (at least if judged in bad faith) risk financial penalties. In comparison, FDA has no legal power to decide on penalties or fines for noncompliance.

Paediatric research is a priority collaboration area as defined within the FDA-EMA confidentiality agreement. The two agencies are committed to a regular information exchange on:

- product-specific paediatric development (PIPs, written requests, deferrals) and waivers from the obligations to perform such paediatric development (which may include discussions on trial design issues)
- general issues related to paediatric development (including sharing early-stage draft guidance documents of paediatric relevance)
- safety issues, particularly in relation to reporting adverse drug reactions (ADRs) occurring in children and exchange of ADR database statistics

There is a strong desire by industry for a means to obtain coordinated feedback from FDA and EMA on paediatric research proposals in the future. An obvious difficulty to overcome is the EU expectation for early submissions of PIPs, including for drugs intended for non-life-threatening diseases.

References

1. Regulation (EC) No 1901/2006 of the European Parliament and of the Council of 12 December 2006 on medicinal products for paediatric use and amending Regulation (EEC) No 1768/92, Directive 2001/20/EC, Directive 2001/83/EC and Regulation (EC) No 726/2004. EC website. http://ec.europa.eu/health/files/eudralex/vol-1/reg_2006_1901/reg_2006_1901_en.pdf. Accessed 11 April 2012.
2. Regulation (EC) No 1902/2006 of the European Parliament and of the Council of 20 December 2006 amending Regulation 1901/2006 on medicinal products for paediatric use. EC website. http://ec.europa.eu/health/files/eudralex/vol-1/reg_2006_1902/reg_2006_1902_en.pdf. Accessed 11 April 2012.
3. Directive 2001/20/EC of the European Parliament and of the Council of 4 April 2001 on the approximation of the laws, regulations and administrative provisions of the Member States relating to the implementation of good clinical practice in the conduct of clinical trials on medicinal products for human use. EUR-Lex website. http://eur-lex.europa.eu/LexUriServ/LexUriServ.do?uri=OJ:L:2001:121:0034:0044:en:PDF. Accessed 11 April 2012.
4. *Communication from the Commission 2008/C 243/01—Guideline on the format and content of applications for agreement or modification of a paediatric investigation plan and requests for waivers or deferrals and concerning the operation of the compliance check and on criteria for assessing significant studies.* EUR-Lex website. http://eur-lex.europa.eu/JOHtml.do?uri=OJ:C:2008:243:SOM:EN:HTML. Accessed 11 April 2012.
5. CPMP/ICH/2711/99, *ICH Topic E11, Clinical investigation of medicinal products in the paediatric population* (January 2001). EMA website. www.ema.europa.eu/docs/en_GB/document_library/Scientific_guideline/2009/09/WC500002926.pdf. Accessed 11 April 2012.
6. Directive 2004/27/EC of the European Parliament and the Council of 31 March 2004 amending Directive 2001/83/EC on the Community code relating to medicinal products for human use. EUR-Lex website. http://eur-lex.europa.eu/LexUriServ/LexUriServ.do?uri=OJ:L:2004:136:0034:0057:EN:PDF. Accessed 11 April 2012.
7. Op cit 4.
8. Op cit 5.

9. Regulation (EC) No 469/2009 of the European Parliament and of the Council of 6 May 2009 concerning the supplementary protection certificate for medicinal products (replacing Regulation (EEC) No 1768/92). EUR-Lex website. http://eur-lex.europa.eu/LexUriServ/LexUriServ.do?uri=OJ:L:2009:152:0001:0010:en:PDF. Accessed 11 April 2012.
10. Regulation (EC) No 726/2004, as amended, of the European Parliament and the Council of 31 March 2004 laying down Community procedures for the authorisation and supervision of medicinal products for human and veterinary use and establishing a European Medicines Agency. EC website. http://ec.europa.eu/health/files/eudralex/vol-1/reg_2004_726_cons/reg_2004_726_cons_en.pdf. Accessed 11 April 2012.
11. Op cit 6.
12. EMA/PDCO/179892/2011 Rev. 1, *Questions and answers on the procedure of PIP compliance verification at EMA* (3 March 2011). EMA website. www.ema.europa.eu/docs/en_GB/document_library/Regulatory_and_procedural_guideline/2009/09/WC500003916.pdf. Accessed 11 April 2012.
13. Op cit 10.
14. Commission Regulation (EC) No 658/2007 of 14 June 2007 concerning financial penalties for infringement of certain obligations in connection with marketing authorisations granted under Regulation (EC) No 726/2004 of the European Parliament and of the Council. EC website. http://ec.europa.eu/health/files/eudralex/vol-1/reg_2007_658/reg_2007_658_en.pdf. Accessed 11 April 2012.
15. *Communication from the Commission 2009/C 28/01—Guidance on the information concerning paediatric clinical trials to be entered into the EU Database on Clinical trials (EudraCT) and on the information to be made public by the European Medicines Agency (EMEA), in accordance with Article 41 of Regulation (EC) No 1901/2006* (4 February 2009). EC website. http://ec.europa.eu/health/files/eudralex/vol-10/2009_c28_01/2009_c28_01_en.pdf. Accessed 11 April 2012.
16. European Commission. *Ethical considerations for clinical trials on medicinal products conducted with the paediatric population, Recommendations of the ad hoc group for the development of implementing guidelines for Directive 2001/20/EC relating to good clinical practice in the conduct of clinical trials on medicinal products for human use* (Final 2008). EC website. http://ec.europa.eu/health/files/paediatrics/docs/paeds_ethics_consultation20060929_en.pdf. Accessed 11 April 2012.
17. EMEA/CHMP/SWP/169215/2005, *Guideline on the need for non-clinical testing in juvenile animals of pharmaceuticals for paediatric indications* (24 January 2008). EMA website. www.ema.europa.eu/docs/en_GB/document_library/Scientific_guideline/2009/09/WC500003306.pdf. Accessed 11 April 2012.
18. EMEA/181377/2006, *Concept paper on the impact of brain immaturity when investigating medicinal products intended for neonatal use* (2 June 2006). EMA website. www.ema.europa.eu/docs/en_GB/document_library/Scientific_guideline/2009/09/WC500003800.pdf. Accessed 11 April 2012.
19. EMEA/CHMP/114218/2006, *Concept paper on the impact of lung and heart immaturity when investigating medicinal products intended for neonatal use—Draft 1* (18 November 2005). EMA website. www.ema.europa.eu/docs/en_GB/document_library/Scientific_guideline/2009/09/WC500003802.pdf. Accessed 11 April 2012.
20. EMEA/CHMP/PEG/194605/2005, *Concept paper on the impact of liver immaturity when investigating medicinal products intended for neonatal use—Draft* (20 July 2005). EMA website. www.ema.europa.eu/docs/en_GB/document_library/Scientific_guideline/2009/09/WC500003803.pdf. Accessed 11 April 2012.
21. CPMP/PEG/35132/03, *Discussion paper on the impact of renal immaturity when investigating medicinal products intended for paediatric use* (16 December 2004).EMA website. www.ema.europa.eu/docs/en_GB/document_library/Scientific_guideline/2009/09/WC500003807.pdf. Accessed 11 April 2012.
22. EMEA/CHMP/EWP/147013/2004/Corr, *Guideline on the role of pharmacokinetics in the development of medicinal products in the paediatric population* (28 June 2006). EMA website. www.ema.europa.eu/docs/en_GB/document_library/Scientific_guideline/2009/09/WC500003066.pdf. Accessed 11 April 2012.
23. CHMP/EWP/83561/2005, *Guideline on the clinical trials in small populations* (27 July 2006). EMA website. www.ema.europa.eu/docs/en_GB/document_library/Scientific_guideline/2009/09/WC500003615.pdf. Accessed 11 April 2012.
24. EMEA/CHMP/PhVWP/235910/2005–rev. 1, *Guideline on conduct of pharmacovigilance for medicines used by the paediatric population* (25 January 2007). EMA website. www.emea.europa.eu/docs/en_GB/document_library/Scientific_guideline/2009/09/WC500003764.pdf. Accessed 11 April 2012.
25. EMEA/CHMP/PEG/194810/2005, *Reflection paper: Formulations of choice for the paediatric population* (28 July 2006). EMA website. www.ema.europa.eu/docs/en_GB/document_library/Scientific_guideline/2009/09/WC500003782.pdf. Accessed 11 April 2012.

Chapter 6

Advertising and Promotion

By Elisabethann Wright and Alexander Roussanov

OBJECTIVES

❑ Understand the legal framework of the EU on advertising of medicinal products and the marketing codes of conduct of pharmaceutical industry associations

❑ Learn about the ongoing review of EU law on information to patients

❑ Understand the differences between national rules on promotion of medicinal products in EU Member States versus EU regulations

❑ Become familiar with EU Directive 2001/83/EC, as amended, laying out, among other things, EU rules on promotion and advertising of medicinal products

DIRECTIVES, REGULATIONS AND GUIDELINES COVERED IN THIS CHAPTER

❑ Directive 2001/83/EC of the European Parliament and of the Council of 6 November 2001 on the Community code relating to medicinal products for human use, as amended,[1] providing the current European regulations on advertising of medicinal products for human use

❑ Directive 2006/114/EC of the European Parliament and of the Council of 12 December 2006 concerning misleading and comparative advertising[2]

❑ Directive 2005/29/EC of the European Parliament and of the Council of 11 May 2005 concerning unfair business-to-consumer commercial practices in the internal market[3]

❑ Directive 2010/13/EU of the European Parliament and of the Council of 10 March 2010 on the coordination of certain provisions laid down by law, regulation or administrative action in Member States concerning the provision of audiovisual media services[4]

❑ World Health Organization (WHO) Ethical Criteria for Medicinal Drug Promotion, 1988[5]

❑ International Federation of Pharmaceutical Manufacturers Association (IFPMA) Code of Pharmaceutical Marketing Practices, updated 2006[6]

❑ Code of Practice on the promotion of prescription-only medicines to, and interactions with, healthcare professionals (EFPIA), Update 2007[7]

❑ Association of British Pharmaceutical Industry (ABPI) Code of Practice for the Pharmaceutical Industry, Update 2012[8]

Introduction

The advertising and promotion of medicinal products in the EU is highly regulated on a number of levels. Directive 2001/83/EC of the European Parliament and of the Council of 6 November 2001 on the Community code relating to medicinal products for human use, as amended, provides

Chapter 6

the general rules applicable in the EU on advertising of medicinal products for human use (the *Community Code*). The directive's provisions are transposed into the national laws of the 27 EU Member States. Compliance with the rules on promotion and advertising of medicinal products is monitored and enforced at the national level by EU Member States' Competent Authorities.

Practical experience in the EU suggests that the interpretation of the provisions of the *Community Code* on the advertising and promotion of prescription-only medicinal products is not always an easy or straightforward task. National laws implementing the provisions of the *Community Code*, as well as their enforcement by the Member States' Competent Authorities, do not seem to be uniform across the EU.

Addressing the issue, the Court of Justice of the European Union (CJEU) delivers guidance and interpretation of the provisions of the *Community Code*, when requested by EU Member States' national courts, to enhance the uniform application of EU law across all Member States.

The EU legislature, aware of the differing interpretations of the provisions of the *Community Code* that govern the promotion and advertising of prescription-only medicinal products, initiated a proposal for reform of those provisions. The proposed changes and clarifications became the object of some controversy among EU Member States, EU institutions, industry, patient organisations and a wide range of other stakeholders. Due to this controversy, the European Commission withdrew its initial proposal and presented a new proposal attempting to accommodate the positions expressed by the EU Member States and the European Parliament. The discussions on the new amended proposal are still ongoing, and the outcome remains uncertain.

In this context of extensive regulation and legal uncertainty, EU and national pharmaceutical industry associations, as well as other international organisations, have found it necessary to develop voluntary codes of practice to guide their members in complying with these regulations.[5–7] These codes supplement the EU and national laws and regulations. The codes are updated regularly, often based on harmonisation standards established at the European level. Some national codes also are enforced by independent industry bodies that monitor companies' compliance.

ABPI Code and Enforcement

The original self-regulatory code on the promotion of prescription medicines was the UK Association of the British Pharmaceutical Industry (ABPI) Code, first issued in 1958. It preceded the establishment of international codes and most EU Member States' national codes. It also preceded the adoption of Council Directive 92/28/EEC of 31 March 1992 on the advertising of medicinal products for human use in EU Member States (now repealed and replaced by the *Community Code*). The latest revision of the ABPI Code came into force on 1 January 2012. Compliance of the association's members with the ABPI Code of Practice is overseen by the Prescription Medicines Code of Practice Authority (PMCPA). PMCPA's tasks include review of complaints about compliance with the ABPI Code governing promotional materials and activities undertaken by pharmaceutical companies. PMCPA also provides advice and guidance on the ABPI Code, conciliation between pharmaceutical companies and scrutiny of samples of advertising for compliance with the code. PMCPA arbitration results and decisions are available on the PMCPA website.[9] The PMCPA decisions provide useful insight and guidance on the interpretation and implementation of the provisions of both the *Community Code* and the ABPI Code regarding the promotion and advertising of prescription-only medicinal products.

WHO Ethical Criteria for Medicinal Drug Promotion

In May 1988, the 41st World Assembly of the World Health Organization (WHO) adopted Resolution WHA41.17, after having considered an executive board report concerning ethical criteria for medicinal drug promotion, based on a draft prepared by an international group of experts.[10]

The ethical criteria for medicinal drug promotion are primarily to support and encourage healthcare improvement through the rational use of drugs. The WHO international working group's criteria constitute general principles for ethical standards that governments could adapt as appropriate to their health system's political, economic and cultural situation. Criteria are not obligatory, and governments may adopt legislation and other means to support the general principles. Other groups may adopt self-regulating practices. Other codes, such as those of the International Federation of Pharmaceutical Manufacturers Association (IFPMA) and the European Federation of Pharmaceutical Industries and Associations (EFPIA), have been developed from this foundation.

International Federation of Pharmaceutical Manufacturers Association (IFPMA)

Founded in 1968, IFPMA represents the research-based pharmaceutical industry. Its members, either directly or through regional organisations, are pharmaceutical industry associations from more than 60 countries worldwide.

The IFPMA *Code of Pharmaceutical Marketing Practices*, adopted voluntarily in 1981, has been updated several times[11] in accordance with founding member objectives to promote and support ethical medicinal product promotion principles. The latest update of the IFPMA Code was adopted in 2011 and becomes effective on 1 September 2012. The IFPMA Code defines the acceptable baseline marketing practice standard. IFPMA member pharmaceutical companies are encouraged to develop their own codes of practice. Some are based on IFPMA's Code, but have been elaborated to include more-specific requirements to suit individual needs and activities.

European Federation of Pharmaceutical Industries and Associations (EFPIA)

EFPIA was founded in 1978, and its members are Europe's national pharmaceutical industry associations. It represents EU pharmaceutical manufacturers that undertake research and development and manufacture medicinal products. EFPIA represents the industry before EU institutions, but also communicates with other relevant stakeholders on both the EU and national levels. In addition, it provides advice and support to national industry associations regarding national and EU matters. EFPIA's mission is to foster a policymaking climate that enables the EU pharmaceutical industry to meet the Community's present and future healthcare expectations.[12]

The *European Code of Practice on the Promotion of Medicines*, adopted in 1991 by the European pharmaceutical industry, has since been revised several times (last updated in June 2011).[13] It sets out minimum standards that individual member associations must meet to ensure their own national codes meet European code standards. Annex B of this code also contains guidelines for Internet websites available to healthcare professionals, patients and the public in the EU. In the absence of specific rules adopted on an EU level regarding the provision of information on medicinal products to the general public in the EU, this could serve as a useful guidance for industry in providing information to the general public in the EU via Internet websites.

The *Community Code*

The *Community Code*, as amended, includes the current EU rules on promotion and advertising of medicinal products for human use. The relevant provisions are contained within Titles VIII and VIIIa of the code (Articles 86–100).

Article 86 defines "advertising of medicinal products" as including "any form of door-to-door information, canvassing activity or inducement designed to promote the prescription, supply, sale or consumption of medicinal products." The article enumerates activities that are considered to constitute advertising. Beyond the obvious advertising to the general public and healthcare professionals and visits by sales representatives, advertising includes supply of samples, sponsorship of promotional meetings or scientific events and the provision of any kind of inducement (gifts, offers or promises of any benefits or bonuses in money or in kind) except where their value is minimal.

The specific implementation and clarification of what is considered "minimal value," as well as the conditions under which the provision of gifts, samples and sponsorship are acceptable, are defined by EU Member States' national legislation and the industry's national and EU-level codes of conduct.

The *Community Code* prohibits the advertising of medicinal products for which a marketing authorisation in the EU has not been granted. The promotion and advertising to the general public of authorised medicinal products available on a prescription-only basis also are banned, as are the promotion and advertising of medicinal products containing substances defined as psychotropic or narcotic by international convention.

EU Member States are required to prohibit the direct distribution of medicinal products to the public by industry for promotional purposes. They also are permitted by the *Community Code* to prohibit the advertising and promotion in their territories of medicinal products whose cost may be reimbursed by national health insurance systems.

The prohibition on promoting prescription-only medicinal products to the general public does not apply to vaccination campaigns approved by the EU Member States' authorities and implemented by industry. The *Community Code* also permits advertising to the general public of medicinal products intended and designed for use without the intervention of a medical practitioner for diagnostic purposes or for the prescription or monitoring of treatment, with the advice of the pharmacist, if necessary.

The *Community Code* requires that any advertising of a medicinal product comply with the information contained in the Summary of Product Characteristics (SmPC). The properties of the medicinal product must be presented in an objective way and should not be exaggerated. Advertising should encourage the rational use of the medicinal product and should not be misleading.

As a reference, the EU *Directive on misleading and comparative advertising* (Directive 2006/114/EC) defines "misleading advertising" as "any advertising which in any way, including its presentation, deceives or is likely to deceive the persons to whom it is addressed or whom it reaches and which, by reason of its deceptive nature, is likely to affect their economic behavior or which, for those reasons, injures or is likely to injure a competitor."

Excluded from the scope of the definition of advertising of medicinal products provided by the *Community Code* (and often subject to other provisions of the *Community Code* and other relevant legislation and guidance) are the following:
- labelling and accompanying package leaflets
- correspondence possibly accompanied by material of a nonpromotional nature
- factual, informative announcements and reference material relating, for example, to pack changes, adverse-reaction warnings as part of general drug

precautions, trade catalogues and price lists, provided they include no product claims
- human health or disease information, provided there is no reference, even indirectly, to medicinal products

Pharmaceutical companies are permitted to sponsor or implement disease awareness campaigns under strict conditions established by Member States' national laws and industry's codes of conduct. Such campaigns should neither refer directly or indirectly to any medicinal products nor be used as a means for direct or indirect promotion of medicinal products.

Required Information in Advertising for a Medicinal Product

Articles 89 and 91 of the *Community Code* describe the minimum information to be included in advertising materials and how it should be presented to either the general public or healthcare professionals. Article 90 describes elements that should not be included in the advertising of a medicinal product to the general public.

Advertising materials intended for the general public should clearly indicate that the product is a medicinal product. They should not suggest that the medicinal product will enhance health, that results are guaranteed, that the medicinal product has no side effects or that the safety of the medicinal product is better than or equivalent to that of another treatment or medicinal product. Materials should not overpromise and should not use alarming or misleading terms or representations. The advertisements should not suggest that not taking the medicinal product could affect health (except for approved vaccination campaigns).

Advertising to the general public should not give the impression that medical consultation or intervention is unnecessary. The advertising materials should not lead to self-diagnosis, or offer or suggest diagnosis or treatment by mail.

Medicinal product advertising to the general public should never be directed exclusively or principally at children. It should not contain recommendations by scientists, healthcare professionals, celebrities or public figures that could encourage the consumption of the product.

Multimedia Advertising (Television and the Internet)

The *Audiovisual Media Services Directive* (Directive 2010/13/EU) prohibits audiovisual commercial communication for prescription-only medicines in several articles (Articles 9.1(f); 10.3; 11.4(b)). Article 21 of the directive also prohibits teleshopping of medicinal products.

The Internet has revolutionised and enhanced worldwide access to product information. This information includes direct-to-consumer marketing of pharmaceutical products originating from regions where it is allowed by national regulations. It is impossible to isolate European patients from Internet direct-to-consumer advertising, although one natural barrier is the fact that many EU consumers do not have a good command of English. Indeed, the dubious quality of the information available on the Internet and the inequality of information access were prime drivers for proposed amendments to the *Community Code* regarding the provision of information to patients, as discussed below.

Under EU law, the promotion of medicinal products on the Internet falls within and should comply with the relevant provisions of the *Community Code*, the directive on misleading and comparative advertising and the *Audiovisual Media Services Directive*.

In many EU Member States, existing laws and regulations allow product-specific information to be provided only to healthcare professionals. Publicly available information on pharmaceutical companies' websites is often disease-specific or related to patient education initiatives. Publication of product-specific information or promotion on these websites requires appropriate access controls and password protection to ensure that only healthcare professionals can access it. As an alternative, some Member States, such as Sweden and the UK, provide product-specific information to the general public on websites set up by the authorities or through private-public partnerships with industry. However, such initiatives are the exception.

In 2004, EFPIA proposed guidelines for company-sponsored websites[14] providing information on medicinal products. However, the guidelines, inspired by the Swedish approach, have not been adopted or implemented in most EU countries. The concept described in the guidelines could be seen as conflicting with the provisions of the national laws of a number of EU Member States that prohibit the provision of information to the general public on prescription-only medicinal products by pharmaceutical companies.

Community Code Shortcomings and the Interpretation of the Court of Justice

A number of elements are not very clear in the provisions of the *Community Code* regarding the promotion of medicinal products. This lack of clarity has led to somewhat differing and conflicting transpositions in EU Member States' national laws.

One particular issue is the absence of a clear definition of what constitutes information on medicinal products provided to patients and where the line should be drawn between information and promotion. As discussed above, Sweden and the UK consider that information on prescription-only medicinal products can be provided to the general public without infringing the prohibition provided in the *Community Code* on advertising and promotion of these products, if this is done in controlled environments. However, this view is not shared by other EU Member States.

In a 2009 ruling,[15] CJEU affirmed that any reference to the properties and/or availability of a medicinal product could qualify as "advertising" and could, potentially, influence consumers' behaviour and encourage consumption of the product. In the same judgment, CJEU also stated that such information provided by an independent third party would be considered advertising of the specific medicinal product. According to the court, the absence of legal, commercial or other links between the manufacturer of a medicinal product and a third party disseminating information on the product does not exclude the activities of the third party from the scope of the definition of "advertising."

In another recent case,[16] CJEU had the opportunity to clarify whether the prohibition in the *Community Code* on providing inducements to healthcare professionals to prescribe medicinal products applies to a national health authority policy providing financial incentives to healthcare professionals to prescribe a specific medicinal product. According to CJEU, the provisions of the *Community Code* imposing restrictions on the promotion and advertising of medicinal products apply only to pharmaceutical companies and independent third parties. CJEU held that those provisions do not apply to EU Member States' national health authorities responsible for ensuring that the provisions of the *Community Code* are applied and also charged with defining public health policy priorities, in particular the rationalisation of the expenditure of national public funds allocated to that policy.

In its most recent ruling[17] regarding the promotion of medicinal products and the provision of information to the general public in relation to prescription-only medicinal products, CJEU ruled that pharmaceutical companies are permitted to provide objective and nonpromotional information to patients and the general public in the EU concerning prescription-only medicinal products authorised to be placed on the EU Market. This information includes "faithful" and "literal" reproduction of the approved packaging of the medicinal product, the patient information leaflet and the SmPC.

Reform of the Rules of the *Community Code* Regarding the Provision of Information to Patients

As discussed above, a number of elements of the provisions of the *Community Code* regarding the promotion of medicinal products remain unclear and prone to different interpretations. Further, technological advances, the increasing availability of Internet information resources, and the developing interest of EU patients in their health and choice of treatment require adaptation of the existing rules to take those elements into account.

As required by the *Community Code*, in 2007, the European Commission conducted a public consultation and presented a report to the European Parliament and the Council on the provision of information on prescription-only medicinal products to patients, particularly on the Internet, the risks involved and benefits for patients. A follow-up public consultation on the key elements of a legal proposal on information to patients was launched by the Commission in February 2008.

Feedback received during the public consultations and the subsequent European Commission report acknowledge that information provided by EU Member States' authorities currently varies considerably. The information provided through the Internet may not always be of appropriate quality. Currently, EU citizens in different Member States have unequal access to information and are exposed to risks related to unreliable or even illegal sources of information available to the general public on the Internet.

In December 2008, the European Commission presented a legal proposal regarding the provision of information to patients to ensure good-quality, objective, reliable and nonpromotional information on prescription-only medicinal products to citizens and to harmonise the rules in EU Member States.

The aim of the proposal is to allow pharmaceutical companies to provide reliable, good-quality, accurate nonpromotional information to patients regarding prescription-only medicinal products. The information provided would be limited to the scope of the summary of product characteristics.

The initial proposal was very contentious. The European Commission faced opposition from certain EU Member States, members of the European Parliament and a number of EU patient and consumer organisations. As a result, the European Commission withdrew its initial proposal and in October 2011 adopted a revised proposal for the new EU rules regarding the provision of information to patients in relation to prescription-only medicinal products. The revised proposal takes into account the amendments adopted by the European Parliament in relation to the Commission's initial proposal. The Commission confirmed that the proposal was reviewed from a patient perspective.

A key element of the new proposal is the definition of advertising of medicinal products. The proposed definition includes activities undertaken by the Marketing Authorisation Holder (MAH) either directly or indirectly through a third party acting on its behalf or following its instructions. Activities undertaken by independent third parties are not included. Moreover, factual, informative announcements and reference material, adverse-reaction warnings, trade catalogues and price lists are no longer automatically excluded from the definition of advertising. This applies even if these materials do not include medicinal product-related claims.

The proposal includes criteria concerning information to be provided to the general public. It also addresses information that must be provided by to the general public by the MAH, as well as the information the MAH could provide to the general public voluntarily. In addition, the proposal addresses the channels for provision of information to the general public and the pre- and post-vetting mechanisms involving the European Medicines Agency (EMA) and Competent Authorities of the EU Member States.

The legislative process is expected to resume in 2012 with discussions in the European Parliament's Committee on Environment, Public Health and Food Safety. The proposal remains highly controversial, and it is challenging to predict when and in what form it would be adopted by the Council and the European Parliament.

National Laws and Regulations

The EU has a unique institutional and political framework for regulating medicinal products. Regulatory oversight is ensured by the 27 EU Member States' Competent Authorities, and this number could expand in the future with the potential accession of new EU Member States, arguably adding complexity to the organisational structure.

Each EU Member State Competent Authority is responsible for ensuring that the provisions of the *Community Code* are applied in its national territory. As discussed above, the implementation of the provisions of the *Community Code* in national law varies from country to country. However, a number of core rules are enforced uniformly in all EU Member States. The advertising of nonauthorised medicinal products, the advertising of prescription-only medicinal products to the general public and the misleading advertising of medicinal products are prohibited throughout the EU.

It would appear that most EU Member States would not require the pre-vetting of promotional materials. However, some national authorities may. For example, the UK Medicines and Healthcare products Regulatory Agency (MHRA) usually requests pre-vetting when:
- a newly licenced product, subject to intensive monitoring, is placed on the market
- a product is reclassified, e.g., from prescription-only to over-the-counter
- a product's previous advertising breached the regulations

Pre-use vetting may also be requested by MHRA when a medicinal product has been granted an authorisation for a new indication or in case of safety concerns. The practice shows that the promotional materials of newly authorised medicinal products are also pre-vetted by MHRA.

In Germany, medicinal product advertising is governed primarily by the *Law on Advertising in the Field of Healthcare* (*Heilmittelwerbegesetz* (*HWG*)), last amended 26 April 2006. German law does not require promotional materials to be submitted to the authorities for review or pre-vetting. Intentional breaches of the rules of the *HWG* on misleading advertising constitute a criminal offence. Sanctions include imprisonment and heavy fines. In addition, the violating company runs the risk of having cease and desist claims, or even damage compensation claims, filed against it by competitors, their associations or consumer protection associations. A violation of the provisions also constitutes a violation of the *Unfair Competition Act (Gesetz gegen den unlauteren Wettbewerb* (*UWG*)). Industry is vigilant regarding competitor activity since a clear process for redress is made available by national law. Misleading advertising could be also sanctioned by the industry "Voluntary Self-regulation of the Pharmaceutical Industry" organization (*Freiwillige Selbstkontrolle für die Arzneimittelindustrie e.V* (FSA)). FSA arbitrators can impose fines up to €250,000.

The advertising of medicinal products in France is governed by provisions of the *French Public Health Code* (*PHC*). Any advertising material for a medicinal product should be submitted to the French National Agency for the Safety of Medicinal Products and Healthcare Products (*Agence nationale de sécurité du médicament et des produits de santé (ANSM)*). Direct-to-consumer advertising materials for nonprescription medicinal products should be approved by ANSM. Until recently, MAHs were not required to submit materials intended for healthcare professionals to ANSM for prior approval. The requirement was to submit promotional materials to ANSM eight days after their first use. However, following a recent reform of the *PHC*, promotional materials intended for healthcare professionals must be submitted to ANSM for prior approval. Breaches of the rules on promotion of medicinal products are considered criminal offences and sanctioned by fines, prohibition of sale, confiscation of the respective medicinal product and destruction of the promotional materials. French law also provides competitors with ways to bring civil proceedings in the commercial courts in cases of illegal advertising and unfair competition.

In Italy, advertising of medicinal products is governed by sections 113-128 of the Legislative Decree of 24 April 2006, No. 219. Advertising is subject to the regulatory authority's prior approval. Advertising to the general public is permitted only for over-the-counter medicinal products. Advertising materials intended for the general public must be approved by the Italian Medicines Agency (*Agenxia Italiana del Farmaco* (AIFA)) during a 45-day assessment period. If no objection is raised by AIFA during this period, the materials are deemed approved. Exceptions are made for reproductions of the product image accompanied by the full text of the indications, contraindications, special notices for its use, interactions, etc. Advertising materials intended for healthcare professionals (other than reproductions of the product's SmPC) must be submitted to AIFA and cannot be used until 10 days have elapsed following the submission. AIFA can prohibit or suspend the distribution of such materials at any time.

This in no way an exhaustive list of Member State differences, but serves to highlight the nuances of the EU and the importance of understanding Community laws and individual Member State laws and regulations.

Summary

- The main rules on promotion of medicinal products in the EU are provided by the *Community Code*, which is implemented in national laws and enforced by EU Member States, resulting in a complex regulatory framework.
- The *Community Code* leaves room for a number of uncertainties that lead to diverging implementation in EU Member States. To address this, CJEU delivers judgments intended to ensure uniform interpretation of the provisions of the *Community Code*. The EU legislature has also undertaken (ongoing) legislative reform.
- Direct-to-consumer advertising of prescription-only medicinal products in the EU is not permitted. The provision of information regarding such products is also excluded in practice in many EU Member States.
- National legislation, as well as national, European and international industry associations' codes of conduct, together with WHO's Ethical Criteria for Drug Promotion, complement the provisions of the *Community Code* and set out the framework applicable in the EU on promotion and advertising of medicinal products.

References

1. Directive 2001/83/EC of the European Parliament and of the Council of 6 November 2001 on the Community code relating to medicinal products for human use (codifying former directives relating to medicinal products for human use). EUR-Lex website. http://eur-lex.europa.eu/LexUriServ/LexUriServ.do?uri=OJ:L:2001:311:0067:0128:en:PDF. Accessed 18 May 2012.
2. Directive 2006/114/EC of the European Parliament and of the Council of 12 December 2006 concerning misleading and comparative advertising (repealing Directive 84/450/EEC and codifying (consolidating) all the amendments to it in a single legal act). EUR-Lex website. http://eur-lex.europa.eu/LexUriServ/LexUriServ.do?uri=OJ:L:2006:376:0021:0027:EN:PDF. Accessed 18 May 2012.
3. Directive 2005/29/EC of the European Parliament and of the Council of 11 May 2005 concerning unfair business-to-consumer commercial practices in the internal market and amending Council Directive 84/450/EEC, Directives 97/7/EC, 98/27/EC and 2002/65/EC of the European Parliament and of the Council and Regulation (EC) No 2006/2004 of the European Parliament and of the Council (*Unfair Commercial Practices Directive*). EUR-Lex website. http://eur-lex.europa.eu/LexUriServ/LexUriServ.do?uri=OJ:L:2005:149:0022:0039:EN:PDF. Accessed 18 May 2012.
4. Directive 2010/13/EU of the European Parliament and of the Council of 10 March 2010 on the coordination of certain provisions laid down by law, regulation or administrative action in Member States concerning the provision of audiovisual media services. EUR-Lex website. http://eur-lex.europa.eu/LexUriServ/LexUriServ.do?uri=OJ:L:2010:095:0001:0024:EN:PDF. Accessed 18 May 2012.
5. World Health Organization. *Ethical Criteria for Medicinal Drug Promotion*. Geneva, Switzerland: World Health Organization; 1988. WHO website. http://whqlibdoc.who.int/publications/1988/924154239X_eng.pdf. Accessed 18 May 2012.
6. International Federation of Pharmaceutical Manufacturers Association (IFPMA). *Code of Pharmaceutical Marketing Practices*, Update 2012. IFPMA website. www.ifpma.org/fileadmin/content/Publication/2012/IFPMA_Code_of_Practice_2012_new_logo.pdf. Accessed 18 May 2012.
7. The European Federation of Pharmaceutical Industries and Associations (EFPIA).*Code of Practice on the promotion of prescription-only medicines to, and interactions with, healthcare professionals*, Update 2012. EFPIA website. www.efpia.eu/content/default.asp?PageID=559&DocID=11731. Accessed 18 May 2012.
8. Association of British Pharmaceutical Industry (ABPI) Code of Practice for the Pharmaceutical Industry, Update 2012. ABPI website. www.abpi.org.uk/our-work/library/guidelines/Pages/code-2012.aspx. Accessed 18 May 2012.
9. Prescription Medicines Code of Practice Authority (PMCPA) PMCPA website. www.pmcpa.org.uk/. Accessed 18 May 2012.
10. Op cit 5.
11. Op cit 6.
12. Op cit 7.
13. Ibid.
14. *Guidelines for Internet web sites available to health professionals, patients and the public in the EU*. EFPIA website. www.efpia.eu/Content/Default.asp?PageID=559&DocID=7539. Accessed 20 May 2012.
15. Court of Justice of the European Union Case C-421/07 Damgaard from 2 April 2009, ECR [2009] I-02629. EUR-Lex website. http://eur-lex.europa.eu/LexUriServ/LexUriServ.do?uri=CELEX:62007J0421:EN:NOT. Accessed 20 May 2012.
16. Court of Justice of the European Union Case C-62/09 Association of the British Pharmaceutical Industry from 22 April 2010, ECR [2010] I-03603. EUR-Lex website. http://eur-lex.europa.eu/LexUriServ/LexUriServ.do?uri=CELEX:62009J0062:EN:NOT. Accessed 20 May 2012..
17. Court of Justice of the European Union Case C-316/09 MSD Sharp & Dohme GmbH v. Merckle GmbH, from 5 May 2011, not yet published.

Chapter 7

Enforcement and National Authorities

Updated by Martha Anna Bianchetto, PharmD, MBA

OBJECTIVES

❑ Understand the basic regulations relevant to enforcement

❑ Examine examples of enforcement action in practice

❑ Review the involvement of third parties and the role of national authorities

❑ Explore EU-wide enforcement and Member States' national enforcement

REGULATIONS AND GUIDELINES COVERED IN THIS CHAPTER

❑ Directive 2001/83/EC of the European Parliament and of the Council of 6 November 2001 on the Community code relating to medicinal products for human use

❑ Commission Regulation (EC) No 540/95 of 10 March 1995 laying down the arrangements for reporting suspected unexpected adverse reactions which are not serious, to medicinal products for human or veterinary use authorised in accordance with the provisions of Council Regulation (EEC) No 2309/93 (now Regulation (EC) No 726/2004), whether arising within the Community or in a third country

❑ Regulation (EC) No 726/2004 of the European Parliament and of the Council of 31 March 2004, laying down Community procedures for the authorisation and supervision of medicinal products for human and veterinary use and establishing a European Medicines Agency

❑ Guideline on the Requirements for Quality Documentation Concerning Biological Investigational Medicinal Products in Clinical Trials (Draft)

❑ Note For Guidance on Virus Validation Studies: The Design, Contribution and Interpretation of Studies Validating the Inactivation and Removal of Viruses (EMEA/CHMP/BWP/398498/05)

❑ Guideline on Strategies to Identify and Mitigate Risks for First-In-Human Clinical Trials with investigational Medicinal Products (EMEA/CHMP/SWP/28367/07, current version)

❑ Regulation (EU) No 1235/2010 of the European Parliament and of the Council of 15 Dec 2010 amending, as regards pharmacovigilance of medicinal for human use, Regulation (EC) No 726/2004 on Community procedures for authorisation and supervision of medicinal products for human and veterinary use and establishing a European Medicines Agency and Regulation (EC) No 1394/2007 on advanced therapy medicinal therapy (published 31 December 2010 and applicable from July 2012)

Regulatory Affairs Professionals Society

Chapter 7

- Directive 2010/84/EU of the European Parliament and of the Council of 15 December 2010 amending, as regards pharmacovigilance, Directive 2001/83/EC on the Community code on medicinal products (published 31 December 2010 and applicable from July 2012)

- European Commission, The Rules Governing Medicinal Products in the European Union, Volume 9A, Guidelines on Pharmacovigilance for Medicinal Products for Human Use

- Regulation (EU) No 1235/2010 amending Regulation (EC) No 726 regarding pharmacovigilance (entering into force 2 July 2012)

- Directive 2010/84/EC amending Directive 2001/83/EC regarding pharmacovigilance (entering into force 2 July 2012)

- ICH Pharmacovigilance-related guidelines (E2 series)

- Council Directive 93/42/EEC of 14 June 1993 concerning medical devices amended by Directive 2007/47/EC

- Council Directive 90/385/EEC of 20 June 1990 concerning active implantable medical devices amended by Directive 2007/47/EC

- Directive 98/79/EC of the European Parliament and of the Council of 27 October 1998 on in vitro diagnostic medical devices

- Commission Decision 2010/227/EU on the European Databank on Medical Devices (Eudamed) of 19 April 2010

- Guidelines on Medical Devices, IVD Medical Device Borderline and Classification Issues–A Guide for Manufacturers and Notified Bodies (MEDDEV.2.1471 Rev. 2, January 2012)

- European Commission, Guide to the Implementation of Directives based on the New Approach and the Global Approach–European Communities (2000)

- Directive 2001/20/EC of the European Parliament and the Council of 4 April 2001 on the approximation of the laws, regulations and administration provisions of the Member States relating to the implementation of good clinical practice in the conduct of clinical trials on medicinal products for human use

- Commission Directive 2005/28/EC of 8 April 2005 laying down principles and detailed guidelines for good clinical practice as regards investigational medicinal products for human use, as well as the requirements for authorisation of the manufacturing or importation of such products (*GCP Directive*)

Introduction

"Enforcement" can be defined as the action taken by a regulatory authority to protect the public from products of suspect quality, safety and efficacy, or to ensure that products are manufactured in compliance with appropriate laws, regulations and standards, as well as manufacturer commitments made as part of the product marketing approval. A "regulatory authority" is a government agency or entity that exercises a legal right to control product use or sale within its jurisdiction. It may take enforcement action to ensure that products marketed within its jurisdiction comply with legal requirements.

The legal basis for enforcement in Europe lies in numerous directives, regulations, decisions and guidelines that emanate from the European Commission. To become enforceable, directives are transposed into national legislation; however, European Commission regulations are directly binding on EU Member States. Decisions directly bind the addressee of the decision only, while guidelines are nonbinding instruments to specify and detail the provisions laid down in European Commission directives and regulations.

Provisions on sanctions, remedies and enforcement are left to national law. Enforcement itself is undertaken by individual regulatory authorities, which have established means of exchanging information on any confirmed problem reports, corrective actions, recalls, rejected import consignments and other product regulatory and enforcement problems.

This chapter covers enforcement basics in two sections. The first section discusses the provisions for pharmaceutical and biologic product enforcement. The second reviews enforcement as it is described in the directives and applied by national Competent Authorities to medical devices and in vitro diagnostics.

The legislative approval process generally is understood by the regulatory community. However, unexpected events occur, and it is important to understand their consequences and the options in such situations. This chapter enables the reader to identify the relevant regulations to find the best strategy to resolve problems.

Pharmaceuticals and Biological Products

Enforcement

Pharmaceutical regulatory compliance is enforced by inspection and backed up by both legislation that grants statutory powers and such criminal sanctions as monetary fines and/or imprisonment for noncompliance. Enforcement areas include manufacture and quality control, preclinical and clinical testing, storage and distribution, promotion and pharmacovigilance. European legislation provides the legal basis of enforcement, which is delegated to the Member States for national implementation.

There are preapproval provisions for a medicinal product's manufacturer, distributor or wholesaler, dealer or marketer. A document specifying the terms and conditions of its issuance governs the approval. That document is the manufacturer's authorisation or license, the wholesale dealer's authorisation or license or the Marketing Authorisation (MA).

Member State regulatory authorities undertake enforcement at a national level for:
- manufacturer, including Good Manufacturing Practice (GMP) compliance and GMP certification
- clinical trials, including Good Clinical Practice (GCP) compliance
- special regulations for advanced therapies medicinal products[1]
- special regulations for biological products
- advertising compliance
- label and leaflet compliance
- pharmacovigilance requirements

In addition to handling enforcement at the national level, Competent Authorities have established several means of exchanging information on confirmed problem reports, corrective actions, recalls, rejected import consignments, and other product regulatory and enforcement problems on a European level to harmonise the enforcement in their day-to-day business.

Manufacture Including GMP Compliance

Using the UK as an example, enforcement of the *Medicines Act* of 1968 and associated medicines legislation is controlled through the Medicines and Healthcare products Regulatory Agency (MHRA) (often in liaison with other organisations such as the Royal Pharmaceutical Society of Great Britain (RPSGB)). One of the ways in which MHRA regulates compliance is by conducting on-site inspections. The GMP Inspectorate (part of MHRA's Inspection, Enforcement and Standards Division) inspects companies that manufacture or wholesale medicinal products and their operations to verify their compliance with the EU GMP and Good Distribution Practice (GDP) guidelines. In particular, the inspections can include:

- the principles of GMP and/or GDP
- compliance with the provisions of the licence/accreditation as granted and/or varied third-country manufacturing sites in support of UK product licences that name them
- manufacturer named in the centralised marketing application or applications at the request of the European Medicines Agency (EMA) or other Member States

In addition, the National Biological Standards Board exercises certain controls over biological substances' purity and potency.

Another enforcement method is batch recall for quality defects. MHRA uses an internationally agreed classification system for recalls based on the expected risk presented to the public by the defective product:

Class 1

Class 1 defects are potentially life-threatening or could pose a serious health risk. Warning about any defects in this class must be made through the rapid alert system. Examples include:
- wrong product (label information and package contents are different)
- correct product but wrong strength, with serious medical consequences
- microbial contamination of a sterile injectable or ophthalmic product
- chemical contamination, with serious medical consequences
- product mix-up (rogues) involving more than one container
- wrong active ingredient in a multi-component product, with serious medical consequences

Class 2

Class 2 defects could cause mistreatment or harm to the patient, but are not life-threatening or serious. Warnings about these defects should be made through the rapid alert system, but only to Member States and MHRA partners to which the batch has likely been distributed (including parallel import/distribution).

Examples include
- mislabelling (e.g., wrong or missing text or figures)
- missing or incorrect information (leaflets or inserts)
- chemical/physical contamination (significant impurities, cross-contamination, particulates)
- mix-up of products in containers (rogues)
- specification noncompliance (e.g., assay, stability, fill/weight)
- insecure closure with serious medical consequences (e.g., cytotoxics, child-resistant containers, potent products)

Class 3
Class 3 defects are unlikely to cause harm to the patient, and the recall is carried out for other reasons, such as:
- noncompliance with the MA or specification
- faulty packaging (e.g., wrong or missing batch number or expiry date)
- faulty closure/contamination(e.g., microbial spoilage, dirt or detritus, particulate matter)

MHRA also issues "Caution In Use" notices, called Class 4 alerts, where there is no patient threat or serious defect likely to impair product use or efficacy. These generally are used for minor defects in packaging or other printed material.

MHRA's Defective Medicines Report Centre (DMRC) plays an important role in enforcing medicines' quality. DMRC receives and assesses reports of suspected defective medicines and coordinates necessary assessment action. Manufacturers and importers must report to MHRA any medicinal product quality defect that could result in a recall or restricted supply. Other medicinal product users and distributors also are encouraged to do this. DMRC is accessible 24 hours a day, every day of the year.

Another way in which MHRA regulates compliance is by medicine testing. This is undertaken by the MHRA's Medicines Testing Unit (or is contracted out to the Royal Pharmaceutical Society's Medicines Testing Laboratory in Edinburgh). MHRA has a continuous program of sampling and analysing medicinal products marketed in the UK that aims to confirm the quality of these products. Each year 2,000–2,500 samples are analysed. UK pharmacopoeial activity is also carried out within the Inspection and Standards Division of MHRA by the Pharmacopoeial Secretariat Group and the British Pharmacopoeia Laboratory Unit.

Liaison with the European Commission and Member States is undertaken by informing EMA of any enforcement action taken within the UK and providing observations on any European Commission notifications about enforcement action taken in other Member States.

Clinical Trials Including GCP Compliance
For clinical trials in the European Union, it is necessary to submit applications to conduct clinical trials to the Competent Authorities for approval. This procedure must be completed separately in each Member State in which the clinical trial is to take place. Together with available guidelines for virus validation and the guideline strategies to identify and mitigate risks for first-in-human clinical trials with investigational medicinal, *The Guideline on the Requirements for Quality Documentation Concerning Biological investigational Medicinal Products in Clinical Trials* aims to ensure that harmonised requirements for the documentation is submitted throughout the European Community. GCP compliance inspection is another important regulatory authority role. In the UK, MHRA's Inspection, Enforcement and Standards Division has established a GCP Inspectorate. This unit assesses the compliance of organisations with UK and EU legislation, e.g., the *Clinical Trial Directive,* relating to the conduct of clinical trials in investigational medicinal products. The regulatory authority also conducts GMP compliance inspections of units preparing packaging products to be used in clinical trials.

Special Enforcement of Biologics
Special medicines inspectors are responsible for inspecting biological and biotechnological manufacturing sites. In addition, certain biological substance purity and potency controls should be in place.

Advertising Compliance
Council Directive 2001/83/EC, Articles 56–100, as amended, lays down the roles for medicines advertising in Europe. Article 99 gives penalty application and enforcement powers directly to the individual Member States: "Member States shall take the appropriate measures to ensure that the provisions of this title are applied and shall determine in particular what penalties shall be imposed should the provisions adopted in the execution of the Title be infringed."

Pharmacovigilance Requirements
Historically, the EU legal framework of pharmacovigilance for medicinal products has been provided by Council Regulation (EEC) No 726/2004[2] with respect to centrally authorised medicinal products and Directive 2001/83/EC with respect to nationally authorised medicinal products (including those authorised through the Mutual Recognition and Decentralised Procedures).

In addition, detailed guidelines, definitions, standards and information regarding the precise execution of pharmacovigilance-related procedures are found in a number of guidance documents, principally, *The Rules Governing Medicinal Products in the European Union, Volume 9A, Guidelines on Pharmacovigilance for Medicinal Products for Human Use*[3] and in the International Conference on Harmonisation's pharmacovigilance-related guidelines (E2 Series).

The basic legal texts are supplemented by Commission Regulation (EEC) No 540/95, which regulates the procedures concerning "suspected unexpected non-serious adverse reactions."

New legislation introduced in 2010 will take effect in July 2012 and will strengthen and rationalise the system for monitoring medicinal product safety. Regulation (EU) No 1235/2010 of the European Parliament and of the Council of 15 December 2010 amending, as regards pharmacovigilance of medicinal products for human use, Regulation (EC) No 726/2004, and Directive 2010/84/EU of the European

Parliament and of the Council of 15 December amending, as regards pharmacovigilance, Directive 2001/83/EC, will improve safety and public health through better prevention, detection and assessment of adverse reactions to medicines. They will allow patients to report adverse drug reactions directly to Competent Authorities. Additionally, reporting of adverse reactions will be broadened to cover, for example, medication errors and overdose.

For more information on the new *Pharmacovigilance Regulation* and *Pharmacovigilance Directive*, see Chapter 25.

Offenses Enforced By Criminal Sanctions

Many requirements subject to enforcement action are supported by criminal sanctions. Breaches of compliance deemed offenses include:
- marketing a product in a way that is not in accordance with the MA
- manufacturing, distributing or marketing a product without a valid MA
- holding an MA but failing to adapt to technical and scientific advances or other required changes
- failure to have a Qualified Person (QP) responsible for pharmacovigilance
- failure to report a suspected adverse event as required
- marketing a product with noncompliant labelling or a noncompliant package leaflet

Penalties for the above offenses range from a fine to imprisonment, depending on severity and the EU Member State's sanction system (e.g., in Germany, imprisonment for up to three years).

Moreover, Regulation (EEC) No 726/2004, Article 84(39) empowers the European Commission, at EMA's request, to impose financial penalties on Marketing Authorisation Holders. Commission Regulation (EC) No 219/2009 of 11 March 2009 implements the procedure to adopt maximum financial penalty amounts, collection conditions and methods.

Medical Devices and In Vitro Diagnostics Devices

Enforcement

The basis for selling medical devices and in vitro diagnostic devices (IVDs) in the EU is the CE Mark. Directive 2007/47/EC,[4,5] which amends Directive 90/385/EC on active implantable medical devices, and Directive 93/42/EEC on medical devices, which address the following:
- changes in Essential Requirements that medical devices must satisfy in order to be lawfully placed on the market
- corresponding assessment procedures
- device classification

Directive 2007/47/EC entered into force on 11 October 2007. According to the second subparagraph of Article 4(1) of the directive, the Member States "shall apply [transposition measures] from 21 March 2010.

The *Active Implantable Medical Devices Directive* (*AIMDD*), *Medical Devices Directive* (*MDD*) and *In Vitro Diagnostics Directive* (*IVDD*) and general guideline documents provide enforcement legislation for Member States.[6]

European Database

Each medical device directive lays out the framework for European enforcement. The *IVDD* (Directive 98/79/EC) amended previous directives to require the development of a European database accessible to Competent Authorities to enable them to perform their duties, including enforcement. In light of this requirement, the database was established on 10 April 2010 via Commission Decision 2010/227/EU on the European Databank on Medical Devices (Eudamed). Eudamed's aim is to strengthen medical device market surveillance and transparency by providing Member State Competent Authorities with fast access to information on manufacturers and Authorised Representatives, on devices, certificates, vigilance and clinical investigation data. Eudamed also is intended to contribute to a uniform application of the *AIMDD*, *MDD* and *IVDD*, particularly in relation to registration requirements.

Depending on the applicable directive, Eudamed contains data on:
- manufacturer, Authorised Representative and device registration
- certificates issued, modified, supplemented, suspended, withdrawn or refused
- the Vigilance Procedure
- clinical investigations

This system:
- establishes connectivity between the Competent Authorities and Eudamed, hosted by the European Commission (Directorate General Enterprise & Industry)
- loads, extracts and modifies data
- compiles reports and queries on Eudamed
- uses already existing components
- is modular, so its component can be re-used for similar purposes linked to directives covered in other domains

Eudamed is a secure web-based portal acting as a central repository for information exchange between national Competent Authorities and the European Commission and is not publicly accessible. Eudamed use has been obligatory since May 2011.

The Enforcement Framework of the Directives

In this section, the enforcement framework of the directives is demonstrated using the *IVDD* as an example. The *MDD* and *AIMDD* contain comparable provisions.[7]

The *IVDD* amends previous medical device directives and outlines a new enforcement framework.[8]

The following articles regulate enforcement:[9]
- Article 8: Safeguard Clause
- Article 11: Vigilance Procedure
- Article 13: Particular health monitoring measures
- Article 15: Notified Bodies
- Article 17: Wrongly affixed CE marking
- Article 18: Decisions in respect of refusal or restriction[10]

Article 8: Safeguard Clause

The strongest article regarding Competent Authorities' market surveillance responsibilities is Article 8, the so-called Safeguard Clause. The article provides Competent Authorities the means to act quickly on any events and information related to devices that may compromise the health and/or safety of patients, users or, where applicable, other persons or property, even though the directive's requirements have been met. It requires Competent Authorities to take appropriate interim measures to withdraw such devices from the market, or prohibit or restrict their placement on the market or entry into service.

The clause allows Member States to restrict products from their markets quickly. The wording regarding Competent Authorities' obligations to prove that the product is not compliant is vague. This article could lead to a situation where products introduced on the EU market correctly would be restricted in certain Member States.

This clause applies when a product fails to meet the Essential Requirements due to shortcomings in harmonised standards. Therefore, a product in full compliance with the regulations (application of harmonised standards) for which safety concerns exist could be restricted or removed from the market.

In such a case, the European Commission enters into consultation with the concerned parties. Possible outcomes are:
- The European Commission agrees with the measures taken and informs all relevant parties. If the concerns are related to shortcomings of standards, a procedure to update such documents may be initiated.
- The European Commission disagrees and takes immediate action to inform the Concerned Member State and manufacturer.

If the Safeguard Clause is applied to a product, the market damage is done once the Competent Authority restricts the sale. Manufacturers should be aware of this clause when dealing with regulators. Overall, this clause is very powerful and is applied by Member States primarily to high-risk products.

Article 11: Vigilance Procedure

Postmarket surveillance, as executed by the manufacturer, is not to be confused with the Competent Authorities' market surveillance activities. The manufacturer's obligation is to implement systemic procedures to monitor and review device experience once the product is CE marked and placed on the market.

Article 11 stipulates Competent Authorities' requiring Member States to centrally record and evaluate information brought to their attention (by manufacturer or other sources) concerning incidents defined in the directive. Some Member States require medical practitioners and medical institutions—and even members of the public—to report directly to them. In other countries, such reporting is not mandatory but is promoted. If the authority becomes aware of incidents, it shall inform the manufacturer or its Authorised Representative. The Vigilance Procedure is being used more and more by distributors and manufacturers who find issues with competitors' products, notify the authorities and consequently advance their own products. Competent Authorities are aware of this practice and will follow up on reports. Reporting incidents is mandatory, and failure to do so is punishable by fines or criminal sanctions in some countries.

Competent Authorities are obligated to evaluate incidents; however, the directive stipulates that, if possible, the evaluation should be carried out in conjunction with the manufacturer. Most Competent Authorities liaise closely with manufacturers.

Competent Authority nonconformity or incident evaluations may result in mandated corrective actions by the manufacturer. In such an instance, the European Commission and relevant Member States shall be informed. The notification procedure is not described in the directives; however, if a Global Harmonization Task Force (GHTF) proposal is applied, other GHTF members—such as the US Food and Drug Administration, Health Canada, etc.—will be informed.

Article 13: Particular health monitoring measures

This article empowers Member States to implement product or product group sanctions as they see fit to ensure health and safety protection and/or ensure that public health requirements are observed. Information shall be distributed to the European Commission and other Member States.

Article 15: Notified Bodies

Article 15, Sections 5 and 6 regulate the Notified Bodies'(NBs) actions in the case of noncompliance. Even though an NB has no enforcement power, it is part of the system and, upon request, is obligated to notify the Competent Authority of withdrawn, suspended, issued or refused certificates.

Noncompliance can be encountered at different stages, resulting in the following situations:
- Before a certificate is issued, where the NB finds the manufacturer's Conformity Assessment Procedure (CAP) not to be compliant with the directive, the manufacturer can implement corrective actions. The products are not approved and, therefore, not available on the EU market. It should be noted that enforcement is not applicable prior to entering the market. As long as no certificate is issued and the manufacturer makes corrections, there is no requirement to notify an authority. However, the manufacturer must complete the CAP with the NB because a signed statement that no other NB is employed for the particular product is part of the NB application. In case of disputes regarding the regulation, the Competent Authority may be consulted. However, if the NB refuses to award a certificate it shall, upon request, inform other NBs and Competent Authorities. The clause is in place to prevent manufacturers from shopping among NBs.
- When a certificate is already in place, the NB cites compliance following its assessment. If deviations are considered critical, the NB determines whether additional review activities (e.g., an audit) are necessary. None of these necessarily triggers Competent Authority notification, provided the manufacturer satisfactorily implements corrective actions. However, if the manufacturer fails to achieve compliance by implementing appropriate corrective measures, resulting in a withdrawn or suspended certificate, the NB is obligated to follow Article 15 and must inform its Competent Authority.

NBs understand their role as assessment procedure partners, but should not be confused with consultants. This relationship is difficult to manage, but as long as the NB and manufacturer each clearly understand one another's responsibilities, the need to inform the Competent Authority should be avoided easily. For example:
- Sterility validation data are out of compliance and the products have been distributed. The NB identifies a quality system breakdown where no internal corrective actions have been initiated, resulting in a critical situation. The deviation is noted and the NB reviews any corrective actions to be implemented. Part of the corrective action might obligate the manufacturer to inform Competent Authorities about this matter (e.g., in case of near accidents or a recall). The NB has no reason to inform the authorities.

The situation would be different if the manufacturer's corrective actions were unacceptable to the NB or were not implemented properly. If the manufacturer does not take further corrective action to resolve the situation, the NB must withdraw, suspend or restrict the certificate. This is particularly important when the health and safety of patients, users and others are in danger. Then, the Competent Authority is responsible for imposing any necessary sanctions on the manufacturer.

Article 17: Wrongly affixed CE Mark
Article 17, Section 1(a) states that the manufacturer must correct the infringement of wrongly affixed CE Marks under conditions imposed by the Member State. What the Member State might impose is not clear; the situation varies from country to country and certainly depends on the arrangement. In addition to product restrictions, local penalties exist to enforce any conditions imposed. Those may include fines or even imprisonment. Should a manufacturer not end the infringement, Section 1(b), which references Article 8, will take effect.

Article 17, Section 2 pertains when the CE Mark is placed on products to which the directive is not applicable. For example, some authorities consider tooth whiteners to be cosmetic products and have restricted their marketing because the *Cosmetic Directive* prohibits a high concentration of a certain ingredient. Other authorities consider tooth whiteners to be medicinal substances and apply national regulations. Some NBs certified tooth whiteners under the *Medical Devices Directive* because there was a clear statement regarding the intended use, based on a medical indication. The product was considered a medical device in Class 2a. There are no provisions in place to restrict the product if the wrong directive is applied.

Article 18: Decisions in respect of refusal or restrictions
Under this article, a Competent Authority that refuses to permit or restricts a product being placed on the market or forces its withdrawal must inform the manufacturer or its Authorised Representative of available remedies in that Member State. The manufacturer should be allowed to present its position before action is taken but, if there is any urgency, the authority may act without consultation.

This article protects the manufacturer against unjustified actions, giving the manufacturer the opportunity to oppose any restriction imposed on its product. The manufacturer should always ask what possible options are available. This clause is not used very often, and authorities work closely with manufacturers to resolve any critical issues.

Summary
The legal basis for enforcement is covered in the scope of numerous directives, regulations, guidelines and decisions that emanate from the European Commission. To become enforceable, the directives are enacted via national regulation. European Commission regulations are directly binding on EU Member States.

Member State Competent Authorities enforce the regulation of biologics and medicinal products through national legislation and guidelines on preparing clinical trial applications, MAAs and distributor/wholesaler or marketer agreements, pharmacovigilance reporting and compliance. Compliance is enforced by inspections and backed up by both legislation that grants statutory powers and such criminal sanctions as monetary fines and/or imprisonment for noncompliance.

Enforcement areas include manufacture and quality control, preclinical and clinical testing, storage, distribution and procurement. European legislation provides the legal basis of enforcement, which is delegated to the Member States for national application. Member States' regulatory authorities undertake compliance enforcement at a national level for GMP, GLP and GCP issues; and through special regulations for advanced therapy medicinal products and biologics, advertising/promotion and labelling requirements.

The medical device articles reviewed in this chapter are the main source of enforcement activities. They describe potential Competent Authority actions and obligations to inform other parties; however they do not specify specific actions to be taken. Enforcement decisions and consequences involved are left up to individual Member States.

The directives merely state that the individual Member States shall be granted sufficient power to enforce the regulation. Sanction details are specified in individual Member States' transposition of the directives.

This approach has changed the medical device regulatory environment. Some EU countries had little or no regulation prior to implementing these new requirements, while others had to change their established regulatory processes significantly. Both the regulatory bodies and the manufacturers had to find and define their roles under the new rules. As more products are covered, there will be increasing market surveillance by Competent Authorities and more extensive application of described articles.

Nonetheless, with the mandate to use the Eudamed database and the associated access to crucial data for medical devices, the EU created an instrument to facilitate the surveillance process in every Member State.

References

1. Amended by Directive 2002/98/EC, 2003/63/EC, 2004/24/EC, 2004/27/EC, Regulation (EC) No 1901/2006, Regulation (EC) No 1394/2007 on advanced therapy medicinal products, by Directive 2008/29/EC on implementing powers conferred on the Commission, by Directive 2009/53/EC, and by Directive 2009/120/EC.
2. Commission Regulation (EC) No 540/95 of 10 March 1995 laying down the arrangement for reporting serious suspected unexpected adverse reactions which are not serious, to medicinal products for human or veterinary use authorised in accordance with the provisions of Council Regulation (EEC) 2309/93(now Regulation No (EC 726/2004), whether arising in the Community or in a third country. EUR-Lex website. http://eur-lex.europa.eu/LexUriServ/LexUriServ.do?uri=CELEX:31995R0540:en:HTML. Accessed 2 May 2012.
3. European Commission, Guide *Eudralex: The Rules Governing Medicinal Products in the European Union, Volume 9A, Guidelines for Pharmacovigilance for Medicinal Products for Human Use* (September 2008). EC website. http://ec.europa.eu/health/files/eudralex/vol-9/pdf/vol9a_09-2008_en.pdf. Accessed 2 May 2012.
4. Council Directive 90/385/EEC of 20 June 1990 on the approximation of the laws of the Member States relating to active implantable medical devices, as amended by Directive 93/68/EEC and Directive 2007/47/EC. EUR-Lex website. http://eur-lex.europa.eu/LexUriServ/LexUriServ.do?uri=CELEX:31990L0385:en:HTML. Accessed 2 May 2012.
5. Council Directive 93/42/EEC of 14 June 1993 concerning medical devices, as amended by Directive 2000/70/EC, Directive 2001/104/EC and Directive 2007/47/EC. EUR-Lex website. http://eur-lex.europa.eu/LexUriServ/LexUriServ.do?uri=CONSLEG:1993L0042:20071011:en:PDF. Accessed 2 May 2012.
6. European Commission, Medical Devices Regulatory Framework. EC website. http://ec.europa.eu/health/medical-devices/regulatory-framework/index_en.htm. Accessed 1 May 2012.
7. European Commission, *Guide to the implementation of directives based on the New Approach and the Global Approach* (2000). EC website. http://ec.europa.eu/enterprise/policies/single-market-goods/files/blue-guide/guidepublic_en.pdf. Accessed 2 May 2012.
8. Directive 98/79/EC of the European Parliament and of the Council of 27 October 1998 on in vitro diagnostic medical devices. EUR-Lex website. http://eur-lex.europa.eu/LexUriServ/LexUriServ.do?uri=CONSLEG:1998L0079:20031120:en:PDF. Accessed 2 May 2012.
9. Council Directive 90/385/EEC of 20 June 1990 on the approximation of the laws of the Member States relating to active implantable medical devices, as amended by Directive 2007/47/EC. EUR-Lex website. http://eur-lex.europa.eu/LexUriServ/LexUriServ.do?uri=CELEX:31990L0385:en:HTML. Accessed 2 May 2012.
10. Op cit 5.

Chapter 8

The European Medical Devices Legal System

Updated by Erik Vollebregt

OBJECTIVES

- Gain insight into the European legislative process
- Understand the basic legal requirements for medical devices
- Become aware of the available guidance concerning the requirements for medical devices

LAWS, REGULATIONS AND GUIDANCE COVERED IN THIS CHAPTER

- Consolidated version of the Treaty on European Union and the Treaty on the Functioning of the European Union
- Decision No 768/2008/EC of the European Parliament and of the Council of 9 July 2008 on a common framework for the marketing of products, and repealing Council Decision 93/465/EEC
- Regulation (EC) No 765/2008 of the European Parliament and of the Council of 9 July 2008 setting out the requirements for accreditation and market surveillance relating to the marketing of products and repealing Regulation (EEC) No 339/93
- Council Directive 90/385/EEC of 20 June 1990 on the approximation of the laws of the Member States relating to active implantable medical devices
- Council Directive 93/42/EEC of 14 June 1993 concerning medical devices
- Directive 98/79/EC of the European Parliament and of the Council of 27 October 1998 on *in vitro* diagnostic medical devices
- Commission Decision 2010/227/EU of 19 April 2010 on the European Databank on Medical Devices (Eudamed)
- Commission Decision 2002/364/EC of 7 May 2002 on common technical specifications for in vitro diagnostic medical devices
- Commission Decision 2009/886/EC of 27 November 2009 amending Decision 2002/364/EC on common technical specifications for in vitro diagnostic medical devices
- Commission Directive 2005/50/EC of 11 August 2005 on the reclassification of hip, knee and shoulder joint replacements in the framework of Council Directive 93/42/EEC concerning medical devices
- Commission Directive 2003/12/EC of 3 February 2003 on the reclassification of breast implants in the framework of Directive 93/42/EEC concerning medical devices

- Guidance from the Commission in the form of MEDDEV documents, consensus statements and interpretative documents

- Guidance from the Notified Body Operations Group (NBOG)

Introduction

The European legal system has changed over the years through successive treaties. The last of these, the *Treaty of Lisbon*, came into force on 1 December 2009. The basic principles of European law can be found in a consolidated version of the *Treaty on European Union* and the *Treaty on the Functioning of the European Union*,[1] hereafter the "*Treaty*," as amended by the *Treaty of Lisbon*.

Although the EU has many institutions similar to those of a sovereign state, its legal nature is nevertheless very different. Its members retain much more sovereignty than would be the case in a federation such as the US. These differences can be best understood in the context of the European legislative process and the interplay between European and national law.

Legislative Process

Article 288 of the *Treaty* defines the legal acts used in the EU. Regulations, directives and decisions are legally binding, whereas recommendations and opinions are not.

A "regulation" is directly applicable in all Member States.

A "directive" must be transposed into national law and administrative provisions. The Member State is free to decide on the nature and contents of the texts adopted nationally, but it must achieve the results intended by the directive. Failure to do so may result in an infringement procedure against the Member State, which may lead to a judgment against it in the Court of Justice of the European Union (CJEU).

A "decision" applies to those to whom it is addressed.

Normally, regulations, directives and decisions are jointly adopted by the European Parliament and the Council based upon a proposal from the European Commission in the "co-decision procedure." This legislative procedure is defined in Article 294 of the *Treaty*. These joint acts can be used to delegate to the Commission the power to adopt legally binding acts in specific cases.

The ordinary legislative procedure is illustrated in **Figure 8-1**.

The basis upon which the Council will make its decisions is subject to a transitional period that ends in March 2017.[2]

Until 31 October 2014, for acts of the European Council and of the Council requiring a qualified majority, members' votes shall be weighted as shown in **Table 8-1**.

From 1 November 2014, the qualified majority is defined as at least 55% of the members of the Council, comprising at least 15 of them and representing Member States comprising at least 65% of the population of the EU. A blocking minority must include at least four Council members, failing which the qualified majority shall be deemed attained.

Between 1 November 2014 and 31 March 2017, when an act is to be adopted by qualified majority, a member of the Council may request that it be adopted in accordance with the qualified majority as defined before 1 November 2014.

The "New Approach" Regulatory Philosophy

Medical devices directives are based on the "New Approach" regulatory philosophy. In the early days of the European Communities, product-related directives contained much technical detail. The first directive on medicinal products[3] in 1965 is a good example of such an approach and one that is still used for medicinal product legislation.[4] Similar style regulations later were instituted for food and cosmetics.

When 1993 was selected as the date for creating a single market, a key challenge was drafting the product-oriented directives needed to eliminate technical barriers to trade that would hinder the free movement of goods in that single market. Indeed, if products were required to conform to different technical standards and regulations in each EU Member State, selling products in Europe would be a very expensive and complicated proposition. To speed up this process of creating a single market—and backed by a line of case law from the European Court of Justice that obligated Member States to mutually recognise products that comply with technical requirements in their Member State of origin—it was decided to abandon the approach

Table 8-1. European Council Weighted Votes

France	29	Italy	29
Poland	27	Romania	14
Belgium	12	Greece	12
Portugal	12	Bulgaria	10
Denmark	7	Ireland	7
Slovakia	7	Estonia	4
Luxembourg	4	Malta	3
Germany	29	United Kingdom	29
Spain	27	Netherlands	13
Czech Republic	12	Hungary	12
Austria	10	Sweden	10
Finland	7	Lithuania	7
Cyprus	4	Latvia	4
Slovenia	4		

The European Medical Devices Legal System

Figure 8-1. EU Legislative Procedure

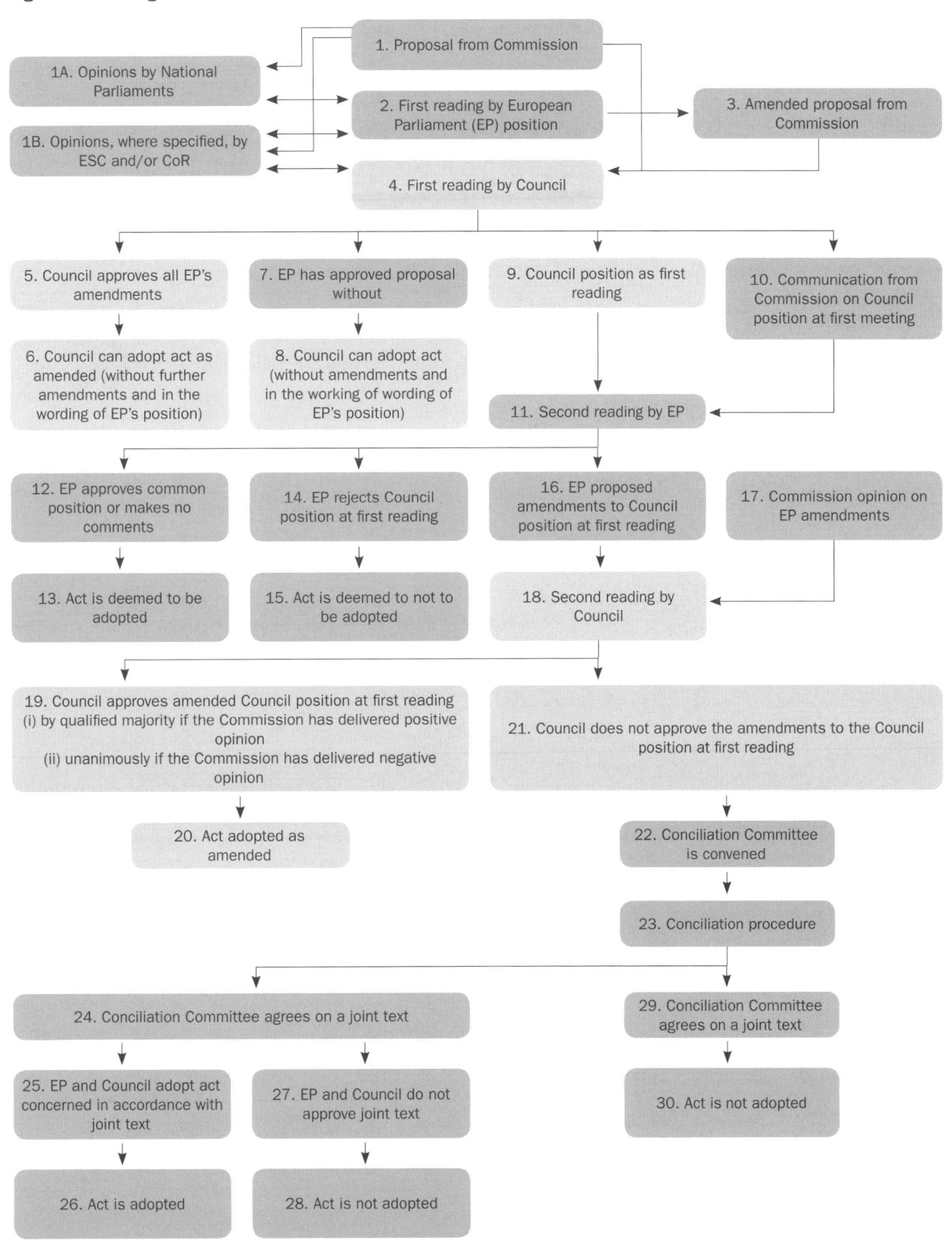

1. Proposal from Commission
   - 1A. Opinions by National Parliaments
   - 1B. Opinions, where specified, by ESC and/or CoR
2. First reading by European Parliament (EP) position
3. Amended proposal from Commission
4. First reading by Council
5. Council approves all EP's amendments
6. Council can adopt act as amended (without further amendments and in the wording of EP's position)
7. EP has approved proposal without
8. Council can adopt act (without amendments and in the working of wording of EP's position)
9. Council position as first reading
10. Communication from Commission on Council position at first meeting
11. Second reading by EP
12. EP approves common position or makes no comments
13. Act is deemed to be adopted
14. EP rejects Council position at first reading
15. Act is deemed to not to be adopted
16. EP proposed amendments to Council position at first reading
17. Commission opinion on EP amendments
18. Second reading by Council
19. Council approves amended Council position at first reading
    (i) by qualified majority if the Commission has delivered positive opinion
    (ii) unanimously if the Commission has delivered negative opinion
20. Act adopted as amended
21. Council does not approve the amendments to the Council position at first reading
22. Conciliation Committee is convened
23. Conciliation procedure
24. Conciliation Committee agrees on a joint text
25. EP and Council adopt act concerned in accordance with joint text
26. Act is adopted
27. EP and Council do not approve joint text
28. Act is not adopted
29. Conciliation Committee agrees on a joint text
30. Act is not adopted

Regulatory Affairs Professionals Society

Chapter 8

Figure 8-2. Flow Chart for the Conformity Assessment Procedures Provided for in Directive 93/42/EEC on Medical Devices

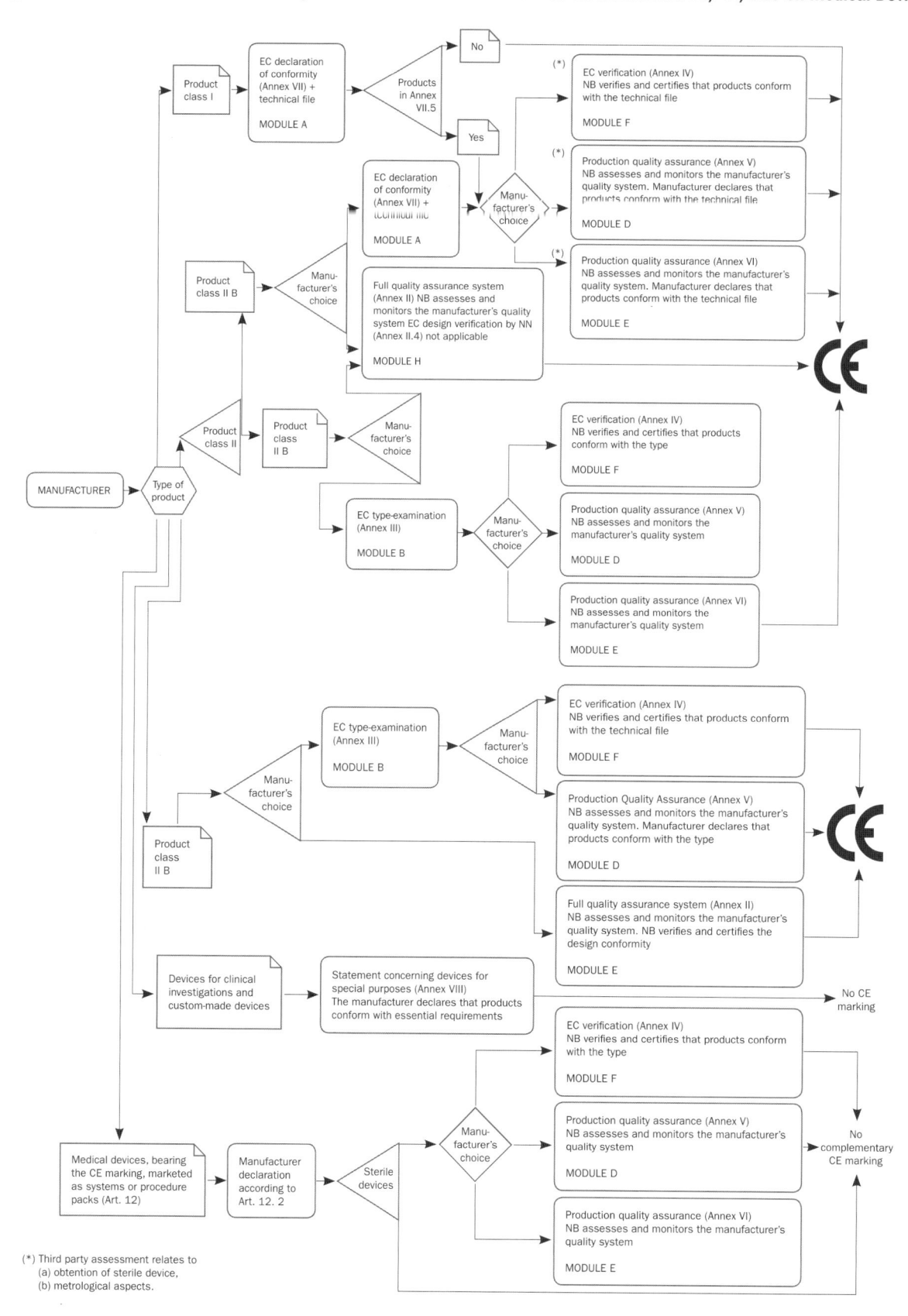

(*) Third party assessment relates to
(a) obtention of sterile device,
(b) metrological aspects.

of detailed technical legislation and use the so-called New Approach to legislation.

Table 8-2 illustrates the areas where the New Approach is used.[5]

All the key medical devices directives can be found in this list, as well as some that may be jointly applicable (e.g., machinery in case of medical devices that also fall within the scope of the *Machinery Directive*). The European Commission has issued guidance on how to deal with devices that fall within the scope of two New Approach directives with respect to overlap with the *Personal Protection Equipment Directive*[6] and the *Machinery Directive*.[7]

The European Commission has issued a guidance document that explains the New Approach concepts in greater detail: the *Guide to the implementation of directives based on the New Approach and the Global Approach* (2000), the "Blue Guide." The Blue Guide explains the New Approach to technical harmonisation and standardisation in great detail. The New Approach established the following principles for legislative harmonisation:

- Legislative harmonisation is limited to Essential Requirements that products placed on the Community market must meet, if they are to benefit from free movement within the Community.
- The technical specifications of products meeting the Essential Requirements set out in the directives are laid down in harmonised standards.
- Application of harmonised or other standards remains voluntary, and the manufacturer may always apply other technical specifications to meet the requirements.
- Products manufactured in compliance with harmonised standards benefit from a presumption of conformity with the corresponding essential requirements.

Key Principles of the "New Approach" Applied to Medical Devices

The New Approach principles discussed above are applied in the medical devices directives as follows.

Compliance With Essential Requirements

- The manufacturer must demonstrate that its products comply with the Essential Requirements. The key objective is to prove that the benefits to the patient outweigh the risks.
- The Essential Requirements are very general in content, but detailed technical explanations are found in voluntary harmonised standards.
- Demonstrated compliance with a harmonised standard creates a presumption of compliance with the corresponding Essential Requirements.

Verification of Compliance

- The manufacturer carries out conformity assessment following its choice of the procedures provided in the medical devices directive that applies to its device (technical file, quality systems).
- Depending upon their risk classification, some products and/or quality systems are certified by a Notified Body (NB).

Compliance is certified by affixing the CE Mark and by a declaration of conformity once the manufacturer is convinced it has achieved compliance with a technical file that adequately demonstrates compliance with the Essential Requirements and a quality system appropriate for the device's risk profile. Schematic overviews of the procedures for arriving at a declaration of conformity for a medical device ("conformity assessment") are provided in Annex 8 of the Blue Guide and are useful tools for determining the requirements in a specific case. Conformity assessment is addressed in detail in Chapter 12.

No Member State can oppose the placing on its market of a CE-marked product unless it has reason to believe that the device is unsafe (principle of safeguard), is a threat to health and safety (precautionary principle) or the CE marking is wrongly affixed (failure to comply with the legal requirements).

It is important to understand that achieving CE marking is, in many cases, just the beginning of compliance, not an end point. The medical devices directives impose a cyclical process of "clinical evaluation" on the manufacturer (**Figure 8-5**), aimed at continuous improvement and clinical substantiation of the device in its technical file. This was recently clarified further in the MEDDEV 2.12/2 rev. 2 guideline, *Post Market Clinical Follow-up Studies*, which sets out EU guidance on postmarketing clinical follow-up studies and how the manufacturer and NB should work together toward the common goal of improving a device's clinical substantiation.[8]

Annex X, point 1.1 of Council Directive 93/42/EEC, the *Medical Devices Directive* (*MDD*), and Annex VII, point 1.1 of Council Directive 90/385/EEC, the *Active Implantable Medical Devices Directive* (*AIMDD*), describe the process of clinical evaluation. As a general rule, clinical evaluation requires collection of clinical data to establish the device's conformity with the Essential Requirements in Annex I concerning its characteristics and performance under normal conditions of use, the evaluation of side-effects and the acceptability of the benefit:risk ratio. Clinical evaluation involves, where appropriate, taking into account any relevant harmonised standards under the *MDD*, a defined and methodologically sound procedure based on a critical evaluation of:

either
- the relevant scientific literature currently available relating to the device's safety, performance, design characteristics and intended purpose, where:
  o there is demonstration of the device's equivalence to the device to which the data relate and
  o the data adequately demonstrate compliance with the relevant Essential Requirements.

or
- the results of all clinical investigations conducted
- the combined clinical data

For implantable devices and Class III devices, clinical investigations shall be performed unless reliance on existing clinical data can be justified.

The terms "clinical evaluation" and "clinical investigation" should be clarified. Clinical evaluation is, in essence, the process of evaluating clinical evidence to support safety and performance. Clinical investigation refers to clinical trials, which may be conducted as part of the clinical evaluation to substantiate safety and performance aspects that cannot be corroborated by reference to literature. Clinical evaluation is described in more detail in Chapter 11.

Manufacturers are obligated to monitor and collect information on the experience gained with the device's use and may need to conduct postmarketing clinical follow-up (PMCF) studies[9] as part of their postmarketing surveillance obligations. Adverse events must be reported as part of the vigilance obligations, which form part of the overarching postmarketing surveillance obligations. More importantly, manufacturers must evaluate this usage experience by assessing whether the earlier determination of the benefit:risk relationship is still valid, for example by initiating PMCF studies.[10] If it is not, and no corrective action is taken, the CE marking would be invalid and the device would be on the market illegally.

The fundamentals of the New Approach have been revised by two key 2008 legal texts.[11,12] Their practical implication for the medical device industry is to tighten the accreditation of NBs and create special requirements for certain economic operators (distributors, importers and Authorised Representatives). The implementation of the new principles is likely to take several years before the potential of these texts to change the regulatory landscape is exhausted.

Agencies

European Medicines Agency
The European Medicines Agency (EMA)[13] is responsible for the scientific evaluation of medicines and thus plays a central role in the approval of pharmaceutical products in the EU. It is also responsible for the Committee for Advanced Therapies (CAT) that deals with advanced therapy medicinal products (ATMPs), e.g., tissue engineering products. It may deal with medical devices when these are combined with medicinal products or ATMPs, which must be evaluated by EMA. There is no equivalent institution for medical devices in the EU. However, ongoing discussion about revising the medical devices regulatory framework in the EU has prompted discussion about setting up a separate institution for medical devices or granting EMA competence to regulate them.

Member States and Other Relevant Countries
Member States must transpose the requirements of directives into their national laws and then enforce these requirements. The *MDD* states:

"Member States shall take all necessary steps to ensure that devices may be placed on the market and/or put into service only if they comply with the requirements laid down in this Directive when duly supplied and properly installed, maintained and used in accordance with their intended purpose."[14]

This general responsibility for enforcement also breaks down into specific responsibilities:
- centrally evaluate adverse incidents (adverse events)
- register manufacturers or their Authorised Representatives
- assess clinical trial applications
- act as a Competent Authority for NBs

Member States typically carry out this responsibility through a national Competent Authority. Most often, there is a common authority for medicinal products and devices (e.g., the Medicines and Healthcare products Regulatory Agency (MHRA) in the UK, Agence nationale de sécurité du médicament et des produits de santé (ANSM) in France and the Irish Medicines Board (IMB) in Ireland), although the organisation may be split internally along drug and device lines.

There are significant differences among the Member States due to the availability of resources and historical experience. A small country like Malta or Luxembourg typically will embed the Competent Authority function in an institution that has much wider responsibilities than just medical devices.

Many countries will delegate some Competent Authority responsibilities to a regional level. Often, this is due to a pre-existing federalist approach to administration (e.g., the system of *Länder* in Germany, Autonomous Communities in Spain and cantons in Switzerland). Probably the most complex situation exists in Germany where the 16 *Länder* (states) may further assign responsibilities to the district level. It is estimated that, in reality, the German "Competent

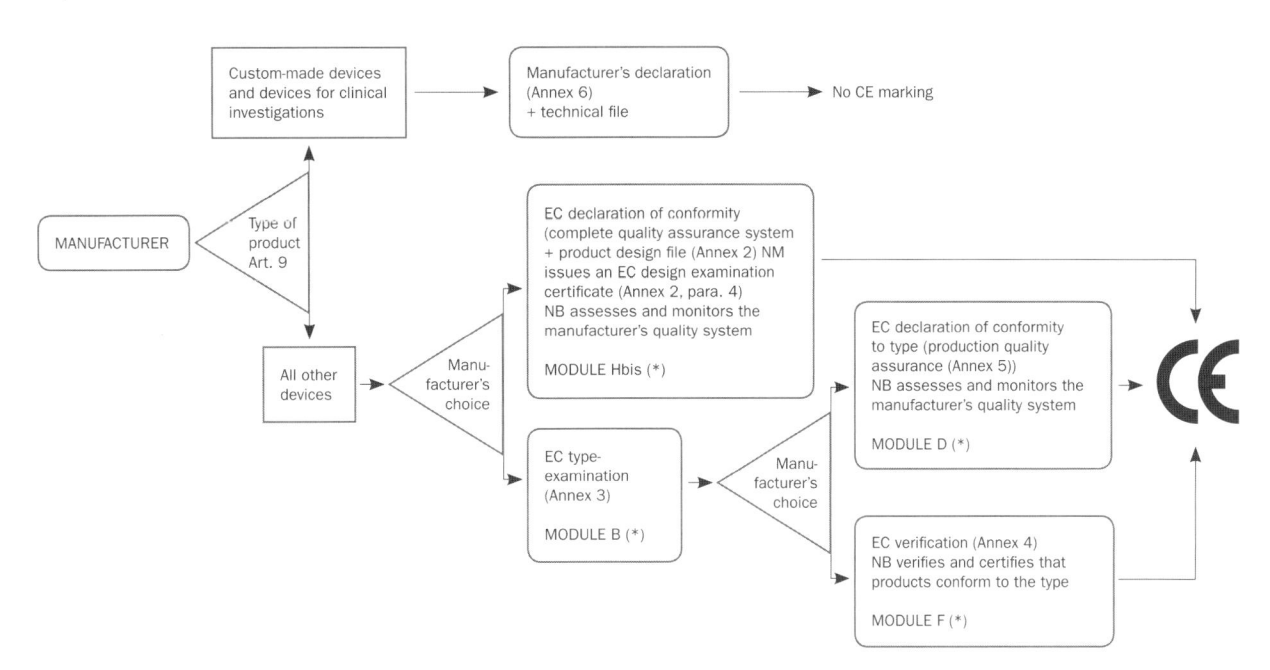

Figure 8-3. Flow Chart for the Conformity Assessment Procedures Provided for in Directive 90/385/EEC on Active Implantable Medical Devices

Authority" consists of some 80 different administrative units.

There are 27 Member States. To this total must be added the three countries of the European Economic Area (Iceland, Liechtenstein and Norway) that apply the medical devices directives. Switzerland and Turkey have specific agreements with the EU that impact medical device regulatory compliance.

A list of these countries and their relevant Competent Authorities as well as their website addresses is provided in **Table 8-3** (the information is given in English and the country's official language(s)).

Several countries are being considered for membership in the EU: Bosnia-Herzegovina, Croatia, FYROM (Former Yugoslav Republic of Macedonia), Kosovo, Serbia and Turkey. Candidate countries often adopt regulations similar to those in the EU.

Notified Bodies (NBs)

NBs are certification organisations. They owe their official name to the fact that they are notified by the Member States to the Commission. They operate on a mandate from the Member State that notifies them to the Commission and must fulfil the requirements of *MDD* Annex XI.

NBs are responsible for assessing manufacturers' compliance with the requirements of European medical device law, attesting to compliance by granting certificates and then monitoring that compliance through periodic audits. The nature of an NB's involvement depends on the product's class. For instance, in the case of a Class III device, an NB will examine the product design and audit the quality system. An NB will not get involved in a Class I device unless it is sterile and/or has a measuring function, and then the NBs scrutiny is limited to those aspects.

Member States' control over the NBs has gradually tightened. This is particularly evident in the New Approach laws issued in 2008[15] that set out specific requirements for NB accreditation.

There are approximately 80 NBs in the EU. Many also have offices outside Europe (e.g., in the US) that carry out audit tasks and sales promotion. Most have prior histories as independent testing houses, and a few are government institutions.

The Commission maintains a list of all NBs that also includes information on their areas of competence (http://ec.europa.eu/enterprise/newapproach/nando/).

The NBs have set up a collective organisation known as NB-MED. The Commission website describes the role of NB-MED:[16]

- to share experience and exchange views on application of conformity assessment procedures with the aim of contributing to a better understanding and consistent application of requirements and procedures
- to draft technical recommendations on matters relating to conformity assessment and build a consensus
- to advise the Commission, at its request, on subjects related to application of the medical devices directives

Figure 8-4. Flow Chart for the Conformity Assessment Procedures Provided for in Directive 98/79/EC on In Vitro Diagnostic Medical Devices

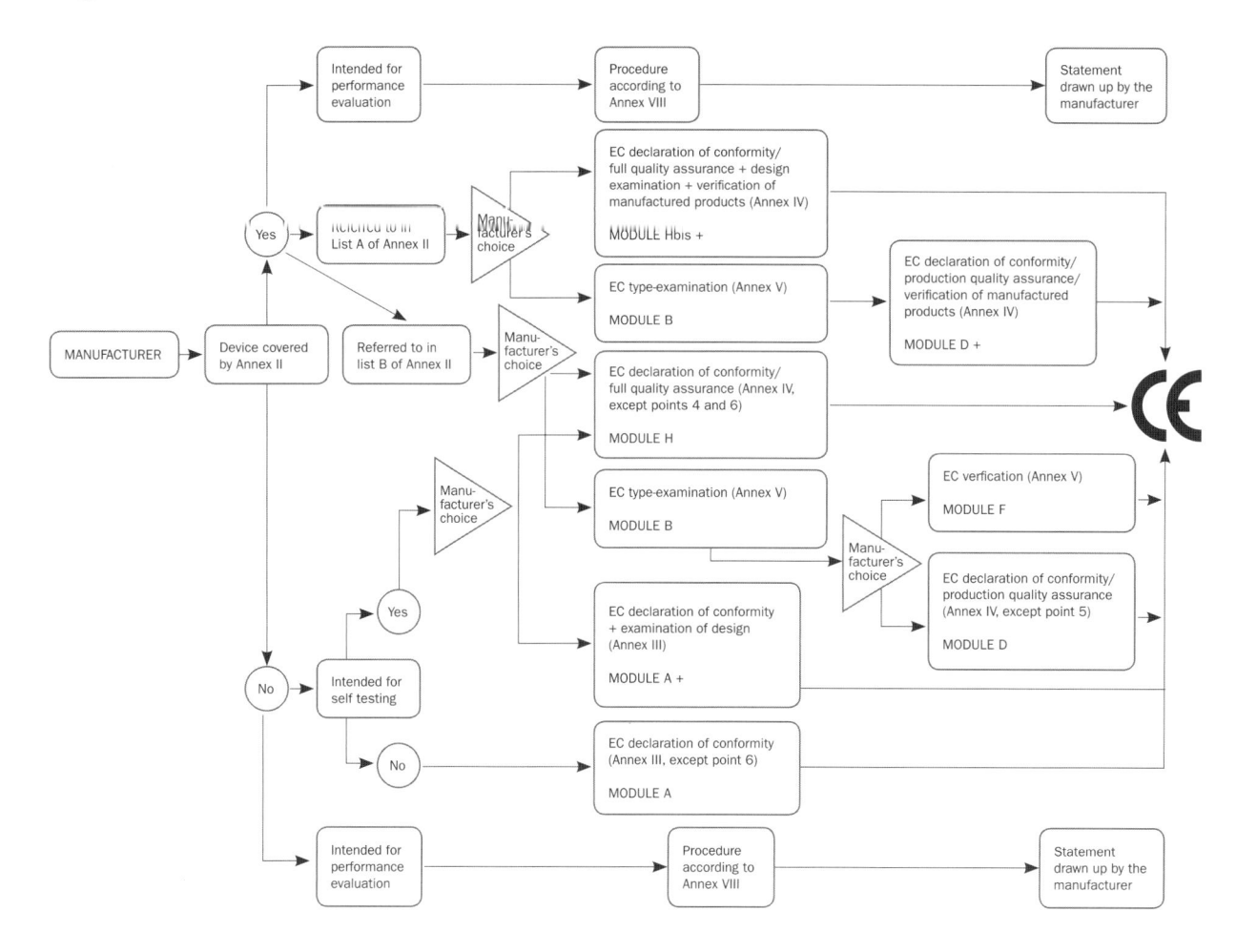

- to consider, and if necessary, draft reports on ethical aspects of NBs' activities
- to ensure consistency with standardisation work at a European level
- to keep informed of harmonisation activities at a European level

A core group of NBs (BSI, DEKRA/KEMA, LNE/G-MED, TÜV Rheinland and TÜV SÜD) has adopted a self-regulatory code for their work under the *MDD* and the *AIMDD*. In addition to a general statement and principles of conduct, the code contains rules on:
- implementation and monitoring of the Code of Conduct
- qualification and assignment of NB assessment personnel
- minimum time for NB assessments
- sampling of Class IIa and IIb technical files
- design dossier reviews
- rules for subcontracting
- rules for certification decisions

The authoring NBs aim to address the current weaknesses in the NB system with this code, particularly by ensuring "a harmonised quality of work amongst the participating Notified Bodies, to gain trust in this work in public perception as well as from political and policy stakeholders, to contribute to ensure the trustworthiness of the system amongst international partners of the European Union and to support the reputation of the participating Notified Bodies."

Standardisation Organisations

There are three main standardisation organisations in Europe:
- The European Committee for Standardization (CEN) develops standards related to general

compliance and specific nonactive (nonpowered) medical devices (www.cen.eu).
- The European Committee for Electrotechnical Standardization (CENELEC) develops standards on electromedical devices (www.cenelec.eu).
- The European Telecommunications Standards Institute (ETSI) develops standards for information and communications technologies (www.etsi.org).

To the extent possible, international standards of the International Organization for Standardization (ISO) and the International Electrotechnical Commission (IEC) are adopted in Europe.

The Commission publishes lists of harmonised standards that provide a presumption of conformity with the requirements of the directives at http://ec.europa.eu/enterprise/policies/european-standards/harmonised-standards/index_en.htm.

Economic Operators

Manufacturers and Authorised Representatives

The medical devices directives provide definitions of manufacturers and Authorised Representatives and set out requirements for both, as discussed in more detail below. They do not mention importers and distributors; these, however, are identified in requirements set out in the New Approach texts.

Importers and Distributors

European medical device law neither provides definitions of importers and distributors nor attributes any role in the compliance system to them. The New Approach texts identify them as economic operators with specific responsibilities, especially in the area of market surveillance, and provide the following definitions:
- "'importer' shall mean any natural or legal person established within the Community who places a product from a third country on the Community market"[17]
- "'distributor' shall mean any natural or legal person in the supply chain, other than the manufacturer or the importer, who makes a product available on the market"[18]

The New Approach texts would, in particular, make importers, and to a lesser extent distributors, responsible for verifying that the products they handle are in compliance with European requirements. It is unclear to what extent these requirements are applicable in the medical device field. From a practical point of view, they would need to be implemented by appropriate measures. Some evidence of this can be found in national requirements. It is possible that when the medical devices directives are revised again,

Table 8-2. New Approach Areas

Reference	Products Covered
2009/105/EC	Simple pressure vessels
2009/48/EC	Safety of toys
89/106/EEC	Construction products
89/686/EEC	Personal protective equipment
2009/23/EC	Non-automatic weighing instruments
90/385/EEC	Active implantable medical devices
2009/142/EC	Appliances burning gaseous fuels
92/42/EEC	Hot-water boilers
93/15/EEC	Explosives for civil uses
93/42/EEC	Medical devices
94/9/EC	Equipment and protective systems intended for use in potentially explosive atmospheres
94/25/EC	Recreational craft
94/62/EC	Packaging and packaging waste
95/16/EC	Lifts
97/23/EC	Pressure equipment
98/79/EC	In vitro diagnostic medical devices
99/5/EC	Radio equipment and telecommunications terminal equipment
2000/9/EC	Cableway installations designed to carry persons
2004/22/EC	Measuring instruments
2004/108/EC	Electromagnetic compatibility
2006/42/EC	Machinery
2006/95/EC	Low voltage equipment

the role of the importer and distributor in market surveillance will be considered.

Healthcare Establishments

The medical devices directives do not assign any clear responsibilities to healthcare establishments. This area is still regarded as the prerogative of national law. As medical technology becomes more complex, it is increasingly obvious that users have a significant burden of responsibility to learn how to operate, maintain and integrate modern devices into the systems of the healthcare establishment. Another trend is manufacturing of devices by healthcare establishments for their own use. New regulations are emerging in these areas at the national level.

Institutional Cooperation and Consensus Building

The national Competent Authorities meet at least twice a year under the chairmanship of the Member State holding the presidency of the European Council (changes every six months).

Chapter 8

Table 8-3. EU Member States and Affiliated Countries Competent Authorities

Member State	Competent Authority
Austria Österreich	Austrian Federal Office for Safety in Health Care Medicines and Medical Devices Agency Federal Ministry of Health Bundesamt für Sicherheit im Gesundheitswesen AGES PharmMed www.basg.at/medizinprodukte/
Belgium België/Belgique	MDD AIMDD Federal Agency for Medicines and Health Products (Federaal Agentschap voor Geneesmiddelen en Gezondheidsproducten/Agence Fédérale des Médicaments et des Produits de Santé) www.fagg-afmps.be/ IVDD Scientific Institute Public Health, (Wetenschappelijk Instituut Volksgezondheid/ Institut scientifique de Santé Publique) www.wiv-isp.be/
Bulgaria България	Drug Agency Изпълнителна Агенция по Лекарствата www.bda.bg/
Czech Republic Česká republika	State Institute for Drug Control Státní ústav pro kontrolu léčiv (SÚKL) www.sukl.cz/index.php
Cyprus Κύπρος	Cyprus Medical Devices Competent Authority Αρμόδια Αρχή για τον Ιατροτεχνολογικό Εξοπλισμό www.moh.gov.cy
Denmark Danmark	Danish Medicines Agency Lægemiddelstyrelsen www.medicaldevices.dk
Estonia Eesti	Health Board, Medical Devices Department Terviseamet www.terviseamet.ee
Finland Suomi	Valvira – National Supervisory Authority for Welfare and Health Valvira – Sosiaali- ja terveysalan lupa- ja valvontavirasto www.valvira.fi/
France	National Agency for the Safety of Medicinal Products and Healthcare Products Agence nationale de sécurité du médicament et des produits de Santé (ANSM) www.ansm.sante.fr
Germany Deutschland	Federal Institute for Drugs and Medical Devices Bundesinstitut für Arzneimittel und Medizinprodukte (BfArM) www.bfarm.de For some IVD aspects Paul-Ehrlich-Institute Paul-Ehrlich-Institut www.pei.de

Member State	Competent Authority
Greece Ελλάδα	National Organization for Medicines Εθνικός Οργανισμός Φαρμάκων http://eof1.eof.gr
Hungary Magyarország	Department for Medical Devices, Office of Health Authorisation and Administrative Procedures Orvostechnikai Főosztály, Egészségügyi Engedélyezési és Közigazgatási Hivatal www.eekh.hu
Ireland Éire	Irish Medicines Board Bhord Leigheasra na hÉireann www.imb.ie
Italy Italia	Ministry of Health, Directorate General of Medicines and Medical Devices Ministero della Salute Direzione Generale dei Farmaci e Dispositivi Medici www.salute.gov.it/dispositivi/dispomed.jsp
Latvia Latvija	State Agency of Medicines Zāļu valsts aģentūra www.zva.gov.lv
Lithuania Lietuva	The State Health Care Accreditation Agency under the Ministry of Health Valstybinė akreditavimo sveikatos priežiūros veiklai tarnyba prie Sveikatos apsaugos ministerijos (VASPVT) www.vaspvt.gov.lt/
Luxembourg	Health Ministry, Division for Therapeutic Medicine Ministère de la Santé, Division de la Médecine Curative www.ms.public.lu
Malta	Consumer and Industrial Goods Unit, Malta Competition and Consumer Affairs Authority Awtorita' Maltija Dwar L-Istandards www.msa.org.mt/
Netherlands Nederland	Farmatec (e.g., device registrations) www.farmatec.nl Health Care Inspectorate (e.g. clinical investigations, vigilance) Inspectie voor de Gezondheidszorg (IGZ) www.igz.nl/
Poland Polska	Office for Registration of Medicinal Products, Medical Devices and Biocidal Products Urząd Rejestracji Produktów Leczniczych, Wyrobów Medycznych i Produktów Biobójczych http://en.urpl.gov.pl/
Portugal	Infarmed – National Authority of Medicines and Health Products INFARMED-Autoridade Nacional do Medicamento e Produtos de Saúde www.infarmed.pt

Member State	Competent Authority
Romania România	Ministry of Health Ministerul Sănătății www.ms.ro/
Slovak Republic Slovenská republika	State Institute for Drug Control, Medical Devices Section Štátny ústav pre kontrolu liečiv, Sekcia zdravotníckych pomôcok www.sukl.sk
Slovenia Slovenija	Agency for Medicinal Products and Medical Devices of the Republic of Slovenia Javna agencija Republike Slovenije za zdravila in medicinske pripomočke (JAZMP) www.jazmp.si
Spain España	Spanish Agency for Medicines and Medical Devices Agencia Española de Medicamentos y Productos Sanitarios www.aemps.es/
Sweden Sverige	Medical Products Agency Läkemedelsverket www.lakemedelsverket.se/
United Kingdom	Medicines & Healthcare products Regulatory Agency (MHRA) www.mhra.gov.uk
EEA countries	
Iceland Island	Directorate of Health Landlæknisembættið www.landlaeknir.is/
Liechtenstein	Office of Public Health Amt für Gesundheit www.ag.llv.li/
Norway Norge	Health Directorate Helsedirektoratet www.helsedirektoratet.no/
Countries that have agreements with the EU with implications for medical devices	
Switzerland Suisse-Schweitz-Swizzera	Swissmedic – Swiss Agency for Therapeutic Products Institut suisse des produits thérapeutiques Schweizerisches Heilmittelinstitut Istituto svizzero per gli agenti terapeutici www.swissmedic.ch
Turkey Türkiye	Ministry of Health General Directorate of Pharmacy and Pharmaceuticals Sağlık Bakanlığı İlaç ve Eczacılık Genel Müdürlüğü www.iegm.gov.tr/

Working Groups Established by the Commission

The Commission has established several working groups that develop guidance on European compliance requirements and related areas. These are described in **Table 8-4**.[19]

Representation of the Industry: European Trade Associations

There are many trade associations in Europe. Some are more active than others in the process of developing consensus among the Commission, the Member States, the NBs and industry regarding interpretation of regulatory requirements. **Table 8-5** lists European industrial trade associations.

Eucomed is the largest of these trade associations and represents all areas of medical device technology except electromedical equipment and in vitro diagnostics. It is a federation of corporate members, European product-specific associations and national associations.

EUROM's membership extends beyond medical device manufacturers, which are placed in a sub-group—the EUROM VI committee.

Medical Device Laws

The key directives that provide the bulk of European medical device law cover:
- active implantable medical devices (90/385/EEC)[20]
- medical devices (93/42/EEC)[21]
- in vitro diagnostic medical devices (98/79/EC)[22]

These are supplemented by several additional measures in the form of Commission directives and decisions.

Scope of the Medical Devices Directives

The scope of the medical devices directives is determined by a number of important concepts, which are discussed in the following.

Medical Devices and Active Implantable Medical Devices

The definitions of the products they regulate are perhaps the most important concepts to discuss in terms of scope of the medical devices directives. A correct definition of the product is important from the start, because it determines the regulatory strategy that a manufacturer will pursue to bring the product to the market. An incorrect product classification can be very costly and significantly delay the market entry of a product.

The core concept for the three medical devices directives is the concept of "medical device" in the *lex generalis* directive 93/42. If a product falls within the scope of that definition, it falls within the scope of one of the three medical devices directives. The next step is to determine if

Regulatory Affairs Professionals Society

Chapter 8

Table 8-4. European Commission Working Groups and Their Activities

Closed groups: European Commission services and national Competent Authorities participate (industry and Notified Bodies are normally excluded)

Competent Authority (CA) meetings

Chair: Member State holding the EU presidency

The Member State holding the rotating presidency of the EU traditionally organizes a meeting at which the national Competent Authorities of the Member States, candidate countries and EFTA and the European Commission discuss policy issues.

Compliance and Enforcement Group (COEN)

Chair: Sweden

COEN focuses on the scope and coordination of the enforcement activities by Member States and considers how communications and cooperation between Member States can be made more effective and efficient.

Notified Body Operations Group (NBOG)

Chair: Germany

NBOG aims to improve the overall performance of NBs, primarily by identifying and promulgating examples of best practice to be adopted by both NBs and organisations responsible for their designation and control.

It reviews recommendations issued by the NB-MED group (in which all the EU NBs participate) and acts as a "Mirror Group" that follows GHTF work on certification bodies.

An NB representative can be invited to participate as appropriate, depending upon the issue discussed.

Open groups: Members are national Competent Authorities, industry (trade associations), NBs, standardisation bodies and Commission services.

Medical Devices Expert Group (MDEG)

Chair: European Commission

Umbrella group for other working groups in the field that also coordinates and oversees their activities. It adopts MEDDEV guidance documents.

MDEG also meets in closed session (with only Commission representatives and Member State Competent Authorities) to discuss confidential implementation issues.

Vigilance (adverse incidents)

Chair: European Commission

The group exchanges guidance, discusses actual cases, reviews current reporting practices and prepares input for the Eudamed database. The Vigilance group also acts as the GHTF-Study Group 2 Mirror Group.

Classification and Borderline

Chair: European Commission

The group discusses borderline (is a specific product a medical device?) and classification cases. Often, this results in an entry into the Commission's *Manual on Borderline and Classification*.

The group typically uses an "Enquiry Template" to communicate questions to all Member States and gather responses. Responses are collated and presented at the meeting by the Member State originator, including its proposed consensus opinion based upon the responses.

IVD Technical Group

Chair: France

The group supplies technical and specific input, for example by drafting CTS documents to the Commission, MDEG and other working groups and also provides input on the interpretation and uniform implementation of the *IVDD*.

Working Group on Clinical Investigation and Evaluation (CIE)

Chair: Austria

The group develops and promotes homogenous interpretation and implementation of European requirements on clinical evaluation and investigation, including postmarket clinical follow-up (PMCF). It monitors the EU and international regulatory environment and technical standardisation in the clinical area.

It serves as the European Mirror Group for GHTF SG 5.

Electronic Labelling Working Group

Chair: European Commission

The group prepares guidance on the circumstances and manner in which Instruction For Use (IFU) and other information required for the safe and proper use of medical devices can be provided, including any limitations and safeguards that should be applied. Such guidance will form the basis for possible Community measures on e-labelling.

New & Emerging Technologies Working Group (NET)

Chair: Portugal

The group identifies new and emerging technologies that may challenge the adequacy of existing regulatory requirements for devices. Where shortcomings are identified, the group makes recommendations to MDEG about addressing these challenges by guidance or by regulatory changes. It also informs MDEG about relevant scientific trends.

Eudamed Working Group

Chair: European Commission

The group advises on all issues related to the implementation of the Eudamed database.

NB-MED

Chair: The Netherlands

The group advises the Commission, at its request, on subjects related to application of the medical device directives. It considers, and if necessary, draft reports on ethical aspects of notified bodie's activities. It ensures consistency with standardization work at European level. Finally the group keeps informed on harmonisation activities at European level.

a *lex specialis* applies because the medical device falls within the scope of the *AIMDD* because it is an active implantable medical device or of the *In Vitro Device Directive* (*IVDD*) because it is an in vitro diagnostic medical device.

The definition of medical device in Article 1 (2) (a) of Directive 93/42/EEC is:

"any instrument, apparatus, appliance, software, material or other article, whether used alone or in combination, including the software intended by its manufacturer to be used specifically for diagnostic and/or therapeutic purposes and necessary for its proper application, intended by the manufacturer to be used for human beings for the purpose of:
- diagnosis, prevention, monitoring, treatment or alleviation of disease,
- diagnosis, monitoring, treatment, alleviation of or compensation for an injury or handicap,
- investigation, replacement or modification of the anatomy or of a physiological process,
- control of conception,

and which does not achieve its principal intended action in or on the human body by pharmacological, immunological or metabolic means, but which may be assisted in its function by such means"

This definition contains a number of defining elements:
- "instrument, apparatus, appliance, software, material or other article"—Basically, anything can be a medical device, including software. Software can constitute a medical device by itself if it does not come pre-installed on a medical device (e.g., on an MRI scanner). A new MEDDEV was recently released to assist with determining whether stand-alone software falls within the scope of the medical devices directive.[23]
- "intended by the manufacturer […] for the purpose of"—This denotes the device's "intended purpose," one of the core concepts of the medical devices directives. The device's intended purpose determines the scope of the conformity assessment and Essential Requirements it has to meet, much like the indications for a medicinal product. The intended purpose is defined in the directive as "the use for which the device is intended according to the data supplied by the manufacturer on the labelling, in the instructions and/or in promotional material." Advertising or using the device outside the scope of the intended purpose as expressed in the CE declaration of conformity and the underlying technical file would constitute off-label advertising and off-label use. Placing a medical device on the market for anything other than the intended use is illegal.
- "for human beings"—Veterinary medical devices (unlike veterinary medicinal products) are not regulated as medical devices.
- "which does not achieve its principal intended action in or on the human body by pharmacological, immunological or metabolic means, but which may be assisted in its function by such means"—This element determines the borderline between medicinal products and medical devices; the principle intended action of a medical device must not be that of a medicinal product (action in or on the human body by pharmacological, immunological or metabolic means are the core elements from the definition of medicinal product in Directive 2001/83/EEC). However, a medical device may be assisted in its function by such means. For example, bone cement containing antibiotics has a mechanical/chemical primary mode of action (harden to keep a prosthesis in place) and that function is assisted by pharmacological means (antibiotics to prevent infection). MEDDEV 2.1/3 rev.3, *Borderline products, drug-delivery products and medical devices incorporating, as integral part, an ancillary medicinal substance or an ancillary human blood derivative*[24] and the Commission's *Manual on Borderline and Classification in the Community Regulatory Framework for Medical Devices*[25] both contain important and practical guidance on how to decide whether a specific product is a medical device or a medicinal product. In addition, the CJEU's case law on pharmacological, immunological or metabolic means concepts is highly relevant,[26] as the scope of these concepts not only positively determines what is a medicinal product but also negatively determines what constitutes a medical device.

Article 1(5) of the *MDD* further excludes from the directive's scope, apart from medicinal products:
- human blood, blood products, plasma or blood cells of human origin, or devices that incorporate, at the time of placing on the market, such blood products, plasma or cells, with the exception of devices incorporating a medicinal product derived from human blood or human plasma
- transplants or tissues or cells of human origin or products incorporating or derived from tissues or cells of human origin, with the exception of devices incorporating a medicinal product derived from human blood or human plasma
- transplants or tissues or cells of animal origin, unless a device is manufactured utilising animal tissue which is rendered nonviable or nonviable products derived from animal tissue

Table 8-5. European Industrial Trade Associations

Trade association	Acronym	Website
European Coordination Committee of the Radiological, Electromedical and Healthcare IT Industry	COCIR	www.cocir.org
European Association of Authorized Representatives	EAAR	www.eaarmed.org/
European Diagnostic Manufacturers Association	EDMA	www.edma-ivd.eu/
European Hearing Instrument Manufacturers Association	EHIMA	www.ehima.com
Eucomed		www.eucomed.be/
European Federation of Precision Mechanical and Optical Industries	EUROM	www.eurom.org/
European Federation of National Associations and International Companies of Contact Lens (and Lens Care) Manufacturers	EUROMCONTACT	www.euromcontact.org/
Federation of the European Dental Industry	FIDE	www.fide-online.org/

Other MEDDEVs that address the scope of the *MDD* can be found in section 2.1, "Scope, field of application, definition" on the MEDDEV guidance page of the European Commission website.[27]

Once a product is deemed a medical device, it needs to be determined whether it is an active implantable medical device or an in vitro diagnostic medical device.

The definition of active implantable medical device consists of two partial definitions, the first of which is nested in the second:

- "active medical device"' means any medical device relying for its functioning on a source of electrical energy or any source of power other than that directly generated by the human body or gravity
- "active implantable medical device" means any active medical device which is intended to be totally or partially introduced, surgically or medically, into the human body or by medical intervention into a natural orifice, and which is intended to remain after the procedure

A typical example of an active implantable medical device is a pacemaker. Suppose, however, that a company invented an implantable pacemaker that is powered by body heat alone. This would not constitute an active implantable device but rather an implantable device covered by the *MDD*, the general medical devices directive. Section 2.1 on the European Commission's MEDDEV guidance page contains specific MEDDEVs that clarify the scope of application of the *AIMDD*.

The definition of an in vitro diagnostic medical device is:

"any medical device which is a reagent, reagent product, calibrator, control material, kit, instrument, apparatus, equipment or system, whether used alone or in combination, intended by the manufacturer to be used in vitro for the examination of specimens, including blood and tissue donations, derived from the human body, solely or principally for the purpose of providing information:
- concerning a physiological or pathological state, or
- concerning a congenital abnormality, or
- to determine the safety and compatibility with potential recipients, or
- to monitor therapeutic measures."

The directive provides that specimen receptacles are considered to be in vitro diagnostic medical devices. "Specimen receptacles" are those devices, whether or not they use vacuum systems, specifically intended by their manufacturers for the primary containment and preservation of specimens derived from the human body for the purpose of in vitro diagnostic examination. Further, products for general laboratory use are not in vitro diagnostic medical devices unless such products, in view of their characteristics, are specifically intended by their manufacturer to be used for in vitro diagnostic examination. In vitro diagnostic devices are discussed in more detail in Chapter 13. The scope of application of the *IVDD* is clarified in MEDDEV 2.14/1 rev.1, *Borderline issues*, of January 2004, which can be found on the European Commission website's MEDDEV page.[28]

Accessory

An accessory in the meaning of the *MDD* is "an article which whilst not being a device is intended specifically by its manufacturer to be used together with a device to enable it to be used in accordance with the use of the device intended by the manufacturer of the device." Article 1(1) of the directive provides that "for the purposes of this Directive, accessories shall be treated as medical devices in their own right." An accessory may be a disposable that could also be made by a manufacturer other than the device manufacturer. In that case, the accessory, even if it is not a medical device in itself, still needs to comply with all the requirements for medical devices under the directive.

Placing on the Market

One of the core concepts of the medical devices directives is the concept of "placing on the market."[29] Placing a device on the market is only allowed after CE marking has been affixed lawfully on the device, based on a valid declaration of conformity. Placing on the market is defined as "the first making available in return for payment or free of charge of a device other than a device intended for clinical investigation, with a view to distribution and/or use on the Community market, regardless of whether it is new or fully refurbished."

This concept begs the question when a device is actually placed on the market, in particular whether a medical device may already be considered as being placed on the market when the manufacturing process is finished, or whether additional steps need to be taken prior to its distribution or use. The latter is the case. The Commission clarified this in an interpretative notice, to the effect that "placing on the market takes place when the product is transferred from the stage of manufacture with the intention of distribution or use on the Community market."[30] This transfer does not merely happen when the device is placed in the warehouse or stocks of the manufacturer, or is has not been released by customs. However, in certain circumstances, a device that physically is still in the manufacturer's warehouse can be considered as placed on the market. For example, this may be the case when the product's ownership or another right already has been transferred to a distributor or an end user but the product is still stored by the manufacturer on their behalf. In addition, the Blue Guide clarifies that a device really must have left the manufacturer's production process in order for it to be placed on the market, and is not yet placed on the market if it is "transferred to a manufacturer for further measures (for example assembling, packaging, processing or labelling)."[31] A device that is only displayed at trade fairs, exhibitions or demonstrations is not placed on the market either,[32] which explains why these devices are not allowed to bear CE marking.[33]

Putting Into Service

Putting into service is another core concept similar to placing on the market and having a valid CE Mark is a condition for a device to be put into service. It is defined as "the stage at which a device has been made available to the final user as being ready for use on the Community market for the first time for its intended purpose."[34] The Blue Guide clarifies that putting into service "takes place at the moment of first use within the Community by the end user."[35] This concept applies to a device that is not placed on the market as a fully functional device but is assembled in the place where it will be used, e.g., a bigger device like an MRI scanner.

Custom-made Devices

Two categories of medical devices are exempt from the full conformity assessment requirements underlying CE marking: custom-made devices and devices intended for clinical investigation. Both of these device categories are made in small volumes and often constitute devices that are mature prototypes. While these devices do not have to undergo full conformity assessment, they must fulfil the requirements set out in *MDD* Annex VIII and may not bear CE marking.

A custom-made device is any device specifically made in accordance with the written prescription of a duly qualified medical practitioner or any other person authorised by virtue of his professional qualifications to do so that gives, under the responsibility of the prescriber, specific design characteristics and is intended for the sole use of a particular patient.[36]

Mass-produced devices that need to be adapted to meet the specific requirements of the medical practitioner or any other professional user are not considered to be custom-made devices (see additional information under the definition of "manufacturer" below).

Custom-made devices require compliance with the Essential Requirements for medical devices set out in Annex I, and description of a quality system that ensures that the devices are manufactured in accordance with the description of the device as set out in Annex VIII, point 2.1. This description consists of:

1. manufacturer's name and address
2. data allowing identification of the device in question
3. statement that the device is intended for exclusive use by a particular patient, together with the patient's name
4. name of the medical practitioner or other authorised person who wrote the prescription and, where applicable, the name of the clinic concerned
5. specific product characteristics as indicated by the prescription

Figure 8-5. Clinical Evaluation Cycle

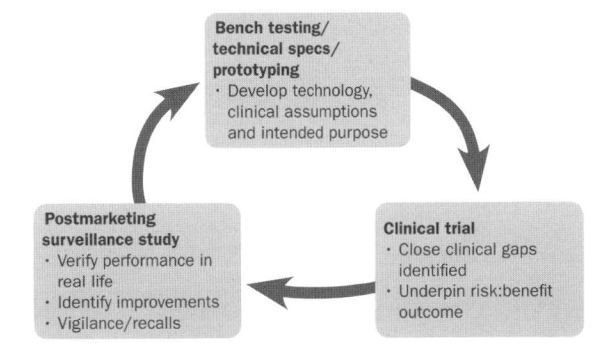

Chapter 8

Table 8-6. MEDDEV Guidance Documents

Code	Title	Date
	2.1. Scope field of application definition	
MEDDEV 2.1/1	*Definitions of "medical devices," "accessory" and "manufacturer"*	April 1994
MEDDEV 2.1/2 rev. 2	*Field of application of directive "active implantable medical devices"*	April 1994
MEDDEV 2.1/2.1	*Field of application of directive "active implantable medical devices"*	February 1998
MEDDEV 2.1/3 rev. 3	*Borderline products, drug-delivery products and medical devices incorporating, as an integral part, an ancillary medicinal substance or an ancillary human blood derivative—December 2009*	December 2009
MEDDEV 2.1/1	*Interface with other directives—Medical devices/Directive 89/336/EEC relating to electromagnetic compatibility and Directive 89/686/EEC relating to personal protective equipment (For the relation between the MDD and Directive 89/686/EEC concerning personal protective equipment, please see the Commission services interpretative document of 21 August 2009)*	March 1994
MEDDEV 2.1/5	*Medical devices with a measuring function*	June 1998
MEDDEV 2.1/6	*Qualification and Classification of standalone software*	January 2012
	2.2 Essential Requirements	
MEDDEV 2.2/1 rev. 1	*EMC requirements*	February 1998
MEDDEV 2.2/3 rev. 3	*"Use by" date*	June 1998
MEDDEV 2.2/4	*Conformity assessment of In Vitro Fertilisation (IVF) and Assisted Reproduction Technologies (ART) products*	January 2012
	2.4 Classification	
MEDDEV 2.4/1 rev. 9	*Classification of medical devices*	June 2010
	2.5 Conformity assessment procedure	
	General rules	
MEDDEV 2.5/3 rev. 2	*Subcontracting quality systems related*	June 1998
MEDDEV 2.5/5 rev. 3	*Translation procedure*	February 1998
MEDDEV 2.5/6 rev. 1	*Homogenous batches (verification of manufacturers' products)*	February 1998
	Conformity assessment for particular groups of products	
MEDDEV 2.5/7 rev. 1	*Conformity assessment of breast implants*	July 1998
MEDDEV 2.5/9 rev. 1	*Evaluation of medical devices incorporating products containing natural rubber latex*	February 2004
MEDDEV 2.5/10	*Guideline for Authorised Representatives*	January 2012
	2.7 Clinical investigation, clinical evaluation	
MEDDEV 2.7/1 rev. 3	*Clinical evaluation: Guide for manufacturers and notified bodies*	December 2009
Appendix 1:	*Appendix 1: Clinical evaluation on coronary stents*	December 2008
MEDDEV 2.7/2	*Guide for Competent Authorities in making an assessment of clinical investigation; notification*	December 2008
MEDDEV 2.7/3	*Clinical investigations: serious adverse event reporting and SAE reporting form*	December 2010
MEDDEV 2.7/4	*Guidelines on Clinical investigations: a guide for manufacturers and notified bodies*	December 2010
	2.10 Notified Bodies	
MEDDEV 2.10/2 rev. 1	*Designation and monitoring of Notified Bodies within the framework of EC Directives on Medical devices and Annexes 1–4*	April 2001
	2.11 Products using materials of biological origin	
MEDDEV 2.11/1 rev. 2	*Application of Council Directive 93/42/EEC taking into account the Commission Directive 2003/32/EC for Medical Devices utilising tissues or derivatives originating from animals for which a TSE risk is suspected and Annex 1*	January 2008
	2.12 Market surveillance	
MEDDEV 2.12/1 rev. 7	*Medical devices vigilance system* *Manufacturer Incident Report; How to use the MIR, Field Safety Corrective Action*	March 2012
MEDDEV 2.12/2 rev. 2	*Clinical Evaluation—Postmarket Clinical Follow-up studies*	January 2012
	2.13 Transitional period	
MEDDEV 2.13 rev. 1	*Commission communication on the application of transitional provision of Directive 93/42/EEC relating to medical devices (As regards the transitional regime of Directive 2007/47/EC, see the Interpretative Document of the Commission's services of 5 June 2009)*	August 1998
	2.14 IVD	
MEDDEV 2.14/1 rev. 2	*Borderline and Classification issues: A guide for manufacturers and notified bodies*	January 2012
MEDDEV 2.14/2 rev. 1	*Research Use Only products*	February 2004
MEDDEV 2.14/3 rev. 1	*Supply of Instructions For Use (IFU) and other information for In-vitro Diagnostic (IVD) Medical Devices*	January 2007
	Form for the registration of manufacturers and devices In Vitro Diagnostic Medical Device Directive, Article 10	January 2007
MEDDEV 2.14/4	*CE marking of blood based in vitro diagnostic medical devices for vCJD based on detection of abnormal PrP*	January 2012
	2.15 Other guidances	
MEDDEV 2.15 rev. 3	*Committees/Working Groups contributing to the implementation of the Medical Device Directives*	December 2008

6. statement that the device in question conforms to the essential requirements set out in Annex I and, where applicable, indicating which Essential Requirements have not been fully met, together with the grounds

The manufacturer has to retain the documentation, indicating manufacturing site(s) and allowing an understanding of the product's design, manufacture and performance, including the expected performance, so as to allow assessment of conformity with the requirements of the directive.

The procedural aspects of ensuring compliance with the rules for a custom-made device are set out in detail in the consensus statement, *Guidance Statement for Manufacturers of Custom-Made Medical Devices*.[37]

Device Intended for Clinical Investigation

As explained above, clinical evaluation of devices as described in *MDD* Annex X may include clinical investigation. Further, as is true for custom-made devices, devices intended for clinical investigation do not have to meet the requirements for full conformity assessment but are not allowed to bear a CE Mark as they might be confused with devices that have undergone full conformity assessment.

In relation to the requirements for devices for clinical investigation see section 6.9 of ISO 14155:2011, which states:
1. Access to investigational devices shall be controlled and the investigational devices shall be used only in the clinical investigation and according to the clinical investigation plan (CIP).
2. The sponsor shall keep records to document the physical location of all investigational devices from shipment of investigational devices to the investigation sites until return or disposal.

Manufacturer

The manufacturer is an important entity in the EU medical devices directives, because this is the individual with all the regulatory obligations in the current EU legal framework for medical devices. The manufacturer is defined as "the natural or legal person with responsibility for the design, manufacture, packaging and labelling of a device before it is placed on the market under his own name, regardless of whether these operations are carried out by that person himself or on his behalf by a third party." This definition essentially means the manufacturer is the party who places devices on the market in the EU under his own name. If the manufacturer has no presence in the EU, he must appoint an Authorised Representative (see below) that function as contact point for the authorities in his stead.

In addition to this definition, which covers the traditional Original Equipment Manufacturer (OEM), the manufacturer obligations also apply to certain post-sale commercial activities with a risk profile similar to that of manufacturing a device. Therefore, the individual who assembles, packages, processes, fully refurbishes and/or labels one or more ready-made products and/or assigns an intended purpose as a device to them with a view to their being placed on the market under his own name must meet the same obligations as a manufacturer.

Assembly or adaptation to the intended purpose of devices already on the market for an individual patient does not constitute assembly regulated like manufacturing. Typical examples are adaptation of glasses by opticians and fitting of dental implants by dentists. The device's intended purpose is the line of demarcation: if the adaptation is such that it brings the device outside its original intended purpose, the party that assembles or adapts does constitute a manufacturer. For example, if a hospital configures software provided for a specific intended purpose (e.g., monitor all cardiac monitors in a ward) to make it suitable for monitoring other devices not included in the intended purpose (e.g., infusion or food pumps), this configuration would make the hospital the manufacturer, provided the other requirement of "placing on the market under its own name" is met.

Authorised Representative

MDD Article 14 provides that where a manufacturer who places a device on the market under his own name does not have a registered place of business in a Member State, he shall designate a single Authorised Representative in the EU. *MDD* Article 1(2)(j) defines the Authorised Representative as any natural or legal person established in the Community who, explicitly designated by the manufacturer, acts and may be addressed by authorities and bodies in the Community instead of the manufacturer with regard to the latter's obligations under the directive. Some of the Authorised Representative's responsibilities include informing the Competent Authority of the Member State in which he has his registered place of business of the registered place of business and provide a description of the devices concerned for Class I devices, custom-made devices, the composition of systems and procedure packs, and the sterilisation of systems and/or procedure packs.

The mutual responsibilities and a clarification of the medical devices directives' requirements are set out in detail in MEDDEV 2.5/10, *Guideline for Authorised Representatives*,[38] dated January 2012. This MEDDEV contains useful guidance on the agreement between the Authorised Representative and the manufacturer and supervision of its implementation by the manufacturer's NB. It emphasises the expectations of Member States' authorities that the Authorised Representatives take an independent position towards its manufacturer and even actively report persistent nonconformities to the authorities and rescind its agreement with a manufacturer.[39]

Chapter 8

Implementing Legislation
- Eudamed—European Databank on Medical Devices[40]
- Common Technical Specifications on IVDs[41,42]
- Medical devices manufactured utilising tissues of animal origin

Reclassification
- Reclassification of hip, knee and shoulder joint replacements[43]
- Reclassification of breast implants[44]

Interpretation of Medical Device Law

Interpretation by Courts

CJEU provides the ultimate interpretation of European law. At this point, however, there is very little case law to provide significant interpretation in the field of medical devices.

National courts may also interpret national and European medical device law because the medical devices directives must be implemented in national law. It is possible that courts in different Member States may come to different conclusions on similar issues. For example, courts may decide differently in respective Member States about whether a particular product is a medical device or a medicinal product.

If the national court is uncertain about a point of European law, it can request a preliminary ruling from CJEU. For example, the first request for a preliminary reference about the borderline of medical devices with medicinal products is pending at the CJEU at the time of writing of this chapter.[45]

Commission Guidance

The Commission provides interpretation in the form of guidance (MEDDEV documents),[46] consensus statements[47] and interpretative documents.[48]

The MEDDEV guidance documents are adopted by the Medical Devices Expert Group (MDEG), which is chaired by the Commission and whose members are representatives of national Competent Authorities, standardisation bodies, European trade associations and NBs. MEDDEV documents are not legally binding, but they represent the consensus of the MDEG members. Often, they are prepared by working groups composed of various members of MDEG. The national Competent Authorities, therefore, generally accept compliance with MEDDEV guidance as indicating compliance with the areas of directives that they cover.

Table 8-6 lists MEDDEV guidances from the Commission's website.[49]

The Commission has also issued statements it has prepared that MDEG has endorsed, which are listed in **Table 8-7**.

Table 8-8 lists interpretative documents issued by the Commission.

Additional guidance can be found from specific MDEG working group websites.

The Notified Body Operations Group (NBOG) issues guidance on NBs (see **Table 8-9**).[50]

The Commission as an Arbitrator

The Commission does not have any clear powers to make decisions in conflicts of interpretation. However, it does provide a forum for building consensus. MEDDEVs and consensus statements are one way of doing this. The Commission also holds closed meetings with representatives of national Competent Authorities where issues of interpretation are discussed. These meetings are confidential, so the outcomes of the discussions usually do not reach the public domain.

There is a quasi-informal process called the "Helsinki procedure." A national Competent Authority can request other national Competent Authorities to provide an opinion on a specific borderline or classification issue. If consensus is not reached in this manner, which is frequently the case, the matter is passed on for consideration to the Commission's Working Group on Classification and Borderline. This group draws its members from MDEG, so it also has representatives of industry and other stakeholders. When consensus is achieved within this group, the results are published in the *Manual on Borderline and Classification*.[51]

Guidance From Other Sources

Many European stakeholders provide guidance.

NBs are grouped in the European Association of Notified Bodies for Medical Devices (Team-NB), which issues guidance relevant to the operations of NBs. Team-NB has issued almost 200 guidance documents that can be found on its website.[52]

Trade associations often issue position papers that, in a sense, can be considered guidance, although there are no guarantees that such opinions would be accepted by Competent Authorities. Eucomed is the most prolific

Table 8-7. European Commission Consensus Statements

Guidance Notes for Manufacturers of Class I Medical Devices (December 2009)
Guidance Notes for Manufacturers of Custom-made Medical Devices (June 2010)
Guidance Document on Directive 2005/50/EC (December 2006)
IVD Trisomy 21 (December 2006)
IVD Rare Blood Groups (December 2003)

publisher of documents that provide an interesting perspective on EU medical device law.[53]

Guidance From Member States
All national Competent Authorities have their own websites that, in most cases, provide links to national laws and regulations as well as guidance and often adverse incident- and enforcement-related information. The vast majority of the information available is in the Member State's national language, but English language content is increasing. The European Commission maintains a list of national Competent Authorities that includes links to the websites of most of them.[54] For the non-linguists, a useful site is that of the UK Competent Authority, MHRA,[55] as it provides a wealth of guidance. However, there is no guarantee that the national Competent Authorities of other Member States would always agree with MHRA on everything.

Significance of Technical Standards
The Essential Requirements and some other directive requirements are very general, but for many of them, solutions have been provided in harmonised technical standards. Compliance with such standards gives rise to a presumption of compliance with the corresponding requirements of the directives.

The general trend is to adopt international standards developed by the International Organization for Standardization (ISO)[56] and the International Electrotechnical Commission (IEC).[57]

European technical standards are adopted by the European Committee for Standardization (CEN)[58] and the European Committee for Electrotechnical Standardization (CENELEC),[59] if possible based on international standards and otherwise based purely on European work. These standards are made available through the national members of these organisations, e.g., the British Standards Institution.[60]

National Enforcement
The European Commission has no enforcement powers with respect to compliance with the medical devices directives. Member States are responsible for enforcement, as stated, for instance, in Article 2 of the *MDD*:

> "Article 2 Placing on the market and putting into service Member States shall take all necessary steps to ensure that devices may be placed on the market and/or put into service only if they comply with the requirements laid down in this Directive when duly supplied and properly installed, maintained and used in accordance with their intended purpose."

Each Member State is free to carry out enforcement in the medical device area as it deems best. The texts transposing the requirements of the European directives into national

Table 8-8. Interpretive Documents Issued by the European Commission

Interpretative document of the Commission's services on placing on the market of medical devices (16 November 2010)
Interpretation of the Customs Union Agreement with Turkey in the field of medical devices (11 February 2010)
Decision No 1/2006 of the EC-Turkey Association Council of 15 May 2006 on the implementation of Article 9 of Decision No 1/95 of the EC-Turkey Association on implementing the final phase of the Customs Union
Statement of Turkey-EC Customs Union Joint Committee on the implementation of Article 1 of Decision 1/2006
Interpretation of the relation between the revised Directives 90/385/EEC and 93/42/EEC concerning (active implantable) medical devices and Directive 2006/42/EC on machinery (21 August 2009)
Interpretation of the relation between the revised Directive 93/42/EEC concerning medical devices and Directive 89/686/EEC on personal protective equipment (21 August 2009)
Interpretative document of the Commission's services implementation of Directive 2007/47/EC amending Directives 90/385/EEC, 93/42/EEC and 98/8/EC (5 June 2009)
Interpretation of the medical devices directives in relation to medical device own brand labellers (4 February 2008)

law often set out enforcement methods and the penalties for violations of the law.

In practice, it is clear that many national Competent Authorities have only limited resources to carry out market surveillance and enforcement: for instance, Luxembourg cannot expend the same effort as France. Even the major Member States do not have unlimited resources. Market surveillance and enforcement efforts, therefore, tend to be more reactive than systematic. Adverse incidents and complaints by competitors tend to trigger action by national Competent Authorities. New information released by FDA or other non-European authorities also may elicit a response. In addition, there is increased interaction between the Member States, e.g., monitoring one another's websites and profiting from contacts made at European Competent Authority and expert meetings.

After the Poly Implant Prothese scandal involving breast implants in 2011, there is a call for more centralised enforcement of medical devices law, which is likely to find its way in the regulation currently in preparation (see below).

Evolution of the Legal System
The *MDD* was amended five times between 1993 and 2007. Most of the significant changes have been based on a better understanding of medical device safety and compliance dynamics. For instance, the role of clinical evaluation has increased considerably, and more pressure has been put on NBs to be stricter in their certification and periodic audits.

More effort is expended in trying to understand the impact of accelerating technological development on the regulatory framework. The Commission has set up a New

Table 8-9. NBOG Documents

Number	Title	Publication
NBOG BPG 2006-1	Change of Notified Body	November 2008
NBOG BPG 2009-1	Guidance on Design-Dossier Examination and Report Content	March 2009
NBOG BPG 2009-2	Role of Notified Bodies in the Medical Device Vigilance System	March 2009
NBOG BPG 2009-3	Guideline for Designating Authorities to Define the Notification Scope of a Notified Body Conducting Medical Devices Assessment	March 2009
NBOG BPG 2009-4	Guidance on Notified Body's Tasks of Technical Documentation Assessment on a Representative Basis	July 2009
NBOG BPG 2010-1	Guidance for Notified Bodies auditing suppliers to medical device manufacturers	March 2010
NBOG BPG 2010-2	Guidance on Audit Report Content	March 2010
NBOG BPG 2010-3	Certificates issued by Notified Bodies with reference to Council Directives 93/42/EEC, 98/79/EC, and 90/385/EEC	March 2010
NBOG Checklists		
Number	Title	Publication
NBOG CL 2010-1	Checklist for audit of Notified Body's review of Clinical Data/Clinical Evaluation	March 2010
NBOG Forms		
Number	Title	Publication
NBOG F 2009-1	Notification form—Directive 93/42/EEC	December 2009
NBOG F 2009-2	Notification form—Directive 90/385/EEC	August 2009
NBOG F 2009-3	Notification form—Directive 98/79/EC	August 2009
NBOG F 2010-1	Certificate Notification to the Commission and other Member States	March 2010

& Emerging Technology Working Group to scan developments that might challenge the regulatory framework. The initial focus was on nanotechnology, but more recently, there has been a new focus on other potentially revolutionary technologies such as optogenetics and synthetic biology.

The EU is presently in the process of reviewing the *AIMDD* and the *MDD*, which was initially referred to as the "Recast," and later as the "Review" or "Revision." The review will, according to statements of the Commission,[61] concentrate on three main areas:

1. Adaption of the rules to technical and scientific progress, including adaptation to scope:
    - closing the regulatory gap between tissue-engineered products falling under the pharmaceuticals legislation and the tissues and cells legislation should be filled
    - implantable or invasive products used for aesthetic purposes, which are similar to medical devices, should be subject to the same requirements as devices
    - reprocessing single-use devices needs to be addressed to ensure a high level of protection of patients and public health
    - genetic tests that provide information about the predisposition of a person to a medical condition or a disease fall under the regulations on in vitro diagnostics
    - review of existing rules to ensure that developments in the sector are duly taken into account during the benefit:risk analysis—for example, the interoperability and compatibility between devices and their environment and the assessment of nanomaterial in devices
2. Effective enforcement across the EU:
    - oversight of NBs is conducted rigorously and in accordance with the same high standards across the EU
    - corrective action to safety issues occurring in the postmarket phase should be taken in a timely and consistent manner throughout the EU
3. Increased transparency, sustainability and efficient management of the system:
    - a single registration of devices placed on the EU market and a system that will allow their traceability through the supply chain
    - a mechanism for borderline products to determine the regulatory status of a product at the EU level with the involvement of all relevant sectors
    - more structured access to external clinical and scientific expertise that will allow for the

- provision of expert advice in the pre- and postmarket phase to manufacturers, NBs, Competent Authorities and the Commission
- enhanced coordination between national authorities that lives up to the principles of the internal market and allows burden-sharing and avoids duplication of work
- enhanced coordination must be provided at the EU level, either through a "European Agency for Health Products" that would integrate the current EMA and a new department for medical devices, or by the Commission itself

The EU is expected to publish the first official proposal at the end of the second quarter of 2012, after which it will enter the European legislative process and may lead to an adopted act around 2014, which may be expected to enter into force around 2015 or 2016.

Summary

European laws are proposed by the Commission and debated and adopted by the Council (representing the Member State governments) and the European Parliament (representing the citizens). They take the form of directly applicable decisions and regulations as well as directives which must be transposed into national law.

Medical devices are regulated primarily by means of New Approach directives. These contain very general requirements that are explained in detail in harmonised technical standards. Compliance is denoted by CE marking, which allows the device to be placed on the market in all EU Member States and some other countries that have specific agreements with the EU.

A significant amount of guidance has been issued by the Commission and other key players. Member States' Competent Authorities are responsible for enforcing compliance. These enforcement actions as well as national court decisions provide further interpretation of the law. Ultimate responsibility for interpretation of the law rests with CJEU.

References

1. The consolidated versions of these texts can be found at http://eur-lex.europa.eu/LexUriServ/LexUriServ.do?uri=OJ:C:2010:083:FULL:EN:PDF. *Official Journal of the European Union*, Volume 53. 30 March 2010. EudraLex website. Accessed 2 April 2012.
2. Consolidated version of the Treaty on European Union—Protocols—Protocol (no 36) on transitional provisions. EUR-Lex website. http://eur-lex.europa.eu/LexUriServ/LexUriServ.do?uri=CELEX:12008M/PRO/36:EN:HTML. Accessed 2 April 2012.
3. Council Directive 65/65/EEC of 26 January 1965 on the approximation of provisions laid down by law, regulation or administrative action relating to medicinal products. EUR-Lex website. http://eur-lex.europa.eu/LexUriServ/LexUriServ.do?uri=CELEX:31965L0065:EN:HTML. Accessed 2 April 2012.
4. Directive 2001/83/EC of the European Parliament and of the Council of 6 November 2001 on the Community code relating to medicinal products for human use. EC website. http://ec.europa.eu/health/files/eudralex/vol-1/dir_2001_83_cons/dir2001_83_cons_20081230_en.pdf. Accessed 2 April 2012.
5. Adapted from "New Approach Standardisation in the Internal Market." EC website. www.newapproach.org/Directives/DirectiveList.asp. Accessed 2 April 2012.
6. European Commission. *Interpretation of the relation between the revised Directive 93/42/EEC concerning medical devices and Directive 89/686/EEC on personal protective equipment*, 21 August 2009. EC website. http://ec.europa.eu/health/medical-devices/files/guide-stds-directives/interpretative_ppe_2009_en.pdf. Accessed 2 April 2012.
7. European Commission. *Interpretation of the relation between the revised Directives 90/385/EEC and 93/42/EEC concerning (active implantable) medical devices and Directive 2006/42/EC on machinery*, 21 August 2009. EC website. http://ec.europa.eu/health/medical-devices/files/guide-stds-directives/interpretative_machinery_2009_en.pdf. Accessed 2 April 2012.
8. European Commission. MEDDEV 2.12/2 rev.2. *Guidelines on Post Market Clinical Follow-up*. May 2004. EC website. http://ec.europa.eu/health/medical-devices/files/meddev/2_12-2_05-2004_en.pdf. Accessed 2 April 2012.
9. Ibid.
10. Ibid.
11. Decision No 768/2008/EC of the European Parliament and of the Council of 9 July 2008 on a common framework for the marketing of products, and repealing Council Decision 93/465/EEC. EUR-Lex website. http://eur-lex.europa.eu/LexUriServ/LexUriServ.do?uri=OJ:L:2008:218:0082:0128:en:PDF. Accessed 3 April 2012.
12. Regulation (EC) No 765/2008 of the European Parliament and of the Council of 9 July 2008 setting out the requirements for accreditation and market surveillance relating to the marketing of products and repealing Regulation (EEC) No 339/93. EUR-Lex website. http://eur-lex.europa.eu/LexUriServ/LexUriServ.do?uri=OJ:L:2008:218:0030:0047:en:PDF. Accessed 2 April 2012.
13. European Medicines Agency. EMA website. www.ema.europa.eu. Accessed 4 April 2012.
14. Article 2 of Council Directive 93/42/EEC of 14 June 1993 concerning medical devices (*MDD*). EUR-Lex website. http://eur-lex.europa.eu/LexUriServ/LexUriServ.do?uri=CONSLEG:1993L0042:20071011:en:PDF. Accessed 3 April 2012.
15. Op cit 11.
16. Working groups and taskforces. EC website. http://ec.europa.eu/health/medical-devices/dialogue-parties/working-groups/index_en.htm. Accessed 4 April 2012.
17. Op cit 12.
18. Ibid.
19. Op cit 16.
20. Council Directive of 20 June 1990 on the approximation of the laws of the Member States relating to active implantable medical devices (90/385/EEC). EUR-Lex website. http://eur-lex.europa.eu/LexUriServ/LexUriServ.do?uri=CONSLEG:1990L0385:20071011:en:PDF. Accessed 3 April 2012.
21. Council Directive 93/42/EEC of 14 June 1993 concerning medical devices. EUR-Lex website. http://eur-lex.europa.eu/LexUriServ/LexUriServ.do?uri=CONSLEG:1993L0042:20071011:en:PDF. Accessed 3 April 2012.
22. Directive 98/79/EC of the European Parliament and of the Council of 27 October 1998 on in vitro diagnostic medical devices. EUR-Lex website. http://eur-lex.europa.eu/LexUriServ/LexUriServ.do?uri=CONSLEG:1998L0079:20090807:en:PDF. Accessed 3 April 2012.
23. European Commission. MEDDEV 2.1/6. *Guidelines on the Qualification and Classification of Stand Alone Software Used in Healthcare Within the Regulatory Framework of Medical Devices*, January 2012. EC website. http://ec.europa.eu/health/medical-devices/files/meddev/2_1_6_ol_en.pdf. Accessed 2 April 2012.
24. European Commission. *MEDDEV 2.1/3 rev 3. Guidelines Relating to the Application of the Council Directive 90/385/EEC on Active*

Implantable Medical Devices, December 2009. EC website. http://ec.europa.eu/health/medical-devices/files/meddev/2_1_3_rev_3-12_2009_en.pdf. Accessed 2 April 2012.
25. European Commission. *Manual on Borderline and Classification in the Community, Regulatory Framework for Medical Devices, Version 1.11*, December 2011. EC website. http://ec.europa.eu/health/medical-devices/files/wg_minutes_member_lists/borderline_manual_ol_en.pdf. Accessed 2 April 2012.
26. See, for example, the BIOS Naturprodukte (Case C-27/08 BIOS Naturprodukte GmbH v Saarland. EUR-Lex website. http://eur-lex.europa.eu/LexUriServ/LexUriServ.do?uri=OJ:C:2009:153:0010:0011:EN:PDF) and Hecht Pharma (C 140/07 HechtPharma v Bezirksregierung Lüneburg. EUR-Lex website. http://eur-lex.europa.eu/LexUriServ/LexUriServ.do?uri=CELEX:62007CJ0140:EN:HTML) cases. Court of Justice of the European Communities. Accessed 2 April 2012.
27. Index of MEDDEV guidance documents. EC website. http://ec.europa.eu/health/medical-devices/documents/guidelines/index_en.htm. Accessed 2 April 2012.
28. Ibid.
29. Article 1 (2) (h) in the *MDD*. EUR-Lex website. http://eur-lex.europa.eu/LexUriServ/LexUriServ.do?uri=CONSLEG:1993L0042:20071011:en:PDF and *AIMDD*. EUR-Lex website. http://eur-lex.europa.eu/LexUriServ/LexUriServ.do?uri=CELEX:31990L0385:en:HTML, article 1 (2) (i) in the *IVDD*. EUR-Lex website. http://eur-lex.europa.eu/LexUriServ/LexUriServ.do?uri=CONSLEG:1998L0079:20031120:en:PDF. Accessed 2 April 2012.
30. European Commission. *Interpretative document of the Commission's services on placing on the market of medical devices*, 16 November 2010. EC website. http://ec.europa.eu/health/medical-devices/files/guide-stds-directives/placing_on_the_market_en.pdf. Accessed 2 April 2012.
31. European Commission. *Guide to the implementation of directives based on the New Approach and the Global Approach*. Blue Guide, p. 19. EC website. http://ec.europa.eu/enterprise/policies/single-market-goods/files/blue-guide/guidepublic_en.pdf. Accessed 2 April 2012.
32. See article 4 (3) MDD. EUR-Lex website. http://eur-lex.europa.eu/LexUriServ/LexUriServ.do?uri=CONSLEG:1993L0042:20071011:en:PDF. Accessed 2 April 2012.
33. Article 1 (2) (i) MDD. EUR-Lex website. http://eur-lex.europa.eu/LexUriServ/LexUriServ.do?uri=CONSLEG:1993L0042:20071011:en:PDF. Accessed 2 April 2012.
34. Op cit 19.
35. Op cit 17.
36. Article 1 (2) (d) MDD. EUR-Lex website. http://eur-lex.europa.eu/LexUriServ/LexUriServ.do?uri=CONSLEG:1993L0042:20071011:en:PDF. Accessed 2 April 2012.
37. *Guidance for Manufacturers of Custom-made Medical Devices*, January 2010. EC website. http://ec.europa.eu/health/medical-devices/files/guide-stds-directives/notes-for-manufactures-custom-made-md_en.pdf. Accessed 2 April 2012.
38. European Commission. Guidelines for Authorised Representatives, January 2012. EC website. http://ec.europa.eu/health/medical-devices/files/meddev/2_5_10_ol_en.pdf. Accessed 2 April 2012.
39. Ibid.
40. Commission Decision of 19 April 2010 on the European Databank on Medical Devices (Eudamed) (2010/227/EU). EUR-Lex website. http://eur-lex.europa.eu/LexUriServ/LexUriServ.do?uri=OJ:L:2010:102:0045:0048:en:PDF. Accessed 3 April 2012.
41. Commission Decision of 7 May 2002 on common technical specifications for in vitro-diagnostic medical devices (2002/364/EC). EUR-Lex website. http://eur-lex.europa.eu/LexUriServ/LexUriServ.do?uri=OJ:L:2002:131:0017:0030:en:PDF. Accessed 3 April 2012.
42. Commission Decision of 27 November 2009 amending Decision 2002/364/EC on common technical specifications for in vitro diagnostic medical devices (2009/886/EC). EUR-Lex website. http://eur-lex.europa.eu/LexUriServ/LexUriServ.do?uri=OJ:L:2009:318:0025:0040:en:PDF. Accessed 3 April 2012.
43. Commission Directive 2005/50/EC of 11 August 2005 on the reclassification of hip, knee and shoulder joint replacements in the framework of Council Directive 93/42/EEC concerning medical devices. EUR-Lex website. http://eur-lex.europa.eu/LexUriServ/LexUriServ.do?uri=OJ:L:2005:210:0041:0043:en:PDF. Accessed 3 April 2012.
44. Commission Directive 2003/12/EC of 3 February 2003 on the reclassification of breast implants in the framework of Directive 93/42/EEC concerning medical devices. EUR-Lex website. http://eur-lex.europa.eu/LexUriServ/LexUriServ.do?uri=OJ:L:2003:028:0043:0044:en:PDF. Accessed 3 April 2012.
45. C-219/11 BrainProducts Gmbh v. Bio Semi V.O.F. and Others and C-109/12 Laboratoires Lyocentre v. Lääkealan turvallisuus- ja kehittämiskeskus/ Sosiaali- ja terveysalan lupa- ja valvontavirasto.
46. Op cit 14.
47. European Commission. Consensus Statements. EC website. http://ec.europa.eu/health/medical-devices/documents/consensus-statements/index_en.htm. Accessed 3 April 2012.
48. European Commission. Interpretative Documents. EC website. http://ec.europa.eu/health/medical-devices/documents/interpretative-documents/index_en.htm. Accessed 3 April 2012.
49. Op cit 45.
50. Notified Body Operation Group website. www.nbog.eu/2.html. Accessed 3 April 2012.
51. Op cit 13.
52. Team-NB public documents. European Association of Notified Bodies for Medical Devices website. www.team-nb.org//index.php?option=com_docman&task=cat_view&gid=17&Itemid=38. Accessed 3 April 2012.
53. Eucomed videos, images and documents. Eucomed website. www.eucomed.org/media-centre. Accessed 3 April 2012.
54. List of Contact Points Within the National Competent Authorities. EC website. http://ec.europa.eu/health/medical-devices/links/contact_points_en.htm. Accessed 3 April 2012.
55. Medicines and Healthcare products Regulatory Agency website. www.mhra.gov.uk/index.htm#page=DynamicListMedicines. Accessed 3 April 2012.
56. International Organization for Standardization website. www.iso.org/iso/home.htm. Accessed 3 April 2012.
57. International Electrotechnical Commission website. www.iec.ch/. Accessed 3 April 2012.
58. European Committee for Standardization website. www.cen.eu/cen/Pages/default.aspx. Accessed 3 April 2012.
59. European Committee for Electrotechnical Standardization website. www.cenelec.eu/. Accessed 3 April 2012.
60. British Standards Institution website. www.bsigroup.com/. Accessed 3 April 2012.
61. Dalli J. Driving Innovation in European Healthcare. Presented at the Eucomed MedTech Forum 2011, Brussels, 12 October 2011.

Chapter 9

Classification of Medical Devices

Updated by Rodney Ruston, RAC, FRAPS

OBJECTIVES

❑ Understand the difference between classes, categories and special devices

❑ Gain insight into the basic concepts and application of classification rules

❑ Learn how to find further guidance information

❑ Become aware of wider issues relating to classification

DIRECTIVES, REGULATIONS AND GUIDELINES COVERED IN THIS CHAPTER

❑ Council Directive 90/385/EEC of 20 June 1990 on the approximation of the laws of the Member States relating to active implantable medical devices

❑ Council Directive 93/42/EEC of 14 June 1993 on medical devices

❑ Directive 98/79/EC of the European Parliament and of the Council of 27 October 1998 on *in vitro* diagnostic medical devices

❑ Commission Directive 2003/12/EC of 3 February 2003 on reclassification of breast implants in the framework of Directive 93/42/EEC concerning medical devices

❑ Commission Directive 2005/50/EC of 11 August 2005 on reclassification of hip, knee and shoulder joint replacements in the framework of Directive 93/42/EEC concerning medical devices

❑ Borderline products, drug-delivery products and medical devices incorporating, as an integral part, an ancillary medicinal substance or an ancillary human blood derivative (MEDDEV 2.1/3 rev 3 December 2009)

❑ Medical devices with a measuring function (MEDDEV 2.1/5 June 1998)

❑ Guidelines on the qualification and classification of stand alone software used in healthcare within the regulatory framework of medical devices (MEDDEV 2.1/6 January 2012)

❑ Classification of medical devices (MEDDEV 2.4/1 rev 9 June 2010)

❑ Guidelines On Medical Devices: IVD Medical Device Borderline and Classification issues. A Guide For Manufacturers And Notified Bodies (MEDDEV 2.14/1 rev 2 January 2012)

❑ Manual on borderline and classification in the community regulatory framework for medical devices, European Commission (Version 1.12 (04-2012))

Regulatory Affairs Professionals Society

Introduction

There are thousands of different types of medical devices presenting varying levels of risk to patients. It would not be feasible to implement the same high level of regulatory control over them all. Since medical devices were first regulated, different attempts have been made to design categorisation or classification systems to ensure that appropriate control mechanisms are applied based on perceived risks and protection of public health. The solution adopted in the EU is a rule-based system that gauges the increasing vulnerability of a human being to a device based on factors such as the device's degree of invasiveness, its local or systemic effect and the duration of its use.

Categories and Classes

Although each of the three medical devices directives applies varying requirements to the devices it covers on the basis of criteria that, in some cases, relate to risk, only the *Medical Devices Directive* (*MDD*) contains a true classification system. This classification system is a four-category system with subcategories. The full classification hierarchy is
- Class I
- Class I (with a measuring function)
- Class I (sterile)
- Class IIa
- Class IIb
- Class III

The *Active Implantable Medical Devices Directive* (*AIMDD*) does not have a risk classification system, but products covered under it are subject to a compliance regime that is very close to the one applied in the *MDD* for Class III devices.

The *In Vitro Diagnostics Directive* (*IVDD*) differentiates between products for professional and patient use and defines the latter, called a "device for self-testing," as "any device intended by the manufacturer to be able to be used by lay persons in a home environment."[1] It also lists certain reagents and related materials thought to carry higher risks in its Annex II. So there are effectively four classes (in this case, in descending order of perceived risk):
- Annex II, List A
- Annex II, List B
- Self testing
- All others

All three directives contain provisions for a further type of medical device, which is called an "accessory." In the *MDD* and *IVDD*, this is defined as "an article which whilst not being a device is intended specifically by its manufacturer to be used together with a device to enable it to be used in accordance with the use of the device intended by the manufacturer of the device." In the *MDD* and *IVDD*, accessories are classified independently, and therefore are not necessarily in the same class as the applicable device. The *AIMDD* is slightly different in that every accessory is also an active implantable medical device.

Lastly, there exist special categories of devices outside the classification system. All three directives recognise certain categories of devices that are subject to requirements different from those for devices intended for CE marking and placing on the market. These special categories and their definitions as they appear in the *MDD* are:
- "Custom-made device," defined as: "any device specifically made in accordance with a duly qualified medical practitioner's written prescription which gives, under his responsibility, specific design characteristics and is intended for the sole use of a particular patient."[2]
- "Device intended for clinical investigation," defined as: "any device intended for use by a duly qualified medical practitioner when conducting investigations..."[3]
- Device authorised nationally "in the interest of protection of health." This category is not defined, but is usually understood to be a situation where the device is not CE marked, but there is a real clinical need for it on compassionate grounds. Some of these devices may be orphan devices.

The same or similar concepts exist in the *AIMDD* and *IVDD*.

The Classification Process in the *MDD*

The manufacturer determines the appropriate class for its device using the classification principles and rules contained in *MDD* Annex IX, based on the device's intended purpose. It is important to understand that anything said about the device by the manufacturer and its agents may be construed as forming part of the intended purpose. The *MDD* provides the following definition:

"'intended purpose' means the use for which the device is intended according to the data supplied by the manufacturer on the labelling, in the instructions and/or in promotional materials."[4]

Basic Principles of Application

MDD Annex IX contains certain basic principles that need to be understood before applying the classification rules.

The intended purpose must be achieved by a describable mode of action supported by scientific evidence. All modes of action present must be considered. The manufacturer cannot pick and choose, e.g., ignore a specific mode of action of the device that contributes to the intended purpose in order to claim the device falls into a lower class than it should.

The manufacturer must consider all the rules. Often, two or more rules may apply to the device. In such a case, the highest possible classification applies. The same principle applies for devices that can be used on different parts of the body or have multiple purposes, i.e., the application resulting in the highest possible class applies.

Individual devices that are used in a system—e.g., an extracorporeal blood circulation system containing an oxygenator, a pump and tubes—can be classified in their own right or the system can be classified as a whole, in which case the item that is in the highest class is used as the class for the whole system.

Key Concepts of Classification

The EU classification system is based on an understanding of human vulnerability in terms of certain key device characteristics and uses: time period, degree of invasiveness, use of a source of energy, biological activity and incorporation of drugs. These concepts tend to have a common sense relationship with risk, e.g., the more invasive a device and the longer it is used, the higher the risk.

Time

The duration of use of the device is categorised in terms of "normally intended continuous use:"[5]

- transient use: less than 60 minutes
- short-term use: not more than 30 days
- long-term use: more than 30 days

These are time periods of use as envisaged by the manufacturer. If an individual decides to use a device beyond the time parameters defined by the manufacturer, this would not affect the device's classification.

The concept of "continuous use" is defined as:
"An uninterrupted actual use of the device for the intended purpose. However where usage of a device is discontinued in order for the device to be replaced immediately by the same or an identical device this shall be considered an extension of the continuous use of the device."[6]

Invasiveness

Invasiveness obviously involves penetration of the body as confirmed by the general definition of an "invasive device:"
"A device which, in whole or in part, penetrates inside the body, either through a body orifice or through the surface of the body."[7]

There is a significant difference between invasiveness through a body orifice and surgical invasiveness, which involves piercing the body surface.

"Body orifice" is defined as:

"Any natural opening in the body, as well as the external surface of the eyeball, or any permanent artificial opening, such as a stoma."[8]

"Surgically invasive device" is defined as:
"An invasive device which penetrates inside the body through the surface of the body, with the aid or in the context of a surgical operation.

For the purposes of this Directive devices other than those referred to in the previous subparagraph and which produce penetration other than through an established body orifice, shall be treated as surgically invasive devices."[9]

A surgically invasive device is not necessarily something that would involve surgery. For instance, needles used for injections are regarded as surgically invasive. Surgically invasive devices may be introduced through a temporary, surgically created opening, e.g., implants. Medical gloves are another example of an invasive device.

The classification system recognises two specific subtypes of surgically invasive devices: implants and reusable surgical instruments. This distinction has been made to separate implants, which are thought to be high risk and classified in Class IIb or III, from reusable surgical instruments, which are regarded as low risk and are therefore in Class I.

This illustrates an important principle of risk classification. A scalpel can cause significant trauma if used badly, but this is outside the manufacturer's control, whereas a patient can die from a poorly designed heart valve, something for which the manufacturer would bear responsibility. Risk classification therefore relates to risk factors that the manufacturer can influence, but not those that are outside the manufacturer's control.

An "implantable device" is defined as:
"Any device which is intended:
—to be totally introduced into the human body or,
—to replace an epithelial surface or the surface of the eye,
by surgical intervention which is intended to remain in place after the procedure."[10]

Any device intended to be partially introduced into the human body through surgical intervention and intended to remain in place after the procedure for at least 30 days is also considered an "implantable device."

"Reusable surgical instrument" is defined as an:
"Instrument intended for surgical use by cutting, drilling, sawing, scratching, scraping, clamping, retracting, clipping or similar procedures, without connection to any active medical device and which can be reused after appropriate procedures have been carried out."[11]

The classification system identifies two areas of the body that are regarded as particularly vulnerable: the central circulatory and nervous systems. The "central circulatory system" is defined as:

"arteriae pulmonales, aorta ascendens, arcus aorta, aorta descendens to the bifurcatio aortae, arteriae coronariae, arteria carotis communis, arteria carotis externa, arteria carotis interna, arteriae cerebrales, truncus brachiocephalicus, venae cordis, venae pulmonales, vena cava superior, vena cava inferior."[12]

The "central nervous system" is defined as: "brain, meninges and spinal cord."[13]

Use of Energy

Energy is regarded as a risk factor because of its potential for systemic effects and the difficulty in restricting the energy to a specific location. Thus the concept of "active device" was created, which is defined as:

"Any medical device, the operation of which depends on a source of electrical energy or any source of power other than that directly generated by the human body or gravity and which acts by converting this energy. Medical devices intended to transmit energy, substances or other elements between an active medical device and the patient, without any significant change, are not considered to be active medical devices."[14]

The critical element of this definition is the concept of conversion of energy, which must produce a significant change. Such a significant change is understood to occur when the nature, level and/or density of energy changes. The effect of resistance in a wire is not regarded as a significant change. The conversion can occur in the device itself, e.g., electrical energy converted to thermal energy, or at the interface between the device and tissue, e.g., the conversion produced by the electrical scalpel blade.

Biological Activity

If a device is intended to have a biological effect or is absorbed, this action tends to push a device into a higher class.

While absorption is generally accepted as normal for some types of devices, a biological mode of action is more difficult to understand as a medical device-like action as opposed to a medicinal (drug) mode of action. The following definition clarifies this point:

"A material is considered to have a biological effect if it actively and intentionally induces, alters or prevents a response from the tissues that is mediated by specific reactions at a molecular level."[15]

"Absorption" is defined as:

"degradation of a material within the body and the metabolic elimination of the resulting degradation products from the body."[16]

Drug/Device Combinations

Integration of a drug into a medical device for an ancillary purpose makes the device a drug/device combination in Class III in most cases. If, however, the manufacturer can demonstrate that the drug substance is not liable to act on the human body, then it does not become the determinant factor in the device's class. Such "pure device" drug/device combinations can even be in Class I.

Software

Software is classified in the same way as any other medical device or accessory, except for the following principles:
- Stand alone software is considered an active medical device.
- Software that drives a device or influences the use of a device falls automatically into the same class. This can be true for both embedded and standalone software.

The European Commission issued guidance on the classification of standalone software, MEDDEV 2.1/6, January 2012. Please note this document is a guidance and is not legally binding.

Classification Rules (Annex IX)

The *MDD* classification rules are grouped into sections as follows:
- Rules 1–4 noninvasive devices
- Rules 5–8 invasive devices
- Rules 9–12 additional rules for active devices
- Rule 13–18 other special rules
  - devices incorporating ancillary action medicinal products and human blood derivatives
  - devices used for contraception or the prevention of the transmission of sexually transmitted diseases
  - devices intended specifically to be used for disinfecting, cleaning, rinsing
  - devices specifically intended for recording x-ray diagnostic images
  - devices manufactured utilising animal tissues or derivatives rendered nonviable
  - blood bags

Following is a typical example of a classification rule:
"Rule 6
All surgically invasive devices intended for transient use are in Class IIa unless they are:

- —intended specifically to control, diagnose, monitor or correct a defect of the heart or of the central circulatory system through direct contact with these parts of the body, in which case they are in Class III,
- —reusable surgical instruments, in which case they are in Class I,
- —intended specifically for use in direct contact with the central nervous system, in which case they are in Class III,
- —intended to supply energy in the form of ionising radiation, in which case they are in Class IIb,
- —intended to have a biological effect or to be wholly or mainly absorbed, in which case they are in Class IIb,
- —intended to administer medicines by means of a delivery system, if this is done in a manner that is potentially hazardous taking account of the mode of application, in which case they are in Class IIb."

Guidance on Classification

The European Commission has issued a number of guidance documents on classification, including the references at the beginning of this chapter.

Although this guidance is helpful, it is important to remember that it is not legally binding.

Classification Disputes

The manufacturer initially determines the device's class using the classification rules. If the Conformity Assessment Procedure requires the intervention of a Notified Body, the two parties must agree on the classification. If there is a disagreement that cannot be resolved between them, the Notified Body will normally go to its Competent Authority to request a solution.

A national Competent Authority may feel unsure about the classification of a specific device. It has the option of submitting its view to a review by the national Competent Authorities of other EU Member States (the so-called "Helsinki procedure"). Often, this results in diverging views expressed by the national Competent Authorities. Such cases usually are brought to the Commission's Working Group on Borderlines and Classification. If it is resolved, the solution is entered in the *Manual on Borderline and Classification*.

Classification decisions by Competent Authorities can be challenged by the manufacturer in the national courts. If the national court feels that the matter involves interpretation of a point of European law that should be resolved first, it can request a preliminary ruling from the Court of Justice of the European Union. At the time of writing, no such cases had occurred.

Reclassification Process

Although the classification rules have worked successfully since the initial adoption of the *MDD*, it is recognised that situations may arise when the rules do not produce an optimal classification result. The *MDD* contains a clause that allows changes that do not require a full legislative process:

"Where a Member State considers that the classification rules set out in Annex IX require adaptation in the light of technical progress and any information which becomes available under the information system provided for in Article 10, it may submit a duly substantiated request to the Commission and ask it to take the necessary measures for adaptation of classification rules. The measures designed to amend non-essential elements of this Directive relating to adaptation of classification rules shall be adopted in accordance with the regulatory procedure with scrutiny referred to in Article 7 (3)."[17]

Summary

The medical device classification system adopted in the EU is based on a set of rules and principles of application listed in *MDD* Annex IX. There are 18 rules that assign devices into one of the risk classes: I, IIa, IIb and III. The manufacturer applies them to its own products, taking into account the intended purpose of each device. The resulting classification determines the conformity assessment options available.

References

1. Directive 98/79/EC of the European Parliament and of the Council of 27 October 1998 on in vitro diagnostic medical devices (*IVDD*). EUR-Lex website. http://eur-lex.europa.eu/LexUriServ/LexUriServ.do?uri=CONSLEG:1998L0079:20031120:en:PDF. Accessed 3 May 2012.
2. Council Directive 90/385/EEC of 20 June 1990 on the approximation of the laws of the Member States relating to active implantable medical devices (*AIMDD*). EUR-Lex website. http://eur-lex.europa.eu/LexUriServ/LexUriServ.do?uri=CELEX:31990L0385:en:HTML. Accessed 3 May 2012.
3. Council Directive 93/42/EEC of 14 June 1993 concerning medical devices (*MDD*). EUR-Lex website. http://eur-lex.europa.eu/LexUriServ/LexUriServ.do?uri=CONSLEG:1993L0042:20071011:en:PDF. Accessed 3 May 2012.
4. *MDD*, Article 1.2(e).
5. *IVDD*, Article 1.2(d).
6. *MDD*, Annex 1, Section 13.1.
7. *MDD*, Article 1.2(g).
8. *MDD*, Annex IX, Section 1.1.
9. *MDD*, Annex IX, Section 2.6.
10. *MDD*, Annex IX, Section 1.2.
11. Ibid.
12. Ibid.
13. Ibid.
14. *MDD*, Annex IX, Section 1.3.
15. *MDD*, Annex IX, Section 1.7.
16. *MDD*, Annex IX, Section 1.8.
17. *MDD*, Annex IX, Section 1.4.

Chapter 10

Technical Requirements for Conformity Assessment

Updated by Rodney Ruston, RAC, FRAPS

OBJECTIVES

- Understand the technical requirements that need to be met in order to demonstrate conformity with the Essential Requirements of the European medical device directives

- Understand the role of European and international standards in the conformity assessment process

- Understand documentation requirements

REGULATIONS AND GUIDELINES COVERED IN THIS CHAPTER

- Council Directive 93/42/EEC of 14 June 1993 concerning medical devices

- Council Directive 90/385/EEC of 20 June 1990 on the approximation of the laws of the Member States relating to active implantable medical devices

- Council Directive 98/79/EC of 27 October 1998 on the approximation of the laws of the Member States relating to *in vitro* diagnostic medical devices

Essential Requirements

For CE marking of every type of medical device, it is necessary to demonstrate conformity with all relevant Essential Requirements contained in Annex I of the applicable European medical devices directive. Notified Bodies (NBs) will expect to see a checklist, listing all the Essential Requirements and indicating, for each one, how conformity has been demonstrated or why it is not relevant. A checklist is also required for Class I devices that are self-certified and, in such cases, provides the assurance needed to underpin the certificate of conformity.

The Essential Requirements have been devised with care and attention to detail and are the result of a systematic approach to specifying necessary and appropriate regulatory requirements. Therefore, they demand an equally ordered approach by those who wish to demonstrate compliance. Only by showing systematically how each of the Essential Requirements has been met can a manufacturer declare conformity and affix the CE Mark. Similarly, when a manufacturer has to make a compliance statement prior to commencing a clinical investigation (an "Annex VIII Statement"), an Essential Requirements checklist is indispensable in providing the signatory with the confidence that a truthful declaration has been made. Even prior to that, the checklist is a valuable tool for gap analysis during design verification.

Technical details should not be included in the Essential Requirements checklist, but standards for which compliance has been claimed should be cited and all documents providing evidence of conformity should be referenced. Such documents must be available in the Technical File (see below). An example of part of an Essential Requirements checklist is provided in **Table 10-1**.

In some way, all Essential Requirements address one of two issues: safety or performance. All the basic principles on which the directives are based are summarised within the first three Essential Requirements. These principles are:
- Devices must not compromise the patient or user's clinical condition or safety.

- Risks must be acceptable when weighed against the benefits to the patient.
- Risks must be eliminated or minimised in line with the state of the art.
- Devices must perform as intended by the manufacturer.

These concepts are difficult to quantify, but the manufacturer needs to demonstrate that it has assessed the risks and benefits of its device and that the balance is appropriate.

The remaining Essential Requirements are permutations on this theme relevant to specific circumstances or device attributes. These are:
- chemical, physical and biological properties
- infection and microbial contamination
- construction and environmental properties
- devices with a measuring function
- protection against radiation
- devices connected to or equipped with an energy source
- information supplied by the manufacturer

Use of Standards

A standard is a consensus document. The Global Harmonization Task Force (GHTF) sees international consensus standards as a tool for harmonising regulatory processes to assure medical devices' safety, quality and performance. The International Standards Organization (ISO) defines a "standard" as a document, established by consensus and approved by a recognised body, which provides, for common and repeated use, rules, guidelines or characteristics for activities or their results, aimed at the achievement of the optimum degree of order in a given context. It further notes that standards should be based on the consolidated results of science, technology and experience and aimed at the promotion of optimum benefit to the community.

The consensus described in the standard was reached by the members of the committee that wrote it, as influenced by the comments of those who participated in the consultation phases. The way standards-writing bodies are constituted and carry out their tasks, therefore, affects the quality of a standard, which should be an important factor in the extent to which a particular standard is used. It is good practice to consider objectively the extent to which the use of a standard ensures compliance with the Essential Requirements and identify any aspects of conformity assessment that need to be addressed by other means. This chapter, therefore, presents some general observations about the nature of standards and the way they are generated. First, however, it is important to consider the critical role that standards play in the European system of medical device regulation.

Regulatory Status of European Standards

The nature and role of standards in the regulatory process is explained in recitals at the beginning of the medical device directives. Because the Essential Requirements of the directives are designed to cover a wide variety of aspects of safety and performance of a wide variety of products, it is recognised that they cannot provide the level of technical detail required to address everything that is relevant to conformity assessment. It is the role of standards to provide this level of detail. The basis for this arrangement lies in the "New Approach" to European regulation, adopted in 1985, based on the principle that the establishment of an internal European market with free movement of goods and services is critically dependent on technical harmonisation. Dismantling the barriers to trade that previously existed within Europe required a mechanism to ensure technical equivalence of goods in terms of safety and critical performance. The European standards bodies were given the task of drawing up technical specifications to meet the Essential Requirements of the various New Approach directives. Inherent in the New Approach is the expectation that compliance with such specifications provides a presumption of conformity with the Essential Requirements.

In practice, this means the European Commission "mandates" the European Standardisation Committee (CEN) or Electrotechnical Commision (CENELEC) to develop the standards considered necessary for demonstrating compliance with the Essential Requirements in one or more of the directives. CEN (or CENELEC) develops a relevant document, normally through cooperation with ISO. Typically, an international standard is developed by a working group within an ISO technical committee and published by European national standards bodies as a dual EN/ISO standard. Not all European standards are harmonised, however. Once the standard has been approved for publication as a European standard, advisors to CEN review it to verify that it is adequate for the task of conformity assessment. If it is, a reference to the standard is published in the *Official Journal of the European Communities* (*OJ*). This process is termed "harmonisation" and the resulting document is known as a harmonised European standard. Lists of harmonised standards are available from the European Commission website (www.europa.eu) and are periodically published in the *OJ*.[3]

An annex in the European version of each harmonised standard indicates the Essential Requirements for which the standard is deemed relevant. By referencing such information and showing compliance with the requirements of the standard, a manufacturer can claim conformity with specific Essential Requirements. This should not be seen as a box-checking exercise; it is necessary to confirm that the standard is indeed appropriate and adequate for demonstrating full compliance. The process is set out in Article 5 of the *MDD*. In summary, a harmonised standard is deemed

Technical Requirements for Conformity Assessment

Table 10-1. Essential Requirement Check List: Example (*MDD* (Directive 93/42/EEC), as amended—Annex I)

	Requirements	A—N/A	Standard/Rationale	Reference to Documents
I.	General Requirements			
1	The devices must be designed and manufactured in such a way that, when used under the conditions and for the purposes intended, they will not compromise the clinical condition or the safety of patients, or the safety and health of users or, where applicable, other persons, provided that any risks which may be associated with their intended use constitute acceptable risks when weighed against the benefits to the patient and are compatible with a high level of protection of health and safety. This shall include: • reducing, as far as possible, the risk of use error due to the ergonomic features of the device and the environment in which the device is intended to be used (design for patient safety), and • consideration of the technical knowledge, experience, education and training and, where applicable, the medical and physical conditions of intended users (design for lay, professional, disabled or other users).	A	Risks to patients and users have been controlled through application of X-XXX-XXX, risk management and analysis procedure, which complies with EN/ISO 14971-2007. A clinical evaluation was carried out in line with European Commission guidance document MEDDEV 2.7.1 Rev.3.	Risk analysis report XXXX. Clinical evaluation report XXXX.
2	The solutions adopted by the manufacturer for the design and construction of the devices must conform to safety principles, taking account of the generally acknowledged state of the art. In selecting the most appropriate solutions, the manufacturer must apply the following principles in the following order: • eliminate or reduce risks as far as possible (inherently safe design and construction) • where appropriate, take adequate protection measures including alarms if necessary, in relation to risks that cannot be eliminated • inform users of the residual risks due to any shortcomings of the protection measures adopted	A	Risk management procedure (X-XXX-XXX), which complies with EN/ISO 14971-2007, includes specification of safety requirements (safety by design, alarms, etc.) and labelling requirements for residual risks.	Risk analysis report XXXX.

necessary and sufficient to carry the presumption of conformity with the Essential Requirements of the relevant European directive.

It is not obligatory to use harmonised standards to demonstrate compliance with the Essential Requirements. It is up to a manufacturer to show compliance through any means considered appropriate. Manufacturers may choose to use an ISO standard where no harmonised CEN standard exists. Alternatively, national or in-house standards (e.g., standard operating procedures (SOPs)) can be used. In any event, SOPs should contain a justification for the methods chosen and include references to the applicable standards, indicating the degree to which compliance with each standard is required. Wherever alternative routes to harmonised standards are used, questions from Competent Authorities and NBs can arise, and a justification for the departure from the norm will be required. The justification should cover the reasons why a harmonised standard is not used and why the methods chosen are appropriate and adequate for the job.

The Nature of Consensus

The purpose of the standards-writing process is to produce a document that is a clear statement of the technical state of the art, particularly with regard to expectations of safety and performance. It is not by accident, therefore, that participants in a working group are called "experts." They should be put forward for membership on the working group by their national standards body because of their high level of relevant expertise. Most of the necessary expertise resides within industry; therefore, it is not surprising that standards committees are dominated by industry representatives.

A criticism often levelled at the standards-writing process is the inadequate or inappropriate level of input from regulatory agencies. Most European Competent Authorities rarely participate in ISO working groups. The comparative lack of relevant technical expertise within Competent Authorities is one reason; another is the perception that it is not the role of the regulatory agency to develop the consensus. It is, however, the agency's role to object when it considers a standard inadequate, and the means is provided by Paragraph 3 of Article 5 of the *MDD*. Where Competent Authorities do participate, they often help to direct the focus of a standard toward its role in conformity assessment. Conversely, US Food and Drug Administration (FDA) officials involved in standards writing often have a high level of technical expertise but participate with the understanding that their agency is not obliged to adopt the standard as a regulatory component. Officials from Japan, China and Korea tend to combine both technical expertise and reliance on standards in their regulations and are increasingly important players in the process.

In addition to technical expertise, therefore, the standards writer must have a keen appreciation of the role the standard will play in the regulatory process and the nuances

Regulatory Affairs Professionals Society

Table 10-2. Hierarchy of Compliance Documents for Technical Documentation

Directive	Directive 90/385/EEC	Directive 93/42/EEC	Directive 98/79/EC
Level 1 Essential Requirements	✓	✓	✓
Level 2 Common Technical Specifications (CTS)	Not applicable		✓
Level 3 Harmonised Standards	✓	✓	✓
Level 4 EU Commission MEDDEV documents	✓	✓	✓
Level 5 Other international, national and nationally accepted standards	✓	✓	✓
Level 6 Industry and company created standards	✓	✓	✓

of language used in standards. For example, there is a critical difference between a normative (or mandatory) requirement (i.e., "shall") and guidance ("should"). There is a responsibility to ensure that the requirements are sufficient to ensure safety and essential performance but are not unnecessarily onerous or restrictive. The wider purpose of a standard is to assist industry and commerce, so it is a delicate balancing act. The user of the standard should also appreciate these points.

In the 20 years since medical device standards were first written with a defined European regulatory purpose in mind, there have been, on the whole, significant improvements in the quality of the standards. In the past, there have been standards that were deemed unsuitable for harmonisation, but that situation should be less likely today. The process is monitored by national standards committees, Competent Authorities, industry groups and other interested and affected parties, and this oversight helps to identify problems and ensure that the product is fit for its purpose. Using a harmonised standard is thus the most convenient and safest way to demonstrate conformity with the Essential Requirements.

Identifying and Referencing Applicable Standards

Generic standards, relevant to all devices or a wide range of product types, are termed "horizontal" (or Level 1) standards. Examples are standards on quality systems, risk management, biological safety and sterilization. "Semi-horizontal" (Level 2) standards contain requirements applicable to a range of similar products, such as endovascular devices or surgical instruments. "Vertical" (Level 3) standards apply to single product types or a range of closely related products, such as vascular stents or surgical scalpels.

National standards bodies, from which standards can be purchased, provide searchable listings on their websites. These generally provide enough information to determine the scope of the standard cited. A list of harmonised standards can be found on the European Commission website (http://ec.europa.eu/enterprise/policies/european-standards/harmonised-standards/index_en.htm)). A search of these sources should reveal all the standards that may be applicable to a product.

There are a number of places within the technical documentation where it is necessary to list all standards that have been applied, in full or in part, to the product. This list is important in the Investigator's Brochure for a premarket clinical investigation and for the Essential Requirements checklist. This requirement is often applied as an afterthought and interpreted as a simple list of all the standards that are relevant and to which some degree of compliance can be shown. A slap-dash approach here can lead to significant problems or delays in regulatory approval. However, the objective of this regulatory requirement is to allow a precise indication of the extent to which conformity with the Essential Requirements can be presumed through the application of harmonised standards. Unless the extent of compliance with a standard is clearly specified, conformity cannot be established in this way.

It makes sense to map out the way conformity will be established early in the product development process. The Essential Requirements checklist is a good place to start such planning. The standards that are potentially relevant can be mapped against the checklist and reviewed to establish whether they are indeed applicable or whether alternative or additional means of conformity assessment are necessary. Whenever a standard is used for the presumption of conformity, any departure from complete compliance should be noted and its significance to compliance with the relevant Essential Requirements taken into account. The reports that are cited alongside references to the applicable standards in the Essential Requirements checklist should clearly indicate any aspect of noncompliance with a standard, the reasons for this and the alternative measures that have been taken to ensure full compliance with the Essential Requirements.

Table 10-2 summarises the hierarchy for using the above sources in creating the Technical Documentation.

Technical Documentation

A number of terms are used to describe the collection of documents that describe how a manufacturer has demonstrated the conformity of its product with the Essential Requirements. The directives speak of technical documentation as a generic term and mention the "design dossier" in the context of NB review, where applicable (i.e., for devices requiring design examination, mainly Class III products). However, there is no definition of this term in the directives. Design dossier should be used to refer to those parts of the "technical file" (also not defined in any directive) that are put together and made available to the NB for review. Technical documentation has to be kept available by the manufacturer or its Authorised Representative for review by the Competent Authority, and there are a number of circumstances where the NB has to examine it.

There are no rules about the technical file's format or location. The documents that make up the technical file are relevant to regulatory compliance and are thus considered critical to product quality. They, therefore, need to be part of the manufacturer's controlled documentation system.

Like their location, the contents of a technical file are indeterminate. However, Annex VII Secton 3 of the *MDD* contains a useful guide. As a minimum, the file must contain everything that can be referenced via the Essential Requirements checklist and anything else relevant to product design and regulatory compliance. Regrettably, there is a blurring of the borders between what should be in the technical file and what should be in the Quality System. This blurring is resulting in double auditing, as matters formerly considered to be the province of the Quality System are now requested in the technical file, e.g., inspection techniques at the manufacturing stage, of which sterilisation procedures are a classic example. Typical contents of a technical file are:

- product identification and regulatory classification
- literature reviews
- design input assumptions and calculations
- design history
- design and manufacturing specifications
- quality plan and rationale for quality control measures
- process validation and design verification reports
- verification of packaging and product stability
- labelling (including information provided with the device)
- postmarket surveillance data and/or plan
- Essential Requirements checklist
- risk management file (including risk management plan and report)
- clinical evaluation report

Relevant SOPs and standards are also referenced by the Essential Requirements checklist and are important elements of conformity assessment. They show how compliance has been achieved and are of interest to assessors. Thus, although they do not contain results relevant to the product, they may be relevant to the technical file.

Guidance on the technical documentation needed to meet the requirements of the medical devices directives is provided by a "recommendation" document produced by the European Association of Medical Device Notified Bodies (NB-MED).[8] The primary purpose of this guidance is to document the consensus view of the Notified Bodies' Recommendations Group on appropriate Conformity Assessment Procedures. However, the document notes that it is also of relevance to Competent Authorities and manufacturers. Although published in 2000, this guidance is still definitive. However, in interpreting its contents, attention should be paid to more recent changes in conformity assessment expectations, for example in the area of clinical evaluation and postmarket clinical follow-up. The NB-MED recommendation contains information on the following topics which, where applicable, should be considered required components of the technical file:

- content of technical documentation
- general description of the device
- description of the device's intended use and operation
- devices incorporating a medicinal substance
- devices incorporating nonviable materials of animal origin
- devices requiring special consideration
- description of the methods of manufacture
- description of accessories, adaptors and other devices or equipment and other interfaces intended to be used in combination with the device
- classification of the device under the relevant directive
- identification of technical requirements
- solutions adopted to fulfil the Essential Requirements
- standards applied
- results of risk analysis
- specification of materials and manufacturing processes (including special processes)
- specifications, drawings and circuit diagrams for components, sub-assemblies and the complete product, software and packaging
- specification of checks, tests and trials intended to be carried out as part of routine production
- performances and compatibilities intended by the manufacturer
- labelling, including any instructions for use
- identification of "shelf-life" reflected by any "use by" date or other "lifetime" of the device
- bench testing results

- clinical data
- documentation and reporting of design changes
- Declaration of Conformity
- application for conformity assessment
- declaration that no other NB is used in conformity assessment
- NB decisions and reports
- manufacturer's undertaking on procedure to review postproduction experience
- recommended structure of the technical documentation
- availability of the technical documentation
- language of the technical documentation

The Place of the Predicate Device

It is important to underscore the fact that the EU regulatory processes for medical devices do not require comparison to a predicate device. Each new submission is required to ensure the data supplied demonstrate conformity with the Essential Requirements. It is not acceptable to produce data that demonstrate the "new" device has the same or better characteristics than a device already on the market.

There are two reasons for this approach. First, no one knows what devices are on the market in the EU. There is neither a central EU database nor any Member State-specific databases. This makes it impossible to find a predicate device. Neither can a predicate device be used that has been cleared under a different legal jurisdiction, since the conditions, verifications and validations used under that jurisdiction are not known to the EU authorities. And full harmonisation of product assessments is not yet available, despite 20 years of GHTF. The second reason for this approach is that it mandates a return to basic principles for each device, and therefore prevents 'drift' where Device B is just so slightly different from Predicate A; Device C is slightly different from Predicate B, etc.

The advantage of this approach is that it is easier to place new devices on the market. The disadvantage is for "me-too" devices, where, despite being equal in every way, the new device must be submitted to exactly the same testing. This can be very difficult, especially in relation to preclinical work, where governments place limits on repeat work with animals.

Summary

This chapter discusses:
- the relationship between the Essential Requirements, harmonised standards and other publicly available documents
- the central roles of the Essential Requirements checklist in the compilation of technical files
- outline of the contents of a techncial file
- predicate devices and the technical file

References

1. Council Directive 93/42/EEC of 14 June 1993 concerning medical devices. EUR-Lex website. http://eur-lex.europa.eu/LexUriServ/LexUriServ.do?uri=CONSLEG:1993L0042:20071011:en:PDF. Accessed 20 May 2012.
2. Council Directive 90/385/EEC of 20 June 1990 on the approximation of the laws of the Member States relating to active implantable medical devices. EUR-Lex website. http://eur-lex.europa.eu/LexUriServ/LexUriServ.do?uri=CELEX:31990L0385:en:HTML. Accessed 20 May 2012.
3. For example: *Official Journal of the European Union*; C 183/15–C 183/43; 7.7.2010. EUR-Lex website. http://eur-lex.europa.eu/LexUriServ/LexUriServ.do?uri=OJ:C:2010:183:FULL:EN:PDF. Accessed 20 May 2012.
4. IEC 56/629/CD Dependability management—Part 3-13: Application Guide—Project risk management. International Electrotechnical Commission, Geneva (1998).
5. See Annex C of ISO 14971:2007.
6. See Annexes D and E of ISO 14971:2007 for guidance and a discussion of the relevant concepts.
7. See Annex D.8 of ISO 14971:2007.
8. NB-MED/2.5.1/Rec5 Rev4: Technical Documentation.
9. Williams DF. "Fundamental aspects of biocompatibility." *Biocompatibility*, 1, CRC Press, 1980; and Williams DF. "Definitions in Biomaterials." *Progress in Biomedical Engineering*, 4, 1-72, 1987.
10. Tinkler J J B. *Biological safety and European medical device regulations*. Quality First International Press, London, England; 2000.
11. ISO 10993-1:2009 Biological evaluation of medical devices: Evaluation and testing within a risk management process.
12. ISO/TR 15499 Guidance on the conduct of biological evaluation within a risk management process.
13. ISO 10993-17, Method for the establishment of allowable limits for leachable substances.
14. ISO 10993-7, Ethylene oxide sterilization residuals.
15. See Annex C of ISO 10993-18, Chemical characterization of materials.
16. MHRA Guidance Note 5: *Guidance on Biocompatibility Assessment*, 2006, updated February 2011. MHRA website. www.mhra.gov.uk/home/groups/es-era/documents/publication/con007509.pdf. Accessed 20 May 2012.

Chapter 11

Clinical Evaluation of Medical Devices

By Rodney Ruston, RAC, FRAPS

OBJECTIVES

- Understand the requirement for clinical evaluations in the EU

- Understand the literature review route for providing a clinical evaluation

- Understand the clinical investigation route for providing a clinical evaluation

- Provide references to key laws, guidance and standards required for clinical evaluations

- Provide guidance on the roles of the EU regulatory organisations in the clinical evaluation process

- Understand the differences in clinical evaluations between medical devices, active implantable medical devices and in vitro diagnostic medical devices

LAWS, GUIDELINES AND STANDARDS COVERED IN THIS CHAPTER

- Council Directive 90/385/EEC of 20 June 1990 on the approximation of the laws of the Member States relating to active implantable medical devices, Article 10 and Annexes 6 and 7

- Council Directive 93/42/EEC of 14 June 1993 concerning medical devices, Article 15 and Annexes VIII and X

- Council Directive 98/79/EC on *in vitro* diagnostic medical devices, Article 9 and Annex VIII

- Clinical Evaluation: A Guide for Manufacturers and Notified Bodies, MEDDEV 2.7.1 Rev.3 (December 2009)

- Guide for competent authorities in making an assessment of clinical investigation Notification, MEDDEV 2.7.2 Rev 1 (December 2008)

- Guidelines on clinical investigation: A guide for manufacturers and Notified Bodies, MEDDEV 2.7.4 Rev1 (December 2010)

- Clinical Investigations: Serious Adverse Event Reporting Under Directives 90/385/EEC AND 93/42/EEC, MEDDEV 2.7.3 (December 2010)

- Post market clinical follow-up studies: A guide for manufacturers and Notified Bodies, MEDDEV 2.12.2 Rev2 (January 2012)

- Checklist for audit of Notified Body's review of Clinical Data/Clinical Evaluation, NBOG CL 2010-1 (March 2010)

- Guidance for Manufacturers on Clinical Investigations to be Carried out in the UK, MHRA Guidance Bulletin No1. (February 2012)

Chapter 11

- EN 14155-1:2011, Clinical Investigation of medical devices for human subjects—Good Clinical Practice

- EN 13612:2002, Performance evaluation of in vitro diagnostic medical devices

Clinical Evaluation

All three EU directives on medical devices (*Active Implantable Medical Devices Directive* (*AIMDD*), *In Vitro Diagnostic Directive* (*IVDD*) and *Medical Devices Directive* (*MDD*)) require the manufacturer to demonstrate that the device to be placed on the market in the EU and EEA:
- performs to its intended purpose
- is such that when used according to its stated purpose, the benefits from its use outweigh the residual risks
- conforms to the Essential Requirements laid out in Annex 1 (*AIMDD*)/Annex I (*MDD* and *IVDD*)

Both the *MDD* and the *AIMDD* require a clinical evaluation to demonstrate conformity to the Essential Requirements: "Demonstration of conformity with the essential requirements must include a clinical evaluation" (*AIMDD*, Annex 1, 5a, and *MDD* Annex I, 6a). The scope of that clinical evaluation depends on the device class and the clinical data available.

Figure 11-1 is a clinical evaluation flow diagram for all types of devices, whether active implantable medical devices (Class I, IIa, IIb and III) or in vitro diagnostic medical devices.

The first step is to determine whether clinical data are appropriate to demonstrate conformity to the Essential Requirements. Although this point is the first in this flow diagram, it is the last point in Section 1 of Annex X (*MDD*) or Annex 7 (*AIMDD*). The definition of "clinical data" is reproduced in **Table 11-1**. Based on that definition, clinical data have two key features:
1. they must be generated from the use of the device and
2. they must be sourced from clinical investigations or other clinical experience

So, data generated from preclinical work are not clinical data. Data generated from bench assessments, tests and validations are not clinical data. Grasping this definition of clinical data is crucial in a world where the term can be used somewhat indiscriminately.

The first question/decision box in the flow diagram is: "Is demonstration of conformity with Essential Requirements based on clinical data appropriate?" Clearly, clinical data cannot be generated if the device does not come into contact or act directly on the patient. (Inserting "act directly on" covers, for example, therapeutic or diagnostic devices that act on the patient through electromagnetic radiation such as ultrasound, infra-red, laser, ultra-violet, alpha, beta, gamma, neutron and other particle radiation). Devices that do not contact the patient directly would include all in vitro diagnostic devices; washer-disinfectors, disinfection fluids for devices and a number of Class I devices; and various accessories for both medical and active implantable medical devices. This list is not exhaustive.

If the use of clinical data is not appropriate, then "adequate justification for any such exclusion has to be given based on risk management output and under consideration of the specifics of the device/body interaction, the clinical performances intended and the claims of the manufacturer" (*MDD*, Annex X, 1.1d, *AIMDD*, Annex 7, 1.5). Obviously such a justification must be clearly documented.

For devices for which clinical data have been shown to be "not appropriate," the directive prescribes performance evaluation, bench testing and preclinical evaluation alone. As written, all three methods are prescribed for clinical evaluation data. However, whether that is careless drafting (it does occur) or an actual prescription is open to question. Since a logical exception from clinical data has been provided in the directive, which is of far greater impact, it seems reasonable to assume that exceptions can be made for one or more of the lesser "performance evaluation, bench testing and preclinical evaluation," noting that it is difficult to differentiate between performance evaluation and bench testing. Performance evaluation is a subset of bench testing.

For in vitro diagnostic medical devices, requirements for performance evaluation are set out in the harmonised standard EN 13612:2002. As with every harmonised standard, compliance is not mandatory in order to meet the directive's legal requirements. However, compliance with the harmonised standard is deemed presumption of conformance with the directive. Furthermore, if the harmonised standard is not used, then "duly justified reasons" must be given for not using it (*IVDD*, Article 5, last two paragraphs).

The next action required on the flow chart is: "Undertake a Literature Review." As written in the directives, it would appear that the manufacturer may carry out either a literature review or a clinical investigation, or both as a clinical evaluation. At this point the flow chart deliberately takes a different route. It requires a literature review or a literature review and a clinical investigation. The point here is, in practice, no clinical investigation should be considered or attempted without a literature review. A review is a requirement for the justification for the clinical investigation design (EN 14155, A.3 and Clause 5.3).

Having completed the literature review, the next step is prescribed in both the *AIMDD* and *MDD*, and concerns implantable devices (active, Class IIa, Class IIb) and all devices in Class III. For these devices there is a first check question before moving to answering the question on the adequacy of the literature review: "Is it duly justified to

Figure 11-1. Clinical Evaluation Flow Diagram for all Device Types (including in vitro diagnostic devices)

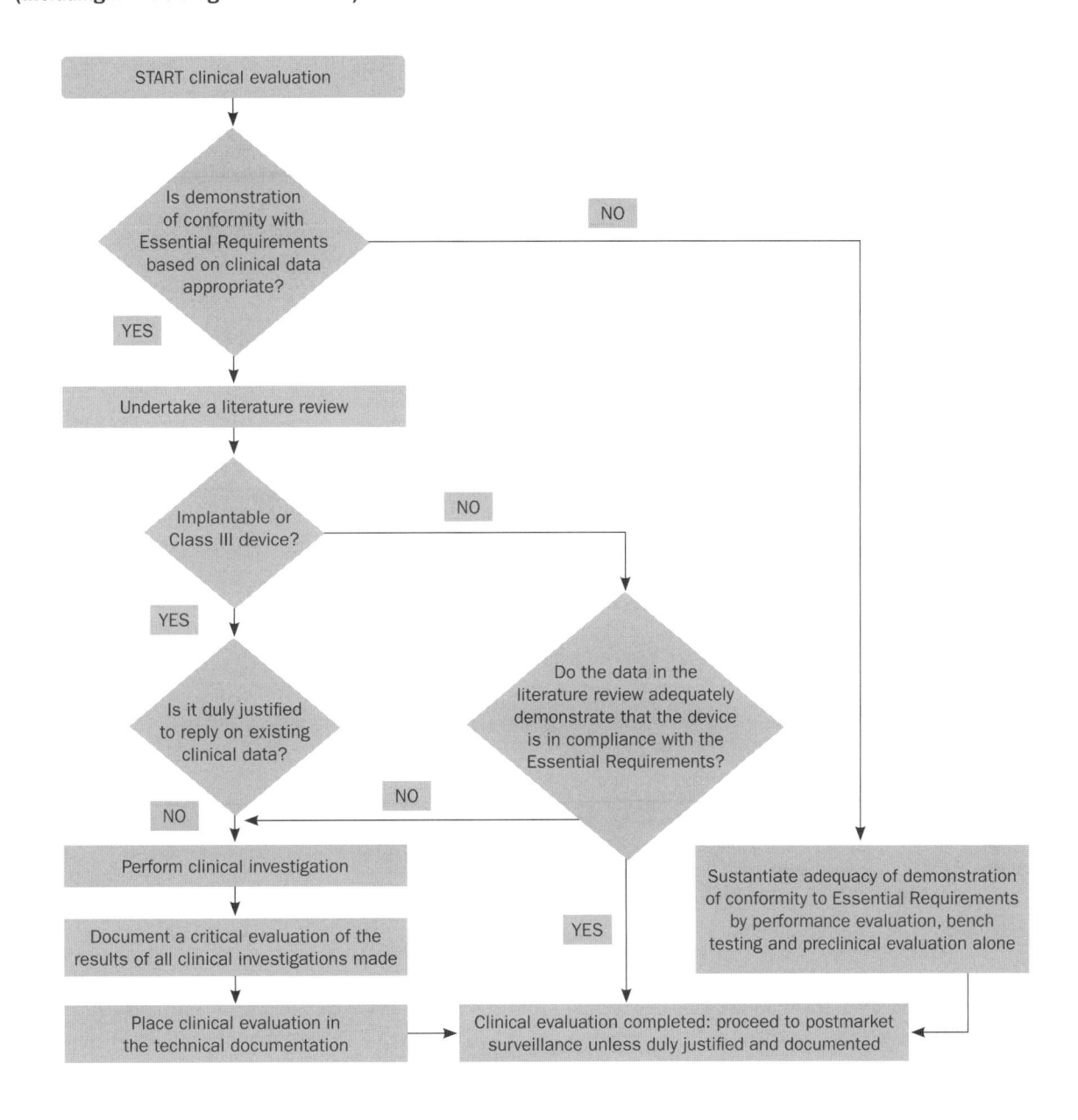

```
START clinical evaluation
          │
          ▼
Is demonstration of conformity with
Essential Requirements based on clinical
data appropriate?
  │ YES                    │ NO ─────────────────────┐
  ▼                                                   │
Undertake a literature review                         │
          │                                           │
          ▼                                           │
Implantable or Class III device?                      │
  │ YES          │ NO ──────────┐                     │
  ▼                             ▼                     │
Is it duly justified to    Do the data in the         │
rely on existing           literature review          │
clinical data?             adequately demonstrate     │
  │ NO          │           that the device is in     │
  │             │           compliance with the       │
  │             │           Essential Requirements?   │
  │             │            │ NO        │ YES        │
  ▼             ▼            ▼           │            ▼
Perform clinical investigation           │   Sustantiate adequacy of demonstration
          │                              │   of conformity to Essential Requirements
          ▼                              │   by performance evaluation, bench
Document a critical evaluation of the    │   testing and preclinical evaluation alone
results of all clinical investigations made
          │                              │            │
          ▼                              ▼            │
Place clinical evaluation in   →  Clinical evaluation completed: proceed to postmarket
the technical documentation       surveillance unless duly justified and documented  ←
```

rely on existing clinical data?" (*AIMDD*, Annex 7, 1.2 and *MDD* Annex X, 1.1a). If the answer is yes, compliance with the Essential Requirements as demonstrated by the literature review must be documented for all devices.

Clinical Evaluation: A Guide for Manufacturers and Notified Bodies, MEDDEV 2.7.1 Rev. 3, contains excellent and detailed guidance on compiling a literature review and should be consulted. It is very difficult to improve upon, and therefore not repeated here.

If, following the literature review, it is concluded that it is not "duly justified to rely on existing clinical data," then the box is "Perform a clinical investigation." However, for further assistance on deciding whether to perform a clinical investigation, the advice from the Medicines and Health product Regulatory Agency's (MHRA) *Guidance for Manufacturers on Clinical Investigations to be Carried out in the UK* is invaluable. It says:

Table 11-1. Abbreviations, Definitions and Terms Used in This Chapter

Adverse event	Any untoward medical occurrence, unintended disease or injury or untoward clinical signs (including abnormal laboratory findings) in subjects, users or other persons, whether or not related to the investigational medical device. (EN 14155)
AIMDD	*Active Implantable Medical Devices Directive* (Directive 90/385/EEC)
Clinical data	Safety and/or performance information generated from the use of a device. Clinical data are sourced from: —clinical investigation(s) of the device concerned; or —clinical investigation(s) or other studies reported in the scientific literature, of a similar device for which equivalence to the device in question can be demonstrated; or —published and/or unpublished reports on other clinical experience of either the device in question or a similar device for which equivalence to the device in question can be demonstrated. (*MDD*)
Clinical evaluation	Assessment and analysis of clinical data pertaining to a medical device to verify the clinical safety and performance of the device when used as intended by the manufacturer.
Clinical evidence	The clinical data and the clinical evaluation report pertaining to a medical device.
Clinical investigation	Any systematic investigation or study in or on one or more human subjects, undertaken to assess the safety and/or performance of a medical device. (EN 14155).
Clinical Investigation Plan (CIP)	Document that states the rationale, objectives, design and proposed analysis, methodology, monitoring, conduct and recordkeeping of the clinical investigation. (EN 14155)
Ethics Committee	Independent body whose responsibility it is to review clinical investigations in order to protect the rights, safety and well-being of human subjects participating in a clinical investigation.
ICH	International Conference on Harmonisation of Technical Requirements for Registration of Pharmaceuticals for Human Use (International Conference on Harmonisation)
IVDD	*In Vitro Diagnostics Medical Devices Directive* (Directive 98/79/EC)
Literature review	Critical evaluation of the relevant scientific literature currently available relating to the safety, performance, design characteristics and intended purpose of the device where: —there is demonstration of equivalence of the device to the device to which the data relates, and —the data adequately demonstrate compliance with the relevant essential requirements. (*MDD*, Annex X, 1.1.1; *AIMDD* Annex 7, 1.1.1)
MDD	*Medical Devices Directive* (Directive 93/42/EEC)
Notification Date	Date on which application to carry out a clinical investigation arrives at a Competent Authority.
Performance evaluation	Investigation of the performance of a medical device based on data already available and/or performance evaluation studies.
Performance evaluation study	Investigation of an in vitro diagnostic medical device intended to validate performance claims under the anticipated conditions of use.

"A clinical investigation of a non-CE-marked medical device should at least be considered in the following circumstances:
- the device is an implantable or Class III medical device;
- the introduction of a completely new concept of device into clinical practice where components, features and/or methods of action, are previously unknown;
- where an existing device is modified in such a way that it contains a novel feature particularly if such a feature has an important physiological effect; or where the modification might significantly affect the clinical performance and/or safety of the device;
- where a device incorporates materials previously untested in humans, coming into contact with the human body or where existing materials are applied to a new location in the human body or where the materials are to be used for a significantly longer time than previously, in which case compatibility and biological safety will need to be considered;
- where a device, either CE-marked or non-CE-marked, is proposed for a new purpose or function;
- where in vitro and/or animal testing of the device cannot mimic the clinical situation;
- where there is a new manufacturer especially of a high-risk device."

The Clinical Investigation

MDD Annex X, 2 (*AMIDD* Annex 7, 2) describes the elements of a clinical investigation. These are further amplified in the *Harmonised Standard on Clinical Investigations*, EN

14155. In fact, along with the European Commission's MEDDEV documents, the Notified Body Operations Group (NBOG) documents and Global Harmonization Task Force (GHTF) documents, a large body of information is available. There are also drug regulatory documents from the International Conference on Harmonisation (ICH) that can be applied.

With the above plethora of information, this chapter will concentrate on the process, rather than the detailed content of a clinical investigation. **Figure 11-2** is a flow diagram of the clinical investigation process. For simplicity, some details have been omitted from the flow diagram. The following paragraphs describe the process, with box numbers on **Figure 11-2** to identify which part of the process is being described. (There are not comments for every box.)

Please note that all activities in this section on clinical investigation related to submission to the Competent Authorities can be carried out by the manufacturer's Authorised Representative.

Box 1

The first step (Box 1) is to create a Clinical Investigation Plan (CIP). Descriptions of the expected contents of such a plan are given in EN 14155 and other documents listed at the beginning of this chapter. This plan should not be merely some initial ideas or thoughts, but the final plan. (However, there are occasions where an outline plan may be useful in order to gauge probable reaction.) Although the directive does not require the Notified Body (NB) to be involved at this early stage of a clinical investigation, it is good practice to set up a consultation with the chosen NB about the proposed investigation. An NB is not able to prescribe advice, but short of that, a good NB can prevent pitfalls.

Box 2

Box 2 is only needed if the protocol calls for clinical investigation centres in Member States whose language is different to the original protocol. Translations take resources (time and money).

While the CIP is awaiting approvals from Ethics Committees (in some cases, four to six months), it is time to ensure that the devices for clinical investigations meet the requirements of *MDD* Annex VIII, 2.2, 3.2 and 4 (*AIMDD* Annex 6, 2.2, 3.2 and 4).

Box 4

Ethics Committees across Member States could request changes to the protocol. Because of cultural differences, e.g., in southern Europe compared to northern, these changes could be in opposition to each other, creating difficulties for reconciliation into a single CIP.

Box 5

The directive talks about a "Notification Date," without specifying that Competent Authorities are required to acknowledge receipt. This means the CIP submission should be sent to the Competent Authorities via a shipping method that records the delivery date and requires a signature for delivery. Note that Member States use their own application forms for the submission. Also, some Member States evaluate the submission at no charge. Others charge a fee based on the class of device in the clinical investigation.

Boxes 7 and 8

The directive is not clear on when the sponsor can begin the clinical investigation. It seems to give the Competent Authorities the option of not replying at all and, therefore, clearance by default; or, even if there are no objections, sending a letter granting permission, stating 'no objections—you are permitted to proceed.' One difficulty that can arise is a rejection by one Member State and acceptance by another. The same problems can occur as were identified in describing Box 4: the cultural difference between southern and northern Europe; what is perfectly acceptable in one zone is not acceptable in the other.

Box 9

During the clinical investigation, there are two document outputs that contain data. The Case Report Forms, which contain the data collected from each subject on which information to be reported to the sponsor is recorded. Second are the Adverse Incident Forms. The latter are submitted to the Competent Authorities using the MEDDEV 2.7.3, *Clinical Investigations: Serious Adverse Event Reporting Under Directives 90/385/EEC and 93/42/EEC*, as opposed to general postmarket vigilance reporting. Reportable events must be reported at the same time to all national Competent Authorities where the clinical investigation has commenced, using the summary tabulation featured in MEDDEV 2.7.3's appendix. (A list of clinical investigation contact points within the national Competent Authorities is published on the Commission's homepage).

Although not specifically mentioned in the directives, any changes to the CIP should be recorded, with a justification why they were or were not reported to the Competent Authorities.

Box 10

It is important to advise the Competent Authorities of the completion of the clinical investigation, or the reason for an early termination.

Chapter 11

Figure 11-2. The Clinical Investigation Process

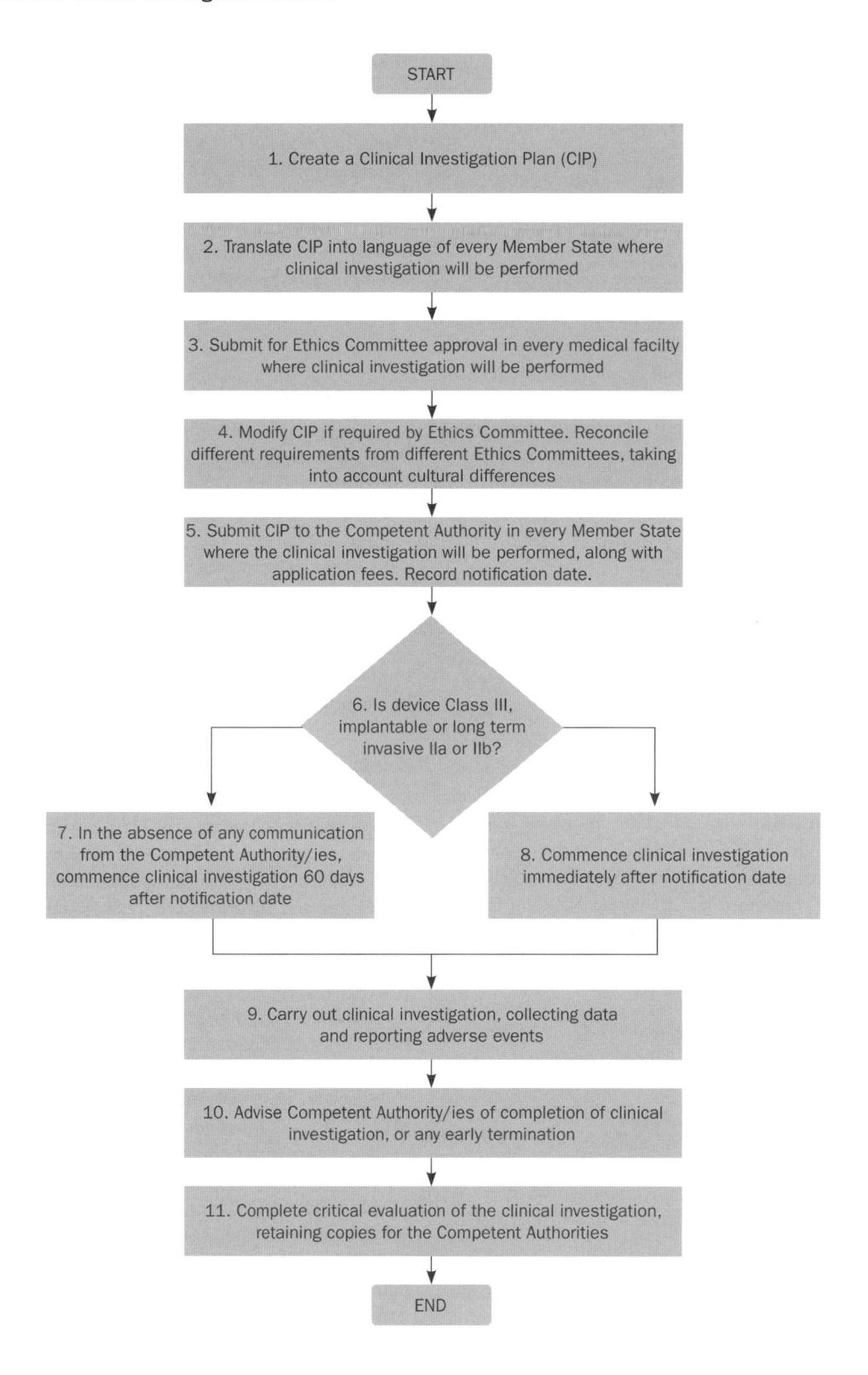

START

1. Create a Clinical Investigation Plan (CIP)

2. Translate CIP into language of every Member State where clinical investigation will be performed

3. Submit for Ethics Committee approval in every medical facilty where clinical investigation will be performed

4. Modify CIP if required by Ethics Committee. Reconcile different requirements from different Ethics Committees, taking into account cultural differences

5. Submit CIP to the Competent Authority in every Member State where the clinical investigation will be performed, along with application fees. Record notification date.

6. Is device Class III, implantable or long term invasive IIa or IIb?

7. In the absence of any communication from the Competent Authority/ies, commence clinical investigation 60 days after notification date

8. Commence clinical investigation immediately after notification date

9. Carry out clinical investigation, collecting data and reporting adverse events

10. Advise Competent Authority/ies of completion of clinical investigation, or any early termination

11. Complete critical evaluation of the clinical investigation, retaining copies for the Competent Authorities

END

Box 11

This is one step that can be missed. The manufacturer is required to make a "critical evaluation" of the clinical investigation. This is not merely a report on the "success of the clinical investigation" but an in-depth analysis of why it was successful, and what unforeseen factors could have either made it successful or created conditions for early termination.

The final stage of clinical evaluation is the requirement to actively update the information with data obtained from postmarket surveillance. This requirement is fixed to the extent that "it must be duly justified and documented" where postmarket clinical follow-up is not deemed necessary (*MDD*, Annex X, 1.1c, *AIMDD*, Annex 7, 1.4).

Summary

Under the medical devices directives, a clinical evaluation is required for all classes of devices. Clinical evaluation can be through performance, bench testing and preclinical work. It can be through a literature review. It can be through a clinical investigation. Finally, it can be through a mixture of all three methodologies. What is not in doubt is that it must be carried out.

This chapter supplies all the necessary references in legal texts, guidelines and standards for executing a clinical evaluation. It also describes the steps to take to reach a position of completing a compliant clinical evaluation.

Chapter 12

Conformity Assessment Procedures' Quality System Requirements

Updated by Claudia Ising, RAC

OBJECTIVES

❑ Understand the Conformity Assessment Procedures and the similarities between directives

❑ Understand the flexibility of the Conformity Assessment Procedures in relation to the risk classes

❑ Understand the involvement of Notified Bodies

❑ Understand the relationship of the Conformity Assessment Procedures to the quality system standard

❑ Understand the role of an Authorised Representative in Conformity Assessment Procedures

DIRECTIVES, REGULATIONS AND GUIDELINES COVERED IN THIS CHAPTER

❑ Council Directive 90/385/EEC of 20 June 1990 on the approximation of the laws of the Member States relating to active implantable medical devices

❑ Council Directive 93/42/EEC of 14 June 1993 concerning medical devices

❑ Directive 98/79/EC of the European Parliament and of the Council of 27 October 1998 on *in vitro* diagnostic medical devices

❑ Directive 2000/70/EC of the European Parliament and of the Council of the 16 November 2000 amending Council Directive 93/42/EEC as regards medical devices incorporating stable derivates of human blood or human plasma

❑ Directive 2002/98/EC of the European Parliament and of the Council of 27 January 2003 setting standards of quality and safety for the collection, testing, processing, storage and distribution of human blood and blood components and amending Directive2001/83/EC

❑ Commission Directive 2003/12/EC of 3 February 2003 on the reclassification of breast implants in the framework of Directive 93/42/EEC concerning medical devices

❑ Commission Directive 2005/50/EC of 11 August 2005 on the reclassification of hip, knee and shoulder joint replacements in the framework of Council Directive 93/42/EEC concerning medical devices

❑ Directive 2007/47/EC of the European Parliament and of the Council of 5 September 2007 amending Council Directive 90/385/EEC on the approximation of the laws of the Member States relating to active implantable medical devices, Council Directive 93/42/EEC concerning medical devices and Directive 98/8/EC concerning the placing of biocidal products on the market

Chapter 12

- ❑ Decision 93/465/EEC Council Decision of 22 July 1993 concerning the modules for the various phases of the conformity assessment procedures and the rules for the affixing and use of the CE conformity marking, which are intended to be used in the technical harmonization directives

- ❑ Decision No 768/2008/EC of the European Parliament and of the Council and of 9 July 2008 on a common framework for the marketing of products, and repealing Council Decision 93/465/EEC

- ❑ EN ISO 13485 Medical Devices—Quality management systems—Requirements for regulatory purposes (2003)

- ❑ Guidelines for conformity assessment of In Vitro Fertilisation (IVF) and Assisted Reproduction Technologies (ART) products, MEDDEV 2.2/4 (January 2012)

- ❑ Guideline for Authorised Representatives, MEDDEV 2.5/10 (January 2012)

- ❑ Commission Regulation (EU) No 207/2012 of 9 March 2012 on electronic instructions for use of medical devices

Introduction

It must be understood that the European system relies on medical device manufacturers' ability to comply with the requirements applicable to them and their products. The articles of each directive describe the requirements, and the annexes may be considered the *a la carte* menu on how to apply the requirements. Article 9 of the *Active Implantable Medical Devices Directive* (*AIMDD*), Article 11 of the *Medical Devices Directive* (*MDD*) and Article 9 in the *In Vitro Devices Directive* (*IVDD*) outline the requirements of Conformity Assessment Procedures (CAPs) available to the manufacturer. Those articles refer to a specific annex or combination of annexes a manufacturer may apply based on the medical device's classification. The CAPs include quality system- and product-related aspects. The selection of annexes allows the application of a specific CAP, which may emphasise one aspect over the other.

The overall goal of the various CAPs is to ensure that a medical device used under proper conditions and for its intended purpose will not compromise the patient's clinical condition or safety, provided that any risks are acceptable when weighed against the benefit of the device throughout its lifetime.

General Aspects

The *AIMDD*, *MDD* and *IVDD* provide a variety of CAP choices. However, the procedures are comparable due to the fact that they have been created based on Council Decision of 22 July 1993 concerning the modules for the various phases of the conformity assessment procedures and the rules for the affixing and use of the CE conformity marking, which are intended to be used in the technical harmonization directives (93/465/EEC). This decision was replaced by Decision No 768/2008/EC of the European Parliament and of the Council of 9 July 2008 on a common framework for the marketing of products, and repealing Council Decision 93/465/EEC, which reinforces the Global Approach.[1] All directive updates will follow this new decision. The description of the general CAPs still applies within this decision; therefore, the elements will remain the same in the future.

Another aspect that makes the conformity assessment similar across the various directives is the so-called New Approach, which addresses technical barriers among Member States (Directive 98/34/EC of the European Parliament and of the Council of 22 June 1998 laying down a procedure for the provision of information in the field of technical standards and regulations).[2] This has led to the implementation of harmonised standards or common technical specifications. All New Approach directives use modules, which can be variously applied to demonstrate conformity assessment.

In general, all CAPs require the preparation of technical documentation (**Table 12-1**) that refers to, among other things, the Essential Requirements, which are described in the first annex of each directive.

Product-related aspects vary simply due to the type of products, but the quality system standard for medical devices is currently EN ISO 13485, which may be applied for all quality system-related requirements.

All CAPs require manufacturer vigilance and postmarket surveillance after the product has been delivered or installed.

At the time of updating this chapter, there are movements in the EU to combine the three medical devices directives into one regulation. This proposal seems to find support from the various stakeholders for the *AIMDD* and the *MDD* but not the *IVDD*. However, the combination of all directives is certainly possible, taking each speciality into consideration. An example of combining the legislations may be seen with the German transposition of all three directives in one law, the *Medizinproduktegestz* (*MPG*).

It is important for manufacturers that have different medical devices to relate the requirements of the directives to one another. For example, an in vitro medical device kit manufacturer may have to include a medical device within the kit, and therefore the CAP selected by the manufacturer should satisfy the requirements of both the *IVDD* and *MDD*. However, understanding the *IVDD* requirement

Figure 12-1. CAPs for Active Implantable Medical Devices

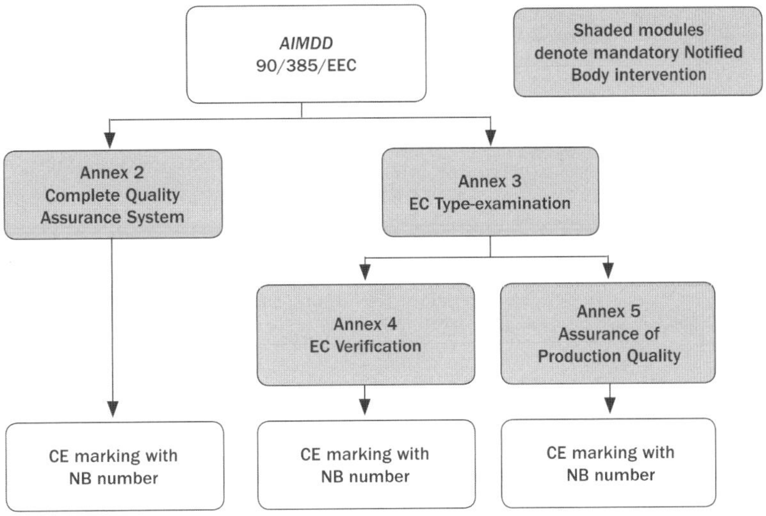

```
                    AIMDD                    Shaded modules
                  90/385/EEC              denote mandatory Notified
                                              Body intervention
          ┌──────────┴──────────┐
          ▼                     ▼
       Annex 2              Annex 3
   Complete Quality      EC Type-examination
   Assurance System            │
          │              ┌─────┴─────┐
          │              ▼           ▼
          │          Annex 4      Annex 5
          │        EC Verification  Assurance of
          │                         Production Quality
          ▼              ▼              ▼
    CE marking with  CE marking with  CE marking with
      NB number       NB number        NB number
```

allows a manufacturer to apply that knowledge to the *MDD*, taking particular differences into consideration.

In 2012, a new guidance (MEDDEV 2.7) was published on products used during in vitro fertilisation and artificial reproductive technology (IVF/ART products). These products may qualify as medicinal products or medical devices, depending on their principal mode of action. When IVF/ART products meet the definition of medical devices, they should be classified according to the rules of *MDD* Annex IX. For more information, see the *Manual on Borderline and Classification in the Community*.[3]

CAPs in Relation to the Risk Class

The selection of the various CAPs is limited to those foreseen for a particular risk class.

The *AIMDD* was the first directive and covers a particular type of medical device, e.g., pacemakers, as indicated in directive's name. This directive also applies to all accessories for those products.

Due to the limited application to one type of medical device, the compliance routes described are particular for these types of high-risk products.

Medical devices covered under the *MDD* are divided into four different risk classes (I, IIa, IIb and III). In vitro diagnostic medical devices are also divided into four different risk classes (Annex II list A and B, devices for self-testing and all other devices). The higher the risk class, the more controls are applied and, therefore, the CAPs vary significantly from the lowest to the highest risk class. Certain aspects of the selected CAP must be reviewed by a Notified Body (NB), which issues a certificate of conformity on those aspects only.

CAP According to the AIMDD

As previously noted, the *AIMDD* is only applicable for particular types of high-risk medical devices. The CAPs outlined are very limited for these products and an NB is always involved. The European Conformity (CE) mark shall always show the NB number. **Figure 12-1** shows the three CAP choices available to a manufacturer.

The CAPs may be compared with those for *MDD* Risk Class III products. The terms vary slightly but the similarity is obvious when comparing **Figure 12-1** with **Figure 12-5**.

CAPs for the MDD and IVDD

In the two other medical device directives, a variety of products are covered with various compliance routes available to the manufacturer. The various CAPs are presented below according to the risk classes.

IVF/ART products follow CAPs for the *MDD*. Some IVF/ART products are considered Class III according to rule 13, due to the incorporation of a medicinal product(s). For these products, the CAP should be conducted under point 7.4 of *MDD* Annex I.

MDD Risk Class I (e.g., Wheelchairs, Orthoses)

A very limited assessment procedure according to Annex VII of the *MDD* is applied to Risk Class I devices. The technical documentation must be in place and available for Competent Authority inspection. An NB is not involved and, therefore, no NB number will accompany the CE Mark (**Figure 12-2**).

Stricter rules apply to Risk Class I devices that have a measuring function or are sterile. For those products, Annex VII requires the manufacturer to also apply Annex II, IV, V or VI. The manufacturer has the choice and shall involve an NB to certify only those specific aspects.

Table 12-1. Conformity Assessment Documentation

MDD Directive 93/42/EEC	AIMDD Directive 90/385/EEC	IVDD Directive 98/79/EEC
Annex III Section 7 7.2. Other notified bodies may obtain a copy of the EC type-examination certificates and/or the supplements thereto. The Annexes to the certificates must be made available to other notified bodies on reasoned application, after the manufacturer has been informed. 7.3. The manufacturer or his authorised representative must keep with the technical documentation copies of EC type-examination certificates and their additions for a period ending at least five years after the last device has been manufactured. In the case of implantable devices, the period shall be at least 15 years after the last product has been manufactured. **Annex IV Section 7** The manufacturer or his authorised representative must, for a period ending at least five years, and in the case of implantable devices at least 15 years, after the last product has been manufactured, make available to the national authorities: • the declaration of conformity • the documentation referred to in Section 2 • the certificates referred to in Sections 5.2 and 6.4 • where appropriate, the type- examination certificate referred to in Annex III **Annex V Section 5.1** 5.1. The manufacturer or his authorised representative must, for a period ending at least five years, and in the case of implantable devices at least 15 years, after the last product has been manufactured, make available to the national authorities: • the declaration of conformity • the documentation referred to in the fourth indent of Section 3.1 • the changes referred to in Section 3.4 • the documentation referred to in the seventh indent of Section 3.1 • the decisions and reports from the notified body as referred to in Sections 4.3 and 4.4 • where appropriate, the type- examination certificate referred to in Annex III **Annex VI Section 5.1** Administrative provisions 5.1. The manufacturer or his authorised representative must, for a period ending at least five years, and in the case of implantable devices at least 15 years, after the last product has been manufactured, make available to the national authorities: • the declaration of conformity • the documentation referred to in the seventh indent of Section 3.1 • the changes referred to in Section 3.4 • the decisions and reports from the notified body as referred to in the final indent of Section 3.4 and in Sections 4.3 and 4.4 • where appropriate, the certificate of conformity referred to in Annex III.	**Annex 2 Section 6.1** For at least 15 years from the last date of manufacture of the product, the manufacturer or his authorised representative shall keep available for the national authorities: • the declaration of conformity • the documentation referred to in the second indent of Section 3.1, and in particular the documentation, data and records referred to in the second paragraph of Section 3.2 • the amendments referred to in Section 3.4 • the documentation referred to in Section 4.2 • the decisions and reports of the notified body referred to in Sections 3.4, 4.3, 5.3 and 5.4 **Annex 3 Section 7.3** The manufacturer or his authorized representative shall keep with the technical documentation a copy of the EC type-examination certificates and the supplements to them for a period of at least 15 years from the manufacture of the last product. **Annex 4 Section 6.5** The manufacturer or his authorized representative shall ensure that he is able to supply the notified body's certificates of conformity on request. **Annex 6 Section 3** The manufacturer shall undertake to keep available for the competent national authorities: 3.1. For custom-made devices, documentation, indicating manufacturing site(s) and enabling the design, manufacture and performances of the product, including the expected performances, to be understood, so as to allow conformity with the requirements of this directive to be assessed. The manufacturer shall take all necessary measures to see that the manufacturing process ensures that the products manufactured conform to the documentation referred to in the first paragraph. 3.2. For devices intended for clinical investigations, the documentation shall also contain: • a general description of the product and its intended use • design drawings, manufacturing methods, in particular as regards sterilization, and diagrams of parts, sub-assemblies, circuits, etc. • the descriptions and explanations necessary for the understanding of the said drawings and diagrams and of the operation of the product • the results of the risk analysis and a list of the standards laid down in Article 5, applied in full or in part, and a description of the solutions adopted to satisfy the essential requirements of the directive where the standards in Article 5 have not been applied	**Article 9(7)** The manufacturer must keep the declaration of conformity, the technical documentation referred to in Annexes III to VIII, as well as the decisions, reports and certificates, established by notified bodies, and make them available to the national authorities for inspection purposes for a period ending five years after the last product has been manufactured. Where the manufacturer is not established in the Community, the obligation to make the aforementioned documentation available on request applies to his authorised representative.

MDD Directive 93/42/EEC	AIMDD Directive 90/385/EEC	IVDD Directive 98/79/EEC
Annex VII Section 2 The manufacturer must prepare the technical documentation described in Section 3. The manufacturer or his authorised representative must make this documentation, including the declaration of conformity, available to the national authorities for inspection purposes for a period ending at least five years after the last product has been manufactured. In the case of implantable devices, the period shall be at least 15 years after the last product has been manufactured. **Annex VIII Section 4** The information contained in the declarations concerned by this Annex shall be kept for a period of time of at least five years. In the case of implantable devices, the period shall be at least 15 years.	• if the device incorporates, as an integral part, a substance or human blood derivative referred to in Section 10 of Annex 1, the data on the tests conducted in this connection, which are required to assess the safety, quality and usefulness of that substance, or human blood derivative, taking account of the intended purpose of the device, • the results of the design calculations, checks and technical tests carried out, etc. The manufacturer shall take all necessary measures to see that the manufacturing process ensures that the products manufactured conform to the documentation referred to in 3.1 and in the first paragraph of this section. The manufacturer may authorize the evaluation, by audit where necessary, of the effectiveness of these measures.	

The 2007 update to the directive added Annex II to the choices. The requirements in Annex II were considered too strict for these low-risk products in the past, but a manufacturer had to apply another CAP (Annex IV, V or VI) if it applied Annex II to other products of higher risk classes. Today, for practical matters, a manufacturer is also able to apply Annex II for Risk Class I products that are sterile or have a measuring function.

It should be noted that the update of the directive in 2010 added the reference to clinical and preclinical data. Therefore, it is evident that clinical data, even for the lowest risk class of products, are mandatory.

MDD Risk Class IIa (e.g., Single-use Surgical Instruments)
Annex VII may be applied to Risk Class IIa products; in addition, the manufacturer shall apply Annex IV, V or VI (**Figure 12-3**). Annex IV covers the verification of products, Annex V covers production quality assurance and Annex VI covers product quality assurance.

The manufacturer also may apply Annex II, full quality assurance system, but without Annex II, Section 4. Section 4 is a design examination required only for Risk Class III products.

These choices allow the manufacturer to select the CAP route it deems most appropriate. A manufacturer with very deep in-house production levels may select Annex II, while a manufacturer with very little production involvement may only apply Annex VII with Annex IV. Annex II relies on the manufacturer's ability to control all aspects of making medical devices, from design to changes to existing products, and an NB will review the whole process. When Annex VII is applied in conjunction with Annex IV, an NB reviews "only" the medical device to the extent that products or a sample of products from a batch are being directly verified against the technical documentation. However, the NB may even test the product, applying harmonised standards.

These two extremes of the CAP choices make it clear that the directive tries to take various business solutions into consideration. The manufacturer must involve an NB with all CAPs.

Since the update in 2007, Annex II, V and VI address the obligation of an NB to assess the technical documentation "for at least one representative sample for each device subcategory for compliance with the provision with this directive." Due to the nature of Annex IV, where the NB will verify the product against the technical documentation, an additional technical file assessment is not foreseen for this CAP.

MDD Risk Class IIb (e.g., Defibrillator, Monitoring Equipment for Vital Physiological Processes)
The CAPs for Risk Class IIb (**Figure 12-4**) deviate only slightly from the ones outlined for devices of Risk Class IIa (**Figure 12-3**). Annex II may be applied in the same manner, but Annex IV, V or VI shall be combined with Annex III. Annex III refers to EC type-examination. This is the procedure where an NB reviews and may even test the type in a very detailed manner. Additional aspects of Annex IV, V and VI ensure that subsequent products shall conform to the type examined by the NB. The NB is involved in all CAPs.

Since the 2007 update, Annex II refers to the obligation of the NB to assess the technical documentation "for at least one representative sample for each generic device group for compliance with the provision of this directive." Due to the combination with Annex III type-examination, it is logical that Annexes IV, V and VI do not refer to such an additional review within these CAPs.

The details for the selection of technical files as well the level of review conducted by the NB were heavily discussed among stakeholders. Guidance was provided by the Notified Body Oversight Group (NBOG). At the time of updating this chapter, NBs may still deviate in regard to this review

Chapter 12

Figure 12-2. CAP for Risk Class I Medical Devices

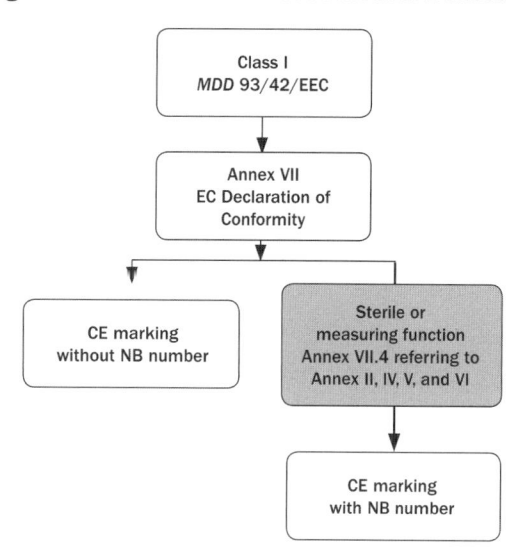

```
        Class I
      MDD 93/42/EEC
            |
            v
        Annex VII
    EC Declaration of
        Conformity
        /        \
       v          v
   CE marking   Sterile or
   without NB   measuring function
   number       Annex VII.4 referring to
                Annex II, IV, V, and VI
                      |
                      v
                  CE marking
                  with NB number
```

process. Therefore, it is recommended that manufacturers communicate with their NBs regarding this additional review level in advance.

MDD Risk Class III (e.g., Circulatory System and Central Nervous System Devices)

In reviewing **Figure 12-5** for Risk Class III products, two aspects are immediately obvious. For Risk Class III products, Annex VI cannot be applied in conjunction with Annex III. Also, Annex II must be applied in its entirety, including Annex II.4, which refers to the design dossier that requires NB review. The NB issues a separate certificate for this aspect.

For Risk Class III products that incorporate medicinal products or human blood derivatives, additional aspects must be considered. For products incorporating medicinal substances, the NB shall consult with one of the Competent Authorities or the European Medicines Agency (EMA). Only EMA shall be involved when products incorporate human blood derivatives. These aspects should be carefully discussed with the NB. Approval depends on a positive outcome of the consultation process between the NB and the agency. These aspects are described in Annex II and Annex III. This means that independent of the CAP selected, equal scrutiny is being applied to these aspects of the product.

IVDD In Vitro Diagnostic Devices (Except those listed in Annex II or devices for self-testing, e.g., HCG test for use in laboratory—professional use)

The *IVDD* annexes contain requirements similar to those of the *MDD* and *AIMDD*. For example, Annex IV refers to the full quality system, as do *MDD* Annex II and *AIMDD* Annex 2. Based on the risk category, the manufacturer may have various choices to achieve compliance, as is the case with the *MDD* and *AIMDD*.

For all devices not listed in *IVDD* Annex II and not for self-testing, the CAP is outlined in Annex III (**Figure 12-6**). The CAP is similar to *MDD* Annex VII for Risk Class I products. However, more-specific quality system aspects are required. As is the case with *MDD* Annex VII, an NB is not involved. Therefore, those products are commonly referred to as Risk Class I, even though the *IVDD* does not utilise a risk class numbering system.

IVDD Self-Testing Products (e.g., HCG test for the lay person)
Self-testing devices offer manufacturers the most choices from which to select (**Figure 12-7**). The manufacturer may apply Annex III in its entirety. Annex III.6 refers to a design dossier and the manufacturer must apply to an NB for the design examination.

Another choice is to apply a full quality assurance system as outlined in Annex IV. Annex IV Sections 4 and 6 are not applied for this risk category. The last option the manufacturer has is to follow Annex V in combination with Annex VI or Annex VII. Annex V refers to the EC type-examination, similar to the procedure outlined in *MDD* Annex III. Annex VI and Annex VII are the procedures that verify that the products produced conform to the type examined by the NB, with Annex VII focusing more on quality aspects. In all instances, an NB is involved.

Products Listed in Annex II List B
The CAPs for Annex II List B (**Figure 12-8**) are similar to those for self-testing devices. However, Annex III is not allowed.

Products Listed in Annex II List A
The products in Annex II List A are considered to be of the highest risk category and, therefore, are the most scrutinised. With the above outlined CAPs for the lower risk classes, certain parts of an annex were not applied. For this risk category, the complete annexes shall be applied (**Figure 12-9**). Furthermore, the choice of CAPs for these products is very limited. With Annex III already not allowed for List B products, now the combination of Annex V and Annex VI is also no longer an option.

The high level of concern regarding these products is made particularly clear by the fact that an NB approves each individual batch with both available CAPs. This may involve actual quality control testing by the NB and the review of manufacturing documentation.

Particulars of the CAPs

This section outlines the main aspects of each particular procedure. Furthermore, it demonstrates the direct correlation of the three medical devices directives to one another and to Decision 768/2008/EC with regard to CAPs. In any case, each directive's particularities must be taken into

Figure 12-3. CAPs for Risk Class IIa Medical Devices

consideration. Certain procedures from the decision were not considered appropriate for all directives and therefore were not applied. In each annex, various additional aspects may apply as outlined above. The decision provides eight assessment procedures or "modules" that cover the design and production phases:
- Module A: Internal production control
- Module B: EC type-examination
- Module C: Conformity to type based on internal production control (Not applicable for the medical devices directives)
- Module D: Conformity to type based on quality assurance of the production process
- Module E: Conformity to type based on product quality assurance
- Module F: Product verification
- Module G: Unit verification (Not applicable for the medical devices directives)
- Module H: Full quality assurance

Internal Production Control (Module A)

With the EC Declaration of Conformity, the main focus is on the technical documentation (**Table 12-2**). The *IVDD* describes further quality system aspects, but an NB is not involved.

EC Type-examination (Module B)

An EC type-examination is product-related, where an NB examines the product and issues an EC type-examination certificate (**Table 12-3**). The device may even be tested directly by the NB. The goal is to verify that the product's

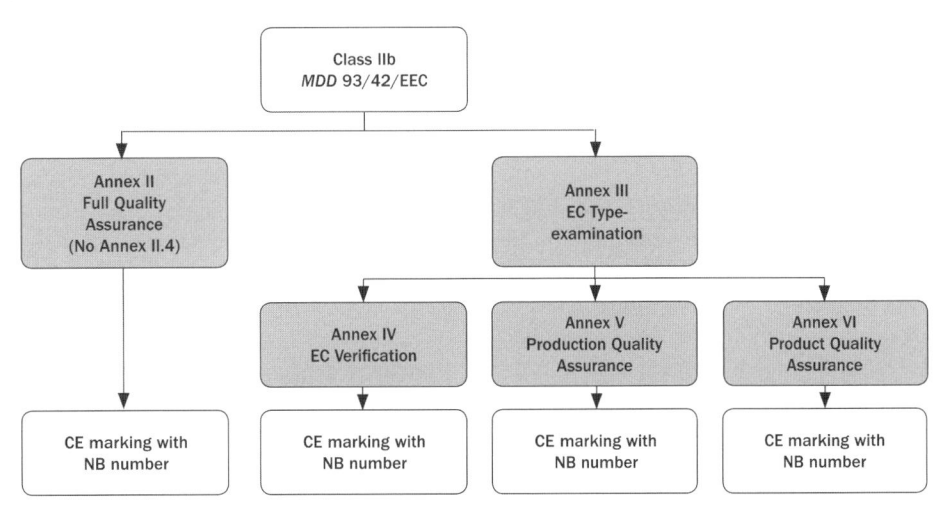

Figure 12-4. CAPs for Risk Class IIb Medical Devices

Chapter 12

Figure 12-5. CAPs for Risk Class III Medical Devices

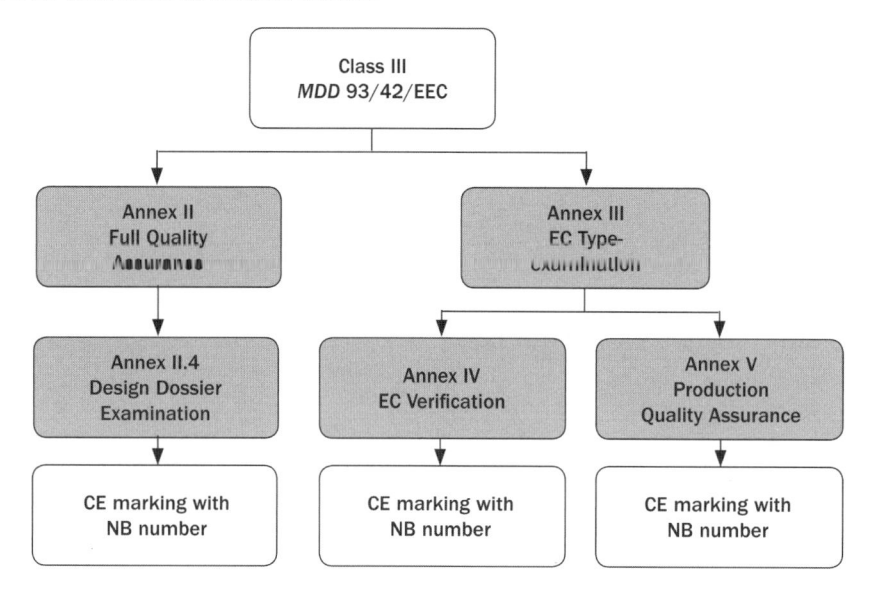

```
                    Class III
                  MDD 93/42/EEC
                        |
        ┌───────────────┴───────────────┐
        ▼                               ▼
    Annex II                        Annex III
  Full Quality                     EC Type-
   Assurance                       examination
        |                               |
        ▼                   ┌───────────┴───────────┐
    Annex II.4              ▼                       ▼
  Design Dossier         Annex IV                Annex V
   Examination         EC Verification         Production
        |                   |               Quality Assurance
        ▼                   ▼                       |
   CE marking with     CE marking with              ▼
    NB number            NB number           CE marking with
                                               NB number
```

design meets the applicable directive's requirements, mainly compliance with that directive's Essential Requirements. The EC type-examination procedure will always be applied with other procedures.

Production Quality Assurance (Module D)

The main goal of the production quality assurance procedure (**Table 12-4**) is to ensure the products are in fact produced and conform to the type described in the EC type-examination certificate. The production shall follow certain requirements that may be fulfilled with the application of the harmonised quality system standard, EN ISO 13485. Since not all aspects of the quality system need to be applied, the exemptions allowed in the standard may be utilised. The production quality assurance procedure is normally applied together with the EC type-examination. However, the *MDD* allows the application with Annex VII for Risk Class IIa products. In that case, the procedure shall ensure the devices produced conform to the technical documentation. An NB is involved.

Product Quality Assurance (Module E)

The main goal of the product quality assurance procedure is to ensure, via final inspection and testing, the products are in fact in conformity with the type described in the EC type-examination certificate (**Table 12-5**). This can be achieved with very limited quality system aspects. The harmonised standard, EN ISO 13485, may be utilised with exemptions not applicable to this procedure. The product quality assurance procedure is normally applied with the EC type-examination. However, the *MDD* allows the application with Annex VII for Risk Class IIa products. In that case, the procedure shall ensure that the devices conform to the technical documentation. An NB is involved. Note that this procedure is not applicable for the *AIMDD* and the *IVDD*.

Product Verification (Module F)

The main goal of the product verification procedure (**Table 12-6**) by the NB is to ensure the devices are in conformity with the type described in the EC Examination Certificate. The verification may be performed on each individual product or a batch of products. The procedure is normally applied with the EC type-examination. However, the *MDD* allows the application with Annex VII for Risk Class IIa products. In that case, the procedure shall ensure that the devices conform to the technical documentation. The NB must carry out appropriate examinations and tests.

Full Quality Assurance System (Module H)

The main goal of this procedure is to ensure the manufacturer applies a full quality assurance system, which includes all aspects of design, manufacture and final product inspection (**Table 12-7**). This may be achieved with the full application of EN ISO 13485. For higher risk classes, the procedure is extended with the examination of the design dossier by the NB. For IVD products, an additional product verification by the NB is being applied within the procedure.

Product Approach or Quality Approach

In reviewing the various procedures, it becomes obvious that a complete CAP may be more focussed on a quality system or on a product. With the EC type-examination, the focus is more product-related, while with the full quality assurance system procedure, the focus is on a quality system approach. All CAPs for a particular risk class shall provide the same level of scrutiny to the products' compliance but, as outlined above, the manufacturer selects the procedure that best fits its business.

Quality System Requirements

The directives refer to certain quality assurance aspects. Those may be fulfilled with the application of harmonised standards. The directives do not stipulate a specific standard to use, and standards are developed independently of the directives. The standards harmonisation process is a faster process than actually updating a particular EU law. This ensures state-of-the-art technical aspects and quality system requirements.

The quality system standards have developed over time. The first standards harmonised and applied were the ISO 9000 series. Today, for medical devices, the EN ISO 13485 quality system standard is the most appropriate. It is important to note that the application of this standard is not mandatory. The manufacturer may apply other quality system standards. However, the application of the harmonised standards conveys the presumption of conformity. In any case, the level of quality control as outlined in the directive shall be achieved. If a different standard is applied, the NB must accept this, but it may be more difficult for the review order to establish compliance with the requirements as outlined in the directives.

The exclusions, which are allowed in EN ISO 13485 for certain quality system aspects, go along with the CAPs. For example, *MDD* Annex II refers to the full quality system, which would mean, in essence, that the complete EN ISO

Figure 12-6. CAP for all In Vitro Medical Devices
(Except devices listed in Annex II and devices for self-testing)

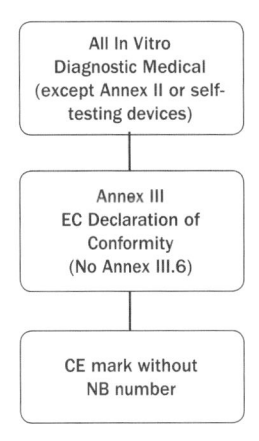

13485 shall be applied. Annex V refers to the production quality system; this would then mean the manufacturer would exclude the particular clause from the standard that refers to design and development. Any exclusion should be carefully reviewed with the NB involved regarding the selected CAP.

NBs

NBs are involved in many stages of the conformity assessment. It is often said that an NB approves products for CE marking. This is a misconception. It should be clearly understood that an NB might have only very limited involvement. However, the level of involvement increases with the risk associated with the product, and most certainly, a product shall not be marketed until the conformity

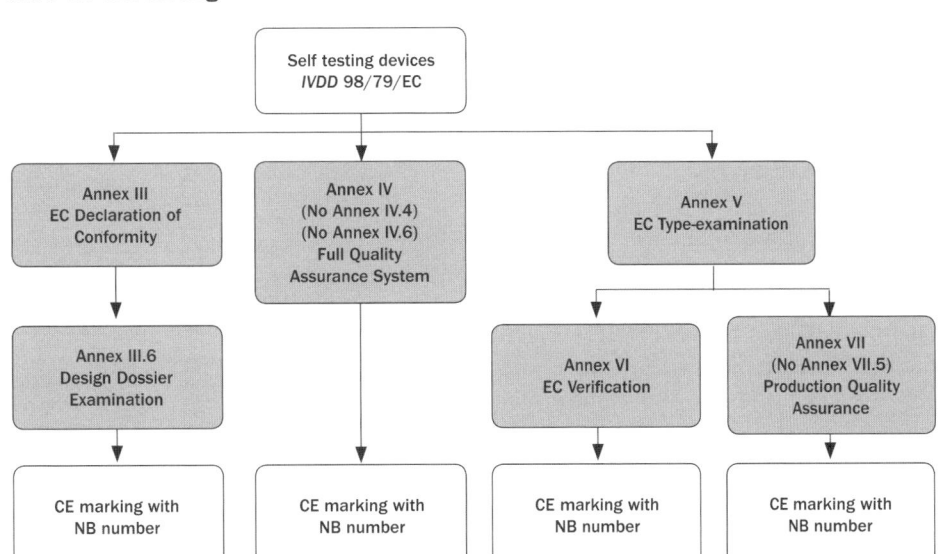

Figure 12-7. CAPs for Self-testing In Vitro Medical Devices

Figure 12-8. CAPs for Annex II List B In Vitro Medical Devices

```
                  Annex II List B devices
                       IVDD 98/79/EC
                    ┌──────┴──────┐
         ┌──────────┤             ├──────────┐
         ▼                                    ▼
    Annex IV                            Annex V
  (No Annex IV.4)                   EC Type-examination
  (No Annex IV.6)                    ┌────┴────┐
 Full Quality Assurance              ▼         ▼
       System                    Annex VI    Annex VII
                              EC Verification (No Annex VII.5)
                                            Production Quality Assurance
         │                          │             │
         ▼                          ▼             ▼
   CE marking with          CE marking with  CE marking with
     NB number                NB number        NB number
```

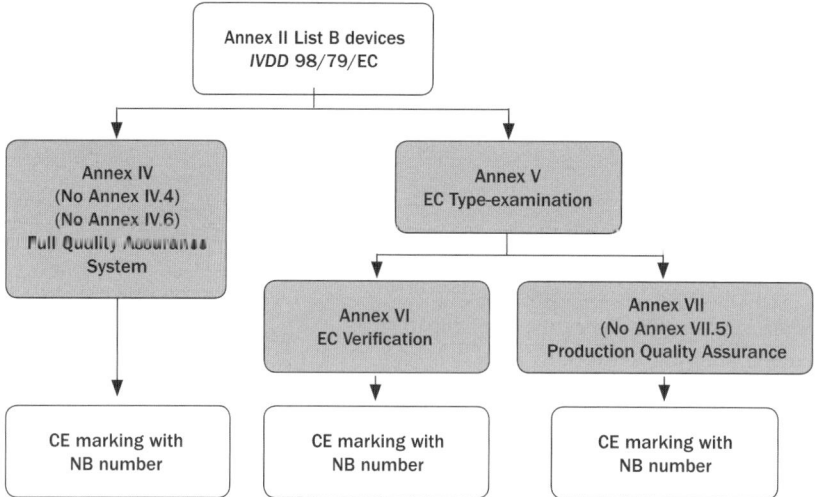

assessment, including issuance of the appropriate certificates by the NB, is completed.

NBs have to fulfil requirements as outlined in the specific directive as well as any additional national requirements. They are approved to be NBs in their countries by their national Competent Authorities. Once approved, they are notified to the European Commission and are published with their scope in the *Official Journal of the European Union*. The national Competent Authorities then further monitor the NB.

An NB may select the specific areas for which it is notified. For example, not all NBs are notified to the Commission for all directives or for all possible CAPs within a directive. Therefore, an NB might not be able to review all CAPs. A manufacturer should check the NBs to find one that can address its particular needs. On the other hand, an NB should not accept an application from a manufacturer for which it cannot provide the required service.

A manufacturer is free to select any NB for its products. Therefore, other relevant aspects may need to be considered, such as timing, price or overall customer service.

Authorised Representatives

Manufacturers who place medical devices on the EU market without having a registered place of business in the territory shall designate an Authorised Representative (AR) to act on their behalf (*AIMDD* Article 10a(2); *MDD* Article 14(2); *IVDD* Article 10.3) (see **Table 12-8**). MEDDEV 2.5/10 details the role of the AR across the devices directives and clearly distinguishes between responsibilities of the manufacturer and the AR.

ARs are involved in many stages of the conformity assessment, representing the manufacturer in specific delegated responsibilities, which should be contractually defined between the manufacturer and the AR.

According to *MDD* Article 11(8), the manufacturer may instruct its designated AR to initiate the procedures provided in Annexes III, IV, VII and VIII:

- lodge conformity assessment applications for EC type-examination (Annex III)
- establish the declaration of conformity to the type described in the EC type-examination certificate (EC Verification: Annex IV)
- establish the Annex VII EC declaration of conformity, including Annex VII, Section 5, in case of products placed on the market in sterile condition and Class I devices with a measuring function

Figure 12-9. CAPs for Annex II List A In Vitro Medical Devices

```
                Annex II List A
                   devices
                 IVDD 98/79/EC
              ┌───────┴───────┐
              ▼               ▼
         Annex IV         Annex V
        Full Quality   EC Type-examination
      Assurance System
              │               │
              ▼               ▼
         Annex IV.4       Annex VII
        Design Dossier  Production Quality
                           Assurance
              │               │
              ▼               ▼
         Annex IV.6      Annex VII.5
         Verification of  Verification of
      manufactured products manufactured products
              │               │
              ▼               ▼
        CE marking with   CE marking with
          NB number         NB number
```

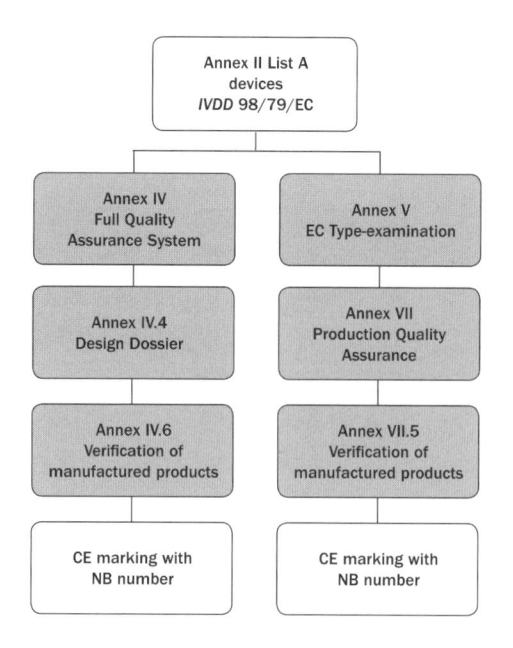

Conformity Assessment Procedures' Quality System Requirements

Table 12-2. Internal Production Control

Decision No 768/2008/EC	AIMDD 90/385/EEC	MDD 93/42/EEC	IVDD 98/79/EEC
Module A	NA	Annex VII	Annex III
Internal production control		EC Declaration of Conformity	EC Declaration of Conformity

Table 12-3. EC Type-examination

Decision No 768/2008/EC	AIMDD 90/385/EEC	MDD 93/42/EEC	IVDD 98/79/EEC
Module B	Annex 3	Annex III	Annex V
EC type-examination	EC type-examination	EC type-examination	EC type-examination

Table 12-4. Production Quality Assurance

Decision No 768/2008/EC	AIMDD 90/385/EEC	MDD 93/42/EEC	IVDD 98/79/EEC
Module D	Annex 5	Annex V	Annex VII
Conformity to type based upon quality assurance of the production process	Assurance of production quality	Production quality assurance	Production quality assurance

Table 12-5. Product Quality Assurance

Decision No 768/2008/EC	AIMDD 90/385/EEC	MDD 93/42/EEC	IVDD 98/79/EEC
Module E	NA	Annex VI	NA
Conformity to type based upon product quality assurance		Product quality assurance	

Table 12-6. Product Verification

Decision No 768/2008/EC	AIMDD 90/385/EEC	MDD 93/42/EEC	IVDD 98/79/EEC
Module F	Annex 4	Annex IV	Annex VI
Conformity to type based upon product verification	EC verification	EC verification	EC verification

Table 12-7. Full Quality Assurance System

Decision No 768/2008/EC	AIMDD 90/385/EEC	MDD 93/42/EEC	IVDD 98/79/EEC
Module H	Annex 2	Annex II	Annex IV
Conformity based upon full quality assurance	Complete quality assurance system	Full quality assurance system	Full quality assurance system

- establish the statement for custom-made devices (Annex VIII Section 2.1)

The *AIMDD* applies Article 9.3 and, where appropriate, procedures provided in Annexes 3, 4 and 6 may be discharged by the manufacturer's AR in the EU:
- lodge conformity assessment applications for EC type-examination (Annex III)

- establish declarations of conformity to the type described in the EC type-examination certificate (EC Verification: Annex IV)
- establish statements for custom-made devices (Annex VI Section 2.1)

IVDD Article 9.6 provides delegation from the manufacturer to its AR to initiate procedures provided in Annexes III, V, VI and VIII:

Chapter 12

Table 12-8. Authorised Representative in Conformity Assessment

AIMDD Directive 90/385/EEC	MDD Directive 93/42/EEC	IVDD Directive 98/79/EEC
Annex 2	Annex II	Annex IV
Article 9(3) "Where appropriate, the procedures provided for in Annexes 3, 4 and 6 may be discharged by the manufacturer's authorised representative established in the Community." See also Annex 2, Section 2 Annex 3, Section 2 Annex 4, Sections 1 and 2 Annex 5, Section 2 Annex 6, Section 1	Article 11(8) "The manufacturer may instruct his authorised representative to initiate the procedures provided for in Annexes III, IV, VII and VIII." See also Annex III, Section 2 Annex IV, Section 1 Annex VII, Section 1 Annex VIII, Section 1	Article 9(6) "The manufacturer may instruct his authorised representative to initiate the procedures provided for in Annexes III, V, VI and VIII." See also Annex III, Section 1 Annex V, Section 2 Annex VI, Section 1 Annex VIII, Section 1

- establish Annex III EC declaration of conformity
- lodge a conformity assessment application for EC type-examination (Annex V)
- establish the declaration of conformity to the type described in the EC type-examination certificate (EC Verification: Annex VI)

Summary

- The medical device directives follow the so-called Global and New Approach promoted for the EU.
- The goal of the various CAPs is to ensure compliance with the Essential Requirements.
- The medical devices directives allow the selection of various CAPs.
- The choice of CAPs is related to the product's risk class.
- Based on the selection, the CAPs may focus either on product- or quality system-related aspects.
- Compliance with CAPs may be achieved with the application of harmonised standards.
- EN ISO 13485 is the harmonised standard to comply with the quality system requirements.
- NBs may be involved with various stages of CAPs.
- NBs are notified to the EU with the scope for which they are allowed to be certified.
- The manufacturer may freely select an NB. Other aspects like cost or service may play a role in the selection of an NB.
- Manufacturers without registered places of business in the EU shall designate an AR that assumes defined functions in the CAPs.

References

1. Decision No 768/2008/EC of the European Parliament and of the Council of 9 July 2008 on a common framework for the marketing of products, and repealing Council Decision 93/465/EEC. EUR-Lex website. http://eur-lex.europa.eu/LexUriServ/LexUriServ.do?uri=OJ:L:2008:218:0082:0128:EN:PDF. Accessed 7 May 2012.
2. Directive 98/34/EC of the European Parliament and of the Council of 22 June 1998 laying down a procedure for the provision of information in the field of technical standards and regulations. EUR-Lex website. http://eur-lex.europa.eu/smartapi/cgi/sga_doc?smartapi!celexplus!prod!DocNumber&lg=en&type_doc=Directive&an_doc=98&nu_doc=34. Accessed 7 May 2012.
3. Manual on Borderline and Classification in the Community: Regulatory Framework for Medical Devices. EC website. http://ec.europa.eu/health/medical-devices/files/wg_minutes_member_lists/version1_4_manual072009_en.pdf. Accessed 7 May 2012.

Chapter 13

In Vitro Diagnostic Medical Devices

Updated by Erik Vollebregt

OBJECTIVES

❑ Summarize the European *In Vitro Diagnostic Medical Devices Directive*

❑ Describe the regulatory process to be followed by IVD manufacturers

❑ Focus on the specific elements in this directive

DIRECTIVES, REGULATIONS AND GUIDELINES COVERED IN THIS CHAPTER

❑ Directive 98/79/EC of the European Parliament and of the Council of 7 December 1998 on in vitro diagnostic medical devices

❑ Directive 93/42/EEC of the European Parliament and of the Council of 14 June 1998 concerning medical devices

❑ MEDDEV 2.14/2 rev.1, IVD Guidance: Research Use Only products, 2004

❑ MEDDEV 2.14/1 rev.2. IVD Guidances: Borderline issues, 2012

❑ MEDDEV 2.12/1 rev. 6. Medical Devices—Guidelines on a medical devices vigilance system, 2009

❑ Summary Technical Documentation (STED) for Demonstrating Conformity to the Essential Principles of Safety and Performance of In Vitro Diagnostic Medical Devices, GHTF

❑ MEDDEV 2.14/3 rev. 1. 2007. IVD Guidances: Supply of Instructions For Use (IFU) and other information for In-vitro Diagnostic (IVD) Medical Devices

❑ MEDDEV 2.14/4. Guideline for the CE marking of blood based in vitro diagnostic medical devices for vCJD based on detection of abnormal PrP, 2012

Introduction

Directive 98/79/EC of the European Parliament and of the Council of 7 December 1998 on in vitro diagnostic medical devices (*IVDD*) became the third in the series of directives on medical devices.[1] It laid out pan-European requirements for in vitro diagnostic medical devices (IVDs), replacing national regulations where they existed. Since 7 December 2003, the end of the transition period, all IVDs in the European Economic Area (EEA) and Switzerland also must comply with the requirements of the *IVDD* and carry the CE Mark.

The *IVDD* has been transposed into the national legislation of each Member State. Although the national transpositions largely follow the *IVDD*, they do contain specific elements with which devices in the respective national territory must comply. The language requirements for IVDs for professional use are a good example of these national differences. Another is the requirement that the label of IVDs for self-testing must be in the local language of the Member State in which the end user resides.

Chapter 13

To gain a full understanding of European regulatory requirements for IVDs, other important documents should be consulted: harmonised standards, guidance documents and, if applicable, the Common Technical Specifications (CTS).

The *IVDD* shares many features with Directive 93/42/EEC of the European Parliament and of the Council of 14 June 1998 concerning medical devices (*MDD*). The *MDD* is treated in more detail in other chapters of this book. This chapter focuses on the particularities of the *IVDD*.

At the time of writing, the European Commission had begun preparing the revision of the *IVDD*. A draft text of this revision is not yet available, but there are indications that the changes will be important.

The Scope of the *IVDD*

The *IVDD* (Art. 1.2.b) defines an *IVD* as follows:

"'in vitro diagnostic medical device' means any medical device which is a reagent, reagent product, calibrator, control material, kit, instrument, apparatus, equipment, or system, whether used alone or in combination, intended by the manufacturer to be used in vitro for the examination of specimens, including blood and tissue donations, derived from the human body, solely or principally for the purpose of providing information:
- concerning a physiological or pathological state, or
- concerning a congenital abnormality, or
- to determine the safety and compatibility with potential recipients, or
- to monitor therapeutic measures."

This definition includes four types of IVDs:
1. higher risk IVDs to diagnose the indications in Annex II list A
2. IVDs to diagnose the lower risk indications in Annex II, list B
3. self tests
4. all other IVDs that diagnose indications not in either of the lists in Annex II

Products for general laboratory use are not in vitro diagnostic medical devices unless such products, in view of their characteristics, are specifically intended by their manufacturer to be used for in vitro diagnostic examination.[2]

The MEDDEV on IVD borderline and classification issues lists a number of illustrative examples of devices that are IVDs or general laboratory equipment, depending on their intended use (see **Table 13-1**).

The definition of IVD also includes kits. Although "kit" is not further defined in the *IVDD*, the IVD borderline MEDDEV clarifies that a kit consists of more than one component, made available together and intended to be used to perform a specific IVD examination. A kit falls within the scope of the *IVDD* if its intended purpose as a combined set falls within the scope of the *IVDD*. This intended purpose for the combination must be classified and assessed for its conformity to the *IVDD* requirements, according to the principal intended purpose of the whole product combination and must be CE marked and labelled under the *IVDD*.[3] A kit can consist of a combination of IVDs that have already been CE marked and medical devices/IVDs that are not yet CE marked, as long as the kit is CE marked for its intended purpose. The kit has to fulfil the requirements regarding the "Information supplied by the manufacturer" separately from the information supplied with CE-marked IVDs and/or medical devices included.[4] In addition, the kit shall not bear an additional CE marking on the outer packaging for the medical devices included in the kit; only the kit itself will be marked.

Medical Device

An assay must first meet the definition of a medical device. This excludes a number of assays, e.g., those intended by their manufacturers to be used for forensic purposes, like detection of biologic agents used in weapons or alcohol tests used for law enforcement purposes.

In addition, the device has to be used for examination. This excludes general purpose lab equipment, unless such products, in view of their characteristics, are specifically intended by their manufacturer to be used for in vitro diagnostic examination.[5]

To Be Used In Vitro

The IVD is used in vitro for the examination of a specimen derived from the human body and where such specimen is never reintroduced into the body. If no specimen is involved, or if the examination takes place in or on the human body (*in vivo*), the devices intended to be used for this examination are not IVDs.[6] By way of examples: a pulse oxymeter emitting light through the fingertip and absorbing infrared light, to measure the oxy/deoxyhemoglobin ratio is not an IVD; neither is a continuous blood glucose monitoring system where the analytical function is carried out at the same time as the continuous specimen collection. Both of these examples are diagnostic medical devices. Devices that involve contact with the human body to obtain continuous specimen collection are not considered to be IVDs.[7]

For the Examination of Specimens, Including Blood and Tissue Donations, Derived From the Human Body

The definition of IVDs states that they are "intended by the manufacturer to be used in vitro for the examination of specimens, derived from the human body." Therefore, if no sample is "derived from the human body," the device is not considered an IVD. Such products shall be qualified

In Vitro Diagnostic Medical Devices

Table 13-1. Examples of General Laboratory Use Products and IVD Medical Devices

	Laboratory Use Product	Covered by *IVDD*
Centrifuges	General centrifuges, cytospin	Hematocrit centrifuge
Pipettes	General purpose pipettes (e.g., single or multiple pipettes, plastic pipettes, Pasteur pipettes)	Blood coagulation pipettes with automatic timing (accessory of coagulometer)
Tubes and flasks	Erlenmeyers, plastic tubes	Blood collection tubes, urine sample containers
Plates	Empty ELISA plates, empty Petri dishes	Coated microtiter plates for the diagnosis of Lyme's disease
Nucleic acid extraction products	DNA and RNA extraction kits that only provide a specimen without an intended IVD detection combination	DNA and RNA extraction kits intended to provide a specimen to be used with an IVD device (validation for at least one combination is to be provided)
General equipment	Scales, balances, microtomes, incubators, sterilisers for laboratory equipment, paraffin embedding machine	
HPLC products	Size-exclusion HPLC columns	HPLC columns for IVD purposes (e.g., HbA1c)
Detection equipment	Mass spectrometer, spectrophotometers, ELISA readers providing raw data that is not readily readable and understandable by the user (e.g., peaks, OD)	McFarland bacteria density testing
Others	Foetal calf serum, cell culture media, fixation solution, mounting media, buffers (e.g., PBS), chemicals (e.g., sulphuric acid, formol, water)	

as medical devices. An example is a non-invasive medical device for the detection of blood glucose by energy emission (e.g., near infra-red energy). This is not an IVD because no specimen derived from the human body is involved, but it is a medical device within the scope of the *MDD*.

Devices for detection of pathological agents in the environment, for example, are not IVDs, and neither are devices for examination of specimens derived from animals.

Specimen Receptacles

Specimen receptacles and accessories to IVDs also are included in the scope of the *IVDD*. Specimen receptacles are those devices, whether utilising a vacuum system or not, specifically intended by their manufacturers for the "primary" containment and "preservation" of specimens derived from the human body for the purpose of in vitro diagnostic examination.[8]

The word "primary" in relation to containment does not necessarily refer to the initial or first container of the specimen, but rather to the container's intended use. A container is regulated as specimen receptacle if it is intended by its manufacturer to mainly come into direct contact with the specimen and could, therefore, affect the specimen.

The word "preservation" does not imply that the receptacle has to contain a specimen preservative, but that the receptacle is intended to protect the specimen, for example, from temperature fluctuations, light, physical breakage, etc. If this is the intended use, it must be clearly indicated on the labelling and any associated promotional literature for the product. The manufacturer also must have evidence and technical documentation to support this use for the product.

If more than one specimen receptacle is involved in the collection, transport and storage of an individual specimen, each such receptacle must have evidence of compliance with the *IVDD*.

Other receptacles in which the specimen may be placed at some point during the analytical process (by aliquoting or otherwise), are not considered "specimen receptacles" within the meaning of the *IVDD* but rather general laboratory equipment.[9]

Products used to obtain specimens from the human body are usually not IVDs if they are used for transfer of a sample from the body rather than primary containment (e.g., plastic pipettes to transfer blood drops from fingers to rapid tests).

Accessories

The accessories rule that applies to IVDs is identical to that for medical devices. An accessory is defined as an "article which, whilst not being an in vitro diagnostic medical device, is intended specifically by its manufacturer to be used together with a device to enable that device to be used in accordance with its intended purpose."[10]

IVDD Article 1(2)(c) states that invasive sampling devices or devices for obtaining specimens that are directly applied to the human body are not considered to be IVD accessories, but are medical devices within the scope of the *MDD* (e.g., needles, lancets, lancing devices, mouthtubes, swabs and urine collection bags for babies).

IVDs for Performance Testing

IVDs that are introduced in European laboratories in order to establish their performance characteristics are also subject to the *IVDD*. Such products cannot carry the CE Mark because their performance characteristics have not yet been established, but otherwise should meet all directive requirements. *IVDD* Annex VIII further details the documentation and notification requirements for performance evaluation of these devices.

Research-only IVDs

Assays intended for research purposes are not subject to the *IVDD*. These assays lack a clinical application and therefore are not medical devices. The *IVDD* neither explicitly defines "Research Use Only" nor defines any requirements for such products. Manufacturers of these reagents should not apply the CE Mark, but clearly label them as "Research Use Only" and should ensure that all the labelling is consistent with the devices' nonclinical purpose. Guidance documents on "Research Use Only"[11] and borderline products[12] further clarify these subjects.

In-House Developed IVDs

It is not unusual for clinical laboratories to develop and produce their own reagents. These so-called "home brew" tests are not subject to the *IVDD*. However, to be exempt, these reagents must be manufactured and used within the same legal entity and in the same geographic location. Moreover, the tests can be run only on specimens from patients from the same health institution. Preamble 11 clearly brings home brew assays "intended to be used in a professional and commercial context" within the *IVDD*'s scope. As a consequence, biotech companies that are, for example, commercialising their often innovative assays as a testing service instead of selling the reagents to other laboratories, will also have to comply with the *IVDD*.

Process to be Followed by the Manufacturer

Short Overview of the Steps

An IVD manufacturer that wishes to place a product on the European market must do the following:
- define its product's classification
- ensure that the product meets the Essential Requirements, preferably complying with harmonised standards and, for Annex II List A products only, complying with the CTS
- ensure that its organization meets the quality system requirements
- implement vigilance procedures
- establish technical documentation, demonstrating compliance with the Essential Requirements and the applied harmonised standards
- draft labelling meeting national language requirements of the target countries
- appoint an Authorised Representative, if it is located outside the EEA or Switzerland
- execute an appropriate Conformity Assessment Procedure (CAP), including Notified Body (NB) certification, if applicable
- sign the Declaration of Conformity and apply the CE Mark to the device
- notify its product to the Competent Authorities in one of the Member States where the product will be placed on the market[13] (if the manufacturer is located outside Europe, this must be done by the Authorised Representative)

These points are described in more detail in this chapter and in other chapters of this book. See **Figure 13-1** for an overview of procedures.

Classification of an IVD

An IVD's classification determines the CAP to be followed and, hence, whether a Notified Body (NB) will be involved in the approval and certification of the product and the quality system, as shown in **Figure 13-1**. The procedure impacts both the cost and the time to market.

The current classification system is risk-based, but instead of defining classification rules, as is the case in the *MDD*, the *IVDD* literally lists the high-risk products in Annex II. This annex contains two lists, List A and List B. List A mentions the highest-risk products. List B mentions the products considered to be high risk but less so than those in List A.

The *IVDD* does not use "Class I, Class II, etc." for products, resulting in rather awkward denominations of the IVD classes. These are likely to be replaced by risk classes similar to those for general medical devices in the revision of the *IVDD* currently in process. Based on Annex II and Articles 1 and 9, the following categories are defined:
- "Annex II List A-products," covering the highest-risk products, which are mainly used in blood transfusion, for the prevention of transmission of HIV and certain types of hepatitis
- "Annex II List B-products," covering products with somewhat less risk
- "Devices for self-testing," covering products to be used by lay persons in their home environment

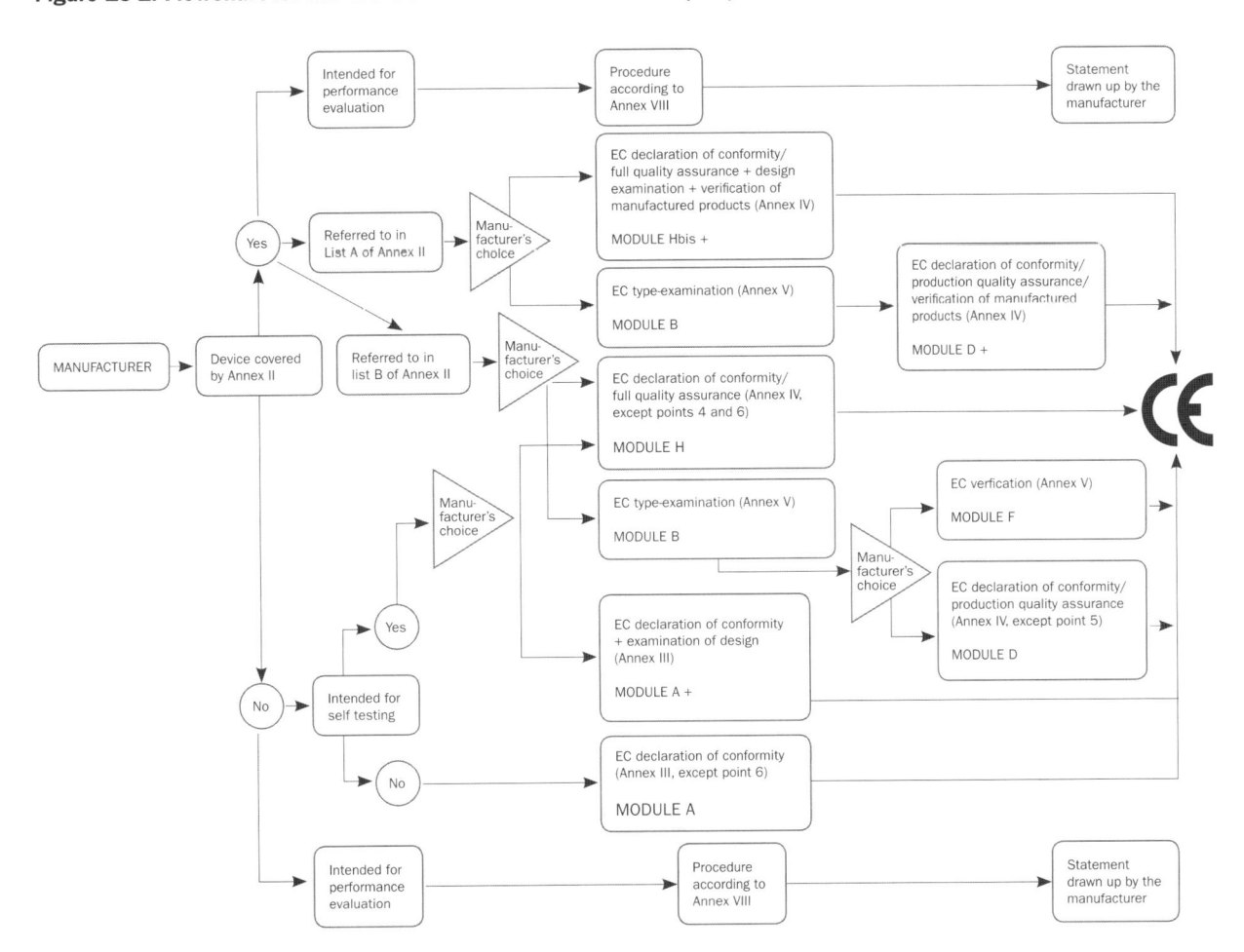

Figure 13-1. Flowchart for the CAPs Provided for in Directive 98/79/EC

Source: Guide to the implementation of directives based on the New Approach and the Global Approach, European Commission.

- "non-Annex II–products for professional use," covering all products not mentioned in the previous classes

Both the classification system and the actual classifications badly need modification to bring them in line with technological and medical advances and also to accommodate future evolutions. Therefore, they probably will be substantially changed in the revised *IVDD*. In the meantime, assays for variant Creutzfeldt-Jakob Disease (vCJD) are likely to be integrated into List A of Annex II.

Following are the lists of highest-risk and high-risk products, as defined in Annex II of the current *IVDD*.

List A

- reagents and reagent products, including related calibrators and control materials, for determining the following blood groups: ABO system, rhesus (C, c, D, E, e), anti-Kell
- reagents and reagent products, including related calibrators and control materials, for the detection, confirmation and quantification in human specimens of markers of HIV infection (HIV 1 and 2), HTLV I and II and hepatitis B, C and D

List B

- reagents and reagent products, including related calibrators and control materials, for determining the following blood groups: anti-Duffy and anti-Kidd
- reagents and reagent products, including related calibrators and control materials, for determining irregular anti-erythrocytic antibodies
- reagents and reagent products, including related calibrators and control materials, for the detection

Chapter 13

and quantification in human samples of the following congenital infections: rubella, toxoplasmosis
- reagents and reagent products, including related calibrators and control materials, for diagnosing the following hereditary disease: phenylketonuria
- reagents and reagent products, including related calibrators and control materials, for determining the following human infections: cytomegalovirus, chlamydia
- reagents and reagent products, including related calibrators and control materials, for determining the following HLA tissue groups: DR, A, B
- reagents and reagent products, including related calibrators and control materials, for determining the following tumour marker: PSA
- reagents and reagent products, including related calibrators, control materials and software, designed specifically for evaluating the risk of trisomy 21
- the following device for self-diagnosis, including its related calibrators and control materials: device for the measurement of blood sugar

Essential Requirements, Harmonised Standards and CTS

Before signing the Declaration of Conformity and affixing the CE Mark, the manufacturer must ensure its product meets the Essential Requirements of *IVDD* Annex I.

Annex I is a long list of requirements that must be met, if applicable. The wording is often rather vague, but many Essential Requirements are supported by harmonised standards. These standards describe in more detail what the regulator expects to achieve compliance with the respective requirement. A manufacturer should carefully identify which Essential Requirements apply to its product and whether any harmonised standards have been published to support these requirements. Compliance with the harmonised standards leads to a presumption of conformity with the Essential Requirements in the respective field.[14]

The high importance and relevance of applying harmonised standards are the same as for medical devices and are explained elsewhere in this book.

Several Essential Requirements and harmonised standards are generic and apply to IVDs and other medical devices alike. A typical and important example is the requirement to manage the risks associated with the use of the device, supported by the harmonised standard ISO14971.[15]

Other Essential Requirements and associated harmonised standards are specific for some IVDs, e.g., the Essential Requirements and harmonised standards for stability testing, for traceability of calibration for quantitative assays, for devices for self-testing and for labelling.

The Essential Requirements cover a variety of subjects, all somehow safety related. They include risk management, analytical and clinical performance, stability, chemical and physical properties, infection and microbial contamination, manufacturing and environmental properties, measuring functions, radiation, electronic safety and electromagnetic compatibility, protection against mechanical and thermal risks, risk for devices for self-testing and information supplied by the manufacturer (labelling).

The CTS[16] are a specific set of requirements published in the *Official Journal of the European Union* and currently only applicable to the Annex II List A products. The name of the document is misleading, since it really contains performance specifications and not technical specifications. The CTS strictly define the minimum performance requirements for the various products in Annex II List A and also describe in detail how they should be established. In addition, they include batch release criteria for these products, as they must be applied by the manufacturer and its NB in charge of batch release.

The purpose of the CTS is to ensure that NBs assess the performance of these highest-risk devices and the quality of the individual batches in a consistent way. The *IVDD* allows CTS to be established for Annex II List B products, too, but these have not yet been developed.

Quality System Requirements and Vigilance Procedures

The *IVDD* imposes quality system requirements on all IVD manufacturers, including those that only place non-Annex II products for professional use on the market.

ISO 13485[17] is the harmonised standard and should be chosen as the quality system model. However, certification against this standard is not mandatory. At the same time, an ISO 13485-certified quality system may show major nonconformities versus the requirements of the *IVDD*.

The quality system should include adequate procedures for handling field safety corrective actions and managing and reporting incidents and other postmarketing surveillance activities in agreement with the *IVDD* and the applicable guidance document.[18]

Technical Documentation and Design Dossier

The manufacturer must be capable of making technical documentation available for all CE-marked IVDs, regardless of their class. This technical documentation must demonstrate compliance with the applicable Essential Requirements and applied harmonised standards. *IVDD* Annex III lists items that should be part of the technical documentation. Not all items are applicable to each device and, conversely, the technical documentation of an IVD may also have to contain information that is not explicitly listed in Annex III.

For Annex II List A products, a design dossier must be submitted to the NB when the Annex IV CAP is chosen. Whereas technical documentation does not have to be one physical file, the design dossier is a single document that addresses all the items required for an effective NB assessment. NBs may make a proposal on the contents of the design dossier. The Summary Technical Documentation (STED) format, developed by Global Harmonization Task Force (GHTF) Study Group 1,[19] may become a model in the future, but its use for IVDs currently is not as widespread as for medical devices.

In practice, manufacturers applying for an NB certificate for Annex II List A or Annex II List B devices or devices for self-testing according to the Annex V CAP may also submit technical documentation structured as a design dossier.

These steps are outlined in **Figure 13-1**.

Labelling, e-Labelling and Language Requirements

Annex I.B.8 spells out the labelling requirements for IVDs, further specified in the ISO 18113 series of harmonised standards.[20] Both sources focus primarily on the contents of the labels and the instructions for use (IFU).

The *IVDD* explicitly demands that the information provided to the users of devices for self-testing be in the national language(s) of the target market, the market in which they reach the end user.[21] The application of this provision remains problematic because not all Member States have implemented this provision and instead rely on the general language requirement that they can require IVDs in general to be labelled in their language.[22] However, for IVDs for professional use, the *IVDD* left the decision on languages to the individual Member States. The Member States published their language requirements in their national transpositions of the *IVDD*. The majority decided to impose their national language(s) for professional IVDs, too. In practice, an IVD manufacturer selling products in all 32 countries covered by the *IVDD* must make IFU available in about 15 languages.

To overcome some of the practical problems resulting from the language requirements, the European Commission published a guidance document[23] defining the conditions for providing IFU by means other than physically sending them with the product itself. Instructions can now be posted on a website. However, strict conditions apply to this "e-labelling" solution. The website must meet certain requirements, and the manufacturer must make a free telephone number available so users can request a mailed or faxed copy.

Devices for self-testing and for point-of-care-testing are excluded from e-labelling. Special requirements apply to instrument manuals.

The language requirements also apply to labels. Use of the symbols from harmonised standard EN 980[24] mitigates the problem.

Conformity Assessment Procedures

The IVD manufacturer must assess the conformity of its products and quality system prior to signing the Declaration of Conformity and affixing the CE Mark to the product. In the case of non-Annex II products for professional use, the manufacturer has sole responsibility for doing this. For other devices, the conformity assessment involves a third-party review by the NB.

In the case of Annex II products, the NB will inspect the product's quality and the conformity of the quality system. In the case of Annex II List A products, the NB also has to release each batch.

Devices for self-testing can be certified by the NB, based on product documentation alone, although the manufacturer can also opt for CAPs including quality system inspections.

Chapter 8 is dedicated to CAPs, and an overview of the CAP for IVDs is shown in **Figure 13-1**.

Authorized Representative, Declaration of Conformity and Registration

Other chapters in this book describe the role of the Authorised Representative and the signing of the Declaration of Conformity.

After signing the Declaration of Conformity and prior to placing the product on the market, the manufacturer and the device(s) must be registered. The manufacturer, or its Authorised Representative in the case of non-European companies, informs the Competent Authority in the country in which it is based about placing the device(s) on the market.

The registration of IVDs is different from the registration of medical devices.

The registration requirement applies to all IVD classes, not only to those that do not require NB involvement. Since the entry into force of the Eudamed database[25] in May 2011, it is no longer necessary to repeat the notification in every country where a product is placed on the market. It is sufficient to notify only the country in which the manufacturer or its Authorised Representative is based.

Only general information is requested for non-Annex II products for professional use; however, information on the performance, NB certificates and labelling must be provided for devices in other classes.

In practice, the large majority of countries accept the "Form for the registration of manufacturers and devices, In Vitro Diagnostic Medical Devices Directive, Article 10,"[26] available on the European Commission's website for this purpose. However, differences between the countries exist with respect to the information to be provided and costs.

Chapter 13

The *IVDD*'s Revision

The *IVDD* is currently under revision. The new version is expected to be published at the end of the second quarter in 2012. A transition period of one to three years is likely to be defined.

No draft is available yet, but from the Public Consultation text,[27] it appears changes are being considered in the following areas:
- the classification of IVDs, which will also impact CAPs
- "home brew" or "in-house" testing
- diagnostic service laboratories
- genetic testing
- point-of-care testing
- demonstrating clinical validity and utility

Other Regulations

IVDs are exempt from other directives, such as those on biocides, machinery, electric safety and electromagnetic compatibility, often because the *IVDD* itself defines requirements that address the safety issues in these directives.

However, other regulations may apply. Relevant examples are:
- regulations on dangerous substances and preparations, which may have an impact on the labelling and may require the availability and distribution of material safety data sheets, such as the REACH regulation[28]
- transport regulations
- Directive 2002/96/EC of the European Parliament and of the Council of 27 January 2003 on waste electrical and electronic equipment
- regulations on radioactive materials
- regulations on animal sourced raw materials

Other regulations and directives also may apply.

Summary
- The *IVDD* shares many features with the *MDD*. The general concept of the regulation, the conformity assessment procedures and the requirements on postmarketing surveillance, vigilance, risk management and technical documentation are identical or very similar. The responsibilities of the manufacturer, the Competent Authorities, NBs and Authorised Representatives are very similar to those defined in the *MDD*.
- Device classification is risk-based. The *IVDD* literally lists the high-risk products in Annex II. This annex contains two lists—List A and List B. Self-testing devices are in a separate category.
- Before signing the Declaration of Conformity and affixing the CE Mark, the manufacturer must ensure that its product meets the Essential Requirements and, preferably, the requirements in the associated harmonised standards. The CTS are additional requirements, only applicable to Annex II, List A products.
- The *IVDD* currently is under revision. Significant changes are expected, e.g., in device classification.

References
1. Directive 98/79/EC of the European Parliament and of the Council of 27 October 1998 on in vitro diagnostic medical devices (*IVDD*). EUR-Lex website. http://eur-lex.europa.eu/LexUriServ/LexUriServ.do?uri=CONSLEG:1998L0079:20031120:en:PDF. Accessed 12 April 2012.
2. *IVDD* Article 1(2)(b). EUR-Lex website. http://eur-lex.europa.eu/LexUriServ/LexUriServ.do?uri=CONSLEG:1998L0079:20031120:en:PDF. Accessed 12 April 2012.
3. *IVDD* Annex I, B, ER 8.4. EUR-Lex website. http://eur-lex.europa.eu/LexUriServ/LexUriServ.do?uri=CONSLEG:1998L0079:20031120:en:PDF. Accessed 12 April 2012.
4. *IVDD* Annex I, B, 8. EUR-Lex website. http://eur-lex.europa.eu/LexUriServ/LexUriServ.do?uri=CONSLEG:1998L0079:20031120:en:PDF. Accessed 12 April 2012.
5. *IVDD* Article 1(2)(b). EUR-Lex website. http://eur-lex.europa.eu/LexUriServ/LexUriServ.do?uri=CONSLEG:1998L0079:20031120:en:PDF. Accessed 12 April 2012.
6. European Commission. MEDDEV 2.14/1 revision 2. *GUIDELINES ON MEDICAL DEVICES IVD Medical Device Borderline and Classification issues A GUIDE FOR MANUFACTURERS AND NOTIFIED BODIES* (January 2012) p. 5. EC website. http://ec.europa.eu/health/medical-devices/files/meddev/2_14_1_rev2_ol_en.pdf. Accessed 12 April 2012.
7. European Commission. MEDDEV 2.14/1 revision 2.*GUIDELINES ON MEDICAL DEVICES IVD Medical Device Borderline and Classification issues A GUIDE FOR MANUFACTURERS AND NOTIFIED BODIES*, p. 13 (January 2012). EC website. http://ec.europa.eu/health/medical-devices/files/meddev/2_14_1_rev2_ol_en.pdf. Accessed 12 April 2012.
8. Article 1(2)(b) IVDD. EUR-Lex website. http://eur-lex.europa.eu/LexUriServ/LexUriServ.do?uri=CONSLEG:1998L0079:20031120:en:PDF. Accessed 12 April 2012.
9. European Commission. MEDDEV 2.14/1 revision 2. *GUIDELINES ON MEDICAL DEVICES IVD Medical Device Borderline and Classification issues A GUIDE FOR MANUFACTURERS AND NOTIFIED BODIES* (January 2012). p. 7. EC website. http://ec.europa.eu/health/medical-devices/files/meddev/2_14_1_rev2_ol_en.pdf. Accessed 12 April 2012.
10. *IVDD* Article 1(2)(c). EUR-Lex website. http://eur-lex.europa.eu/LexUriServ/LexUriServ.do?uri=CONSLEG:1998L0079:20031120:en:PDF. Accessed 12 April 2012.
11. European Commission. MEDDEV 2.14/2 rev.1. *GUIDELINES ON MEDICAL DEVICES IVD Guidance: Research Use Only products A GUIDE FOR MANUFACTURERS AND NOTIFIED BODIES* (February 2004). EC website. http://ec.europa.eu/health/medical-devices/files/meddev/2_14_2_research_only_product_en.pdf. Accessed 12 April 2012.
12. European Commission. MEDDEV 2.14/1 rev.2. *GUIDELINES ON MEDICAL DEVICES IVD Medical Device Borderline and Classification issues A GUIDE FOR MANUFACTURERS AND NOTIFIED BODIES*(January 2012). EC website. http://ec.europa.eu/health/medical-devices/files/meddev/2_14_1_rev2_ol_en.pdf. Accessed 12 April 2012.
13. Since the entry into force of the Eudamed decision IVD manufacturers no longer have to notify the IVD in each member state in which the IVD is placed on the market, see Commission Decision

of 19 April 2010 on the European Databank on Medical Devices (Eudamed), OJ 2010 L102/45. EUR-Lex website. http://eur-lex.europa.eu/LexUriServ/LexUriServ.do?uri=OJ:L:2010:102:0045:0048:EN:PDF. Accessed 12 April 2012.
14. *IVDD* Article 5(1). EUR-Lex website. http://eur-lex.europa.eu/LexUriServ/LexUriServ.do?uri=CONSLEG:1998L0079:20031120:en:PDF. Accessed 12 April 2012.
15. ISO 14971:2009. *Medical Devices—Application of risk management to medical devices.*
16. Commission Decision of 20 December 2011amending Decision 2002/364/EC on common technical specifications for in vitro-diagnostic medical devices (2011/568/EU), OJ 2011 L341/63. EUR-Lex website. http://eur-lex.europa.eu/LexUriServ/LexUriServ.do?uri=OJ:L:2011:341:0063:0064:EN:PDF. Accessed 12 April 2012.
17. ISO 13485:2003. *Medical Devices—Quality management systems—Requirements for regulatory purposes.*
18. European Commission. MEDDEV 2.12/1 rev. 6. *Guidelines on a medical devices vigilance system* (December 2009). EC website. http://ec.europa.eu/health/medical-devices/files/meddev/2_12_1-rev_6-12-2009_en.pdf. Accessed 12 April 2012.
19. Global Harmonization Task Force, Study Group 1. *Summary Technical Documentation (STED) for Demonstrating Conformity to the Essential Principles of Safety and Performance of In Vitro Diagnostic Medical Devices* (March 2011). GHTF website. http://www.ghtf.org/documents/sg1/sg1final_n063.pdf. Accessed 12 April 2012.
20. ISO 18113:2009 (part 1–5). *In vitro diagnostic medical devices—Information supplied by the manufacturer (labelling).* (5 parts have been published).
21. *IVDD* Annex I.B, section 8.1, last paragraph. EUR-Lex website. http://eur-lex.europa.eu/LexUriServ/LexUriServ.do?uri=CONSLEG:1998L0079:20031120:en:PDF. Accessed 12 April 2012.
22. *IVDD* Article 4(4). EUR-Lex website. http://eur-lex.europa.eu/LexUriServ/LexUriServ.do?uri=CONSLEG:1998L0079:20031120:en:PDF. Accessed 12 April 2012.
23. European Commission. MEDDEV 2.14/3 rev. 1. *GUIDELINES ON MEDICAL DEVICES IVD Guidances: Supply of Instructions For Use (IFU) and other information for In-vitro Diagnostic (IVD) Medical Devices A GUIDE FOR MANUFACTURERS AND NOTIFIED BODIES.* EC website. http://ec.europa.eu/health/medical-devices/files/meddev/2_14_3_rev1_ifu_final_en.pdf. Accessed 12 April 2012.
24. European Committee for Standardization. EN 980:2008. *Symbols for use in the labelling of medical devices.* CEN website. www.cen.eu/cen/News/Spotlight%20on%20standards/Archive/Pages/Symbols.aspx. Accessed 12 April 2012.
25. Commission Decision 2010/227/EU of 19 April 2010 on the European Databank on Medical Devices (Eudamed). OJ 2010 L102, 23.4.2010. EUR-Lex website. http://eur-lex.europa.eu/LexUriServ/LexUriServ.do?uri=OJ:L:2010:102:0045:0048:EN:PDF. Accessed 12 April 2012.
26. *IVDD* Article 10, Form for the registration of manufacturers and devices. EUR-Lex website. http://eur-lex.europa.eu/LexUriServ/LexUriServ.do?uri=CONSLEG:1998L0079:20031120:en:PDF. Accessed 12 April 2012.
27. European Commission. *Revision of Directive 98/79/EC of the European Parliament and of the Council of 27 October 1998 on in vitro diagnostic medical devices—Summary of Responses to the Public Consultation* (February 2011). EC website. http://ec.europa.eu/health/medical-devices/files/recast_docs_2008/ivd_pc_outcome_en.pdf. Accessed 12 April 2012.
28. Regulation (EC) No 1907/2006 of the European Parliament and of the Council of 18 December 2006 concerning the Registration, Evaluation, Authorisation and Restriction of Chemicals (REACH), establishing a European Chemicals Agency, amending Directive 1999/45/EC and repealing Council Regulation (EEC) No 793/93 and Commission Regulation (EC) No 1488/94 as well as Council Directive 76/769/EEC and Commission Directives 91/155/EEC, 93/67/EEC, 93/105/EC and 2000/21/EC, OJ L 396, 30.12.2006, p. 1–849. EUR-Lex website. http://eur-lex.europa.eu/LexUriServ/LexUriServ.do?uri=oj:l:2006:396:0001:0849:en:pdf. Accessed 12 April 2012.

Chapter 14

Active Implantable Medical Devices

By Rodney Ruston, RAC, FRAPS

OBJECTIVES

❑ Summarise the EU *Active Implantable Medical Devices Directive*

❑ Describe the regulatory process to be followed by active implantable device manufacturers

❑ Focus on the specific elements in this directive

DIRECTIVES, REGULATIONS AND GUIDELINES COVERED IN THIS CHAPTER

❑ Council Directive 90/385/EEC of 20 June 1990 on the approximation of the laws of the Member States relating to active implantable medical devices

❑ MEDDEV 2.1/2 rev 2, Guidelines relating to the field of application of: The Council directive 90/385/EEC on active implantable medical devices, The Council directive 93/42/EEC on medical devices (April 1994)

❑ NB-MED/2.1/Rec3. Accessories and other parts for Active Implantable Medical Devices, 1996

❑ NB-MED/2.2/Rec2. Treatment of computer used to program Active Implantable Devices, 2000

Introduction

At first, it appears slightly strange that there is a directive (Council Directive 98/385/EEC, *Active Implantable Medical Device Directive* (*AIMDD*)) solely for the small sub-sector of active implantable medical devices (AIMDs). A quick look at the requirements reveals they are simply Class III medical devices. The significant clue as to why there is an *AIMDD* lies in the directive's publication date. Published in 1990, it preceded the *Medical Devices Directive* (*MDD*) by three years.

In the mid- to late 1980s, several EU Member States (or, more correctly for the time, EEC Member States) were contemplating regulatory approval procedures for active implantable devices. Until that time, no EEC Member State had legislation specifically related to medical devices. The active implantable medical device sector was and is fairly close-knit, and news of these Member States' intentions quickly filtered through the whole of the sector.

Although the following may not be an exact historical record, the final result is not in question. The active implantable medical device industry, now alarmed at the spectre of new regulatory approvals in numbers of European countries, approached the Commission to see if there was room within the then recently launched "New Approach" directives for active implantable medical devices. Such a move at the Commission level would set aside the efforts of Member States to publish their own legislation. At the same time, creation of a directive for a small sub-sector of medical devices would act as a useful pilot for a directive to cover the whole sector.

The result was the *AIMDD*.

The *AIMDD* has been something of an "orphan" since its publication. For example, it was somehow left out of the amendments contained in the *In Vitro Diagnostic Devices Directive*. Several amendments to the *MDD* are in that directive, which were directly applicable to the *AIMDD*. The *AIMDD* contained a number of errors that were not corrected until Directive 2007/47/EC, e.g., in clinical investigations,

Table 14-1. Comparison of *AIMDD* and *MDD* Annexes

AIMDD	MDD	Notes
Annex 1	Annex I	Fewer clauses in the *AIMDD* since it covers a narrower field of devices
Annex 2	Annex II	No difference
Annex 3	Annex III	No difference
Annex 4	Annex IV	No difference
Annex 5	Annex V	No difference
Annex 6	Annex VIII	No difference
Annex 7	Annex X	Difference in paragraph numbering only
Annex 8	Annex XI	No difference
Annex 9	Annex XII	No difference
None	Annex VI, VII, VIII, IX	No equivalent in *AIMDD*

the *AIMDD* required the manufacturer to record adverse incidents, but there was no provision for notifying authorities.

Bestowing orphan status on the *AIMDD*, in fact, does it a disfavour. This is because in Article 6(2) it establishes the Committee on Medical Devices. This committee is referenced in both of the later directives on medical devices, the *MDD* (93/42/EEC, Article 7(1), and the *IVDD*, Article 7(1).

The Scope of the *AIMDD*

The *AIMDD* (Art. 1.2.b) defines an AIMD as follows:

"(a) 'medical device' means any instrument, apparatus, appliance, software, material or other article, whether used alone or in combination, together with any accessories, including the software intended by its manufacturer to be used specifically for diagnostic and/or therapeutic purposes and necessary for its proper application, intended by the manufacturer to be used for human beings for the purpose of:
— diagnosis, prevention, monitoring, treatment or alleviation of disease,
— diagnosis, monitoring, treatment, alleviation of or compensation for an injury or handicap,
— investigation, replacement or modification of the anatomy or of a physiological process,
— control of conception,
and which does not achieve its principal intended action in or on the human body by pharmacological, immunological or metabolic means, but which may be assisted in its function by such means;
(b) 'active medical device' means any medical device relying for its functioning on a source of electrical energy or any source of power other than that directly generated by the human body or gravity;
(c) 'active implantable medical device' means any active medical device which is intended to be totally or partially introduced, surgically or medically, into the human body or by medical intervention into a natural orifice, and which is intended to remain after the procedure;"[1]

MEDDEV 2.1/2 rev 2, although published in 1994, remains current, and gives useful guidance on what should or should not be considered as an AIMD. A good example is given in an external infusion pump. It says "an external drug infusion pump, although for long-term or permanent use, which is connected to a catheter "partially introduced" into the body is not considered as an active implantable device."[2]

The other key difference between the *AIMDD* and the other medical devices directives is in the definition of a medical device. The first sentence in the definition of a medical device in the *AIMDD* (Article 1(2)) states:

"'medical device' means any instrument, apparatus, appliance, software, material or other article, whether used alone or in combination, *together with any accessories*, including the software intended by its manufacturer…"[3] (italics used here to accentuate the difference).

This difference means that accessories to active implantable medical devices are themselves classified as active implantable medical devices. It is difficult to understand what, precisely, was in the minds of those who wrote this directive when they included "accessories as active implantable medical devices." The case starts to look somewhat absurd when the Essential Requirement for labelling (Annex 1(14)) requires that "every device must bear…the following particulars…"[4] It then goes on to stipulate that the sterile pack must carry the "method of sterilization…the time limit for implanting the device safely."[5] It is clear that requirement cannot apply to a programmer used for controlling, etc., active implantables. So, how can accessories be "active implantable medical devices"?

Process to be Followed by the Manufacturer

The processes to be followed by the manufacturer are exactly the same as for Class III medical devices under the *MDD*. The advent of amending Directive 2007/47/EC has brought the conformity assessment annexes in the *AIMDD* to exactly the same wording as the *MDD*. These are cross-referenced in **Table 14-1**.

Finally, as with the other directives, CE marking under the *AIMDD* remains a self-declaration by the manufacturer, and not the responsibility of the Notified Body (NB). Of course, as in the other routes to conformity where an NB is required to be involved, the declaration can only be made "on the basis of Notified Body certificate…," but, nevertheless, it is a self-declaration.

Summary

The *AIMDD* was the first medical devices directive. As such, it was a pilot for the remaining medical device directives. It remains a directive, and all active implantable devices and their accessories (which are also classified as "active implantable devices") are regulated through it.

The conformity assessment routes for AIMDs are the same as those for Class III medical devices.

References

1. Council Directive 90/385/EEC of 20 June 1990 on the approximation of the laws of the Member States relating to active implantable medical devices (*Active Implantable Medical Devices Directive (AIMDD)*). EUR-Lex website. http://eur-lex.europa.eu/LexUriServ/LexUriServ.do?uri=CELEX:31990L0385:en:HTML. Accessed 21 May 2012.
2. MEDDEV 2.1/2 rev 2, *Guidelines relating to the field of application of: The Council directive 90/385/EEC on active implantable medical devices, The Council directive 93/42/EEC on medical devices* (April 1994). EC website. http://ec.europa.eu/health/medical-devices/files/meddev/2_1-2___04-1994_en.pdf. Accessed 21 May 2012.
3. Op cit 1.
4. Ibid.
5. Ibid.

Chapter 15

Medical Device Compliance: Postmarket Requirements

Updated by Claudia Ising, RAC

OBJECTIVES

- Obtain an overview of the mechanisms in place to ensure medical device compliance in the postmarket phase

- Review the requirements for manufacturers concerning postmarket surveillance procedures

- Understand the European vigilance system concerning medical devices and the requirements for incident reporting

- Review other measures that are used by Member States' Competent Authorities to control the medical device market

DIRECTIVES, REGULATIONS AND GUIDELINES COVERED IN THIS CHAPTER

- Council Directive 90/385/EEC of 20 June 1990 on the approximation of the laws of the Member States relating to active implantable medical devices

- Council Directive 93/42/EEC of 14 June 1993 concerning medical devices

- Directive 98/79/EC of the European Parliament and of the Council of 27 October 1998 on *in vitro* diagnostic medical devices

- Directive 2001/95/EC of the European Parliament and of the Council of 3 December 2001 on general product safety

- MEDDEV 2.12/1 (Rev. 7) Medical Devices—Guidelines on a medical devices vigilance system, 2012

- MEDDEV 2.12/2 (Rev. 2) Medical Devices—Guidelines on post market clinical follow-up, 2004

- Commission Decision of 19 April 2010 on the European Databank on Medical Devices (Eudamed) 2010/227/EC

- Report on the Functioning of the *Medical Devices Directive*

- Communication from the Commission of 2 July 2003 to the Council and the European Parliament on Medical Devices

Introduction

In the application and enforcement of the European medical device directives, it is essential to have an effective system to collect, analyse and share information about issues concerning devices and any adverse incidents resulting from their day-to-day use. Having an effective information system makes it possible for all interested parties, particularly Member State Competent Authorities, to take action as needed to protect the public.

The medical device directives establish two principal mechanisms for providing feedback about medical devices. The first mechanism arises from the requirement for manufacturers to implement a systematic procedure to review postproduction phase device experience and implement appropriate means to apply any necessary corrective action. This mechanism is commonly referred to as postmarket surveillance. Directive 2007/47/EC of the European Parliament and of the Council of 5 September 2007, amending Council Directive 90/385/EEC on the approximation of the laws of the Member States relating to active implantable medical devices (*AIMDD*) and Council Directive 93/42/EEC concerning medical devices (*MDD*) indicated that postmarket surveillance data are also to be used to update the clinical evaluation report document.

The second mechanism stems from the requirement to notify Competent Authorities when a so-called incident, near incident or recall (Field Safety Corrective Action (FSCA)) occurs. An "incident or recall" is defined as:

a) any malfunction or deterioration in a device's characteristics and/or performance, as well as any inadequacy in the labelling or the Instructions for Use that might lead to or might have led to the death of a patient or user or a serious deterioration in his state of health

b) any technical or medical reason relating to a device's characteristics or performance for the reasons referred to in subparagraph (a), leading to a manufacturer's systematic recall of devices of the same type

The criteria and procedures used by manufacturers, Competent Authorities and all other interested parties to notify and handle incidents and FSCAs/recalls are collectively known as the Medical Devices Vigilance System.

Provisions regarding these two mechanisms are found in various sections of the medical device directives, as summarised in **Table 15-1.**

In each case, the objective is to provide feedback and analysis so the manufacturer and/or Competent Authority can put any subsequent measures into practice.

Relationship Between the *General Product Safety Directive* and the Medical Devices Directives

Other, less-obvious, horizontal directives, such as Directive 2001/94/EC of the European Parliament and of the Council of 3 December 2001 concerning general product safety (*General Product Safety Directive* or *GPSD*), also need to be considered. This directive is intended to ensure a high level of product safety for consumer products; it completes, complements and reinforces the medical device vigilance provisions found in the *AIMDD, MDD* and *In Vitro Devices Directive* (*IVDD*).

Regarding the *MDD*, examples of products falling under the scope of the *GPSD* are adhesive bandages, crutches, condoms, glasses, contact lenses, hearing aids and in vitro diagnostics for self-testing. Medical devices supplied to healthcare professionals and intended to be used by them—even if used on a consumer—generally do not qualify as consumer products. Examples include cardiovascular catheters, laboratory equipment, scalpels and x-ray equipment.

The *GPSD* uses the term "producer," and producers are responsible for placing safe products on the market. Producers are defined as follows: manufacturer of a product when established in the EU, entity presenting as manufacturer by affixing name or trademark, manufacturer's representative or importer of product and other professionals in the supply chain whose activities may affect a product's safety.

The medical device directives cover most producer obligations specified in the *GPSD*. *GPSD* Articles 5.1 and 5.3 may, however, apply regarding producers' general obligation to follow up on product safety after placing devices on the market and to inform Competent Authorities about dangerous products and actions to prevent risk related to custom-made devices, in those cases where they are considered consumer products. Additionally, the medical device directives have no provisions related to distributors' obligations, though the "New Approach" directives define economic operators: manufacturer, Authorised Representatives, importers and distributors. Therefore, aspects of *GPSD* Article 5 relevant for distributors apply to medical device consumer products.

Postmarket Surveillance Procedures

As indicated in the corresponding directive articles, medical device manufacturers are required to implement a systematic procedure to review device experience in the postproduction phase.

This requirement affects all information concerning medical devices that:

- have been appropriately CE marked and put into service
- are not CE-marked:
  o but fall under the directives' scope (e.g., custom-made devices)
  o were placed on the market before the entry into force of the *MDD*
  o where such incidents lead to Corrective Actions(s) relevant to the devices mentioned above

The guidelines cover FSCAs relevant to CE-marked devices offered for sale or in use within the EEA, Switzerland and Turkey.

This system should be both proactive (seeking information) and reactive (collecting and assessing complaints). Possible sources of information and/or experience include:

- customer and user surveys

- adverse incidents (vigilance system)
- user reports and feedback on product aspects
- customer complaints
- customer requirements, contract information and market needs
- patient follow-up after clinical trials or investigations
- services and evaluation reports
- scientific papers in peer-reviewed journals
- reports on similar products by competitors
- compliance-related communications from regulatory agencies
- changes to relevant standards and regulations

The important point is that the manufacturer must implement procedures to collect and analyse this information, then handle and process it appropriately to determine whether any corrective or preventive action is necessary. If incidents, near incidents or FSCAs are detected through this procedure, or if the actions to be taken involve change or correction of devices already placed on the market, the Competent Authorities may need to be informed in accordance with the vigilance system. (It should be noted that the term "near incident" is no longer used since the revision of the European guidance, MEDDEV 2.12/1.)

Procedures for reviewing feedback also are mentioned in standards for medical device quality assurance and management systems. For example, Section 8.2.1 of EN ISO 13485 states that the manufacturer, "shall establish a documented procedure for a feedback system to provide early warning of quality problems and for input to the corrective and preventive action processes" and that, "if national or regional regulations require the organisation to gain experience from the post-production phase, the review of this experience shall form part of the feedback system."

Trend reporting is introduced as part of the medical devices vigilance system with MEDDEV 2.12 (Rev. 7). Manufacturers or their Authorised Representatives are required to report a significant increase or trend in events or incidents that usually are excluded from individual reporting as per 2.12 Rev. 7's Chapter 5.1.3 to the relevant National Competent Authority. The trend report is expected regardless of whether Periodic Summary Reporting has been agreed.

The system for gathering postmarket surveillance information has been identified by the Medical Devices Expert Group as a weak point in the medical device directives; the consensus is that further guidance is needed to promote manufacturer improvement of these systems.

Risk Management in the Medical Device Industry

Risk assessment, risk analysis and risk management are critical phases for any medical device in design, production and postmarket surveillance.

Regulatory bodies and standards development committees prefer a descriptive rather than a prescriptive approach during the standards development process. This seems a sensible way to move forward, as technology changes rather quickly, and prescribing numeric values or specific details for compliance makes the existing standards' versions outdated in regard to any technological advance. Effectively, it means that the onus is on manufacturers to define their own risk-acceptance criteria in accordance with the relevant standards' described guidance to demonstrate compliance.

As part of postmarket surveillance activities, manufacturers need to review developments in regulations and standards. Currently, manufacturers are reasonably well-organised when it comes to generating the initial risk management file. However, they rarely revisit and update these documents from risk perspectives after product release; at times, these documents do not reflect the current status of known issues with which risks may be associated. If a new standard has been implemented, existing products are not necessarily considered unsafe. However, it could be questionable whether a product is still complying with the state-of-the-art principle, and Notified Bodies are likely to address this question in the context of certificate renewal. Implementing new or revised standards stresses the importance of a comprehensive risk management file and emphasises that the file should be a living document that reflects and documents all known product issues from all project phases, including postmarket surveillance. From risk perspectives, manufacturers usually react to a raised complaint or an issue and then try to address the problem. It would be advisable to have a combination of proactive and reactive strategies for managing risks throughout the product lifecycle.

Postmarket Surveillance for AIMDs and MDDs

Additionally, clinical evaluation and its documentation must be actively updated. In general, postmarket clinical follow-up (PMCF) is deemed necessary, as premarket data do not necessarily enable the manufacturer to detect infrequent complications or problems that become apparent only after long-term use. Where PMCF is deemed unnecessary as part of the device's postmarket surveillance plan, this must be duly justified and documented. All of this information should be included in the risk assessment, which is part of the technical file/design dossier. MEDDEV 2.12-2 (Rev. 2) emphasises requirements to update data throughout the product's lifecycle and lays out expectations and requirements for data to remain state of the art in compliance with the initial CE-marked device. Postmarket surveillance plans, required by the manufacturer's quality system, are supposed to help identify and investigate residual risks associated with placing devices on the market.

Medical Devices Vigilance System

Competent Authorities are responsible for establishing and operating a medical devices vigilance system within each Member State. Under *AIMDD* Article 8, *MDD* Article 10 and *IVDD* Article 11, Competent Authorities are responsible for taking all necessary steps to ensure that information concerning incidents is centrally recorded and evaluated. This coordination is facilitated by a central database.

Eudamed is a central database not accessible by the public for information exchange between national Competent Authorities and the European Commission. Eudamed's use became obligatory in May 2011. Within Eudamed, use of a common code, the Global Medical Device Nomenclature (GMDN) code, is encouraged; at the time of updating this chapter, entries can be made without using GMDN code. For IVDs, the regulatory hurdle to file Article 10 notifications in every EU Member State was eliminated with the implementation of Eudamed. **Table 15-1** gives an overview of what data is included in Eudamed across the three medical device directives.

Information and data collected and recorded in this manner are intended to be shared among Competent Authorities, thereby facilitating corrective action earlier than if data were evaluated on a state-by-state basis. This gives the vigilance system considerable relevance for protecting patients', users' and third parties' health and safety. On the basis of the information collected and evaluated, Competent Authorities may decide to disseminate information within the market to prevent incidents.

Extensive guidance on interpreting the directives' requirements concerning vigilance is provided in MEDDEV 2.12/1 (Rev. 7, June 2012). There were significant modifications from Rev. 4 (April 2003) to Rev. 5 (April 2007) and Rev. 6 (December 2009). Revision 7 includes, in addition to general amendments:

- the introduction of European medical device database Eudamed
- transposition and integration of Global Harmonization Task Force (GHTF) international regulatory guidance documents on vigilance and postmarket surveillance into the European context; introduction of EU trend reporting
- new and updated forms: new Report Forms, Annex 6—Manufacturer's Periodic Summary Report and Annex 7—Manufacturer's Trend Report Form and updated Report Forms (Annex 3 and Annex 4)

Revision 7 of this MEDDEV harmonises vigilance system requirements based on the following GHTF guidances:

- SG2-N8 *Guidance on How to Handle Information Concerning Vigilance Reporting Related to Medical Devices*
- SG2-N79 *Medical Devices: Post Market Surveillance: National Competent Authority Exchange Criteria and Report Form*
- SG2-N54 *Global Guidance for Adverse Event Reporting for Medical Devices*

Although not legally binding, this guidance is the result of a general consensus among Competent Authorities, European Commission services and industry representatives and, in the latest revision, GHTF. It is expected, therefore, that the document's recommendations will be closely followed in many Member States.

MEDDEV 2.12/1 (Rev. 7) describes the medical devices vigilance system as a vehicle for adverse incident notification and evaluation. It covers the activities of the European Commission, Competent Authorities, manufacturers, Authorised Representatives, users and others concerned with continued medical device safety. Moreover, the vigilance guidelines clarify actions to be taken once a manufacturer or Competent Authority receives information concerning an incident. The guideline is intended for uniform application of the medical device vigilance system to the *AIMDD*, *MDD* and *IVDD*. The procedures are intended to be the same for all the directives with respect to the vigilance system and refer to incidents that occur within EU Member States and those within the European Economic Area (EEA), Switzerland and Turkey regarding devices bearing the CE Mark. The guidance also applies to incidents involving devices that do not bear the CE Mark when they lead to an FSCA relevant to CE-marked devices.

The vigilance guidance establishes that incident reporting for in vitro diagnostic devices (IVDs) may be comparatively difficult to implement because such devices do not generally come into contact with patients. In those cases, direct harm to patients due to IVDs may be difficult to demonstrate. Any harm is more likely to be indirect—a consequence of a medical decision or action taken on the basis of information provided by the device, such as the following:

- wrong or delayed diagnosis
- inappropriate or delayed treatment
- transfusion of inappropriate substances

The guidance gives special attention to self-test devices because with those products, the medical decision is to be made by the user or patient. The guidance establishes that inadequacies in the information and Instructions for Use of self-test devices may lead to harm and should be carefully reviewed.

Types of Incidents to Be Reported

Three types of incidents must be reported to the Competent Authorities:

- incidents that result in a death

Table 15-1. Eudamed Data Repository

Concern	MDD Directive 93/42/EEC	AIMDD Directive 90/385/EEC	IVDD Directive 98/79/EEC
Vigilance	Data relating to CE certificates issued, modified, suspended, withdrawn or refused Data relating to registration of manufacturers and authorized representatives and devices (excluding custom-made devices) Data obtained in accordance with the vigilance procedure in MDD	Data relating to CE certificates issued, modified, suspended, withdrawn or refused Data obtained in accordance with the vigilance procedure in AIMDD	Data relating to CE certificates issued, modified, suspended, withdrawn or refused Data relating to registration of manufacturers and Authorised Representatives and devices in accordance with Article 10 Data obtained in accordance with the vigilance procedure in IVDD
Clinical Investigations	Annex VIII notification to the EU country where clinical trial is to be conducted. Authority interventions in clinical investigations Notification of (early) termination of clinical investigation to authorities	Annex 6 notification reported in the country where clinical investigation is conducted Authority interventions in clinical investigations Notification of early termination of clinical investigation to authorities	N/A

- incidents that result in a serious deterioration in the state of health of a patient, user or other person
- events that might have led to death or serious deterioration in health but did not, as a result of fortunate circumstances or the intervention of healthcare personnel

The vigilance guidance states specifically that "serious deterioration in the state of health" may include life-threatening illness or injury or the permanent impairment of or damage to a bodily function. The same is true for cases that require medical treatment or surgery to prevent injury or permanent impairment of specific bodily functions.

For events that might have led to death or serious deterioration in health, the reporting duty exists if the event occurred in connection with the use of a medical device and was such that it might lead to death or serious deterioration in health if it occurs again. These events also may occur when testing or examining the device, or the Instructions for Use reveals deterioration in characteristics or shortcomings that could lead to death or serious deterioration in health.

In all cases, the guidance points out that the term "serious deterioration" cannot be conclusively defined in practice because it is subject to evaluative interpretation in each case. When doubt exists as to reporting duty, the guidance establishes that a medical practitioner must be consulted and that, in general, personnel should be predisposed to report.

Criteria for Incident Reporting

When they become aware of a situation that may be considered an incident or near incident, manufacturers are to use three basic criteria to decide whether the Competent Authorities should be notified:

- An event has occurred.
- The manufacturer's device is suspected of being a contributory cause of the incident.
- The event led, or might have led, to one of the following outcomes:
  o death of a patient, user or other person
  o serious deterioration in the state of health of a patient, user or other person

Some additional considerations must be taken into account concerning what may be a "serious deterioration in the state of health," and certain events may be considered exempt from reporting duties even though they meet reporting criteria. Section 5.13 of the vigilance guidance provides criteria for determining such exemptions; examples include:

- deficiencies in devices found by the user prior to use
- events caused by patient conditions
- adverse events related to use of the device after the stated service life or shelf life has expired
- events that did not lead to death or serious deterioration in the state of health because protection against a fault functioned correctly
- events that did not lead to death or serious deterioration in the state of health and when, within a full risk assessment, the risk of death or serious deterioration was quantified and found to be negligible

- expected and foreseeable side effects
- events described in an advisory notice
- specific exemptions granted by a Competent Authority

Manufacturers should carefully consider all circumstances when deciding whether an event should be exempt from reporting duties. All criteria used should be formally documented for possible future reference as evidence that the issue was evaluated and the rationale for the decision.

Medical Device Linked to the Incident

To trigger a reporting duty, a certain link must exist between the event and the use of the medical device. The vigilance guidance recommends that the manufacturer take certain background information into account when the link between the event and the medical device is difficult to establish. Examples of such information are:
- the opinion, based on evidence, of healthcare professionals
- results of the manufacturer's own preliminary assessment
- evidence of previous similar incidents
- other evidence held by the manufacturer

Such a link is assumed to exist in the event of a medical device's malfunction or deterioration in characteristics or performance. Malfunction or deterioration is understood to be the failure of the device to perform its intended purpose when used in accordance with the manufacturer's instructions (e.g., an unpredicted biological effect of the device).

Omission of information or errors and inaccuracies in labelling or Instructions for Use also are considered sufficient grounds for establishing a possible link between the incident and the medical device.

Timeline for Initial Reporting of an Incident

Incidents are to be reported to the Competent Authority immediately, unless there is a justifiable reason for delay. The vigilance guidance establishes the maximum elapsed time from awareness of the event to notification of the Competent Authorities as two calendar days for a serious public health threat, 10 calendar days for death or unanticipated serious deterioration in state of health and 30 elapsed calendar days for other incidents.

In practice, when a death or serious deterioration is reported, the manufacturer has up to 10 days to determine whether the occurrence fulfils the reporting criteria for events. If, within that time, the manufacturer is unable to rule out a device placed on the market under its responsibility as the cause, it must inform the Competent Authorities and submit an initial vigilance report.

Similarly, when the manufacturer receives a report that a death or serious deterioration could have occurred, although fortunate circumstances or the intervention of healthcare personnel precluded death or serious deterioration in state of health relative to a device placed on the market under its responsibility and it cannot rule out the device as the cause within 30 days, it must inform the Competent Authorities and submit an initial vigilance report.

To Whom Should the Initial Report Be Sent?

In general, the report should be made to the Competent Authority in the country where the incident occurred.

In addition, national transpositions of the medical device directives may require that manufacturers inform particular Member State Competent Authorities when planning to take action in response to incidents within that Member State's territory. Manufacturers and individuals responsible for placing medical devices on the market must take this into account when applying Community-wide corrective or preventive actions.

If the manufacturer is located outside the EEA, a suitable contact point within the EEA should be provided in the initial report (European Authorised Representative).

A suggested format for the initial report is included as Annex 3 of MEDDEV 2.12/1 (Rev. 7). This document is now available on the European Commission website. Some Member States have made similar formats available on the Internet to facilitate the administrative procedure and provide specific incident reporting criteria. Also, some Member States require mandatory electronic reporting.

If the initial report is made by means other than mail or fax (e.g., telephone or email), it should be followed as soon as possible by written confirmation. The manufacturer must avoid unduly delaying the report due to incomplete information, and may include a statement to the effect that it is making the report without prejudice and does not imply any admission of liability for the incident or its consequences.

Incident Investigations

Manufacturers are expected to follow up initial incident assessments with an investigation of the surrounding circumstances. Competent Authorities may initiate their own investigations and decide to intervene in the manufacturer's investigation, especially if access to the device associated with the incident may alter it in any way that might affect subsequent analysis. If the manufacturer cannot perform the investigation, the Competent Authorities must ensure that an investigation is carried out and keep the manufacturer informed.

Involved Competent Authorities may monitor the investigation's progress. Monitoring may include requesting follow-up reports from the manufacturer on:

- how many devices are involved and where they have been sold
- the current status of the devices on the market
- how long the devices have been on the market
- details of design changes that have been made

The ability to trace medical devices' distribution is, therefore, vital to providing reliable information on the location and state of use of particular devices or batches in the event of an incident.

For incidents involving notification of more than one Competent Authority, a single coordinating Competent Authority responsible for most communications may be designated.

Following the investigation, the manufacturer should take all necessary action, including consulting with the Competent Authority and performing any recalls. The follow-up to the investigation should conclude with the manufacturer's final report to the relevant Competent Authority illustrating the investigation's outcome. Outcomes may include:
- no action
- additional surveillance or follow-up of devices in use
- dissemination of information to users (e.g., by advisory notice)
- corrective action for future production
- corrective action for devices in use
- device recall/FSCA
- cessation of device commercialisation

Additionally, the Competent Authority may take the following actions:
- gather more information by commissioning independent reports
- make recommendations to the manufacturer to improve information provided with the device
- keep the European Commission and Competent Authorities informed about recalls and other actions to be taken
- consult with the relevant Notified Body (NB) on matters relating to the conformity assessment
- consult with the European Commission if device reclassification is necessary
- provide additional user education
- take any other action to supplement manufacturer action

Competent Authorities also may decide to disseminate information related to reported incidents. Such information may be circulated among Competent Authorities using a Competent Authority Report. Such reports are intended only for other Competent Authorities and the European Commission, and the manufacturer should be informed when they are to be issued. The MEDDEV also mentions the GHTF National Competent Authority Report exchange programme.

Competent Authorities and manufacturers may decide to disseminate information to medical device users. Such information should be directed to specific medical practitioners and healthcare facilities but, in exceptional circumstances, it also may be directed to the public. It is important to coordinate actions by Competent Authorities and manufacturers, especially when preparing and issuing statements to the media, to review the information's possible positive or negative impact.

Following receipt of the manufacturer's final report, the Competent Authority may close the incident file and inform the manufacturer; however, these files are retained by the Competent Authority and the incident may be reopened if circumstances change.

Field Safety Corrective Actions and Field Safety Notices

The manufacturer must notify the Competent Authority of any technical or medical reasons for a device's systematic recall or FSCA. The term "withdrawal" used in the *AIMDD* is interpreted in the same way. Removals from the market for purely commercial reasons are not included and do not require any vigilance reporting.

When implementing an FSCA, the manufacturer must issue a Field Safety Notice (FSN) and send copies of the FSN to the Competent Authorities of the countries in which the FSCA is performed. The Competent Authority responsible for the manufacturer or Authorised Representative (if the manufacturer is not established in the EU) should be notified. For devices with NB involvement in the conformity assessment, the Competent Authority in the state in which the NB is located should also be notified.

Trend Reporting

Trend reporting is introduced in MEDDEV 2.12 (Rev. 7). Manufacturers or their Authorised Representatives are required to report a significant increase or trend in events or incidents that are usually excluded from individual reporting as per Chapter 5.1.3 to the relevant national Competent Authority. A report (using Form 7) should be filed with the relevant national Competent Authority. Manufacturers should have suitable systems in place and proactively scrutinise trends in complaints and incidents occurring with their devices.

The trend report (Annex 7 to MEDDEV 2.12) should be made if there is a significant increase in the rate of:
- already reportable incidents
- incidents that are usually exempt from reporting
- events that are usually not reportable

Chapter 15

Table 15-2. Comparison of Safeguard Clause and Health Monitoring Measures

Concern	Safeguard Clause Mechanism	Health Monitoring Measure
Initiation of the procedures	The Member State must establish (e.g., as a result of vigilance) that a device may compromise health or safety when used as intended.	The Member State must provide sufficient evidence to support reasonable doubt that the medical device offers an adequate level of protection of health and safety.
Parties involved	The European Commission consults with the Member State that invoked the Safeguard Clause and other interested parties.	The European Commission must consult with interested parties and all Member States.
Outcome	If the European Commission confirms that the national measure is justified, Member States are informed and may adopt appropriate national measures.	If the European Commission confirms that the national measure is justified, it develops a measure that must be adopted (uniformly) throughout the Community after Regulatory Committee consultation.

The trend report is expected regardless of whether Periodic Summary Reporting has been agreed.

Relation to Medical Device Global Vigilance

GHTF has been working toward establishing a global vigilance system. With transition from GHTF to the International Medical Device Regulator Forum (IMDRF) in 2012, the remaining tasks are being transferred to the new organisation. The global vigilance approach has many similarities to the European Medical Devices Vigilance System, but it also differs in several ways. For instance, the global system terminology is somewhat different (e.g., it uses the term "adverse event" instead of "incident"). In addition, in contrast to the European manufacturer-oriented reporting system, the global system is wider in scope, encompassing user reports and user errors. To promote systematic notation in global vigilance reporting, a technical specification (ISO TS 19218) has been developed to establish a coding system for adverse event reporting. The new system will facilitate global data exchange among regulatory bodies, thereby providing more-accurate reporting and identification of the involved devices and event types.

Vigilance Versus Manufacturers' Postmarket Duties

Although the processes are interrelated, medical device vigilance must be distinguished from manufacturers' postmarket surveillance duties.

Postmarket surveillance may be understood as a "proactive and reactive" process that involves detecting quality problems through review and analysis of market feedback. The system implemented by the manufacturer to obtain feedback should fulfil the requirements of EN ISO 13485, clause 8.2.1. Reviewing experience gained with medical devices in the postmarket phase is an important element of risk management. Medical device risk management should be implemented in accordance with EN ISO 14971.

Vigilance is a "reactive" process because it involves responding appropriately to reports that a medical device has caused or may cause patient harm, or that the instructions for use are inaccurate or open to misinterpretation. Vigilance procedures are expected to follow MEDDEV 2.12/1 (Rev. 7) even though, as guidance, the provisions may not be enforced by law.

Vigilance is an element of postmarket surveillance. Postmarket surveillance is a process for understanding experience with the device through systematic feedback and review of information from many sources, among them vigilance information. Vigilance is a specific procedure for communicating with Competent Authorities and acting on reported incidents appropriately. Incidents are often detected, for example, through such postmarket surveillance procedures as complaint handling.

Other Provisions for Market Surveillance and Control

The medical devices vigilance system described in MEDDEV 2.12/1 (Rev. 7) is one mechanism Competent Authorities use to control the medical devices market. Various other mechanisms foreseen in the medical device directives are intended specifically to facilitate enforcement of those provisions. Competent Authorities may develop administrative procedures for further market control in their corresponding Member States on the basis of the following regulations:
- requirements that technical documentation be made available for inspection by the Competent Authorities
- ability to extend incident reporting obligations to include users and persons responsible for medical device calibration and servicing
- requirements for a registry containing the names and addresses of all persons responsible for placing medical devices on the market

Therefore, depending on the Member State in question, additional requirements may be in place to enhance market control:
- licence for manufacture, import, assembly and sterilisation activities
- notification of distribution activities, sales activities and sales with individual adaptation of medical devices (e.g., hearing aids)
- regulation of publicity

These methods improve Competent Authorities' awareness of both the products being placed on the market within their territory and the individuals responsible for placing them on the market. Anomalies detected by Competent Authorities through market surveillance include:
- products bearing the medical device CE Mark that are not covered by the medical device directives (e.g., borderline products such as cosmetics and personal protection equipment)
- devices for which the appropriate Conformity Assessment Procedure has not been followed (e.g., Class I sterile devices without intervention by an NB)
- devices including parts that do not bear a CE Mark or that have been given a different intended use by a supplier than that intended by the original manufacturer
- devices whose labelling is not in the required language

A special Market Surveillance Operations Group (MSOG) has been established to improve Member States' coordination on these and other issues relating to market control.

Safeguard Clause

Market control procedures may facilitate information transmittal to Competent Authorities; this information may be used to initiate special measures in accordance with the Safeguard Clause in the medical device directives (*AIMDD* Article 7, *MDD* Article 8 and *IVDD* Article 8). Member States have the right under the Safeguard Clause to take all appropriate interim measures to withdraw a device from the market, or prohibit or restrict its placement on the market, if the device, when correctly installed, maintained and used for its intended purpose, may compromise health or safety. A Member State that takes such measures is obliged to notify the European Commission; it must indicate the reasons for taking the actions and, if the measures are justified, the Commission informs all other Member States. This process, however, does not mean that all other Member States are obliged to adopt similar measures, even though they may be expected to do so.

Health Monitoring Measures

The *IVDD* introduced a new mechanism for Competent Authorities to use in the postmarket phase. Through health monitoring, a Member State may take any necessary and justified transitional measures relative to a given product or group of products if, to protect consumer health and safety or the public health, product availability should be prohibited, restricted or subjected to particular requirements. The Member State then must inform the European Commission and all other Member States. These health monitoring measures are intended to apply a precautionary principle. The Safeguard Clause and health monitoring measures have fundamental differences, summarised in **Table 15-2**.

An example of a measure taken in accordance with the Safeguard Clause is Germany's banning of catgut. In general, it is considered that further guidance is necessary to clarify the conditions under which Member States can use health monitoring measures.

European Databank on Medical Devices—Eudamed

The aim of Eudamed is to strengthen market surveillance and transparency in the medical device field by providing Member State Competent Authorities fast access to information on manufacturers and Authorised Representatives; on devices, certificates, vigilance and clinical investigation data; and to contribute to a uniform application of the directives, particularly in relation to registration requirements.

Eudamed's Role in Postmarket Requirements (Market Surveillance and Vigilance)

The *MDD*, *AIMDD* and *IVDD*, as amended, made provision for a central European databank for medical devices. Mandatory for Member States since May 2011, following the European Commission decision of 19 April 2010 on the European Databank on Medical Devices (Eudamed), the databank allows Competent Authorities to create transparency and coordinate enforcement of the device directives, e.g., for postmarket requirements. The databank is not publicly accessible. The annex to Commission Decision 2010/227/EU lists data minimally required to be entered in various modules following obligations arising from the medical device directives, including:.
- registration of manufacturers, Authorised Representatives and devices
- devices placed on the Community market
- certificates issued, modified, supplemented, suspended, withdrawn or refused
- vigilance procedure data
- clinical investigation data

Eudamed significantly enhances the coordination between Competent Authorities regarding enforcement of the medical device directives and is particularly relevant in facilitating communication within the European Medical Devices Vigilance System. For this reason, the vigilance module was one of the first features put into operation.

Some issues, such as nomenclature, custom-made device inclusion or exclusion, and minor differences between the European Medical Devices Vigilance System and that proposed by GHTF, had led to delays in implementing Eudamed. Nomenclature was covered by ISO 15225 and the Global Medical Device Nomenclature (GMDN), and custom-made devices were excluded from the database.

The GMDN Maintenance Agency maintains web-based nomenclature accessible to manufacturers for a fee (www.gmdnagency.com). While the GMDN code is standard for most Member States, the translation into German encountered delays in changing from using UMDNS code systems.

Summary

- Medical device manufacturers are obliged to implement postmarket surveillance procedures to understand the experience with medical devices in the postproduction phase and provide input to corrective and preventive processes.
- Information feedback and risk management are important postmarket surveillance aspects; they may be implemented in accordance with EN ISO 13485 and EN ISO 14971, respectively.
- Manufacturers are obliged to report incidents and near incidents to the relevant Competent Authorities. In some EU Member States, this reporting obligation is extended to medical device users.
- MEDDEV 2.12/1 (Rev. 7) establishes detailed guidance and criteria for both reportable incidents and procedures manufacturers and Competent Authorities should follow when such incidents occur. Revision 7 implements global harmonisation aspects of postmarket surveillance, vigilance reporting and adverse event reporting
- Vigilance reporting is obligatory when manufacturers implement medical device recalls for technical or medical reasons. Trend reports are expected regardless of agreements to submit periodic safety summaries.
- Postmarket surveillance and vigilance are interrelated processes; each uses information from the other as input.
- Member State Competent Authorities exercise market surveillance using mechanisms to enforce implementation of the medical device directives' provisions.
- Member State Competent Authorities may implement special controls and restrictions under the Safeguard Clause or as health monitoring measures.
- The Eudamed database facilitates regulatory data exchange and enforcement among Competent Authorities, particularly concerning vigilance.

Chapter 16

Medical Device National Particularities

Updated by Claudia Ising, RAC

OBJECTIVES

❑ Understand the importance of national transpositions, in particular the following aspects:

    o   Language requirements for Instructions for Use and labels

    o   Notification to the Competent Authority

    o   National provisions for marketing, sales and distribution organisations and personnel

    o   National provisions in clinical development

(Note this chapter relates primarily to "general" medical devices.)

DIRECTIVES, REGULATIONS AND GUIDELINES COVERED IN THIS CHAPTER

❑ Council Directive 93/42/EEC of 14 June 1993 concerning medical devices

❑ Directive 2007/47/EC of the European Parliament and of the Council of 5 September 2007 amending Council Directive 90/385/EEC on the approximation of the laws of the Member States regarding active implantable medical devices, Council Directive 93/42/EEC concerning medical devices and Directive 98/8/EC concerning the placing of biocidal products on the market

Introduction

After many years of living with a variety of national requirements for the regulation of medical devices—with some countries focusing on the sterility of medical devices and others on electromedical equipment—industry welcomed CE marking for medical devices as "the passport" to Europe. CE marking would cut across all national requirements and provide manufacturers with a single key to unlock the regulatory systems and markets of all EU Member States.

Council Directive 93/42/EEC, the *Medical Devices Directive* (*MDD*), provides a definition of "medical device," a standard classification system and a clear set of Conformity Assessment Procedures for each device class and procedures to follow to establish clinical investigations. However, the scope remains for national particularities in interpreting these areas, as well as the opportunity for Member States to establish requirements in other important areas for doing business with medical devices.

A directive, while a European legal instrument, does not in itself constitute European law. The provisions of a directive come into effect only when they are transposed into the national law of each Member State. While in principle the model of the regulatory system, as represented by the *MDD*, should be transposed identically in each Member State, this is not always the case. The European Commission has the right and duty to review national transposition texts and, if necessary, to take action to eliminate inconsistencies. However, the practicalities are such that administrative features of the national legislation that do not constitute technical barriers to trade are allowed to remain.

This chapter deals with the following aspects of national transpositions, with the aim of clarifying some of the existing national particularities:

- languages for labelling and Instructions for Use (IFU)
- notification to the Competent Authority before placing devices on the market and putting them into service
- activities and qualifications of marketing, sales and distribution organisations and personnel

Other aspects of national transpositions where variations exist, such as vigilance and procedures for initiating clinical investigations, are dealt with elsewhere in relevant chapters of this book.

In summary, it is crucial when doing business in Europe to consider the national laws. Although the text of the directive is often used by manufacturers as the source text when working to achieve CE marking, it is essential to remember that each country is still independent and has its own national laws with which devices are required to comply.

Use of Languages for Labelling and Instructions for Use

EU Member States have the right to require the use of their national language(s) for device labels and IFU when a device reaches the final user. This is stated in *MDD* Article 4.4:

> "Member States may require the information, which must be made available to the user and the patient in accordance with Annex I, point 13, to be in their national language(s) or in another Community language, when a device reaches the final user, regardless of whether it is for professional or other use."

This clause should be examined more closely. Although it is written as a permissive statement (Member States "may," rather than "must" or "should"), almost all Member States and signatory states to the European Economic Area (EEA) do require their national language—see below for details and to verify the current situation, since language requirements are subject to change.

The clause covers information made available to the user and the patient. It does not specifically cover, for example, information provided in service manuals that are not intended for the patient or user.

The scope of the clause is found in *MDD* Annex I, point 13, covering information supplied by the manufacturer that is needed to use the device safely and properly, taking into account the training and knowledge of potential users, and to identify the manufacturer. Information concerning patents or country of origin would, therefore, not be covered.

While Member States would be expected to require information in their national language(s), there are one or two interesting exceptions to this for both information on labels and IFU.

The national language requirements are designed to be triggered when the device reaches the final user. This potentially allows IFU to be added at a later stage in the distribution process. It also suggests that Notified Bodies (NBs) should not concern themselves with whether products have labels and IFU in accordance with the requirements of the countries in which they are intended to be made available. However, NBs should ensure that a process and procedure are in place to ensure that translations, where required, are sufficient to ensure that the device can be used safely and properly, as per *MDD* Annex I Essential Requirement 13.1.

Member States are allowed to impose national language requirements, regardless of whether the device is for professional or other use. In some cases, guidance from Competent Authorities suggests that there is some flexibility for professional use devices.

As stated above, it is imperative to consider the relevant country's national transposition of the *MDD* when placing a product on the market. Some examples of national language requirements follow. These countries were chosen to illustrate the range of different approaches to national language requirements and are examples only. Note also that requirements can change.

Austria

The *MDD* is transposed in Austria by the national law relating to medical devices, *Bundesgesetz betreffend Medizinprodukte* (medical devices law, *Medizinproduktegesetz* (*MPG*)), of 1996, BGBl. Nr. 657/1996, last amended by BGBl. I Nr. 77/2008 and BGBl. I Nr. 143/2009.

The national authority, the Austrian Federal Office for Safety in Health Care, *Bundesamt fuer Sicherheit im Gesundheitswesen* (BASG), is also responsible for medical devices. The former BASG/AGES PharmMed, was renamed to *BASG/Medizinmarktaufsicht* as of 1 February 2012.

The Austrian Inspectorate carries out GXP inspections, as well as inspections of pharmacovigilance systems and Ethics Committees. The inspectorate also monitors advertising according to the *Medicines Act*.

In Austria, the authority responsible for entering clinical investigations into the Eudamed database is BASG, when first notified. In clinical investigations, patient information has to follow specific text and formal requirements, as available at Austrian Ethics Committees (www.ethikkommissionen.at/).

Belgium

The *MDD* is transposed in Belgium by the Royal Decree of 17 March 2009, modifying the Royal Decree of 18 March 1999 relating to medical devices. This decree was published in the *Moniteur Belge* on 27 March 2009. The national language requirement is stated as follows (this is an unofficial English translation from the French language text):

"Art. 18

§ 1. The information provided to the patient in accordance with Annex I, point 13, must at least be drawn up in the national languages.

§ 2 The information provided to professional users in accordance with Annex I, point 13, must at least be drawn up in the national language of the users, unless on a case-by-case basis, and conditional upon due justification, the users make another arrangement with the manufacturer, his authorised representative or the approved distributor of the devices. This agreement is signed by the parties concerned and held available to the Competent Authorities. It must satisfy the requirements of the General Regulation for worker protection, approved by the decrees of the Regent of 11 February 1946 and 27 September 1947."

Active implantable devices are regulated by the Royal Decree dated 15 July 1997 concerning active implantable medical devices amended by the Royal Decree dated 10 December 2002 and by the Royal Decree dated 21 January 2009.

The national authority presents information on medical devices on its website www.fagg-afmps.be/fr/humain/produits_de_sante/dispositifs_medicaux/.

The requirement for patient information is clear—information must be provided in the three national languages of Belgium: French, Flemish/Dutch and German.

In the case of information for professional users, it is possible in specific cases for users and manufacturers (or the Authorised Representative or distributor) to agree to supply information in either just one of these three languages or in a different language, such as English. Caution must be used, however, to ensure that an agreement made, for example, with an individual user is valid and representative for that user's healthcare establishment.

Bulgaria

Legislation amending the law on medical devices, published on 30 December 2008, is the national transposition of *MDD*, as amended. While the *Medical Devices Law* requires IFU and labels of medical devices placed on the market in Bulgaria to be translated into the Bulgarian language, according to the Competent Authority, labels in English are acceptable for devices intended for professional use only.

Czech Republic

Registration of products with the national authority is required, including the GMDN code and the GMDN code description in English.

Denmark

The *MDD* is transposed in Denmark by The Ministry of Health and Prevention's Executive Order No. 1263 of 15 December 2008 concerning medical devices. This order states that the Danish language is required for labelling and the IFU for all medical devices, regardless of the intended user's skills or profession.

According to the Danish Medicines Agency's Medical Devices Department website, www.medicaldevices.dk, the order "does not require that software and service manuals must be provided in Danish. However, it is the manufacturer's responsibility to define which information is necessary for the correct and safe use of the device." The guidance goes on to clarify this statement, as follows:

"Display, buttons and keys

Single words or phrases such as "Load," "Enter," "Page Down," etc., are considered to be symbols. Symbols are not required to be translated, but must be explained in the instructions for use. If the information involves more than two words, and provides information/instruction to the user, this must be in Danish."

Finland

Article 12 of the *Law on Healthcare Products and Equipment* states, "the information accompanying the device must be in Finnish, Swedish or English, unless the information takes the form of generally known direction or warning symbols. Information intended for users or patients to ensure the safe use of the device must be in Finnish and Swedish. The instructions for use and labelling of medical devices intended for self-care must be in Finnish and Swedish."

Thus, in the case of professional use devices, there may be some latitude for providing information in English only. However, the worst-case interpretation of the text is that Finnish and Swedish are required for all information supplied with the device (even for professional use devices), if one assumes that all information provided is for the purpose of ensuring safe use. A manufacturer could make such a decision on the basis of a risk assessment. It is clear that for self-care devices (i.e., patient use devices) both Finnish and Swedish are required.

Netherlands

The language requirement is established in Article 6, Section 2 of the *Dutch Medical Devices Decree*.

All information intended for the patient and/or user of a medical device, e.g., label and IFU, must be in Dutch. There are exemptions to this rule under certain conditions, which are specified in Article 8. These can be found on the website of the *Centraal Informatiepunt Beroepen Gezondheidszorg* (CIBG, Central Health Professions Center) at www.cibg.nl. All three of the following criteria must be met:

- the product is to be used by medical specialists;

- users receive special training in the use of the device in question
- the product is to be used regularly, allowing for a routine to be established

Labelling requirements are described in Part 1, Section 13.3 of the Annex to the *Medical Devices Decree*.

The minimum labelling information requirements are:
- name, street address, postcode, town/city and country of the manufacturers or Authorised Representative's registered office
- the name of the device, its intended purpose and (if possible) an illustration of the device
- further instructions and warnings

Information relating to the safe use of the device must, where possible and useful, be on the device itself, on the individual packaging of each unit or, where circumstances demand, on the sales packaging. If it is not possible to include information on the unit packaging, that information must be included in the IFU accompanying each device or batch of devices.

The packaging of each medical device must include IFU. For Class I and IIa devices, exemption may be granted if the device can be safely used without specific instructions. It is not permitted to issue the instructions solely by means of an alternative channel such as the Internet.

Norway

Norway is worth a mention here since it made a significant change to its national language requirement in 2006 that caused some manufacturers to rapidly source Norwegian translations. The current national language requirement, as per Regulation 2005-12-15 no. 1690, amended and applicable from December 2010, is as follows:

"§2-6: The information as provided for in AIMDD I no. 13, 14 and 15, IVDMDD I part B no. 8, or MDD I no. 13 shall be in Norwegian.

The information can be provided with harmonised symbols, recognised codes or other similar solutions, provided that safe and correct use is ensured.

For medical devices for clinical investigation, languages other than Norwegian can be used as long as this is accepted by the user, but the information which is intended for the patient must nevertheless be in Norwegian.

As long as safe and correct use is ensured, the competent authority can make exceptions from the requirement for Norwegian language."

Prior to a regulation amendment in September 2006, Norwegian was not required for IFU for professional use medical devices. However, pressure from professional users, who noted that Norway was almost unique in offering this flexibility, resulted in the regulation amendment that required all devices for professional use to be supplied with IFU in Norwegian from October 2007.

Switzerland

The multi-lingual country of Switzerland offers some flexibility for professional use devices with some conditions. The Swissmedic website also offers information in English. www.swissmedic.ch/php/modules/leitfaden/leitfaden.html?lang=en.

The *Regulation on Medical Devices* was amended on 24 March 2010 to be effective from 1 April 2010. It contains very detailed information on the national language requirements:

"Article 7 Product information
1. Product information shall be in accordance with:
   a. Classical medical devices: Annex I, Section 13 of the Directive 93/42/EEC;
   b. Active implantable medical devices: Annex 1, Sections 14 and 15 of the Directive 90/385/EEC;
   c. Medical devices for in vitro diagnosis: Annex I, Section 8 of the Directive 98/79/EC;
2. The product information must be written in all three official languages. Symbols which are contained in harmonized standards can replace wording.
3. Product information can be restricted to less than the three official languages, or be in English, provided:
   a. the medical device is supplied exclusively to professionals or where the medical device is a custom-made device or a medical device manufactured in-house;
   b. there is assurance that the user has the necessary professional and linguistic qualifications, and agrees with the language restriction;
   c. the protection of patients, users and third parties is nevertheless ensured; and
   d. effective and intended use is not jeopardized.
4. If requested, additional information shall be given to users in one of the official languages."

The conditional restriction to fewer than the three official languages of Switzerland gives some scope to manufacturers who may wish to make a limited initial introduction of a product to the Swiss market and have not yet prepared instructions for use in French, German or Italian. However, it is unlikely that the restriction will be used widely since French, German and Italian are required respectively for France, Germany/Austria and Italy.

UK

Readers may be surprised to know that the UK does not require its national language for IFU. According to the national transposition text (Statutory Instrument 2008 No. 2936, *The Medical Devices (Amendment) Regulations 2008, Consumer Protection*), information on the packaging and on any label must be in English, regardless of whether the device is for professional or other use. However, IFU can be in English or another Community language, on condition that if the instructions are not in English, any packaging, label or promotional literature carry a clear statement in English stating the language in which the instructions are given. The regulation thus leaves the market to decide whether or not to purchase products where the IFU is not in English and ensures that purchasers are aware of this.

Notification to the Competent Authority Before Placing on the Market or Putting Into Service

Article 14 of the *MDD* established the principle that for certain devices (Class I devices, custom-made devices, and systems and procedure packs) the person involved in placing such products on the market should provide a description of the devices to the Competent Authority of the Member State in which he is established. The purpose of Article 14 is to ensure that national Competent Authorities have a contact for the manufacturer and the means to know what Class I and custom-made devices are being put on the market by entities based in that country. Note that the emphasis of Article 14 is actually the registration of the person concerned. It is that person who makes his existence known to the Competent Authority and, in addition, informs the authority about the products for which he is responsible.

Article 14 was amended in 1998 and currently reads as follows:

"14 Registration of persons responsible for placing devices on the market
1. Any manufacturer who, under his own name, places devices on the market in accordance with the procedures referred to in Article 11 (5) and (6) and any other natural or legal person engaged in the activities referred to in Article 12 shall inform the competent authorities of the Member State in which he has his registered place of business of the address of the registered place of business and the description of the devices concerned.

    For all medical devices of classes IIa, IIb and III, Member States may request to be informed of all data allowing for identification of such devices together with the label and the instructions for use when such devices are put into service within their territory.
2. Where a manufacturer who places a device on the market under his own name does not have a registered place of business in a Member State, he shall designate a single authorized representative in the European Union. For devices referred to in the first subparagraph of paragraph 1, the authorized representative shall inform the competent authority of the Member State in which he has his registered place of business of the details referred to in paragraph 1.
3. The Member States shall on request inform the other Member States and the Commission of the details referred to in the first subparagraph of paragraph 1 given by the manufacturer or authorized representative."

When added in 1998, the second paragraph of 14.2 referred only to Class IIb and III devices. It was expanded to include Class IIa devices by means of Directive 2007/47/EC. Importantly, this is a permissive clause, in that "Member States may request to be informed …" Also, the requirement refers to putting into service (rather than placing on the market), and can therefore be fulfilled by any entity, regardless of location, and is not restricted to companies having a registered place of business in a particular country. Most countries have taken the opportunity to be notified of putting into service. Some examples of national requirements follow.

France

Article R.5211-66 pursuant to Article L.5211-4 of the *Code of Public Health* provides that all data allowing identification of Class IIa, IIb and III devices must be communicated to *Agence nationale de sécurité des médicaments et des produits de santé* (ANSM) when they are put into service within French territory. The data to be communicated to ANSM are: the trade description of the medical device; the name and address of the person submitting the communication; and a specimen of the medical device's labelling and IFU.

The communication must be made at the time of putting the device into service on national territory. The requirement applies to the manufacturer, the Authorised Representative or the distributor. Only one communication per device is needed.

ANSM provides a form in both French and English that can be used for the communication. This is available at http://www.ansm.sante.fr/.

Italy

The Italian Decree of 20 February 2007, updated 21 December 2009, established a new registration system for medical devices that, by allocating a registration number to each device, was intended to improve device traceability. The registration consists of two levels. The notification of medical devices to a database is mandatory for the manufacturer or the Authorised Representative situated in Italy. Entities situated outside Italy must notify Class IIa, IIb and III devices and active implantable medical devices. The next level of notification is to have the devices listed in the *Repertorio*, costing €100 per device listing (note: this fee may yet be repealed). The *Repertorio* is the list of devices available to be sold to the Italian National Health Service.

Although the *Repertorio* was introduced in phases, it has been compulsory for all devices within its scope since 5 May 2010.

The information initially required for registration was comprehensive. This requirement has since been simplified, following a challenge by the European Commission on the basis that the requirement to register Class I devices and systems/procedure kits in Italy was excessive if such devices had already been notified in the country in which the manufacturer or its Authorised Representative was based. However, the modalities for registration are burdensome, as the entity registering must gain access to the database using the online portal and a smart card. Information on the registration process is available at www.salute.gov.it/dispositivi/ and there is also a user manual.

Netherlands

The *Regulation on Medical Devices*, as amended, does not include a Competent Authority request for information on Class IIa, IIb and III devices when they are put into service in the Netherlands. Class I medical devices and in vitro diagnostics (IVDs) need to be registered by the CIBG (www.cibg.nl).

Portugal

In accordance with Article 11.1 of Decree Law no. 145/2009, manufacturers or Authorised Representatives based in Portugal that place Class I and custom-made devices on the market must notify the Competent Authority (Infarmed) of their name and address and all information necessary to identify the devices in question.

When Class IIa, IIb and III devices are put into service in Portugal, Infarmed requests extensive information including:
- name of manufacturer/Authorised Representative/distributor
- device name and type
- description and intended purpose
- Notified Body ID number
- copies of labels and IFU
- date of placing on the market or putting into service in Portugal
- certificates

Note that Class IIa devices were added to this group as a result of the transposition of Directive 2007/47/EC via Article 11.3 of Decree Law no. 145/2009. Notification must be done online and can be done in English. English language guidance is also provided at www.infarmed.pt.

Spain

Article 24 of Royal Decree 1591/2009 of 16 October 2009 establishes that a manufacturer based in Spain, or the Spain-based Authorised Representative of a non-EU manufacturer, must notify the placing on the market of Class I and custom-made devices to the Competent Authority and the Spanish Agency for Medicines and Healthcare Products (AEMPS). Note that prior to 21 March 2010, this notification was made to the Competent Authority in the Autonomous Community where the manufacturer or Authorised Representative was based.

Article 22 of the Royal Decree establishes that any person who makes a Class IIa, IIb or III device available for the first time for distribution and/or use on Spanish territory must communicate this to AEMPS at the time of making the device available.

This requirement applies to any entity, in Spain or elsewhere, putting devices on the Spanish market. The details of the communication to AEMPS are provided in Article 23.1. The communication is to be made electronically via a portal specifically established for the purpose, at www.aemps.es. Prior to making this communication, manufacturers should obtain a password from AEMPS. A fee is required for each product notification.

Activities and Qualifications of Marketing, Sales and Distribution Organisations and Personnel

Distribution is not covered by the *MDD*, with the result that national regulatory systems can include requirements relating to distribution of medical devices. This omission is likely to change in the recast of the *MDD* currently under consideration, since distributors play a key role in moving the product from the manufacturer to the final user. Currently, only a few countries specifically regulate the activities of distributors, some by means of provisions in their national *MDD* transposition text, others by means of other regulatory texts. The following are examples only.

Germany

The federal system foresees delegation of authority to or beyond the state level regarding various aspects of medical device regulation. Manufacturers or Authorised Representatives located in Germany or sponsors for clinical trials may refer to lists of contacts for relevant authorities published by the DIMDI (German Institute for Medical Documentation and Information www.dimdi.de) (see **Table 16-1**).

Premarket

Depending on the medical device type and class, federal or state or both authorities need to be involved in the approval process.

Table 16-1. Relevant Authorities in Germany

Subject	MPG*	Relevant Authority Level	Link
Placing on the market	§§25 and 30	State	www.dimdi.de/static/de/mpg/adress/behoerden/beh-liste.htm
Applications for clinical trials and Leistungsbewertungspruefungen, as well as any changes	§§ 22a to 24	Federal	www.dimdi.de/static/de/mpg/adress/behoerden/klifo-liste-bob.htm
Applications for clinical trials and Leistungsbewertungspruefungen	§§ 22a to 24	State	www.dimdi.de/static/de/mpg/adress/behoerden/klifo-liste.htm
Ethics Commissions	§§ 22	State	www.dimdi.de/static/de/mpg/adress/ethik/ethik-liste.htm
Inspections		State	www.dimdi.de/static/de/mpg/adress/behoerden/index.htm)

MPG – German Medical Devices Law

Code System
UMDNS Code published by DIMDI is applied to medical devices.

Inspection
According to §26 of the *Medical Devices Law* (*Medizinproduktegesetz* (*MPG*)), entities in Germany that carry out activities regarding medical devices, generally including handling and/or distribution of medical devices, are subject to inspection by the authorities.

Medical Devices Advisor
The *MPG* sets out special education and training requirements for persons who advise medical circles about medical devices in a professional capacity. This is described in the *MPG* as follows:

"§31 Medical Devices Adviser
(1) Whoever informs professional circles professionally about medical devices and instructs them in the proper handling of medical devices (Medical Devices Adviser), may only practise this activity, if he has the necessary professional knowledge and experience for informing and where necessary, for the instruction in handling and use of the respective medical devices. Sentence 1 applies also to information provided over the telephone.
(2) Professional knowledge is possessed by,
  1. Anyone who has successfully completed an education in a natural science, medical or technical profession, and who been trained in the respective medical devices, or
  2. Anyone who has gained by means of an activity of at least one year, which in justified cases can be shorter, experience in information and where necessary in the instruction in handling of the respective medical devices.
(3) The medical device adviser is required to provide documentary evidence of the specialist knowledge to the Competent Authorities on demand. He must keep himself up to date on the respective medical devices, in order to be able to advise expertly. The employer must ensure regular training for the medical device adviser.
(4) The medical devices adviser is required to maintain written records of communications from persons belonging to professional circles regarding side effects, mutual influences, malfunctioning, technical defects, contra-indications, counterfeits or any other risks associated with medical devices and to communicate these in writing to the responsible person in accordance with [MPG] § 5 sentences 1 and 2 or their designated persons responsible for safety in writing."

Ireland

In early 2010, the Minister for Health and Children in Ireland announced a proposal to introduce legislation to regulate distributors of medical devices. Such regulation might include:
- registration of distributors with the Competent Authority
- recordkeeping requirements for distributors and retailers
- requirements to ensure distributors have suitable facilities, personnel and equipment to maintain medical device quality during storage, transport and distribution
- requirements to ensure medical devices are CE marked and meet the mandatory labelling requirements when supplied
- requirements for maintaining a quality system in medical device distribution operations

Spain

Royal Decree 1591/2009 of 16 October 2009, regulating medical devices, contains the following provisions relating to distributors.

Article 26 enables the authorities to ask a manufacturer, Authorised Representative, importer or distributor to supply information about a product if there are concerns about it.

Article 26.5 places responsibility on the Spanish distributor to ensure the product meets the decree's requirements and the necessary information has been provided to the authorities prior to distributing the product.

Article 27 states that devices can only be stored in appropriate premises. Distribution and sales entities are subject to vigilance and inspection by the local authorities. Distributors must make a prior notification of their activity. Distribution entities must hold a documented register of all devices distributed. They must also have the services of a "*tecnico responsible*" (responsible technician), who is responsible for maintaining technical health information on the products distributed or put into service.

Other National Particularities

In addition to the above, there is much latitude in the different stages of the medical device lifecycle, from development to use, that can be regulated by national legislation. Reimbursement and purchasing schemes are specifically excluded from the scope of the *MDD*, by virtue of the directive's fourth recital, which states:

> "Whereas the harmonised provisions must be distinguished from the measures adopted by the Member States to manage the funding of public health and sickness insurance schemes relating directly or indirectly to such devices; whereas, therefore, the provisions do not affect the ability of the Member States to implement the abovementioned measures provided Community law is complied with."

No mention is made in the directive of specific sales outlets; hence, the *MDD* does not establish any restrictions on who may dispense medical devices, although restrictions are applied to certain devices in some countries.

Postmarket servicing, credentials of service organisations and availability of spare parts are outside the scope of the *MDD*, while national requirements may exist in some jurisdictions.

Administration, enforcement and penalties are left to the discretion of the individual Member States. Knowledge and understanding of these areas are essential for doing business.

Summary

The *Medical Devices Directive* has harmonised the requirements for safety and performance of medical devices, to create a level playing field across the EU, EEA and beyond, with CE marking recognised as a sign of a safe medical device. However, manufacturers must look beyond CE marking to the national laws and regulations of the countries in which they wish to do business to ensure they are in compliance. Successful manufacturers will familiarise themselves not only with the *MDD* and its national transpositions but also with other regulatory texts dealing with medical devices at the national level. Alternatively, they can entrust themselves to the services of local experts.

Chapter 17

Overview of Authorisation Procedures for Medicinal Products

Updated by Martha Anna Bianchetto, PharmD, MBA

OBJECTIVES

❑ Gain an understanding of the regulatory procedures necessary to grant a medicinal product access to the marketplace

❑ Learn about aspects of compiling a Marketing Authorisation Application in different procedures

❑ Learn about legislation, procedural steps and the Competent Authorities

---

DIRECTIVES, REGULATIONS AND GUIDELINES COVERED IN THIS CHAPTER

❑ Council Directive 65/65/EEC of 26 January 1965 on the approximation of provisions laid down by law, regulation or administrative action relating to medicinal products

❑ Directive 2001/83/EC of the European Parliament and of the Council of 6 November 2001 on the Community code relating to medicinal products for human use, as amended by:

  o Directive 2002/98/EC of the European Parliament and of the Council of 27 January 2003 setting standards of quality and safety for the collection, testing, processing, storage and distribution of human blood and blood components and amending Directive 2001/83/EC

  o Directive 2003/63/EC of the European Parliament and of the Council of 25 June 2003 amending Directive 2001/83/EC of the European Parliament and of the Council on the Community code relating to medicinal products for human use

  o Commission Directive 2004/33/EC of 22 March 2004 implementing Directive 2002/98/EC of the European Parliament and of the Council as regards certain technical requirements for blood and blood components

  o Directive 2004/27/EC of the European Parliament and of the Council of 31 March 2004 amending Directive 2001/83/EC on the Community code relating to medicinal products for human use

  o Directive 2004/24/EC of the European Parliament and the Council of 31 March 2004 amending, as regards traditional herbal medicinal products, Directive 2001/83/EC on the Community code relating to medicinal products for human use

  o Regulation (EC) No 1901/2006 of the European Parliament and of the Council of 12 December 2006 on medicinal products for paediatric use and amending Regulation (EEC) No 1768/92, Directive 2001/20/EC, Directive 2001/83/EC and Regulation (EC) No 726/2004

Regulatory Affairs Professionals Society

Chapter 17

- o   Regulation (EC) No 1394/2007 of the European Parliament and of the Council of 13 November 2007 on advanced therapy medicinal products and amending Directive 2001/83/EC and Regulation (EC) No 726/2004

- o   Directive 2008/29/EC of the European Parliament and of the Council of 11 March 2008 amending Directive 2001/83/EC on the Community code relating to medicinal products for human use, as regards the implementing powers conferred on the Commission

- o   Directive 2009/53/EC of the European Parliament and of the Council of 18 June 2009 amending Directive 2001/82/EC and Directive 2001/83/EC, as regards variations to the terms of marketing authorisations for medicinal products

❑ Commission Regulation (EC) No 1234/2008 of 24 November 2008 concerning the examination of variations to the terms of marketing authorisations for medicinal products for human use and veterinary medicinal products

❑ Commission Regulation (EC) No 1084/2003 of 3 June 2003 concerning the examination of variations to the terms of a marketing authorisation for medicinal products for human use and veterinary medicinal products granted by a competent authority of a Member State

❑ Commission Regulation (EC) No 1085/2003 of 3 June 2003 concerning the examination of variations to the terms of a marketing authorisation for medicinal products for human use and veterinary medicinal products falling within the scope of Council Regulation (EEC) No 2309/93

❑ Regulation (EC) No 726/2004 of the European Parliament and of the Council of 31 March 2004 laying down Community procedures for the authorisation and supervision of medicinal products for human and veterinary use and establishing a European Medicines Agency

❑ The Rules Governing Medicinal Products in the European Union, Volume 2, Notice to Applicants (NTA)

❑ The Rules Governing Medicinal Products in the European Union, Volume 2A, NTA Procedures for Marketing Authorisation

- o   "Chapter 1 Marketing Authorisation" (Updated November 2005),

- o   "Chapter 2 Mutual Recognition" (Updated February 2007)

- o   "Chapter 3 Community Referral" (Updated September 2007)

- o   "Chapter 4 Centralised Procedure" (Updated April 2006)

- o   "Chapter 5 Guideline on the operations of the procedures laid down in Chapters II, III and IV of Commission Regulation (EC) No 1234/2008 of 24 Nov 2008" (Updated February 2010)

- o   "Chapter 6 Community Marketing Authorisation" (Updated version November 2005)

- o   "Chapter 7 General Information" (Updated July 2008)

❑ The Rules Governing Medicinal Products in the European Union, Volume 2B, NTA, Presentation and Content of the Dossier

- o   Common Technical Document—CTD (May 2008)

- o   Module 1.2 Application Form (May 2008)

- o   Questions and Answers (February 2008)

- o   eCTD—electronic Common Technical Document

❑ The Rules Governing Medicinal Products in the European Union, Volume 2C, NTA Regulatory Guidelines

- o   Guideline on Summary of Product Characteristics (SmPC) (September 2009)

- o   Guideline on the Categorisation of New Applications (NA) versus Variations Applications (V) (October 2003)

152   Regulatory Affairs Professionals Society

- ○ Guideline on the packaging information of medicinal products for human use authorised by the Community (February 2008)

- ○ Guideline on the readability of the label and package leaflet of medicinal product for human use, Rev. 1 (12 January 2009)

- ○ Guidance concerning consultation with target patient groups for the package leaflet (May 2006)

- ❑ Guideline on the Investigation of Bioequivalence (August 2010)[1]

- ❑ ICH, M4 Implementation Working Group Questions & Answers (R3) (June 2004)

- ❑ ICH, Organisation of the Common Technical Document for the Registration of Pharmaceuticals for Human Use M4 (January 2004)

- ❑ ICH M2 EWG Electronic Common Technical Document Specification (V 3.2.2, July 2008)

- ❑ EU Module 1 Specification v 1.4 (August 2009)

- ❑ CMDh Best Practice Guide on the Use of the Electronic Common Technical Document (eCTD) in the Mutual Recognition and Decentralised Procedures (June 2010)

- ❑ Guidance for Industry on Providing Regulatory Information in Electronic Format: eCTD electronic Submissions (EU Telematic Implementation Group—electronic submissions (TIGes, v. 1, May 2009))

Introduction

The EU utilises several types of legislative instruments to establish laws and policies, though not all are legally binding.

The legally binding instruments include:
- Regulations are directly enforceable laws, applicable and binding on all Member States; no national legislation is required to give them effect.
- Directives are binding on the Member States, must be transposed and adopted into national regulations within a specified timeframe. They may be effective in a Member State even before that state has enacted the corresponding national law.
- Decisions are binding in their entirety upon those to whom they are addressed (Member States or legal entities, e.g., legal persons or companies.)
- European Pharmacopoeia

Instruments without binding legal effect are:
- guidelines (Notes for Guidance)
- recommendations and opinions
- position papers and concept papers
- notices
- communications
- ICH Notes for Guidance

Although these are not legally binding, they usually are strongly recommended either by the European Medicines Agency (EMA) or Member States' Competent Authorities, and they often have considerable political force.

Guidances, recommendations, opinions and position and concept papers are issued by the Committee for Medicinal Products for Human Use (CHMP), scientific advisory groups and other committees at EMA, as well as by the Coordination Group for Mutual Recognition and Decentralised Procedures–Human (CMDh).

Communications are issued by the European Commission to explain Community law or programmes of actions to governments and economic partners.

Notices are not, strictly, legislation, neither are they are enforceable in law; however, they often take the form of guidelines intended to help relevant bodies or applicants meet the terms of a specific directive.

Move Toward Harmonisation

In the EU, medicinal products are covered by the internal market principle of the free movement of goods. This chapter provides an overview of authorisation procedures that apply to medicinal products in the EU.

Throughout much of the 20th century, individual Member States enacted national legislation that regulated medicinal products for human use. With the adoption of Council Directive 65/65/EEC of 26 January 1965, which stipulated that a medicinal product may only be placed on the market in the EU after a Marketing Authorisation (MA) has been granted, the first major step was taken toward harmonising medicinal product authorisation procedures. Since 1965, the EU pharmaceutical legislation framework has been extended and refined with the objectives of protecting public health and maintaining the free movement of medicinal products.

A final comprehensive document—the *Notice to Applicants* (*NTA*)—was issued by the European Commission in 1986 as part of *The Rules Governing Medicinal Products in the European Union*. The *NTA* is presented in three parts: *Volume 2A* deals with procedures for MAs; *Volume 2B* covers application dossier presentation and content; and Volume 2C contains regulatory guidelines. The *NTA* has been revised several times and represents the current harmonised view of Member States, EMA and the European Commission. It is not legally binding, however, and reference should always be made to the appropriate Community directives and regulations.

In 1995, a new system for authorising medicinal products entered into force. It was based on two separate Community procedures for granting an MA for a medicinal product: the Centralised Procedure was administered through EMA, and Member State Competent Authorities were responsible for the Mutual Recognition Procedure.

In addition, a purely national authorisation was possible for a product that was marketed in only one Member State.

The new pharmaceutical regulations (Directive 2004/27/EC) that came into force in 2005 provided another option to authorise medicinal products within the EU: the Decentralised Procedure. The other procedures (Centralised Procedure and Mutual Recognition Procedure) were maintained, but important changes to them were introduced.

The European MA System for Medicinal Products

Definition of MA

A medicinal product may be placed on the EU market only when an MA (which initially lasts five years and is usually subject to one renewal) has been issued by the regulatory authority of a Member State for its own territory (so-called national authorisation, which can be a purely national authorisation, or can be granted following a Mutual Recognition Procedure or a Decentralised Procedure) or when an authorisation is granted for the entire Community (so-called Community authorisation, following the Centralised Procedure).

The Marketing Authorisation Holder (MAH) must be established in the European Economic Area (EEA), which comprises the 27 Member States plus Norway, Iceland and Liechtenstein.

The MA is granted to a single MAH and includes, when available, the International Nonproprietary Name (INN) of the active substance(s) and, when branded, a single invented name (i.e., the trade name). Companies that wish to market the same medicinal product with a second trade name must submit a separate Marketing Authorisation Application (MAA). The MAH, which may be a natural person or legal entity established in the EEA, is responsible for marketing the medicinal product. The MAH is bound by several obligations and responsibilities, including:
- taking into account any technical and scientific progress to update manufacturing and control operations
- when the MAH is not the manufacturer, signing a written agreement with the manufacturer to guarantee that manufacturing operations comply with dossier rules and conditions (Annex 5.11 to the application form)
- informing authorities of any information brought to the attention of the MAH that could lead to modification of the MA dossier or Summary of Product Characteristics (SmPC) and Product Information Leaflet (PIL)
- submitting the MA renewal application at least six months before the expiration date; usually an MA needs to be renewed only once, five years after the first MA is granted (the consequence of failure to submit the renewal application is a cancellation of the MA)
- paying the relevant fees (MAs, renewals, variations, yearly fees, etc.)
- having a Qualified Person (QP) in charge of pharmacovigilance and a scientific service in charge of each medicinal product's scientific information
- being responsible for medicinal product advertising
- retaining and archiving all medicinal product documentation and, in particular, any documents related to clinical trials
- submitting samples of the product, active pharmaceutical ingredient (API) and the reference product (for generic applications) upon request by the Competent Authority
- for immunological medicinal products and medicinal products derived from human blood or human plasma, submitting samples from each batch of the bulk and/or finished product for examination by a state laboratory or a laboratory designated for that purpose

Since the new legislation came into force in November 2005, the MAH additionally is required to:
- inform the authority that has granted the MA of any new data that may affect the risk:benefit balance of the medicinal product
- inform the authorities of the date of placing the product on the market, volume of sales (in each Member State), medicinal product presentations and cessation of marketing

Additionally, authorisations not used in the territory for a period of three consecutive years become invalid (the sunset clause).

Format for MAAs in the EU

MAAs comprise administrative information and documentation necessary to demonstrate the medicinal product's quality, safety and efficacy.

The Common Technical Document (CTD) went into force in July 2003 in all three regions (Europe, the US and Japan) covered by the International Conference on Harmonisation (ICH). The CTD is an internationally agreed-upon format for preparing a well-structured presentation for applications to be submitted to regulatory authorities in the three ICH regions. It is organised into five modules. The content of Module 1 was defined by the European Commission in consultation with Member State Competent Authorities, EMA and interested parties. Module 1, which consists of administrative data, is not considered a part of the CTD. Modules 2, 3, 4 and 5 are common for all regions.

- Module 1 should provide administrative, regional or national information (e.g., the application form with 22 annexes, proposed summary of product characteristics, labelling and PIL, pharmacovigilance system description, risk management plan).
- Module 2 contains high-level summaries and overviews (the overall quality summary, nonclinical overview and summary and clinical overview and summary) that must be prepared by suitably qualified and experienced persons (i.e., experts). The experts must sign and add brief information on their educational background and specific expertise in a special section in Module 1.
- Module 3 provides chemical, pharmaceutical and biological documentation.
- Module 4 consists of the nonclinical study reports.
- Module 5 consists of the clinical study reports.

The applicant's (open) part of the Active Substance Master File (ASMF) should be included in Section 3.2.S of the quality documentation presented in the CTD format. It is the applicant's responsibility to ensure that the complete ASMF, consisting of the open part and the active substance manufacturer's restricted (closed) part, is supplied to the authorities in CTD format. The ASMF closed part should be supplied directly by the active substance manufacturer, synchronised to arrive at the same time as the MAA (submitted by the applicant). An original, signed Letter of Access (LoA) addressed to the regulatory authority where the application is made must be attached to the ASMF restricted part, and a copy of the LoA must be included in Annex 5.10 of the application form in Module 1. The restricted part of the ASMF should follow the structure of CTD Module 3.2.S. A separate quality summary (2.3.S) for the information included in the restricted part should also be provided as part of the ASMF.

Acronyms and abbreviations should be defined the first time they are used in each module. When preparing product information for Centralised Procedure, Decentralised Procedure and Mutual Recognition Procedure applications (Module 1.3.1), use of the Quality Review of Documents (QRD) convention is mandatory. The QRD working group's mission is to ensure clarity, consistency and accuracy of medicinal product information and its translations. The group has developed product information templates to provide practical advice on how to present product information.

For the National Procedure, Decentralised Procedure and Mutual Recognition Procedure, additional data might be requested, including the following:

- statement of MA transfer signed by both parties (Bulgaria, Greece, Hungary, Portugal, Spain)
- statement on having a QP responsible for pharmacovigilance activities in the national territory where the application is made (Portugal, Romania, Spain)
- packaging size declaration and samples declaration (Hungary, Poland)
- contractual technical agreement between MAH and manufacturer(s) (Spain)

Additional data required by different Member States are specified in Chapter 7 of *NTA Volume 2A*, but it is best practice to check the Competent Authority website or contact the Competent Authority via email a few months or weeks prior to submission of the MAA.

This international format applies to all medicinal product categories (including new chemical entities (NCEs), radiopharmaceuticals, vaccines and herbals) and all application types (standalone and abridged), although some adaptations may be necessary for specific application or product types. It is not designed to indicate what studies are required for successful approval, but rather to indicate appropriate information organisation for the application.

Throughout the CTD, information should be unambiguous and transparent to facilitate review of the basic data and to help reviewers become quickly oriented to the MAA contents. Text and tables should be prepared using margins that allow the document to be printed on A4 paper. The left-hand margin should be sufficiently wide that information is not obscured by binding. Font sizes and styles for text and tables should be large enough to be easily legible, even after photocopying. Times New Roman 12-point font is recommended for narrative text.

eCTD Format and Acceptability

The electronic Common Technical Document (eCTD) is now the standard for submitting MAAs in the Community and most EU Member States. It is the mandatory format for centrally authorised products at EMA. Since January 2010, all National Competent Authorities are obliged to accept the eCTD and/or the Non eCTD electronic format (NeeS). However, acceptability of e-submissions in each Member State is sometimes difficult to determine. Often, there are some local requirements on submitting applications in eCTD format (e.g., in France, Spain, Germany, the UK and the Netherlands). It is highly advisable to check national agencies' guidance documents and websites before submission. Additionally, it is good practice to check the list

Chapter 17

Table 17-1. Standard Timetable for Evaluation of a Centralised Application

Day	Action
1	Start of the procedure
80	Receipt of the Assessment Report(s) or critique from rapporteur and co-rapporteur by CHMP members (including peer reviewers) and EMA. EMA sends rapporteur and co-rapporteur Assessment Report/critique to the applicant, making it clear that this only sets out preliminary conclusions, is sent for information only and does not yet present CHMP's position.
100	Rapporteur, co-rapporteur, other CHMP members and EMA receive comments from CHMP members (including peer reviewers).
115	Receipt of draft list of questions (including the CHMP recommendation and scientific discussion) from rapporteur and co-rapporteur by CHMP members and EMA.
120	CHMP adopts the list of questions, as well as the overall conclusions and review of the scientific data to be sent to the applicant by EMA. **Clock stop.** By Day 120 at the latest, adoption by CHMP of request by GMP/GCP/GLP inspection, if necessary (inspection procedure starts).
121*	Submission of the responses, including revised SmPC, labelling and PIL texts, and restart of the clock.
Evaluation of Responses	
Day	Action
150	Joint Assessment Report from rapporteur and co-rapporteur received by CHMP members and EMA. EMA sends joint Assessment Report to the applicant, making it clear that it only sets out preliminary conclusions, is sent for information only and does not yet represent CHMP's position. Where applicable, inspection to be carried out. EMA/QRD subgroup meeting to review English product information with participation of the applicant (optional) around Day 165.
170	Deadline for comments from CHMP members to be sent to rapporteur and co-rapporteur, EMA and other CHMP members.
180	CHMP discussion and decision on the need for adopting a list of "outstanding issues" and/or an oral explanation by the applicant. If an oral explanation is needed, the clock is stopped to allow the applicant to prepare it. Submission of final inspection report to EMA, rapporteur and co-rapporteur by the inspections team (at the latest by Day 180).
181	Restart of the clock and oral explanation (if needed).
181 to 210	Final draft of English SmPC, labelling and package leaflet sent by applicant to the rapporteur and co-rapporteur, EMA and other CHMP members.
By 210	Adoption of CHMP opinion and CHMP Assessment Report. Adoption of a timetable for the provision of revised product information translations.
Preparation of the Annexes to the Commission Decision	
Day	Action
215 at the latest	Applicant provides EMA with SmPC, Annex II, labelling and package leaflet and Annex A in all EU languages. EMA circulates draft translations to Member States for review.
232 at the latest	Applicant provides EMA with final translations of SmPC, Annex II, labelling and package leaflet in all EU languages, taking account comments received from Member States by Day 229.
By 237	Transmission of opinion and annexes in all EU languages to applicant, EC and Members of the Standing Committee, and Norway, Iceland and Liechtenstein.
By 246	Applicant provides EMA with one final, full-colour "worst-case" mock-up of outer and inner packaging for each pharmaceutical form.
	IMPORTANT NOTE: Once the medicinal product is authorised, and in all cases before the medicinal product is placed on the market, specimens of the final outer and immediate packaging and the package leaflet of all product presentations must be submitted to EMA within a timeframe agreed between the agency and the MAH.

*Target dates for the submission of the responses are published on the EMA website—Presubmission Guidance

Source: *NTA Volume 2A*, Chapter 4

of Member State contact points for e-submissions published on the EMA website.

The eCTD allows the applicant to submit the CTD in electronic format to the authorities and control the application's lifecycle both during the procedure and once the MA has been granted (variations, renewals).

The registration documents in the electronic submission are organised according to version 3.2 of the ICH eCTD specification and the current version of the EU Module 1 specifications. In other words, an eCTD is the submission of (mostly) PDF documents, stored in the eCTD directory structure, accessed through an Internet browser (via index.xml).

Details on the requirements for eCTD submissions can be found in *Guidance for Industry on Providing Regulatory Information in Electronic Format: eCTD electronic submissions*. This document assumes a basic understanding of eCTD applications and reflects the current situation with e-submissions. It is regularly updated to reflect changes in national and European legislation and experience gained during the ongoing applications handled in European procedures described below: Centralised Procedure,

Decentralised Procedure, Mutual Recognition Procedure and National Procedure.

Community Authorisations

Centralised Procedure

Use of the Centralised Procedure is confined to certain categories of medicinal products as described in the annex to Regulation (EC) No 726/2004. EMA is responsible for evaluating MAAs for medicinal products for human and veterinary use in the following categories:
- Those developed by means of the following biotechnological processes:
    - recombinant DNA technology
    - controlled expression of gene coding for biologically active proteins in prokaryotes and eukaryotes, including transformed mammalian cells
    - hybridoma and monoclonal antibody methods

  This category includes any medicinal product containing a proteinaceous constituent obtained by recombinant DNA technology.
- Orphan medicinal products developed pursuant to Regulation (EC) No 141/2000.
- Medicinal products for human use that contain a new active substance that, on the date of entry into force of Regulation (EC) No 726/2004, were not authorised by any Member State for the following therapeutic indications:
    - acquired immune deficiency syndrome (AIDS)
    - cancer
    - neurodegenerative disorder
    - diabetes
    - autoimmune diseases and other immune dysfunctions
    - viral diseases
- Veterinary medicinal products, including those not derived from biotechnology, intended primarily for use as performance enhancers to promote the growth of treated animals or increase yields from treated animals

The definition of "new chemical, biological or radiopharmaceutical active substances" includes the following:
- a chemical, biological or radiopharmaceutical substance not previously authorised as a medicinal product in the EU
- an isomer, a mixture of isomers, a complex or a derivative or salt of a chemical substance previously authorised as a medicinal product in the EU but differing in safety and efficacy properties from that previously authorised chemical substance
- a biological substance previously authorised as a medicinal product in the EU but differing in molecular structure, nature of the source material or manufacturing process
- a radiopharmaceutical substance that is a radionuclide or a ligand not previously authorised as a medicinal product in the EU, or for which the coupling mechanism to link the molecule and radionuclide has not been previously authorised in the EU

A fixed combination of active substances can be considered a new active substance if it has not previously been authorised as a medicinal product in the EU.

An applicant can utilise the Centralised Procedure for other medicinal products if it can show that a product constitutes a significant therapeutic, scientific or technical innovation, or that granting authorisation via the Centralised Procedure is in the interests of patients or animal health at the Community level. This option also may be used for generic medicinal products where the reference product is authorised by the Community.

To maintain coherence and preserve the unity of the single Community market, when the same MAH wishes to place another medicinal product on the market with an active substance that is already the subject of a Community authorisation, the Centralised Procedure should be used, particularly when the new medicinal product's therapeutic indication is within the third level of the Anatomic, Therapeutic, Chemical Classification (ATC) code. However, a generic medicinal product of a reference medicinal product authorised by the Community also may be authorised by the Member States' Competent Authorities in accordance with Directive 2001/83/EC, as amended, under certain conditions. In this case, applicants have a choice between the Centralised Procedure and Decentralised Procedure. This is discussed in more detail in Chapter 21 Generic Medicinal Products.

Applicants are strongly advised to notify EMA of their intended MAA submission date by sending the presubmission request form (Intent to submit MA) to the email address specified on EMA's website. Submission dates must be realistic and accurate so the agency will have sufficient time to appoint the rapporteur and co-rapporteur and their assessment teams for submission evaluation. The deadline for sending the letter of intention to submit the MAA is seven months prior to the intended submission date. Rapporteurs and, if required, co-rapporteurs are appointed from among members and alternate members of CHMP. For Advanced Therapy Medicinal Products (ATMPs), rapporteurs are appointed from among members and alternate members of the Committee for Advanced Therapies (CAT). The rapporteur and co-rapporteur are supported by a team of assessors/experts (assessment team) during the various phases of the application's evaluation. Normally, postauthorisation activities are also assessed by the same group of people.

In cases where the applicant is not certain about some issues regarding the medicinal product that is the subject of the application or if there are some concerns about the product's development, it may seek advice from EMA. Such Scientific Advice and Protocol Assistance may be requested either during a medicinal product's initial development (i.e., before submission of an MAA) or later, during the postauthorisation phase. Scientific Advice is subject to a fee, which varies depending on the scope of the advice; however, some fee reductions and/or waivers are available (e.g., orphan designation or paediatric use).

Since October 2009, EMA accepts only electronic requests for Scientific Advice and Protocol Assistance, including follow-up requests. Applicants should submit their applications only on a CD or DVD.

For more administrative issues and questions, the applicant may request a Presubmission Meeting. The Presubmission Meeting is strongly recommended, even for companies with experience with the Centralised Procedure and when the application is apparently straightforward. Such a meeting can significantly facilitate submission and validation of the MAA. To arrange such a meeting with EMA, the applicant must submit a Presubmission Meeting Request Form (available on EMA's website). The form requires administrative details about the applicant, the contact person and medicinal product information: trade name, active substance(s), INN, proposed ATC code, pharmaceutical forms, strength(s), packaging and pack sizes, proposed indications and posology. Proposed dates for the meeting, the proposed date for submitting the application, a draft summary of product information (SmPC, PIL, labelling) and other relevant draft documentation must also be provided. In addition, the applicant must describe areas it wishes to discuss at the meeting (for example, if the proposed trade name is acceptable, when exactly the rapporteur(s) will be appointed, whether the product is eligible for accelerated assessment, whether the samples have to be submitted together with the application, what fees have to be paid, how to handle multiple applications, whether a risk management system is required, etc.). Following the meeting, the applicant must prepare minutes and send them to EMA for comments within two weeks.

Applications under the Centralised Procedure are made directly to EMA by a person based in the Community and authorised by the applicant and accompanied by a fee payable under Regulation (EC) No 297/95, with further amendments. A conventional, approved form of the dossier (all the documents that comprise the MAA) is described in detail in *NTA Volume 2B*. As noted previously, the mandatory format for the Centralised Procedure is the eCTD.

The application must include proof of establishment in the EEA as well as the following:

- a document identifying the QP responsible in the EEA for pharmacovigilance activities
- a document describing the scientific service in the EEA in charge of information about the medicinal product
- a document identifying the QP in the EEA responsible for batch release and the contact person for product defects and product recalls
- a document describing, in detail, the pharmacovigilance system and, where appropriate, the risk management system, as required in Article 8(ia) of Directive 2001/83/EC, as amended

Once the application is validated (administratively and technically) with a positive outcome, the applicant is informed in writing that the validation has been successfully completed and is given the names of CHMP members to whom full or partial copies of the dossier should be sent for review. Negative outcome of the validation is also provided in written format to the applicant and may result from failure to provide the data, information or clarifications requested or to adhere to the EU CTD format.

Once positively validated, and provided the rapporteur and co-rapporteur have confirmed that they have received the dossier (including any additional information requested during the validation phase), EMA starts the procedure at the monthly starting date published on its website. There is a set timetable for processing of centralised applications, and this stipulates that CHMP must deliver its opinion in not more than 210 days. The standard timetable for MAA evaluation is presented in **Table 17-1**.

For medicinal products that are of major public health interest, particularly from a therapeutic innovation point of view, the applicant may request the accelerated assessment procedure in accordance with Article 14(9) of Regulation (EC) No 726/2004. If the request is accepted by CHMP, the abovementioned standard timetable will be reduced to 150 days.

There are three main possible outcomes to the MAA:
- a negative/unfavourable CHMP opinion
- a conditional opinion (Conditional MA or MA under Exceptional Circumstances)
- a positive opinion

An unfavourable opinion is given when CHMP does not consider the MAA to fulfil the authorisation criteria set out in Regulation (EC) No 726/2004.

A Conditional MA is granted in accordance with Article 14(7) of Regulation (EC) No 726/2004. Under this regulation, CHMP may adopt an opinion recommending that an MA be granted subject to certain specific conditions and obligations that are to be reviewed annually. The list of these obligations shall be made publicly accessible. Such authorisation shall be valid for one year, on a renewable basis.

In accordance with Article 14(8) of Regulation (EC) No 726/2004, in exceptional circumstances and following consultation with the applicant, an authorisation may be granted subject to a requirement for the applicant to introduce specific procedures, particularly concerning the product's safety. Such authorisation must be based on one of the grounds set out in Part II.6 of Annex I to Directive 2001/83/EC. Continuation of the authorisation shall be linked to the annual reassessment of these conditions.

Following positive scientific evaluation by CHMP, the European Commission drafts a decision on a Community MA. An MA granted under the Centralised Procedure is valid for the entire EU market; the medicinal product may be put on the market in all Member States. The European Free Trade Association (EFTA) states—Iceland, Liechtenstein and Norway—have, through the EEA agreement, adopted a complete Community *acquis* (EU laws and objectives) on medicinal products and are consequently parties to the Centralised Procedure, although they still issue national MAs following successful completion of the procedure.

With the positive CHMP opinion, and in accordance with Article 13 of Regulation (EC) No 726/2004, EMA shall publish the CHMP assessment report on the medicinal product, which includes the reasons for its opinion in favour of granting authorisation, after deleting any information of a commercially confidential nature. This document is called the European Public Assessment Report (EPAR). If the opinion is negative, a summary of opinion relating to the negative opinion is published at Day 0 (i.e., the day of adoption of the negative opinion). If a company withdraws the application, this fact also will be published.

Once the MA is granted, it can be subject to:
- Specific obligations (when the Conditional MA or MA under Exceptional Circumstances is granted)—In this case, the applicant is obliged to submit additional data (postauthorisation data) known as "specific obligations" set out in Annex IIC of the Commission Decision.
- Follow-up measures (FUMs)—whether or not for conditional approval or under exceptional circumstances—FUMs can be requested at the initial CHMP opinion or in addition to the CHMP assessment of any submitted additional data/applications.
- Variations (all MAs)—Variations may be required as a result of FUM or specific obligations when these data would require changes to the product information or to the MA (e.g., changes to the Quality Module).

The MAH must indicate realistic target dates for the submission of postauthorisation data in its Letter of Undertaking. If no documents are submitted or in case of non-fulfilment of the obligations, in accordance with Article 14(7) and 14(8) of Regulation (EC) No 726/2004, CHMP will formulate an opinion recommending the "variation/suspension/revocation" of the MA.

The European Commission MA issued under the Centralised Procedure is valid throughout the Community under the same trademark name in all Member States. Medicinal products that have been authorised through the Centralised Procedure shall benefit from the 10-year period of protection referred to in Article 10(1) of Directive 2001/83/EC, as amended. According to this article, this protection can be extended to a maximum of 11 years if, during the first eight years, the MAH obtains an authorisation for one or more new therapeutic indications that, during the scientific evaluation prior to their authorisation, are held to bring a significant clinical benefit in comparison with existing therapies.

In accordance with Article 13(4), the MAH shall inform EMA of the dates of the actual marketing of the product in all Member States, taking into account the various presentations authorised. Any authorisation that is not followed by actual marketing in the Community within three years after authorisation shall cease to be valid. Similarly, when a product previously marketed in the Community is no longer actually present on the market for three consecutive years, the authorisation shall cease to be valid. However, the European Commission, in exceptional circumstances, may grant exemptions from these provisions on duly justified public health grounds.[2]

Mutual Recognition Procedure

The principle of mutual recognition is that an MA in one Member State (Reference Member State (RMS)) must be recognised by the regulatory authorities of other Member States (Concerned Member States (CMS)), unless there are grounds for supposing that the product may present a risk to the public health. The Mutual Recognition Procedure may be triggered by an applicant or a Member State. Under the new legislation, the Mutual Recognition Procedure can be used only when there is already an MA in at least one Member State. If there is no MA in any EU Member State, the Decentralised Procedure should be used (or the Centralised Procedure, if its requirements are met).

The Mutual Recognition Procedure must be used for the following products:
- medicinal products containing new active substances outside the centralised therapeutic areas
- OTC (over-the-counter) products
- homeopathic medicinal products
- generic products (also generic versions of products authorised by the Centralised Procedure before November 2005, with the exception of biotechnology-derived ones)
- "abridged" applications, "well-established use," line extensions of "old Mutual Recognition Procedure"

Chapter 17

Table 17-2. Mutual Recognition Procedure Flowchart

Approximately 90 days before submission to CMS	Applicant requests RMS to update Assessment Report (AR) and assign procedure number.
Day -14	Applicant submits the dossier to CMS; RMS circulates the AR including SmPC, PIL and labelling to CMSs. Validation of the application in the CMSs.
Day 0	RMS starts the procedure.
Day 50	CMS send their comments to RMS and applicant.
Day 60	Applicant sends the response document to CMS and RMS.
Until Day 68	RMS circulates its assessment of the response document to CMS.
Day 75	CMS send their remaining comments to RMS and applicant. A break-out session can be organized between Days 73-80.
Day 85	CMS send any remaining comments to RMS and applicant.
Day 90	CMS notify RMS and applicant of final position (and, in case of negative position, also EMA's CMD secretariat); if consensus is reached, RMS closes the procedure. If consensus is not reached, points of disagreement submitted by CMS are referred to CMDh by RMS within seven days after Day 90.
Day 150	For procedures referred to CMDh: if consensus is reached at the level of CMDh, RMS closes the procedure. If consensus is not reached at the level of CMDh, RMS refers the matter to CHMP for arbitration.
5 days after close of procedure	Applicant sends high-quality national translations of SmPC, PIL and labelling to CMS and RMS.
30 days after close of procedure	Granting of national MAs in the CMS, subject to submission of acceptable translations.

Source: *NTA Volume 2A*, Chapter 2, February 2007; CMDh Flowchart on MRP (May 2007).

As mentioned above, the Mutual Recognition Procedure can be used for standalone and abridged applications, provided the application is legally valid and meets the requirements of Article 28(2) of Directive 2001/83/EC, as amended. Once the procedure has been used, all variations, changes and line extensions (including changes falling under the scope of Annex I and II of Commission Regulation (EC) No 1234/2008) to these medicinal products must use the Mutual Recognition Procedure. The procedure is also applicable for line extensions of existing national MAs under certain conditions mentioned in Commission Communication 98/C229/03, which describes a case in which an applicant initially was granted two different national authorisations in different Member States for the same medicinal product. If, afterward, the same applicant wishes—by lodging applications for changes or variations of the national MAs—to obtain harmonised national authorisations in different Member States, it would not be possible to exclude such a case from the scope of application of the Mutual Recognition Procedure.

For medicinal products with a well-established use demonstrated in accordance with Article 10(a) of Directive 2001/83/EC (bibliographic application), as amended, the Mutual Recognition Procedure is applicable. But when the well-established use is based on data referring to an existing group of products for which no Community authorisation exists, the applicant still has the option to follow independent National Procedures as stated in Commission Communication 98/C229/03.

To fulfil the dossier criterion of identical product prior to a Mutual Recognition Procedure, the applicant must harmonise the already approved national SmPCs. This *a priori* harmonisation can be achieved through coordinated national variation procedures or through the procedure foreseen in Article 30 of Directive 2001/83/EC, as amended.

The Mutual Recognition Procedure is regarded as a two-stage process: first a national approval and then the mutual recognition process. If this second stage fails (due to refusal of one or more Member States to recognise the first approval), there may be a third stage—arbitration (see Community Referral below). If the Member States disagree about the product's quality, safety and efficacy, a scientific evaluation of that matter is carried out by CHMP, leading to a single decision that is binding on all Member States. However, faced with this option, the applicant may decide to withdraw the application, at least in the "problem" countries. The arbitration process is lengthy and unpopular with pharmaceutical companies.

As mentioned above, the first phase of the Mutual Recognition Procedure is in many respects similar to the National Procedure, where the RMS authorises the medicinal product. Those National Procedures significantly differ across Member States and depend on the experience of the national Competent Authority in clinical, regulatory and marketing issues. Those factors have to be taken into account when selecting the RMS. In theory, the national process that results in an MA takes no longer than 210 days. The reality is that a number of factors can lead to substantial delays. The second phase of the procedure—the Mutual Recognition

Procedure itself—follows clear rules and a strict timeline. The procedure starts with the preparation or update of the assessment report by the RMS, which takes 90 days. Once the assessment report is ready and sent to the CMS together with the SmPC, PIL and labelling, the applicant sends the dossier to the CMS and the validation period starts. Usually the validation period takes 14 days, but, in reality, it may take 30 days. With the positive validation, the procedure starts at Day 0. The first comments from CMS are sent on Day 50, and the applicant has 10 days to respond to them (Day 60). Within the next eight days, the RMS prepares the Assessment Report (AR) on the responses and circulates it among the interested parties (Day 68). CMS have until Day 75 to submit their comments on the AR. If a potential serious risk is identified, a break-out session may be arranged, usually around Day 75 (between Day 73 and Day 80). The aim of the break-out session is to create a platform for discussion for the RMS, the CMS and, if necessary, the applicant, to clarify the outstanding issues and achieve consensus through negotiations. Additional comments (if any) may be sent by CMS until Day 85. If consensus is reached, the CMS notify the RMS and applicant of their final position and the RMS closes the procedure. If consensus is not reached, the points for disagreement submitted by CMS are referred to CMDh by the RMS within seven days after Day 90. If consensus is reached at the level of CMDh, the RMS closes the procedure at Day 150. If consensus is not reached at the level of CMDh, the RMS refers the matter to CHMP for arbitration.

Five days after the procedure is finalised, the applicant is obliged to send high-quality translations of the SmPC, PIL and labelling to the RMS and CMS. In accordance with Article 28(5) of Directive 2001/83/EC, as amended, the CMS shall adopt a decision in conformity with the approved AR and grant a national MA within 30 days after acknowledgment of the procedure. In reality, it might take a few months, depending on the national Competent Authority.

For the Mutual Recognition Procedure flowchart, see **Table 17-2**.

The Mutual Recognition Procedure can be used more than once for subsequent applications to other Member States for the same medicinal product ("repeat use"). Repeat use can be used after the completion of either the Mutual Recognition Procedure or Decentralised Procedure. The repeat-use procedure is applicable in the following situations:

- when the application is submitted to a new CMS not involved in the first Mutual Recognition Procedure or Decentralised Procedure
- when the application is resubmitted to a CMS where it was withdrawn during the first procedure ("reapplication")

The repeat-use procedure(s) can be employed until all Member States are involved in the procedure. Before starting the procedure, the applicant should finalise all ongoing procedures (variations, renewals, updating SmPCs, etc.) and update the dossier. The next step is submission of the updated dossier to the RMS and to formally request an update of the AR. For more details see *Procedural Advice on Repeat Use*.[3]

In order to coordinate and facilitate Mutual Recognition Procedure operations, a Mutual Recognition Facilitation Group (MRFG) was established in 1995. The MRFG met monthly and comprised senior representatives from each Member State. Under the new legislation (Directive 2004/27/EC), the MRFG has been renamed the Coordination Group for Mutual Recognition and Decentralised Procedures–Human (CMDh). It is chaired by one of its members for a period of three years, who may be re-elected once. The vice chairperson shall be appointed from among the members of the coordination group by the Member State that has the presidency of the Council of the European Union for the duration of the term of the presidency. The secretariat for this group is provided by EMA. CMDh meets monthly at EMA, and can be joined by observers from the European Commission and EMA. When necessary, in connection with the plenary meeting, breakout sessions related to ongoing procedures may be held. Additional subgroup meetings are organised on specific topics.

The group provides a forum for discussing procedural issues arising from Mutual Recognition Procedures and Decentralised Procedures and resolving problems. It can undertake an overview of individual applications; however, scientific discussions related to individual applications are handled in breakout sessions organised and chaired by the specific RMS. CMDh considers points of disagreement raised by a Member State related to the AR, SmPC, labelling and PIL of a medicinal product on the grounds of "potential serious risk to public health" within Mutual Recognition Procedures and Decentralised Procedures, and facilitates the dialogue between Member States. On an annual basis, CMDh prepares a list of products that must be harmonised among all Member States. Furthermore, this group identifies issues to be referred to the European Commission, the Pharmaceutical Committee, the Heads of Medicines Agencies (HMA) or other regulatory bodies; works closely with the Pharmacovigilance Working Party (PhVWP) of CHMP to ensure best practice of risk management for medicinal products authorised via Mutual Recognition Procedures and Decentralised Procedures; and creates its own Rules of Procedure to be endorsed by the HMA and approved by the European Commission.

More information on the Mutual Recognition Procedure can be found in Directive 2001/83/EC, as amended, the *NTA Volume 2A*, Chapter 2 and the HMA/CMDh website.

Chapter 17

Decentralised Procedure

As already mentioned, the Decentralised Procedure was established by Directive 2001/83/EC, as amended, and has been in force since November 2005. The newly created CMDh group has the same competencies for both the Mutual Recognition Procedure and Decentralised Procedure. In addition, in cases where serious public health issues are still raised by one or more of the participating Member States at the end of the procedure, and despite a withdrawal of the dossier in the CMS, automatic arbitration by EMA and the European Commission is applicable to both Mutual Recognition Procedures and Decentralised Procedures.

The Decentralised Procedure is used for medicinal products for which there is no existing MA in any EU Member State. In accordance with Article 17(2) of Directive 2001/83/EC, as amended, the MA for the same medicinal product cannot be granted in parallel in two or more Member States by separate National Procedures. In such cases, the Decentralised Procedure must be followed. The Decentralised Procedure covers all medicinal products not authorised in the EU (for which the Centralised Procedure is not mandatory). As in the Mutual Recognition Procedure, the applicant can select the RMS and list the CMS. In order to do so, the applicant has to request one Member State to act as the RMS for the particular product by filing the Common Request Form (the most current version of this document can be found on the HMA/CMDh website). Once the RMS has agreed, the date of intended submission is scheduled and a Decentralised Procedure number is assigned. Prior to the submission, the applicant may request a presubmission meeting to familiarise the national Competent Authority with the product and submission details. Usually the presubmission meeting is held three months before the intended submission date. The applicant is encouraged to discuss the necessity of conducting a presubmission meeting with the RMS. On the agreed date, the applicant submits the dossier simultaneously to RMS and CMS (Day -14) and the validation period begins. In theory, it is scheduled for 14 days, but, in practice, can last much longer (sometimes more than 30 days). The validation period depends on national requirements that have to be followed for each CMS and the applicant's ability to meet those requirements on time. As soon as the dossier is submitted, the RMS initiates the procedure in the Communication and Tracking System (CTS) database, so the CMS and RMS are able to communicate on the procedure through the CTS record immediately after receipt of the dossier. CMS are obliged to update the CTS database daily to inform the RMS about the application's validation status. The most common invalidation issues include:

- lack of original, signed documents (e.g., LoA for a person responsible for communication during and after the procedure (Annex 5.4), Manufacturer's Commitment (Annex 5.11)
- improperly written statement on GMP compliance (Annex 5.22)
- lack of some nationally required documents (Application Form not translated into national language (Spain, Greece), technical agreements between the applicant and manufacturer(s), declaration on pack sizes and samples, etc.)
- mistakes in the application form
- wrong format of the submitted dossier (for example, if the dossier is not in the eCTD or NeeS format)
- technical issues related to the eCTD (wrong PDF files, improperly named folders, too many CDs, broken CDs/DVDs, etc.)
- lack of a paper version of administrative documents while submitting an eCTD in some Member States

The applicant has to respond to deficiencies on a daily basis in order to have the submission positively validated by the RMS and CMS. Once this goal is achieved, the procedure is started and Day 0 is assigned. The Decentralised Procedure consists of two steps. Assessment Step I corresponds to the Day 120 period in which the Draft Assessment Report (DAR) is prepared, followed by draft SmPC, labelling and PIL. During Assessment Step I, the Preliminary Assessment Report (PrAR) is prepared by the RMS and circulated to the applicant and CMS. By Day 100, CMS should communicate their comments to the RMS, other CMS and the applicant. Between Day 100 and 105, the RMS consults with the CMS on the comments submitted. If there are no potential serious risks to public health and consensus is reached, the RMS can update the PrAR and prepare the Final Assessment Report (FAR). The procedure is finalised on Day 105 and the national phase can be started.

If consensus is reached that the product is approvable but there are comments that can be easily resolved, the RMS stops the clock and forwards these comments to the applicant on Day 105. After receiving sufficient responses from the applicant, the RMS updates the PrAR, creates the FAR and finalises the procedure on Day 120, followed by national phases in each Member State.

If consensus in not reached, the RMS stops the clock at Day 105 and asks the applicant to answer all remaining issues within the specified timeframe. Usually, the clock stop is scheduled for three months, but its duration can be mutually agreed between the RMS and the applicant (it can be shortened or lengthened in justified cases). The applicant may submit draft responses, including updated SmPC, PIL and labelling proposals, to the RMS for preassessment. In any case, the applicant should reach agreement on the submission date of the final response with the RMS. After submission of the final response and receipt of the list of dispatch dates in all CMS, the RMS restarts the procedure at Day 106. Between Day 106 and 120, the RMS updates the PrAR to prepare the DAR and draft product

Overview of Authorisation Procedures for Medicinal Products

Table 17-3. Decentralised Procedure Flowchart

Pre-procedural Step	
Before Day -14	Applicant discussion with RMS. RMS allocated procedure number; creation in CTS.
Day -14	Submission of the dossier to RMS and CMS. Validation of the application.
Assessment Step I	
Day 0	RMS starts the procedure.
Day 70	RMS forwards the Preliminary Assessment Report (PrAR), SmPC, PIL and labelling to CMS and applicant.
Until Day 100	CMS send their comments to RMS and applicant.
Until Day 105	Consultation between RMS, CMS and applicant. If consensus not reached, RMS stops the clock to allow applicant to supplement the dossier and respond to the questions.
Clock Stop period	Applicant may send draft responses to RMS and agrees to final response submission date with RMS. Applicant sends the final response document to RMS and CMS within a recommended period of three months, which could be extended, if justified.
Day 106	Valid applicant response submission received. RMS restarts the procedure.
Day 106-120	RMS updates the PrAR to prepare Draft Assessment Report (DAR), draft SmPC, draft labelling and draft PIL to CMS and Applicant.
Day 120	RMS may close procedure if consensus is reached. Proceed to national 30-day step for granting MA.
Assessment Step II	
Day 120 (Day 0)	If consensus is not reached, RMS sends the DAR, draft SmPC, draft labelling and draft PIL to CMS and applicant.
Day 145 (Day 25)	CMS send final comments to RMS and applicant.
Day 150 (Day 30)	RMS may close procedure if consensus is reached. Proceed to national 30-day step for granting MA.
Until 180 (Day 60)	If consensus is not reached by Day 150, RMS to communicate outstanding issues with applicant, receive any additional clarification and prepare a short report (Day 180 Report) for discussion at coordination group.
Until Day 205 (Day 85)	Breakout group of involved Member States reaches consensus on the matter (if applicable)
Day 210 (Day 90)	Closure of the procedure including CMS' approval of Assessment Report, SmPC, labelling and PIL, or referral to coordination group. Proceed to national 30-day step for granting MA.
Day 210 (at the latest)	If consensus was not reached at Day 210, points of disagreement will be referred to the coordination group for resolution.
Day 270 (at the latest)	Final position adopted by coordination group with referral to CHMP for arbitration in case of unsolved disagreement.
National Step	
Day 110/125/155/215/275	Applicant sends high-quality national translation of SmPC, labelling and PIL to CMS and RMS.
Day 135/150/180/240	Granting of national MA in RMS and CMS if no referral to the coordination group (national agencies will adopt the decision and issue the MA subject to submission of acceptable translations).
Day 300	Granting of national MA in RMS and CMS if positive conclusion by the coordination group and no referral to CHMP (national agencies will adopt the decision and issue the MA subject to submission of acceptable translations).

Source: *Decentralised Procedure – Member States' Standard Operating Procedure (MRFG, October 2005) & Best Practice Guide for Decentralised and Mutual Recognition (CMDh, Rev. 6 May 2007)*

information (SmPC, labelling, PIL). The DAR and draft informative texts are sent to the applicant and CMS. On Day 120, Assessment Step II is initiated and the RMS starts the 90-day period, corresponding to Day 0 of the 90-day period mentioned in 28(4) of Directive 2001/83/EC. Each CMS should send its final comments on the DAR no later than Day 145 of the procedure (i.e., Day 25 of the 90-day period). If consensus is reached, the RMS prepares the FAR and may close the procedure at Day 150 (i.e., Day 30 of the 90-day period). The procedure continues with the national step if the Member States consider the product approvable.

Between Day 145 and 150, the RMS consults with the CMS to discuss the comments submitted. If consensus is not reached by Day 150, the applicant is informed of outstanding issues by the RMS. The applicant must submit additional clarification by Day 160, including any revised proposal for the SmPC, PIL and labelling, and the RMS prepares a short report and forwards it to the CMS no later than Day 180 (i.e., Day 60 of the 90-day period). This is called a Short Report or Day 180-Report and includes the RMS' proposals for an update of the overview portion of the DAR to derive the FAR.

At the latest, at Day 205 (i.e., Day 85 of the 90-day period), a breakout session may be held at EMA with the involved Member States to reach consensus on major outstanding issues.

At Day 210 (i.e., Day 90 of the 90-day period), the RMS closes the procedure if consensus was reached with all Member States on the outstanding issues. The RMS includes information in the FAR about how major outstanding issues were resolved by discussions via written procedures and by discussion in the CMDh (if applicable). Together with the FAR, which includes the final product release and shelf-life specifications, the final informative texts are attached. If there are any conditions to be fulfilled or any FUMs recommended, they are specified in an End-of-Procedure letter, also attached to the FAR.

Once the procedure is finalised, the applicant must submit high-quality national translations of the SmPC, PIL and labelling to the RMS and CMS within five days.

For the Decentralised Procedure flowchart, see **Table 17-3**.

Applicants can multiply or duplicate their applications via either the Mutual Recognition Procedure or Decentralised Procedure but there is no definition of a "duplicate" in the pharmaceutical legislation. It can be done at the beginning of the procedure, during the procedure (i.e., Day 106 in the Decentralised Procedures) or after the procedure is finalised. The possibility of duplicating the application should be discussed and agreed with the RMS. In general, a duplicate application is defined by the reference to the first MA as follows:
- same dossier (copy of Modules 1, 2, 3, 4 and 5)
- same legal basis according to Directive 2001/83/EC, as amended
- different trade name
- same or different applicant/MAH

Applications for duplicates result in independent MAs that can be varied individually. However, MAHs are strongly encouraged to keep the SmPC, PIL and labelling of the duplicates harmonised whenever possible.[4]

National Authorisations

Each EU Member State's Competent Authority is responsible for granting MAs for medicinal products placed on its market, except medicinal products authorised using Community procedures. Since January 1998, independent National Procedures have been strictly limited to the initial phase of mutual recognition and to medicinal products that are not to be authorised in more than one Member State. Under the new legislation, independent National Procedures are restricted to medicinal products that will be authorised in only one Member State.

Independent National Procedures can continue to be followed for medicinal products with a well-established use demonstrated in accordance with Article 10(a) Directive 2001/83/EC, as amended, and based on data referring to an existing group of products with different SmPCs in the Member States, as long as no Community harmonisation exists on the use of said product's constituent(s). They also can be used for line extensions of authorised medicinal products as long as no *a priori* harmonisation has been achieved.

Different Types of Applications and Legal Basis for the Submission

Complete/Full and Independent Applications

In accordance with Article 8(3) of Directive 2001/83/EC, as amended, a full (standalone) MAA must include:
- physicochemical, biological or microbiological tests
- pharmacological and toxicological tests
- clinical trials

This type of application is compulsory for new chemical entities (new active substances), which are listed at the beginning of this chapter.

Generic Applications for Essentially Similar Medicinal Products (Abridged Applications)

Under Article 10(1) and Part II(2) of Directive 2001/83/EC, as amended, the applicant is not required to provide pharmacological and toxicological test or clinical trial results when the medicinal product is essentially similar to a product that has been authorised in the EU under the previous legislation for not less than six or 10 years (depending on the Member State) and is marketed in that Member State at the time of the application (generic application). The new legislation harmonises the timeframes to an eight-year data protection period (submission) and a 10-year period of marketing protection (approval). This period can be extended to 11 years if, during the first eight, the MAH obtains an authorisation for one or more new therapeutic indications that bring a significant clinical benefit in comparison with existing therapies. The new periods of protection (8–2–1) do not apply to reference medicinal products for which the initial application for authorisation (date of submission of the application, not validation) was submitted before 20 November 2005.[5] For those products, the exclusivity period under the previous legislation applies:
- 10 years for all medicinal products authorised through the Centralised Procedure
- 10 years for all other medicinal products originally authorised in Belgium, Germany, France, Italy, the Netherlands, Sweden, the UK and Luxembourg

- 10 years for all medicinal products authorised following a CHMP opinion in accordance with Article 4 of Directive 87/22/EEC (ex-concertation procedure)
- six years in all other Member States, plus Norway and Iceland

A generic authorisation may be issued for all therapeutic indications and all pharmaceutical forms, strengths and posology already authorised for the reference drug. A generic authorisation may be extended to cover more or other indications, strengths and pharmaceutical forms than the original product if the applicant submits sufficient bridging data.

The European Court of Justice, in its judgment in Case C-368/96 (Medicinal products—MA—Abridged procedures—Essentially similar products), confirmed that if the four conditions listed above are fulfilled, a generic authorisation may be issued for all therapeutic indications, dosage forms, doses and dosage schedules already authorised for the reference drug, even if some of those indications, dosage forms and doses were authorised for a period shorter than six or 10 years (old legislation).

The concept of essential similarity implies the following criteria:
- the same qualitative and quantitative composition of active substances
- the same pharmaceutical form (all oral pharmaceutical forms for immediate release must be regarded as the same pharmaceutical form)
- well- and appropriately demonstrated bioequivalence

In accordance with Article 10.2(b) of Directive 2001/83/EC, as amended, different salts, esters, ethers, isomers, mixtures of isomers, complexes or derivatives of an active substance shall be considered to be the same active substance unless they differ significantly in properties with regard to safety and/or efficacy. In such cases, additional information providing proof of the safety and/or efficacy of the various salts, esters or derivatives of an authorised active substance must be supplied by the applicant. The various immediate-release oral pharmaceutical forms (i.e., tablets and capsules) shall be considered to be one and the same pharmaceutical form for the concept of essential similarity.

For biotechnology products, the concept of essential similarity is difficult to apply.

Generic and informed consent applications (please see below) are linked to the original authorisation granted on the basis of a complete dossier (abridged applications may not refer to an abridged dossier). The original product dossier must be at the disposal of the regulatory authorities.

Generic applications are described in detail in Chapter 21 Generic Medicinal Products.

Hybrid Applications

In accordance with Article 10(3) of Directive 2001/83/EC, as amended, these types of applications may require inclusion in the dossier of the results of the appropriate preclinical tests and/or clinical trials, in cases where:
- the medicinal product does not fall within the definition of a generic medicinal product
- bioequivalence cannot be demonstrated through bioavailability studies
- there are changes in the active substance(s), therapeutic indications, strength, pharmaceutical form or route of administration vis-à-vis the reference medicinal product

Bibliographic Applications (Well-established Use)

According to Article 10(a) of Directive 2001/83/EC, as amended, and Annex I, Part II(1), it is possible to replace pharmacological and toxicological tests or clinical trial results with detailed references to published scientific literature if a medicinal product's constituent(s) has a well-established medicinal use, recognised efficacy and an acceptable safety level. The definition of a Bibliographic Application includes specific criteria associated with the time period over which the use has been established, quantitative aspects of use and scientific interest in the substance's medicinal use. Therefore, different time periods may be necessary to verify well-established use of different substances. In any case, the time period required to establish a well-established use of a medicinal product constituent must not be less than one decade from that substance's first systematic and documented use as a medicinal product in the EU. This applies to any medicinal product or chemical or biological substance for which there is no original/reference medicinal product to which essential similarity can be claimed. This is the case, for instance, for "old" medicinal products whose use is well-established in the medicinal practice, and for known indications, strengths and pharmaceutical forms, in view of the period of time over which they have been used and the information that has been publicly available about their safety and efficacy.

"Well-established use" refers to a specific therapeutic use. If well-known substances are used for entirely new therapeutic indications for which the Annex I requirements to Directive 2003/63/EC cannot be fulfilled, it is not possible to solely refer to a well-established use. Additional data on the new therapeutic indication should be provided together with appropriate safety data.

It must be stressed that such assessment reports as the EPAR for Community MAs, made publicly available by Competent Authorities for reasons of transparency, do not supply sufficient information to meet Directive 2001/83/EC Annex requirements.

Fixed-combination Application

In accordance with Article 10(b) of Directive 2001/83/EC, as amended, and Annex I, Part II(5), fixed-combination applications are possible for medicinal products containing active substances used in the composition of authorised medicinal products (but not to be used in combination for therapeutic purposes). In that case, the results of new preclinical tests or new clinical trials relating to that combination shall be provided in accordance with Article 8(3)(i), but it is not necessary to provide scientific references relating to each individual active substance.

Moreover, any fixed combination may be considered a complete/full, independent application because it is a new and unique medicinal product requiring a separate SmPC.

Informed Consent Applications

Under Article 10(c) of Directive 2001/83/EC, as amended, these applications are appropriate in cases when the medicinal product is essentially similar to a product already authorised in the Member State and the original product's MAH gave the second applicant rights to refer to its approved dossier.

For regulatory authorities, demonstration of informed consent is a formal prerequisite when the application is submitted. Withdrawing the informed consent at a later stage, however, has no direct consequences for the MA's existence or validity.

Mixed Marketing Applications

Annex I, Part II(7) of Directive 2001/83/EC, as amended, specifies that mixed MAAs must present published scientific literature together with original results of tests and trials. Such applications must be submitted and processed following the complete, full and independent MA dossier requirements. These requirements apply to the use of bibliographic references in mixed dossiers both as supporting data for the applicant's own tests and trials or in order to replace any tests or trials in Module 4 and/or 5. All other module(s) are in accordance with the structure described in Part I of the above-mentioned Annex 1.

The Competent Authority will accept the applicant's proposed format on a case-by-case basis.

Herbal Medicinal Products

Regulation (EC) No 726/2004 established the Committee on Herbal Medicinal Products (HMPC). In addition, Directive 2004/24/EC was introduced as part of the new legislation amending Directive 2001/83/EC on the Community code relating to medicinal products for human use with regard to traditional herbal medicinal products. It created a simplified registration procedure ("traditional-use registration") for herbal medicinal products that fulfil certain criteria.[6]

Referrals

European Community Referrals

EU pharmaceutical legislation has created a binding Community arbitration mechanism to achieve cooperation between Member States as needed. The EU legislation, however, recognises the need for urgent, unilateral measures by Member States when necessary to protect the public health and until a definitive action is adopted. In these specific cases, Member States may take temporary national measures suspending a medicinal product's marketing and use. They must inform the European Commission, EMA and other Member States no later than the next working day.

The decision following a referral is applicable only to the specific medicinal products that have been the subject of the referral procedure and to the Member States involved in the procedure.

Mutual Recognition and Decentralised Procedure Referral

Under Articles 29, 32 and 33 of Directive 2001/83/EC, as amended, referral to CMDh may be initiated by the RMS or CMS in the course of a Mutual Recognition Procedure or Decentralised Procedure if a medicinal product's MA presents a potential serious public health risk.

Within the coordination group, all Member States concerned give the applicant an opportunity to present its point of view orally or in writing. If the Member States have not reached agreement within 60 days, CHMP undertakes a scientific evaluation of the matter and issues an opinion, normally within 60 days of receiving the referral. From this opinion, the European Commission drafts a single decision binding the Member States and applicant.

Divergent Decision Referral

This referral may be started by any Member State, the European Commission or the applicant (or MAH), according to Article 30 of Directive 2001/83/EC, as amended, when divergent decisions have been made by Member States related to a particular medicinal product (e.g., suspension or withdrawal of an MA or divergence of the therapeutic indications of an authorised product).

CHMP is called upon to issue an opinion on the area(s) of divergence within 60 days of the procedure's start date. This period can be extended by up to 90 days.

The resulting European Commission decision must be implemented in all Member States concerned (i.e., those in which the particular medicinal product's MA has been granted, refused, suspended or withdrawn).

Community Interest Referral

According to Article 31 of Directive 2001/83/EC, as amended, this referral may be started by Member States, the European Commission or the applicant (or MAH) when Community interests are involved. This latter expression refers particularly to Community public health interests related to a marketed medicinal product for which new quality, safety and efficacy data or new pharmacovigilance information have become available.

CHMP issues a reasoned opinion within 60 days of the referral date. This period may be extended by a further 90 days. A binding decision of the European Commission follows.

Follow-up Referral

This referral may be started by an MAH or Member State, under Articles 35, 26 and 27 of Directive 2001/83/EC, as amended, where an MA has already undergone a Community procedure. A follow-up referral is initiated when a change or variation, suspension or withdrawal of a harmonised MA is necessary to protect the public health, or when mutual recognition by one or more national regulatory authorities of the RMS draft decision on a variation is not possible. This mechanism aims to resolve divergences among Member States after harmonisation is achieved.

CHMP issues a reasoned opinion within 60 days of the referral date. This period may be extended by another 90 days. A binding decision of the European Commission follows.

Summary

- EU laws and policies are established by several types of legislative instruments. Although not all are legally binding, the instruments without binding legal effect in many cases are strongly recommended either by EMA or Member States' Competent Authorities.
- MAAs in the EU can be granted following the Centralised, Decentralised or Mutual Recognition Procedures, or can be a purely national authorisations; authorisations not used in the territory for a period of three consecutive years become invalid (sunset clause).
- The accepted format for MAAs is the Common Technical Document, organised into five modules; Module 1 is not a part of the CTD and consists of administrative application data (including specific national requirements for the CMS).
- The eCTD is a standard for submitting MAAs in the Community and most of the EU Member States. It is the mandatory format for centrally authorised products at EMA.
- The Centralised Procedure can be utilised for orphan and veterinary products, for medicinal products developed by biotechnological processes and for new active substances for specified therapeutic indications.
- Once an MA is granted, it can be subject to: specific obligations (Conditional MA or MA under Exceptional Circumstances), follow-up measures (FUMs) and variations).
- Applicants/MAHs can submit multiple and/or duplicate applications via the Mutual Recognition Procedure or Decentralised Procedure; the possibility to duplicate the application should be discussed and agreed with RMS.
- Several types of applications (standalone or abridged) are specified in Directive 2001/83/EC, with further amendments.
  - For difficult and specific cases, European pharmaceutical legislation has created a binding Community arbitration mechanism to manage cooperation between Member States and/or the applicant/MAH.

References

1. *Guideline on the Investigation of Bioequivalence*, CPMP/EWP/QWP/1401/98 Rev. 1/Corr. Committee for Medicinal Products for Human Use, European Medicines Agency. 1 August 2010. EMA website. www.emea.europa.eu/docs/en_GB/document_library/Scientific_guideline/2010/01/WC500070039.pdf. Accessed 23 May 2012.
2. *The Rules Governing Medicinal Products in the European Union, Notice to Applicants, Volume 2A*, Chapter 4). EC website. http://ec.europa.eu/health/files/eudralex/vol-2/a/chap4rev200604_en.pdf. Accessed 23 May 2012.
3. *Procedural Advice on Repeat-Use*, CMDh/008/2009/Revision 6. Co-ordination Group for Mutual Recognition and Decentralised Procedures—Human. January 2009. HMA website. www.hma.eu/fileadmin/dateien/Human_Medicines/CMD_h_/procedural_guidance/Application_for_MA/RepeatUse_2009_01_Rev6-Clean.pdf. Accessed 23 May 2012.
4. Recommendations on Multiple/Duplicate Applications in Mutual Recognition and Decentralised Procedures, Revision 3. Co-ordination Group for Mutual Recognition and Decentralised Procedures—Human. June 2007. HMA website. www.hma.eu/uploads/media/rec_multiapp.pdf. Accessed 23 May 2012.
5. *The Rules Governing Medicinal Products in the European Union, Notice to Applicants, Volume 2A*, Chapter 1, Section 6.1. EC website. http://ec.europa.eu/health/files/eudralex/vol-2/a/vol2a_chap1_2005-11_en.pdf. Accessed 23 May 2012.
6. "Chapter 2a Specific provisions applicable to traditional herbal medicinal products," Directive 2001/83/EC of the European Parliament and of the Council of 6 November 2001 on the Community code relating to medicinal products for human use, as amended. EUR-Lex website. http://eur-lex.europa.eu/LexUriServ/LexUriServ.do?uri=OJ:L:2001:311:0067:0128:en:PDF. Accessed 23 May 2012.

Chapter 18

Medicinal Product Clinical Trials

Updated by Gautam Maitra

OBJECTIVES

- Understand the Ethics Committees and Health Authority (Competent Authority) requirements for commencing a clinical trial in the EU

- Understand requirements regarding Good Manufacturing Practice and importation of investigational medicinal products

- Understand requirements regarding "postapproval" changes (amendments) to the clinical trial application

- Understand pharmacovigilance and reporting requirements

DIRECTIVES, REGULATIONS AND GUIDELINES COVERED IN THIS CHAPTER

- Directive 2001/20/EC of the European Parliament and of the Council of 4 April 2001 on the approximation of the laws, regulations and administrative provisions of the Member States relating to the implementation of good clinical practice in the conduct of clinical trials on medicinal products for human use[1]

- Commission Directive 2003/94/EC of 8 October 2003 laying down the principles and guidelines of GMP in respect of medicinal products for human use and investigational medicinal products for human use[2]

- Commission Directive 2005/28/EC of 8 April 2005 laying down the principles and guidance for Good Clinical Practice as regards investigational medicinal products for human use, as well as the requirements for authorisation of the manufacture and importation of such paroducts[3]

- The Rules Governing Medicinal Products in the European Union, Volume 10, "Clinical Trials Notice to Applicants." July 2006—First Edition[4]

- Guideline on the requirements to the chemical and pharmaceutical quality of documentation concerning investigational medicinal products in clinical trials (CHMP/QWP/185401/2004/final[5])

- Guideline on strategies to identify and mitigate risks for first-in-human clinical trials with investigational medicinal products (EMEA/CHMP/SWP/28367/07[6])

- The Rules Governing Medicinal Products in the European Union. Detailed guidance for the request for authorisation of a clinical trial on a medicinal product for human use to the competent authorities, notification of substantial amendments and declaration of the end of the trial, CT-1, 2010/C82/01 communication dated 30 March 2010 (This document is based on Article 9(8) of Directive 2001/20/EC and replaces the document ENTR/F2/BL D(2003) dated October 2005.)

Introduction

Medicinal products must have a Marketing Authorisation (MA) granted before they can be sold or supplied to patients. Before this authorisation is granted, information about the product is assessed to ensure the product is safe and effective and is of acceptable quality.

Clinical trials are investigations in humans intended to discover or verify the effects of one or more investigational medicinal products (IMPs). They are undertaken to collect data on new product safety and efficacy. **Table 18-1** provides practical suggestions for the clinical trial process. These trials can be conducted using healthy volunteers or patients, depending on the type of product and its stage of development. Nonclinical safety information will have been obtained before the clinical trial programme commences.

Clinical trials begin with small studies in controlled populations of healthy volunteers or patients and, as data are gathered, then expand to large-scale studies in patients. These large-scale studies often compare the new product to the currently used treatment for the particular indication. As information is obtained, larger numbers of patients are exposed to the new product, and safety data are collected demonstrating the product's safety in the intended patient population.

Clinical trials in the EU formerly were conducted according to each individual Member State's laws, regulations and administrative provisions. Consequently, for many years, regulation was characterised by a wide array of national application and approval processes, combined with a lack of standardisation in applying Good Clinical Practice (GCP) and Good Manufacturing Practice (GMP). However, in April 2001, European Directive 2001/20/EC[7] governing clinical trials came into force with the objective of harmonising these processes and detailing the legal provisions for GCP and GMP across the EU. The aim was to increase and standardise the protection afforded to clinical trial participants. EU Member States were required to integrate these provisions into national legislation no later than 1 May 2004.

Since 1 May 2004, all EU clinical trials must be conducted in accordance with GCP. GMPs also must be applied to the manufacture of IMPs. Any site concerned with a clinical trial, particularly the trial site, the manufacturing site, any laboratory used for analyses and/or the sponsor's premises may be inspected.

Before commencing a clinical trial, the sponsor must submit a valid request for authorisation to conduct the trial to the Competent Authority in the Member State where the trial will be conducted, and must receive either no grounds for nonacceptance or a regulatory approval. Additionally, a single, favourable Ethics Committee opinion is required. Applications to the Competent Authority and Ethics Committee may proceed in parallel or sequentially, depending on the Member State and local guidelines (see **Figure 18-1**).

Legal Basis

Requirements for the conduct of clinical trials in the EU are provided in Directive 2001/20/EC of the European Parliament and of the Council of 4 April 2001 on the approximation of the laws, regulations and administrative provisions of the Member States relating to the implementation of good clinical practice in the conduct of clinical trials on medicinal products for human use (*Clinical Trials Directive*).

The *Clinical Trials Directive* is strengthened by Commission Directive 2005/28/EC of 8 April 2005 laying down principles and detailed guidelines for good clinical practice as regards investigational medicinal products for human use, as well as the requirements for authorisation of the manufacturing or importation of such products (*GCP Directive*).

Clinical trials performed in the EU are required to be conducted in accordance with the *Clinical Trials Directive*. If the clinical trials are conducted outside the EU, but are submitted in an EU Marketing Authorisation Application (MAA), they must follow principles that are equivalent to the provisions of the *Clinical Trials Directive* (cf. Annex I, point 8 of the Directive 2001/83/EC of the European Parliament and of the Council of 6 November 2001 on the Community code relating to medicinal products for human use (*Community Code*)).

These directives are supplemented by several EU guidance documents (available in a single volume from EudraLex, *The Rules Governing Medicinal Products in the European Union*[8]) that provide advice on application format and content of requests to Ethics Committees[9] and Competent Authorities.[10,11] Additionally, *Volume 10* includes guidance documents that cover the European database of clinical trials, EudraCT,[12] monitoring/clinical safety,[13,14] quality of the IMP[15-17] and inspections.[18,19]

These directives and guidance documents provide a general, harmonised framework for trials conducted in the EU, but should always be read in conjunction with relevant Member States' legislation and guidance documents.

In March 2010, the European Commission published Communication 2010/C82/01.[20] This document provides detailed guidance on the request to the Competent Authorities for authorisation of a clinical trial on a medicinal product for human use, the notification of substantial amendments and the declaration of the end of the trial (CT-1) and replaces the document ENTR/F2/BL D(2003) dated October 2005.[21]

Definitions

Definitions are provided in Directive 2001/20/EC, Article 2. These include the definition of a "clinical trial" as any investigation in human subjects intended to:

- discover or verify the clinical, pharmacological and/or other pharmacodynamic effects of one or more IMPs and/or

Table 18-1. Practical Notes for Clinical Trials

1	Obtain the dedicated EudraCT number for the clinical trial.
2	Extract the CTA index, generally available on the website for each Competent Authority.
3	Ensure that all contracts with contract manufacturers and contract research organisations are in place.
4	Ensure that the insurance forms for the clinical trial are signed.
5	GMP, GLP and GCP certificates should be available.
6	Make sure all toxicology studies are conducted under GLP.
7	Select Investigators who are in some way close to the patients; this will help boost patient recruitment.
8	Keep the clinical trial protocol consolidated by including the amendments, simple but not simpler.
9	Ideally, submissions to the Ethics Committee and the Competent Authorities should occur simultaneously, but if possible, try to clear the Ethics Committee hurdle before submitting to the Competent Authorities.
10	It is advisable to liaise with the Competent Authorities whenever possible.
11	Ensure a strong clinical operations team and manage the departmental interfaces with well-defined SOPs.
12	The sponsor should ensure patient safety.
13	Consider the Voluntary Harmonisation Procedure when access to more patients is needed as the process is considered successful.

- identify any adverse reactions to one or more IMPs and/or
- study absorption, distribution, metabolism and excretion of one or more IMPs with the object of ascertaining safety and/or efficacy of the IMPs

The directive covers all clinical trials—Phase I to Phase IV—carried out at one site or multiple sites, in one or more Member States.

An IMP is defined as a pharmaceutical form of an active substance or placebo being tested or used as a reference in a clinical trial. IMPs include products that already have an MA but are used or assembled (formulated or packaged) differently than the authorised form, or are used for an unauthorised indication or to gain further information about the authorised form. On this basis, provided requirement(s) are met, reference products used as comparators should be considered IMPs.

Directive 2001/20/EC applies to all IMPs, including:
- chemical entities
- biotechnology products
- cell therapy products
- gene therapy products
- plasma-derived products
- other extractive products
- immunological medicinal products (such as vaccines, allergens and immune sera)
- herbal medicinal products
- radiopharmaceutical products
- homeopathic products

Products not considered IMPs, as defined in Article 2(d) of the *Clinical Trials Directive*, may be supplied to subjects participating in a trial and used in accordance with the protocol. For instance, some clinical trial protocols require the use of such medicinal products as concomitant or rescue or escape medication for preventive, diagnostic or therapeutic reasons and/or to ensure that adequate medical care is provided for the subject. Medicinal products also may be used in accordance with the protocol to induce a physiological response (i.e., as a challenge agent). These types of medicinal products do not fall within the definition of IMP and may be referred to as "noninvestigational medicinal products" (NIMPs).[22,23] Member States may have their own slightly different interpretations of IMPs and NIMPs, depending on whether the product in question is being used in accordance with the terms of an MA. If necessary, the sponsor should discuss protocol specifics with the Competent Authorities in those Member States in which the study will be conducted prior to submitting a clinical trial application (CTA).

A "sponsor" is defined as an individual, company, institution or organisation that takes responsibility for a clinical trial's initiation, management and/or financing.

According to Article 19 of the directive, the sponsor or sponsor's legal representative must be established in the European Community.

A multicentre clinical trial is conducted according to a single protocol but at more than one site, which may be in one or several Member States and/or in Member States and third countries.

An exemption from the directive's provisions is given for "noninterventional trials," where the medicinal product is prescribed in the usual manner in accordance with

Figure 18-1. Commencement of a Clinical Trial

Ethics Committee and Competent Authority procedures may be run in parallel, depending on the Member State and local regulations.

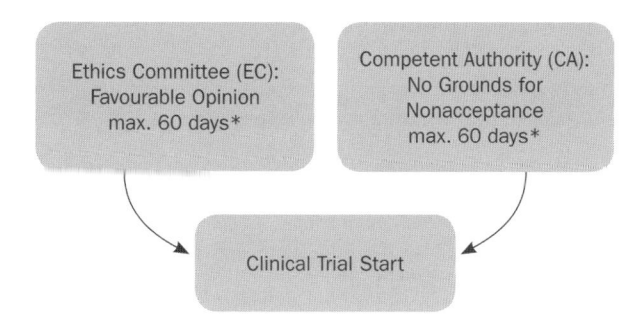

*Standard Products.

MA terms. Certain conditions are included within this definition:
- patient assignment to a particular therapeutic strategy is not decided in advance by a trial protocol but falls within current practice
- medicine prescription is clearly separated from the decision to include the patient in the study
- there is no application of additional diagnostic or monitoring procedures to patients
- there is use of epidemiological methods to analyse collected data

European Clinical Trial Database (EudraCT)

One of the major provisions of Directive 2001/20/EC (Article 11) is the establishment of EudraCT, a European database of all EU clinical trials from 1 May 2004 onwards. The database was set up to provide information on the status of all EU clinical trials and is interfaced with the EudraVigilance Clinical Trial Module for e-submission of adverse events reports (EVCTM).[24] These databases are supported by the European Medicines Agency (EMA) and are available on the Internet through EMA's homepage. Information within the EudraCT database is confidential and, in general, accessible only to Member States' Competent Authorities, EMA and the European Commission. However, a new piece of legislation (Regulation (EC) 1901/2006 as amended, the *Paediatric Regulation*) introduced 26 January 2007, establishes sweeping changes in the regulatory environment for paediatric medicines that are designed to better protect the health of children in the EU. EudraCT was previously not accessible to the public. However, Article 41 of the *Paediatric Regulation* provides the legal basis for publication of information on paediatric clinical trials entered in this database.[25] The regulation also stipulates that details of the results of paediatric clinical trials, including those terminated prematurely, henceforth have to be made public by EMA.

On 4 February 2009, the European Commission published a guidance document[26] on the information concerning paediatric clinical trials to be entered into EudraCT and on the information to be made public by EMA. The *List Of Fields Contained In The 'EudraCT' Clinical Trials Database To Be Made Public* has also been published. As soon as a particular trial is approved in the first EU country, designated public fields from the local application form would be accessible to the public. When additional countries approve the same trial, this information will be also made available. If the CTA is not approved in any country, the information will not be available via the EudraCT database except in the case of paediatric trials. For paediatric studies, even if the CTA is not approved, such information will be made public.[27]

As this chapter was being updated, EudraCT Version 8 was in use, with additional functionality and an updated CTA form. Among the new features:
- the ability to complete and upload notification of a third-country clinical trial as part of a Paediatric Investigation Plan
- redesigned user interface
- a validation program to check and ensure CTA forms have been completed prior to submission
- more extensive validation rules to ensure better quality CTAs
- improved XML comparison rules to assist users in direct comparisons of CTAs
- ability to switch EEA CTAs to third-country clinical trial information and vice versa to improve efficiencies for sponsors
- searchable help system accessible from each page in the application, including a glossary and FAQs
- where specified, help at the level of each field to assist with data entry
- XML conversion utility to convert v7 XMLs to v8 XMLs

A clinical trial sponsor must obtain a unique EudraCT number from the database before submitting a CTA to a Competent Authority or the Ethics Committee. This number identifies the trial protocol, whether the study is being conducted at a single site or at multiple sites in one or more Member States. All clinical trial documentation should include the EudraCT number.

The first step is obtaining an authenticated security code from the database. The security code is valid for only one EudraCT number and expires after 24 hours. Once a security code has been obtained, the second step is getting a EudraCT number. The EudraCT number can be requested by providing the standard information such as the name of the sponsor and the unique protocol code on the EudraCT request form. The assigned EudraCT number is communicated to the sponsor by email. The sponsor should include this information message in the CTA.[28,29]

The EudraCT number is formatted YYYYNNNNNN-CC, where:
- YYYY is the year in which the number is issued
- NNNNNN is a six-digit sequential number
- CC is a check digit

The EudraCT database is also utilised to generate the Ethics Committee and Competent Authority CTA forms (see later section).[30] The CTA form in both XML and PDF formats must be saved to a local computer; it cannot be saved to the EudraCT database. Only Competent Authority personnel are able to save XML application forms to the EudraCT system when they are submitted. EudraCT operates a help desk to support applicants who have questions related to EudraCT (eudract@ema.europa.eu).

Types of Information Available

The EU Clinical Trials Register website launched on 22 March 2011 enables users to search for information that has been included in the EudraCT database.

Users are able to:
- view descriptions of Phase II–IV adult clinical trials with investigator sites in EU Member States and the European Economic Area (EEA)
- view descriptions of paediatric clinical trials with investigator sites in the EU and any trials that are part of a paediatric investigation plan (PIP), including those where the investigator sites are outside the EU
- download up to 20 results (per request) in a text file (.txt)

The details in the clinical trial description include:
- design of the trial
- sponsor
- investigational medicine (trade name or active substance identification)
- therapeutic areas
- trial status (authorised, ongoing, complete)

What Is not Available

The EU Clinical Trials Register website does not:
- provide information on clinical trial results
- provide information on non-interventional clinical trials of medicines (observational studies on authorised medicines)
- provide access to the authorisation document from the national Competent Authority or the opinion document from the relevant Ethics Committee
- provide information on clinical trials for surgical procedures, medical devices or psychotherapeutic procedures
- manage the process for joining any clinical trial published on the website
- provide navigation and web content in languages other than English

Application for Ethics Committee Opinion

The application for an Ethics Committee opinion may be filed by the sponsor, the sponsor's legal representative in the European Community and/or the principal/coordinating investigator for a multicentre trial. A single Ethics Committee opinion is required for each Member State in a multicentre trial. The applicant must submit a valid application with all required documents completed. Full details about required application information are provided in the guideline covering Ethics Committee submissions.[31] Required information varies depending on the Member State where the application is being made. The requirements specific to each Member State are included in guideline attachments 1 and 2.

The Ethics Committee application form may be composed of two modules:
- Module 1 is compulsory and is common for all Member States. This is the application form described in the detailed guidance on the Competent Authority submission and contains information on the administration of the trial, the trial site(s) with principal investigator(s), the trial design and the IMP.[32] This module provides the Ethics Committee with an easy overview of the trial design and an evaluation of the required review expertise. This form, used for application to the Ethics Committee (and the Competent Authority), is generated by the EudraCT database, which can be accessed via EMA's website.
- Module 2 is optional and might consist of a national or local Ethics Committee application form.

Generally, the application for an Ethics Committee opinion contains the following core information:
- confirmation of receipt of the EudraCT number (copy of the email)
- cover letter
- application form composed of module 1 (and 2, if applicable)
- list of Competent Authorities to which the application has been submitted and details of decisions, if available
- informed consent form
- subject information leaflet
- subject recruitment arrangements
- clinical trial protocol with all current amendments

Chapter 18

- protocol summary in the national language
- Investigator's Brochure
- trial facilities
- curriculum vitae of the coordinating/principal investigator
- investigator and sponsor liability insurance or indemnity
- investigator and subject compensation information

An Ethics Committee is required to review a CTA within 60 days of receiving a valid application. The application is considered valid if all the required documents are complete. Some local Ethics Committees set specific dates of the month for the submission of applications; the sponsor/applicant should be familiar with local provisions. Within this period, the committee may send one request for supplementary information to the applicant, during which time the review clock will be stopped.

Longer review periods are permitted for certain specific product types:
- gene therapy and somatic cell therapy, including xenogenic cell therapy
- medicinal products containing genetically modified organisms

For these products, except xenogenic cell therapy, the Ethics Committee may extend the 60-day review period by 30 days. This 90-day review period may be extended by a further 90 days if consultation with an expert group or committee is required to meet national requirements. There is no review period time limit for xenogenic cell therapy.

The European Forum for Good Clinical Practice (EFGCP) is a nonprofit organisation supported by the European Commission. EFGCP promotes GCPs and encourages the practice of common, high-quality standards in all stages of biomedical research throughout Europe and globally. The 2010 update of the EFGCP report identifies relevant aspects of the ethical review process for each EU Member State, plus Norway and Switzerland.[33]

Application for Competent Authority Authorisation

As detailed in Directive 2001/20/EC, Article 9, the sponsor (if based within the EU), or the sponsor's legal representative in the European Community must submit a request for authorisation to conduct a clinical trial to the Competent Authority of the Member State(s) in which the clinical trial is planned.

If the sponsor is not the applicant, a letter from the sponsor authorising action on its behalf should be enclosed in the application.[34] According to Article 9(2) of the *Clinical Trials Directive*, the applicant must submit a valid application with all required documents completed.

Some documents, constituting the core information, are required by all Member States. This core information includes:

- cover letter, with the EudraCT number and sponsor protocol number
- confirmation of receipt of the EudraCT number (copy of the email)
- application form as an XML file (on a CDROM) and a PDF version (paper copy); this form is common to both the Competent Authority and Ethics Committee applications (Module 1), but with different tick boxes (it must be prepared via EMA's website) (as noted above, the CTA form in XML and PDF formats must be saved to a local computer)
- clinical trial protocol with all current amendments: protocol content and format should comply with the GCP guideline (CPMP/ICH/135/95)
- Investigator's Brochure (IB): content, format and procedures for updating the IB should comply with Directive 2005/28/EC, Article 8 and the GCP guideline (CPMP/ICH/135/95) (The approved Summary of Product Characteristics (SmPC) will replace the IB if the IMP is authorised in any Member State, and if it is used according to the terms of the MA.) The IB, as approved by the Competent Authority (or SmPC for approved products), serves as the reference safety information for the assessment of the likelihood of any adverse reaction that might occur during the clinical trial.[35]
- Investigational Medicinal Product Dossier (IMPD) (refer to section below)

Additional information must be provided according to individual Member States' specific requirements.

Sections 2.9 and 2.10 of Commission Communication 2010/C 82/01[36] provide information on all the national requirements and no longer refer to the table mentioned above. By implementing this new information, the European Commission aims to harmonise this procedure across the individual Member States. However, individual EU countries need to adopt these recommendations, which will result in more-consistent and harmonised requirements among the Member States.

The Competent Authority is required to review a valid application within 60 days of receiving it, although individual Member States may apply a shorter period as an internal target. The number of days Concerned Member States (CMS) can take to validate CTAs can vary, and these additional days should be included in the overall timeline for clinical study start-up in a CMS.

The Competent Authority may notify the sponsor before the end of this 60-day review period that it has grounds for acceptance, thus allowing the sponsor to commence the trial.

If the Competent Authority notifies the sponsor of grounds for nonacceptance, the sponsor may, only once, amend the application to take those grounds into account. If the amendments are considered inadequate, the request shall be rejected and the clinical trial may not commence.

For all IMPs except xenogenic cell therapy, the Competent Authority may extend the 60-day review period by 30 days. This 90-day review period may be extended by a further 90 days in the event of consultation with an expert group or committee in accordance with the concerned CMS' requirements. There is no review period time limit for xenogenic cell therapy.

One area in which expert advisory groups may be consulted by Member States is first-in-human (FIH) trials with higher-risk IMPs. Sponsors of FIH trials should take into account the *Guideline on strategies to identify and mitigate for first-in-human clinical trials with investigational medicinal products* (EMEA/CHMP/SWP/28367/07), which was adopted in July 2007.[37] This guideline resulted from experiences in an FIH clinical trial conducted in the UK in 2006, during which six healthy male volunteers experienced severe systemic adverse reactions soon after an intravenous injection of the monoclonal antibody TGN1412. All six volunteers developed a cytokine release syndrome with multi-organ failure and required intensive treatment and supportive measures.

Areas for consideration when determining risk factors for IMPs include mode of action, nature of the target and relevance of animal species and models.

Sponsors are encouraged to seek scientific advice from either EMA or the Competent Authorities in the CMS on whether the IMP in question falls within the higher-risk category. In general, sponsors should consider seeking EMA scientific advice or advice from the CMS throughout clinical development when there appears to be no answer, or lack of appropriate details in the EMA guidelines. Additionally, a sponsor that wishes to deviate from available guidance should obtain advice.[38]

The *Clinical Trials Directive* indicates that written authorisation may be required before commencing clinical trials for the following products:
- medicinal products that do not have an MA and are referred to in Regulation 2309/93/EEC, Annex, Part A[39]
- medicinal products containing an active ingredient that is a biological product of human or animal origin, or contains biological components of human or animal origin, or the manufacturing of which requires such

The sponsor should become familiar with local laws, regulations and guidance documents for written authorisations, as

Figure 18-2. Serious Adverse Event Reporting

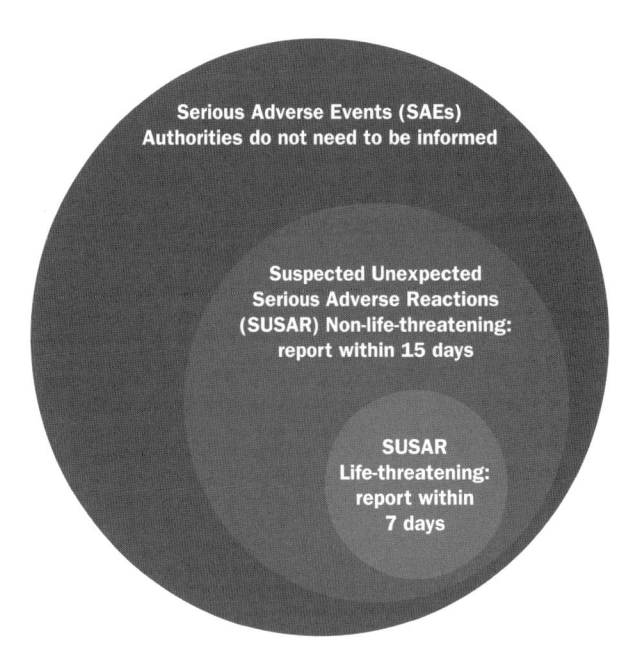

Serious Adverse Events (SAEs) Authorities do not need to be informed

Suspected Unexpected Serious Adverse Reactions (SUSAR) Non-life-threatening: report within 15 days

SUSAR Life-threatening: report within 7 days

an explicit approval letter is not always issued for these types of products. Tacit approval may sometimes be the standard approach, depending on the Competent Authority. Where approval to commence the trial is based on tacit approval, i.e., not receiving grounds for nonacceptance within the specified time limit, it is advisable to prepare a letter for the trial master file indicating all pertinent dates, including the effective date of authorisation.

In certain circumstances, written authorisation from concerned Competent Authorities is mandated before commencing clinical trials. This mandate applies to:
- gene therapy and somatic cell therapy, including xenogenic cell therapy
- medicinal products containing genetically modified organisms

Investigational Medicinal Product Dossier

The Investigational Medicinal Product Dossier (IMPD) must justify the quality of any IMP to be used in the clinical trial, including reference products and placebos. It also must provide data from nonclinical studies and previous clinical use of the IMP, or justify why information is not provided. An overall risk:benefit assessment must be included to justify the protocol provisions for which approval is sought.

A full IMPD submission is required if the IMP information has not been assessed previously as part of an MA in any Member State or as part of a CTA to the concerned Competent Authority.

The IMPD format should follow the Common Technical Document (CTD) headings.[40] However, it is recognised that it will be inappropriate or impossible to provide information under all CTD headings for all IMPs. The dossier requirements depend on many factors, including the nature of the IMP, the stage of development, the population to be treated, the disease's nature and severity and the nature and duration of exposure to the IMP. Where it is necessary to omit data for reasons that are not obvious, scientific justification should be provided.

The applicant may cross-reference the IB for the IMPD's nonclinical and clinical sections. When considering this strategy, the sponsor should take care to ensure the IB contains sufficient information in an appropriate format to enable Competent Authority review. In some instances, it may also be necessary to cross-reference the IMPD submitted by another sponsor held by a CMS. This requires a letter of authorisation from the sponsor that submitted the IMPD.

A simplified IMPD may be submitted if the IMP information has been assessed previously as part of an MAA in any EU Member State or as part of a CTA to the concerned Competent Authority.[41] More detailed guidance on the content of the simplified IMPD has been provided by the European Commission.[42]

For marketed products, where the product is to be used in accordance with the current version of the SmPC, the sponsor may submit the current SmPC version as the IMPD. In that case, the IMP is being used in the same form, for the same indications and with a dosing regimen covered by the SmPC. It also may be used to support studies with dosage regimens outside the SmPC's scope, if justification is provided.

IMPs for a clinical trial must be manufactured in compliance with GMP set out in Directive 2003/94/EC[43] and the guidance on applying those principles set out in Annex 13 (revised July 2003) to the *Community Guide to GMP*.[44] (More details are provided in Chapter 22 Quality Systems and Inspectorate Process—Medicinal Products.) Briefly, Annex 13 has been revised to incorporate provisions of the new *Clinical Trials Directive*, which requires IMP manufacturers to apply GMP both within the EU and for products to be imported for trials. Member States must allow each imported production batch of IMPs to be manufactured and tested in accordance with standards at least equivalent to EU GMPs. Moreover, a Qualified Person must certify the release of each batch of material for clinical trials, including imported material. Key points of the directive include the IMP manufacturing licence, which differs from a manufacturing licence for medicinal products for human use. IMP labelling is covered by Annex 13. According to *Clinical Trials Directive* Article 14, labelling must be in the official language of the Member State in which the trial will be conducted. The sponsor should review the CMS' laws, regulations and administrative provisions as additional provisions beyond Annex 13 may also be applied locally.

Notification of Amendments

Directive 2001/20/EC, Article 10(a)[45] allows amendments to the conduct of a clinical trial after its commencement. Amendments can be classified as nonsubstantial or substantial.

Nonsubstantial amendments to the CTA do not require Ethics Committee or Competent Authority notification. A nonsubstantial amendment does not meet the criteria of substantial amendments (detailed hereafter). Nevertheless, these amendments should be recorded, archived in the trial master file and made available on request for inspection at the trial site.[46] Examples of nonsubstantial amendments are the correction of typographical errors in a protocol; updates to the IB that do not result in a change in the trial's risk:benefit assessment; changes to the chief investigator's research team other than the appointment of key collaborators; and changes in funding arrangements.

Substantial amendments require notification of the Ethics Committee, the Competent Authority or both, depending on the type of change to be introduced. Substantial amendments to the documentation may arise from protocol changes or new information related to the scientific documents submitted with the CTAs to the Competent Authority or Ethics Committee.

In all cases, amendments are regarded as substantial when they are likely to have a significant impact on the:
- subjects' safety or physical or mental integrity
- trial's scientific value
- trial's conduct or management
- IMP's quality or safety

Commission Communication 2010/C82/01 Section 3.4[47] provides examples as guidance for sponsors on the case-by-case decision on whether amendments to protocols, IMPDs and IBs are substantial or nonsubstantial, as assessed by national Competent Authorities. For aspects considered by Ethics Committees as substantial amendments, sponsors should consult Article 8 of the *Clinical Trials Directive*.[48]

More information, including headings for trial aspects that might involve a substantial amendment, is provided in Attachment 5 of the guideline covering submissions to Competent Authorities[49] and in the guideline (CHMP/QWP/185401/2004/final) that covers chemistry and pharmaceutical quality data.[50] This latter guideline, adopted as final in October 2006, defines harmonised requirements for the quality documentation to be submitted throughout the EU for multicentre studies involving different Member States. One topic covered within this guideline is shelf-life extensions, previously an area of great contention.

Substantial amendments to the documentation supporting the trial's initial authorisation should be reported using the Substantial Amendment Form, which is common to both the Ethics Committee and Competent Authority.

This form is provided in Annex 2 of the guideline covering Competent Authority submissions.[51]

In addition, the application should contain:
- a cover letter stating the type of amendment and reasons, EudraCT number, protocol number and amendment number
- a summary of the proposed amendment
- a list of modified documents (identity, version, date)
- pages with previous and new wording, if applicable
- supporting information, including new versions of modified documents
- revised XML file and PDF version of the initial application form with amended data highlighted
- comments on any novel aspect of the amendment

For substantial amendments assessed only by the Competent Authority (e.g., changes to the quality section of the IMPD), the sponsor should also inform the Ethics Committee of the application. Similarly, the sponsor should inform the Competent Authority of any substantial amendment for which only the Ethics Committee is responsible (e.g., changes to the informed consent form). It is sufficient to provide this information by submitting the Notification of Amendment Form (Annex 2) indicating in Section A4 that it is "for information only."

The sponsor may implement a substantial amendment when the Ethics Committee opinion is favourable and the Competent Authority has raised no grounds for nonacceptance. Article 10(a) of the *Clinical Trials Directive* requires an Ethics Committee to give an opinion within 35 days. It does not set a time limit within which the Competent Authority must respond to such a notification. However, as guidance, the amendment may be implemented 35 days after the receipt of a valid notification of an amendment if the Competent Authority has not raised grounds for non-acceptance. Note that the response time may be extended if the Competent Authority consults an expert group or committee.

Urgent safety measures should be taken to protect subjects against any immediate hazard that may affect their safety. *Clinical Trials Directive* Article 10(b) requires a sponsor and investigator to inform the Competent Authority and Ethics Committee of those new events and the measures taken as soon as possible, and as a substantial amendment no more than 15 days later. Such safety measures as temporarily halting the trial may be taken without prior Competent Authority authorisation. However, the trial may not restart in that Member State until a substantial amendment has been submitted. According to Article 12 of the *Clinical Trials Directive*, a Competent Authority may suspend or prohibit a clinical trial where it has objective grounds for considering that the authorisation conditions are no longer met, or has information raising doubts about the trial's safety or scientific validity. Before the Member State reaches its decision, it shall, except where there is imminent risk, ask the sponsor and/or investigator for their opinions within one week, addressing the issues raised. When the Competent Authority suspends a trial, it must inform the other Competent Authorities, concerned Ethics Committees, EMA and the European Commission.

Notification of Adverse Events

According to *Clinical Trials Directive* Article 16, the investigator shall report all serious adverse events (SARs), except those that the protocol identifies as not requiring immediate reporting, to the sponsor immediately. This task also involves reporting of serious events related to NIMPs.

The sponsor should ensure that all relevant information about suspected unexpected serious adverse reactions (SUSARs) for IMPs and NIMPs is recorded and reported as soon as possible to the Competent Authorities and Ethics Committees and, in any case, no later than seven calendar days after the sponsor gains knowledge of such an occurrence. It also must communicate any relevant follow-up information within an additional eight calendar days (Article 17 of Directive 2001/20/EC). All other suspected SUSARs should be reported to the Competent Authority and Ethics Committee as soon as possible, but within a maximum of 15 days of first knowledge by the sponsor (see **Figure 18-2**).

The sponsor is also required to report all SUSARs associated with a comparator product in the concerned clinical trial, even if the comparator product has an MA. If a trial is blinded, the sponsor should break the blinding before reporting a SUSAR to the Competent Authority or Ethics Committee.

An adverse event's causality should be determined by the sponsor, based on the reference document, usually the IB, which is prospectively identified and included in the CTA. Additional guidance for reporting adverse events is provided in the guideline, *Detailed guidance on the collection, verification and presentation of adverse reaction reports arising from clinical trials on medicinal products for human use,* April 2006, Revision 2.[52]

Throughout the duration of the trial, the sponsor submits an Annual Safety Report[53] to the concerned Competent Authorities and Ethics Committees. This Annual Safety Report has three parts:

Part I: an analysis of the subjects' safety in the concerned clinical trial

Part II: a line listing of all suspected SARs (including all SUSARs) that occurred in the concerned clinical trial, including those from third countries

Part III: an aggregate summary tabulation of suspected SARs that occurred in the concerned trial

The Annual Safety Report timetable starts with the date of the first clinical trial authorisation by a Competent

Authority in any EU Member State. This date is designated as the cutoff (data lock point) for data to be included in the Annual Safety Report. The sponsor must submit annual reports within 60 days of the data lock point.

For FIH trials or other short-term studies (e.g., metabolism or pharmacokinetic), the safety report should be submitted to the Competent Authority and Ethics Committee within 90 days of the end of trial, together with the notification of the end of trial, according to Article 10(c) of Directive 2001/20/EC.

If the sponsor conducts several clinical trials with the same IMP, only one Annual Safety Report should be prepared covering the necessary information from all of those trials.

Declaring the End of a Clinical Trial

The end of the clinical trial must be defined in the protocol, and any change to this definition must be notified as a substantial amendment. Generally, it will be the date of the last visit of the last patient participating in the trial. Any exceptions (e.g., date of database lock) should be justified in the protocol and/or on the application form.

The sponsor must submit a Declaration of the End of the Trial Form to the Competent Authority and Ethics Committee when:
- the trial ends in the concerned Member State(s) territory
- the complete trial has ended in all participating centres in all countries within and outside the EU

This form is provided in Annex 3 of the guideline covering submissions to Competent Authorities.[54] In this form, the applicant, on the sponsor's behalf, confirms that a summary (or synopsis) of the clinical trial report will be submitted to the concerned Competent Authority and Ethics Committee as soon as available and within one year after the trial ends in all countries.

The sponsor must notify the concerned Competent Authority and Ethics Committee of the trial's end within 90 days. The Competent Authority is responsible for entering this information into the EudraCT database.

In the event the sponsor stops the study prematurely, before the declared end-of-study date stated in the protocol, it must notify the concerned Competent Authority and Ethics Committee as soon as possible, but within 15 days from when the trial is halted, clearly explaining the reasons.

Further Developments in EU Clinical Trial Procedures

The current system, the legal framework of which is the *Clinical Trial Directive*,[55] has resulted in a lack of harmonisation across the Member States. There is divergence in terms of content, format or language requirements, regulatory review timelines, distribution of duties between the Competent Authorities and the Ethics Committees, as well as evident differences across Member States in the scientific basis of the review. This lack of harmonisation results not only in additional workload and staffing requirements for the companies and the Competent Authorities but also in delayed trial starts and, hence, delayed availability of innovative medicines to patients.

The Impact on Clinical Research of European Legislation (ICREL) project, financed by the EU 7th Framework Programme, measured and analysed the direct and indirect impact of the *Clinical Trials Directive* and related legislation in the EU on all categories of clinical research and on the different stakeholders: commercial and noncommercial sponsors, Ethics Committees and Competent Authorities. The results of this survey were presented and discussed during a conference in Brussels on 2 December 2008, and the conclusions of the meeting are presented in the final report to the European Commission. The indisputably increased administrative burden imposed on the evaluation process and supervision of clinical trial authorisations was reflected by an increase in workforces and related costs, and was even acknowledged by the contributing EU health authorities.[56]

Several interactions between the European Commission, the Heads of Medicines Agencies and EU pharmaceutical associations such as the European Federation of Pharmaceutical Industries and Associations (EFPIA) during 2009–10 addressed the issues of increased complexity, increased administrative burden and conflicting assessments or queries from Member States for the same trials or data sets. The European Commission has also formally collected information from all stakeholders in order to address the challenge of increased administrative burden without real benefit or extra protection to patients.[57]

The outcome of these consultations and the feedback provided by different stakeholders was also published on the European Commission's Public Health website.[58]

These discussions again confirmed that the increased complexity of the clinical trial authorisation process due to local interpretations had not always had a real impact on patient safety. Hence, there was general agreement on the need for simplification and a consistent overall process across the Member States. It is recognised by all stakeholders that the EU clinical trial system needs a complete overhaul. This will be a lengthy process because amendments to the legal framework are required.

Based on these assessments and recommendations, the European Commission is planning to take additional steps. A Communication from the Commission dated March 2010[59] is the first step in this direction.

Activities of the Clinical Trials Facilitation Group

To coordinate the implementation of the *Clinical Trials Directive* across the Member States at an operational and national level, in 2004, the EU Heads of Medicines Agencies created the Clinical Trials Facilitation Group (CTFG).[60] The CTFG's mandate includes:

- sharing of scientific assessment of multi-national clinical trials
- harmonising processes, practices and assessment relating to clinical trials, mainly in the fields of CTAs, clinical trial amendments and safety procedures
- developing data sharing and participating in improvement of information systems
- developing communication with stakeholders and cooperating with other EU working groups

This is another major step toward harmonising clinical trials in Europe.

Voluntary Harmonisation Procedure

The organisation of coordinated assessment of multinational clinical trial authorisation through the Voluntary Harmonisation Procedure (VHP) has been a major objective of the CTFG work plans since 2008. This procedure has been set up within the current clinical trial legal framework.[61]

VHP is a two-step process. The first step is a consolidated scientific assessment of the core clinical trial authorisation package by the health authorities of the applicable Member States. On Day 30 of the procedure, a positive opinion is granted or a request for further information (RFI) is issued if the health authorities have questions relating to the submission. In the latter case, the sponsor has 10 days (by Day 40) to provide a response, with a positive opinion being received at Day 50 or Day 60, depending on whether there are outstanding points for discussion. The second step is a 10-day review of the national documents done on an individual Member State basis.

The main advantages of the VHP process:
- consolidated health authority feedback
- reduced internal resources as there is one round of health authority interaction
- faster clinical trial authorisation approval in some Member States
- parallel preparation of national documentation during initial VHP step
- fixed assessment timelines
- possibility to get uniform trial design in all Member States with no deviations

Potential challenges of the VHP:

- VHP experience currently based on very limited experience across industry
- only one or two counties would accept VHP applications in 2010
- sponsor needs to be able to respond to any RFI within 10 calendar days
- process is still voluntary and the risk exists of Member States' opting out during the process
- CTFG group is not centralised or directly supported by EMA or the European Commission

Based on limited experience with the VHP in 2009 and dialogue with industry, CTFG developed a new version of the VHP that was introduced in early 2010.[62] The procedure was modified to streamline assessment, enlarge the scope of the pilot phase and compress the timelines. In the new process, for each VHP, one of the participating national Competent Authorities takes the lead in the scientific consolidation of the letter. Procedures such as assessment reports and rapporteurships from the Decentralised Procedure are being discussed as possible inclusions in the VHP.

The main changes in version 2 compared to version 1 refer to:
- acceptability of all clinical trials with at least three Concerned Member States
- deletion of the "Pre-procedural step" or "Request for VHP" phase in the procedure
- inclusion of substantial amendments in the scope of the VHP

Through mid-November 2011, 97 applications had been submitted for the VHP: 86 standard VHPs and 11 accelerated VHPs for pandemic influenza vaccines. Of the 86 standard applications, 74 had been completed with a positive outcome. The mean time for a VHP decision was 50.4 days.[63]

VHP offers a short- to medium-term alternative to the purely national system of the management of clinical trials in the EU.

Summary

Implementation of the *Clinical Trials Directive* has been a challenge for all parties involved in conducting clinical trials in Europe, including Ethics Committees, Competent Authorities and pharmaceutical companies. All Member States had implemented the directive's key features and those of the supporting directives by end of 2008. The Heads of Medicines Agencies' Clinical Trial Facilitation Group, which coordinated the implementation of the *Clinical Trials Directive* across all Member States, continues to meet to discuss and resolve ongoing challenges. While the directive has created a general framework for the conduct of clinical trials across Europe, different interpretations of the legislation by Member States have created nuances in implementation. Thus, it is necessary for sponsors to familiarise themselves with local regulations, laws and administrative provisions. Developments in 2009–11 in terms of harmonising some national requirements to reduce the administrative burden and availability of the alternative VHP procedures provide further hope for simplifying the procedures. Nevertheless, the directive has improved the conduct of clinical trials and the harmonisation of core requirements and has provided greater assurance of patient safety and clinical data quality to support the MAA.

References

1. Commission Directive 2001/20/EC of the European Parliament and of the Council of 4 April 2001 on the approximation of the laws, regulations and administrative provisions of the Member States relating to the implementation of good clinical practice in the conduct of clinical trials on medicinal products for human use. EUR-Lex website. http://eur-lex.europa.eu/LexUriServ/LexUriServ.do?uri=CELEX:32001L0020:EN:HTML. Accessed 8 May 2012.
2. Commission Directive 2003/94/EC of 8 October 2003 laying down the principles and guidelines of good manufacturing practice in respect of medicinal products for human use and investigational medicinal products for human use. EC website. http://ec.europa.eu/health/files/eudralex/vol-1/dir_2003_94/dir_2003_94_en.pdf. Accessed 8 May 2012.
3. Commission Directive 2005/28/EC of 8 April 2005 laying down principles and detailed guidelines for good clinical practice as regards investigational medicinal products for human use, as well as the requirements for authorisation of the manufacturing or importation of such products. EC website. http://ec.europa.eu/health/files/eudralex/vol-1/dir_2005_28/dir_2005_28_en.pdf. Accessed 8 May 2012.
4. European Commission. *EudraLex, The Rules Governing Medicinal Products in the European Union*, Volume 10, "Clinical Trials Notice to Applicants" (July 2006—First Edition). EC website. http://ec.europa.eu/health/documents/eudralex/vol-10/. Accessed 8 May 2012.
5. *Guideline on the requirements to the chemical and pharmaceutical quality of documentation concerning investigational medicinal products in clinical trials*, CHMP/QWP/185401/2004/final (London, England: EMEA, 31 March 2006). EC website. http://ec.europa.eu/health/files/eudralex/vol-10/18540104en_en.pdf. Accessed 8 May 2012.
6. *Guideline on strategies to identify and mitigate risks for first-inhuman clinical trials with investigational medicinal products*, EMEA/CHMP/SWP/28367/07 (London, England: EMEA, 19 July 2007). EMA website. http://www.emea.europa.eu/docs/en_GB/document_library/Scientific_guideline/2009/09/WC500002988.pdf. Accessed 8 May 2012.
7. Op cit 1.
8. Op cit 4.
9. European Commission. *EudraLex, The Rules Governing Medicinal Products in the European Union, Detailed guidance on the application format and documentation to be submitted in an application for an Ethics Committee opinion on the clinical trial on medicinal products for human use*, Revision 1 (February 2006). EC website. http://ec.europa.eu/health/files/eudralex/vol-10/12_ec_guideline_20060216_en.pdf. Accessed 8 May 2012.
10. European Commission. *EudraLex, The Rules Governing Medicinal Products in the European Union, Detailed guidance for the request for authorisation of a clinical trial on a medicinal product for human use to the competent authorities, notification of substantial amendments and declaration of the end of the trial*, Revision 2 (October 2005). EC website. http://ec.europa.eu/health/files/pharmacos/docs/doc2005/10_05/ca_14-2005_en.pdf. Accessed 8 May 2012. In March 2010 European commission has published Communication 2010/C82/01 This document provides detailed guidance on the request to the competent authorities for authorisation of a clinical trial on a medicinal product for human use, the notification of substantial amendments and the declaration of the end of the trial (CT-1) and it replaces the document ENTR/F2/BL D(2003) dated October 2005 –[Ref 12]. EUR-Lex website. http://eur-lex.europa.eu/LexUriServ/LexUriServ.do?uri=OJ:C:2010:082:0001:0019:EN:PDF. Accessed 8 May 2012.
11. European Commission. *EudraLex, The Rules Governing Medicinal Products in the European Union, Notice to Applicants—Questions & Answers—Clinical Trial Documents* (January 2005). EC website. http://ec.europa.eu/health/files/pharmacos/docs/doc2006/04_2006/clinical_trial_qa_april_2006_en.pdf. Accessed 8 May 2012.
12. European Commission. *EudraLex, The Rules Governing Medicinal Products in the European Union, Detailed guidance on the European clinical trials database (EUDRACT Database) Amendment describing Deployment of EudraCT—Lot 1 for 1* (May 2004). EC website. http://ec.europa.eu/health/files/eudralex/vol-10/13_cp_and_guidance_eudract_april_04_en.pdf. Accessed 8 May 2012.
13. European Commission. *EudraLex, Communication 2011/C 172/01— Detailed guidance on the collection, verification and presentation of adverse reaction reports arising from clinical trials on medicinal products for human use ('CT3')* (June 2011). EC website. http://ec.europa.eu/health/files/eudralex/vol-10/2011_c172_01/2011_c172_01_en.pdf. Accessed 8 May 2012.
14. European Commission. *EudraLex, The Rules Governing Medicinal Products in the European Union, Detailed guidance on the European database of Suspected Unexpected Serious adverse reactions (Eudravigilance—Clinical Trial Module)* (April 2003). EC website. http://ec.europa.eu/health/files/pharmacos/docs/doc2003/april/cp-guidance-eudravigilance_160403_en.pdf. Accessed 8 May 2012.
15. Op cit 5.
16. European Commission. *EudraLex, The Rules Governing Medicinal Products in the European Union, Guide to Good Manufacturing Practice*, ANNEX 13, "Investigational Medicinal Products" (July 2010). EC website. http://ec.europa.eu/health/files/eudralex/vol-4/2009_06_annex13.pdf. Accessed 8 May 2012.
17. European Medicines Agency. *Community basic format for manufacturing authorisations & Community basic format for manufacturers/importers* (July 2011). EMA website. http://www.emea.europa.eu/docs/en_GB/document_library/Regulatory_and_procedural_guideline/2009/10/WC500004706.pdf. Accessed 8 May 2012.
18. European Commission. *EudraLex, The Rules Governing Medicinal Products in the European Union, Recommendation on the qualifications of inspectors* (July 2006). EC website. http://ec.europa.eu/health/files/eudralex/vol-10/v10_chap4_en.pdf. Accessed 8 May 2012.
19. European Commission. *EudraLex, The Rules Governing Medicinal Products in the European Union. Recommendations on inspection procedures for the verification of Good Clinical Practice Compliance* (July 2006). EC website. http://ec.europa.eu/health/files/eudralex/vol-10/v10_inspection-proc_en.pdf. Accessed 8 May 2012.
20. Op cit 10.
21. Ibid.
22. Ibid.
23. European Commission. *EudraLex, The Rules Governing Medicinal Products in the European Union. Guidance on Investigational Medicinal Products (IMPs) and Noninvestigational Medicinal Products (NIMPs)*. EC website. http://ec.europa.eu/health/files/eudralex/vol-10/imp_03-2011.pdf . Accessed 8 May 2012.
24. Op cit 14.
25. Regulation (EC) 1901/2006 of the European Parliament and of the Council of 12 December 2006, on medicinal products for paediatric use and amending Regulation (EEC) 1768/92, Directive 2001/20/EC, Directive 2001/83/EC and Regulation (EC) No 726/2004. EUR-Lex website. http://eur-lex.europa.eu/LexUriServ/site/en/consleg/2006/R/02006R1901-20070126-en.pdf. Accessed 8 May 2012.
26. Communication from the Commission 2009/C28/01 Guidance on the information concerning paediatric clinical trials to be entered into

the EU Database on Clinical Trials (EudraCT) and on the information to be made public by the European Medicines Agency (EMEA), in accordance with Article 41 of Regulation (EC) No 1901/2006. EC website. http://ec.europa.eu/health/files/eudralex/vol-10/2009_c28_01/2009_c28_01_en.pdf. Accessed 8 May 2012.
27. Information to be made public by the European Medicines Agency (EMEA), in accordance with Article 41 of Regulation (EC) No 1901/2006 (2009/C 28/01). 4 February 2009. EMA website. http://ec.europa.eu/health/files/eudralex/vol-10/2009_02_04_guideline_en.pdf. Accessed 8 May 2012.
28. Op cit 10.
29. Op cit 12.
30. Ibid.
31. Op cit 9.
32. Ibid.
33. *The Procedure for the Ethical Review of Protocols for Clinical Research Projects in the European Union*. EFGCP website. www.efgcp.be/EFGCPReports.asp?L1=5&L2=1. Accessed 8 May 2012.
34. Op cit 10.
35. Op cit 4.
36. Op cit 10.
37. Op cit 6.
38. EMEA/H/4260/01 Ref 4, *Guidance for Companies Requesting Scientific Advice (SA) or Protocol Assistance (PA)*, (London, England: EMEA, 19 January 2007).
39. Council Regulation (EEC) 2309/93 of 22 July 1993 laying down Community procedures for the authorisation and supervision of medicinal products for human and veterinary use and establishing a European Agency for the Evaluation of Medicinal Products. EC website. http://ec.europa.eu/health/files/eudralex/vol-1/reg_1993_2309/reg_1993_2309_en.pdf. Accessed 9 May 2012.
40. Op cit 10.
41. Ibid.
42. European Commission, EudraLex. *The Rules Governing Medicinal Products in the European Union*. Section 87, Table 1, *Volume 10, Clinical Trials Guidelines*. European Commission Public Health website. http://ec.europa.eu/health/documents/eudralex/vol-10/. Accessed 9 May 2012.
43. Op cit 2.
44. Op cit 16.
45. Op cit 1.
46. Op cit 10.
47. Ibid.
48. Op cit 1.
49. Op cit 10.
50. Op cit 5.
51. Op cit 10.
52. Op cit 13.
53. Ibid.
54. Ibid.
55. Op cit 1.
56. Impact on Clinical Research of European Legislation (ICREL), Final Report – Second Version. 15 June 2009. EFGCP website. www.efgcp.be/icrel/?L1=6&L2=0. Accessed 9 May 2012.
57. *Assessment of the Functioning of the "Clinical Trials Directive" 2001/20/EC, Public Consultation Paper*. Brussels, 9 October 2009 (ENTR/F/2/SF D(2009)). EC website. http://ec.europa.eu/health/files/clinicaltrials/docs/2009_10_09_public-consultation-paper.pdf. Accessed 9 May 2012.
58. Responses to the Public consultation paper "Assessment of the functioning of the 'Clinical Trials Directive' 2001/20/EC". EC website. http://ec.europa.eu/health/human-use/clinical-trials/developments/responses_2010-02_en.htm. Accessed 9 May 2012.
59. Op cit 10.
60. Introduction to CTFG website. HMA website. www.hma.eu/78.html. Accessed 9 May 2012.
61. Clinical Trials Facilitation Group's Guidance document for a Voluntary Harmonisation Procedure (VHP) for the assessment of multinational Clinical Trial Applications. HMA website. http://www.hma.eu/fileadmin/dateien/Human_Medicines/01-About_HMA/Working_Groups/CTFG/2010_03_VHP_Guidance_v2.pdf. Accessed 9 May 2012.
62. Ibid.
63. CTFG Activity Report: Period Covered 2010–2011. HMA website. www.hma.eu/fileadmin/dateien/Human_Medicines/01-About_HMA/Working_Groups/CTFG/2010-2011_CTFG_activity_report.pdf. Accessed 8 May 2012.

Recommended Reading

Good Manufacturing Practice, Medicinal Products for Human and Veterinary Use, Annex 13, http://ec.europa.eu/health/files/eudralex/vol-4/2009_06_annex13.pdf (Accessed 12 May 2012)

EU Clinical Trials Register Glossary https://www.clinicaltrialsregister.eu/doc/EU_Clinical_Trials_Register_Glossary.pdf#zoom=100,0,0 (Accessed 12 May 2012)

Chapter 19

Registration Procedures for Medicinal Products

Updated by Gautam Maitra

OBJECTIVES

❑ Understand the establishment and function of the European Medicines Agency

❑ Identify the role of the Committee for Medicinal Products for Human Use

❑ Understand the Centralised Procedure, the Decentralised Procedure and the Mutual Recognition Procedure, and the role of the European Commission and the Reference Member State

---

DIRECTIVES, REGULATIONS AND GUIDELINES COVERED IN THIS CHAPTER

❑ Regulation (EC) No 726/2004 of the European Parliament and of the Council of 31 March 2004 laying down Community procedures for the authorisation and supervision of medicinal products for human and veterinary use and establishing a European Medicines Agency

❑ Commission Regulation (EC) No 1084/2003 of 3 June 2003 concerning the examination of variations to the terms of a marketing authorisation for medicinal products for human use and veterinary medicinal products granted by a competent authority of a Member State

❑ Commission Regulation (EC) No 1085/2003 of 3 June 2003 concerning the examination of variations to the terms of a marketing authorisation for medicinal products for human use and veterinary medicinal products falling within the scope of Council Regulation (EEC) 2309/93

❑ Commission Regulation (EC) No 1662/95 of 7 July 1995 laying down certain detailed arrangements for implementing the Community Parliament and of the Council of decision-making procedures in respect of MAs for products for human or veterinary use

❑ Commission Regulation (EC) No 2141/96 of 7 November 1996 concerning the examination of an application for the transfer of a marketing authorisation for a medicinal product falling within the scope of Council Regulation (EEC) 2309/93

❑ Directive 2001/83/EC of the European Parliament and of the Council of 6 November 2001 on the Community code relating to medicinal products for human use, as amended. Amendments have been introduced by:

  o Directive 2002/98/EC of the European Parliament and of the Council of 27 January 2003 setting standards of quality and safety for the collection, testing, processing, storage and distribution of human blood and blood components and amending Directive 2001/83/EC

Chapter 19

- o Directive 2004/24/EC of the European Parliament and of the Council of 31 March 2004 amending, as regards traditional herbal medicinal products, Directive 2001/83/EC

- o Directive 2004/27/EC of the European Parliament and of the Council of 31 March 2004 amending Directive 2001/83/EC on the Community code relating to medicinal products for human use

- o Regulation (EC) No 1901/2006 of the European Parliament and the Council of 12 December 2006 on medicinal products for paediatric use and amending Regulation (EEC) No 1768/92, Directive 2001/20/EC, Directive 2001/83/EC and Regulation (EC) No 726/2004

- o Regulation (EC) No 1394/2007 of the European Parliament and the Council of 13 November 2007 on advanced therapy medicinal products and amending Directive 2001/83/EC and Regulation (EC) No 726/2004

- o Directive 2008/29/EC of the European Parliament and of the Council of 11 March 2008 amending Directive 2001/83/EC on the Community code relating to medicinal products for human use, as regards the implementing powers conferred on the Commission

- o The current annex is laid down in Commission Directive 2003/63/EC of 25 June 2003 amending Directive 2001/83/EC of the European Parliament and of the Council on the Community code relating to medicinal products for human use.

EU Overview

The EU currently consists of 27 Member States. Its key institutions are the European Parliament, the European Commission, the Court of Justice and the European Council of Ministers. The European Council of Ministers is the EU's supreme body; it meets to debate and decide such specific issues as new legislation (usually proposed by the European Commission). The process relies on expert working groups and the Committee of Permanent Representatives of the EU Ambassadors in Brussels (COREPER). A COREPER agreement results in the measure's adoption by the Council of Ministers. The Economic and Social Committee also may be consulted during the development of new Community legislation.

Members of the European Parliament and the Council of Ministers jointly adopt new EU legislative measures. The European Court of Justice, the EU's highest judicial body, enforces and interprets Community law. The following sections describe the European institutions that play a key role in medicinal product regulation.

The European Commission

The European Commission is the EU civil service; it consists of 44 directorate-generals (DGs) and services and 27 commissioners. The pharmaceutical sector currently is in DG Health and Consumers. Commissioners serve five-year terms and, although they are nominated by national governments, do not represent national interests. Each commissioner is responsible for a specific area.

The Commission's primary roles include proposing, drafting and administering European legislation and monitoring legislative compliance. Regarding the pharmaceutical sector, the Commission's activities include reviewing and consolidating legislation on regulatory activities.

The European Commission also chairs both the Pharmaceutical and Standing Committees. The former is the pharmaceutical sector's policymaking unit; the latter is the Commission's decision-making arm for refusing or granting marketing authorisation (MA).

Committee for Medicinal Products for Human Use

The Committee for Proprietary Medicinal Products (CPMP), established by Directive 75/319/EEC (now codified in Council Directive 2001/83/EC), played a major coordinating role in the European regulatory process. When the current legislation became effective, the committee was renamed the Committee for Medicinal Products for Human Use (CHMP). As the Community's expert scientific committee, CHMP is the arbitrator when Member States cannot reach agreement.

Prior to 1995, when Member States disagreed, CPMP decisions were not binding throughout the EU; therefore, CPMP was legally impotent. The 1995 implementation of the revised registration systems, however, gave CPMP new status in the European regulatory arena, converting its opinions into legally binding decisions by the European Commission through the Standing Committee. This also applies to CHMP opinions.

CHMP has 34 members and a chairman. Each of the 27 EU Member States nominates one member and one alternate after consultation with the European Medicines Agency's (EMA) management board. In addition, Iceland and Norway each nominate a member and an alternate. The committee has co-opted an additional five members with specific areas of complementary expertise. Members are appointed for renewable three-year terms. CHMP provides scientific opinions based on quality, safety and efficacy criteria. Such issues as cost and reimbursement do not fall within CHMP's remit and currently remain national responsibilities. CHMP members are expected to act independently and use their own scientific skill and judgment without being influenced by their own national authorities.

CHMP meetings take place monthly and last for four days. The meeting dates determine the timing of submissions and interactions with CHMP members regarding centralised applications.

European Medicines Agency

The European Agency for the Evaluation of Medicinal Products (EMEA) was established by Council Regulation (EEC) 2309/93, which became effective in February 1995. The current legislation changed the name to European Medicines Agency (EMA). EMA comprises an executive director, management board, six scientific committees—CHMP, the Committee for Veterinary Medicinal Products (CVMP), the Committee for Orphan Medicinal Products (COMP), the Committee on Herbal Medicinal Products (HMPC), the Paediatric Committee (PDCO) and the Committee for Advanced Therapies (CAT)—and a permanent secretariat.

EMA's administrative and technical framework supports all aspects of the current European registration system. It administers products filed via the Centralised Procedure and coordinates Member State resources for medicinal product assessment and supervision. EMA is also responsible for producing assessment reports, European product characteristic summaries and labelling and package leaflets, and publishing European public assessment reports. The agency also plays an increasing role in enforcement and inspection activities, including coordinating manufacturing and testing requirements with Good Laboratory Practices (GLPs), Good Clinical Practices (GCPs) and Good Manufacturing Practices (GMPs). However, EMA is not a law enforcement agency.

EMA is responsible for supervising medicinal products authorised for use within the Community and maintaining all relevant databases. The agency also coordinates national pharmacovigilance centres. In addition, EMA makes significant contributions to relations with non-European regulators and industry, and promotes cooperation between public control laboratories and the European Pharmacopoeia.

The Marketing Authorisation

Medicinal products can be marketed in Europe only when data supporting their quality, safety and efficacy have been evaluated and MAs granted. The initial MA is valid for five years, after which it can be renewed once. Upon renewal, the MA usually is valid for an unlimited period.

Three MA routes are available in Europe (for products authorised in more than one Member State). In the Mutual Recognition Procedure, after the data have been evaluated by the relevant Member State regulatory agency, the initial MA is recognised by other Member States. The Mutual Recognition Procedure, therefore, can result in multiple, identical MAs. The current legislation allows the Mutual Recognition Procedure only for products that already have an MA in at least one Member State.

In the Decentralised Procedure, the evaluation is also performed by one national regulatory agency, but the MA usually is granted in other Member States only after all Member States involved reach agreement.

In the Centralised Procedure, CHMP evaluates a given medical product's data at the European level. This process results in one Community or European MA that is valid throughout all EU Member States. EMA administers the Centralised Procedure; however, the actual licence takes the form of a decision issued by the European Commission.

Regardless of the registration procedure used, the MA is granted to a single party referred to as the Marketing Authorisation Holder (MAH). The MAH must be established within the European Economic Area (composed of the EU Member States plus Iceland, Norway and Liechtenstein). The MA entitles the MAH to market the product in the relevant territory and, in so doing, places many obligations on the MAH. These include maintaining the MA to reflect technical and scientific progress, releasing the product onto the market in accordance with EU law (through a Qualified Person (QP)) and providing pharmacovigilance and scientific information.

European Medicines Regulation—Historical Perspective

The primary purpose of medical product regulation in the EU is to safeguard public health. This purpose is complicated by the fact that the EU is not a single nation but consists of multiple, independent countries, each with its own legislative framework and cultural, medical and political practices. As part of the European Community, each Member State is subject to relevant EU law. Having said that, to facilitate EU processes, each Member State's rights and culture must be respected in drafting any Community-wide legislation. It becomes a balancing act between individual Member States' customs and practices and the creation of a single market with the attendant free movement of goods, the EU's fundamental philosophy.

EU principles apply to all commerce areas, including pharmaceuticals. In an attempt to harmonise this unique market, procedures governing medicinal product regulation and approval have been implemented. Prior to 1995, three MA systems were available in the European Community.

Chapter 19

The first of these was the national MA; as the name suggests, this authorisation was valid in only one Member State.

The national route offered the individual Member State regulatory agencies a significant amount of freedom in terms of how much influence could be exerted on a Marketing Authorisation Application (MAA). This route inevitably resulted in labelling that fully reflected each Member State's local preferences and medical culture and practices. The regulatory situation was referred to as horizontal disharmony, and effectively divided the European market. Because horizontal disharmony is contrary to EU principles, in 1998, national registration procedures were closed for new product registration when approval in more than one Member State was required.

Before 1995, two options for European procedures existed. The first of these was known as the Multistate Procedure and was based on the principle that one Member State's approval of an application should subsequently be recognised by other Member States. Unfortunately, however, this recognition was neither mandatory nor enforceable. A second system of registration also existed specifically for biotechnology and other high-technology products: this was the Concertation Procedure. It was designed to give innovative products rapid, easy access to the pan-European market.

The concertation and multistate systems existed alongside National Procedures, and the three routes were used to various degrees. For the multistate procedure, the lack of recognition between Member States and the fact that decisions were not binding meant that the entire process was cumbersome, resource-intensive and inherently flawed. In the Concertation Procedure, the principal concern related to the length of time it took the Member States to reach consensus on product approval. Instead of speeding market access as intended, the lengthy process inevitably delayed product approval.

European Registration Procedures Between 1995 and 2005

After reviewing the problems of the multistate and concertation registration processes, the European Commission put forward proposals for future MA systems. One aim was to more closely integrate all activities relating to drug registration, including such postlicensing activities as pharmacovigilance and product surveillance. These proposals were adopted, and on 1 January 1995, two new MA procedures became operational.

These procedures governed the granting and management of European MAs (the Centralised Procedure); the Member States' recognition of national MA decisions; and Community-level harmonisation of decisions taken by Member States concerning the MA granting, suspension, withdrawal or amendment (the Mutual Recognition Procedure). Both procedures were described in European legislation, a summary of which is presented in the EU Pharmaceutical Legislative Framework section of this chapter.

The Centralised Procedure effectively replaced the Concertation Procedure and is under EMA's control; the Mutual Recognition Procedure replaced the Multistate Procedure. Applications following the Mutual Recognition Procedure remained under the control of each Member State's Competent Authority. The legal aspects of mutual recognition were described in Council Directive 75/319/EEC on the approximation of provisions laid down by law, regulation or administrative action relating to medicinal products (as amended by Directive 93/39/EEC). This directive has now been replaced by Council Directive 2001/83/EC, as amended.

Current European Registration Procedures

A revised system entered into force in 2005. In addition to the three procedures mentioned above (Centralised Procedure, Mutual Recognition Procedure and National), the Decentralised Procedure was introduced (see **Table 19-1**). The other procedures were maintained but underwent important changes.

The Centralised Procedure, Mutual Recognition Procedure and Decentralised Procedure

The Centralised Procedure

The Centralised Procedure (see **Table 19-2**) is based on the practical experience gained with the old Concertation Procedure. Access to the procedure is limited to certain medicinal product categories. The system is mandatory for biotechnology products, orphan medicinal products and medicinal products containing a new active substance intended to treat acquired immune deficiency syndrome (AIDS), cancer, neurodegenerative disorders, diabetes, auto-immune diseases and other auto-immune dysfunctions and viral diseases. The procedure is optional for other products defined by Council Regulation (EC) No 726/2004.

Centralised Procedure applications are made to EMA. The applications are not reviewed in detail by all of CHMP (although the legislation does not preclude this). Instead, two members of the CHMP, a rapporteur and co-rapporteur, are appointed to scientifically evaluate the data on behalf of other CHMP members. In addition, the committee appoints peer reviewers from among the members of CHMP (including co-opted members) or CHMP alternate members.

The timetable for processing centralised applications, to which CHMP strictly adheres, is outlined in Council Regulation (EC) No 726/2004. CHMP is required to provide its opinion within 210 days from the start of the review.

The CHMP opinion is subsequently transmitted to the European Commission for conversion into a product licence. A centralised community authorisation is valid for

Table 19-1. Procedures to Obtain MA

1. Centralised Procedure: MA for all EU Member States issued by the European Commission
2. Decentralised Procedure: MA in those Member States that were part of the procedure, issued by the national authorities
3. Mutual Recognition Procedure: Concerned Member States (CMS) recognize the MA issued by the Reference Member State (RMS) and issues a national license based on this recognition
4. National Procedure: Only possible in the EU if the product has not been approved or submitted in another EU Member State

the entire EU market, although the MAH is not required by law to market the medicinal product in all Member States.

A product filed through the centralised route normally can have only one trademark. This restriction is considered the centralised route's major downside because it severely restricts co-licensing agreements. It is possible, however, for multiple, parallel applications with different trademarks to be submitted for the same product.

A Centralised Procedure approval results in the publication of a European Public Assessment Report (EPAR), a public summary written in collaboration with the applicant. The EPAR's main function is to improve the transparency of the regulatory process. The application's regulatory history is described in detail. EPAR documents are, therefore, considered helpful to industry in understanding the regulatory process, timing and issues.

Presubmission Activity

A sponsor planning to use the Centralised Procedure may seek Scientific Advice from CHMP well in advance of the actual application. This request must be made in writing to EMA (written guidance for applicants exists).[1] The process is well defined, although the advice itself is not binding on either the applicant or CHMP. Direct discussions with individual national regulatory agencies prior to application submission for formal Scientific Advice may be very helpful, if time allows.

Seven months before the MAA is submitted, EMA must be notified of the intention to submit using the "Presubmission meeting request form." This notification includes an overview of the product and its development programme (quality, nonclinical and clinical) together with a draft table of contents of the application listing the studies performed for each EU Common Technical Document (EU-CTD) heading and the draft product information. Another important document to be provided is a draft MAA Form (EU-CTD Module 1.2), which should be as complete and accurate as possible. Along with the presubmission meeting request form, applicants need to provide a number of documents related to the product and the application. These are listed on the second page of the form. Depending on the topics to be discussed, the applicant should provide additional information (e.g., draft justification for accelerated review).

EMA assigns a project team leader (PTL) to the application. The PTL, who is not a CHMP member, plays an administrative and liaison role; he or she is responsible for coordinating all aspects of the application.

The rapporteur and co-rapporteur are appointed following receipt of the applicant's letter of intent to submit. Once the application is accepted for review, the applicant is informed of the rapporteur and co-rapporteur's names, applicable fees and dossier requirements of all CHMP members.

A product's proposed trade name also will be checked for acceptability in the presubmission phase of a centralised application. Provided the medicinal product is eligible for evaluation under the Centralised Procedure, the applicant should inform EMA of the proposed invented name(s) for its medicinal product at the earliest 18 months prior to the planned MAA submission date. EMA reviews the proposed trade name in consultation with the national Competent Authorities to determine whether it would raise any identifiable public health concerns. EMA guidance is available on this subject. This approach is intended to minimise application delays as a result of difficulties with the proposed trade name.

Application Submission

A Centralised Procedure application is made to EMA. The applicant must be able to provide evidence of EEA establishment as well as documents showing the capacity to fulfil all MAH responsibilities required under Community legislation. The application must include a document identifying the QP for pharmacovigilance and one identifying the medical information service.

For applications that include a manufacturing site located outside the EEA where no mutual recognition agreement is in place, EMA coordinates any necessary pre-authorisation inspections.

The Centralised Procedure submission must be made in electronic format. Since 1 January 2010, electronic Common Technical Document (eCTD) is the only acceptable electronic format for all applications and all submission types.

Table 19-2. Centralised Procedure

Legal Basis	Directive 726/2004/EC
Aim	Obtain a single MA for all EU Member States issued by the European Commission
Mandatory for	• Biotechnology products • Medicinal products for the treatment of AIDS, neurogenerative disorders, cancer and diabetes • Orphan medicinal products • Advanced therapies
	Other products may utilise the Centralised Procedure if they represent a therapeutic, scientific or technological innovation
	Generic or biosimilar products may utilise the Centralised Procedure if the originator product was approved via the Centralised Procedure

Non-eCTD electronic applications are no longer a valid format for submissions. Only one copy (on CD-ROM or DVD) of the application in electronic format should be submitted to the agency. The electronic application should always be accompanied by a cover letter providing information as to its origin and nature, preferably in the "subject" line.

The applicant and EMA arrange the precise submission date, which normally is determined by the next CHMP meeting date. Submission dates are published on the EMA website. The dossier is submitted to EMA and the rapporteur and co-rapporteur. Submission should be made well in advance of the start of the procedure to allow time for validation of the dossier by the EMA secretariat. The date and time of delivery of the dossier to EMA should be arranged between the applicant and the agency. The submission deadlines and full procedural timetables are now published as a generic calendar on EMA's website. At the time of application validation, EMA will send an invoice to the applicant. Following a positive validation, EMA notifies the applicant, who is then responsible for submitting additional copies of the dossier to other CHMP members. At this stage, the applicant is also notified of the review timetable.

Scientific Review of the Application
Scientific evaluation of the dossier is carried out by the assessment team (the rapporteur and co-rapporteur) in the respective Member States. Scientific evaluation must occur within 80 days, after which the preliminary assessment report is circulated to other CHMP members for their comments. The applicant receives a consolidated list of questions from CHMP at Day 120. The clock then stops, usually for a period of up to three months with a maximum period of six months, during which the applicant responds to any issues raised. The response review starts on Day 121. On Day 180, CHMP discusses whether to adopt a list of "outstanding issues" and/or require an oral explanation of these issues by the applicant. If an oral explanation is needed, the clock is stopped until the applicant prepares the oral explanation, which is presented in person on Day 181 (the 60-days procedure). The final CHMP opinion is reached within the legal time frame of 210 days, although in most cases it occurs sooner.

Within five days after the adoption of the CHMP opinion, the applicant must provide EMA and all CHMP members the relevant product information translations for comments. Copies of product information (the Summary of Product Characteristics (SmPC), label and package leaflet) are required in all official EU languages, as well as Norwegian and Icelandic.

If there is a negative or conditional opinion, the applicant has 15 days in which to communicate an intention to appeal. The proviso for an oral explanation during an appeal is not stated in Regulation (EC) No 726/2004. If there is an appeal, the applicant is required to appeal to the same committee that returned the disputed decision (although in most cases, CHMP will elect to appoint a new rapporteur to coordinate the appeal procedure).

The applicant has the option to withdraw the application prior to the adoption of a negative opinion.

As discussed previously, the CHMP opinion represents the committee's scientific consensus and is not, in itself, legally binding. The opinion and relevant annexes are subsequently transmitted to the European Commission for conversion into a Community MA. The applicant must inform EMA of any intention to appeal within 15 days following receipt of the opinion. If there is no appeal, the opinion is forwarded to the European Commission in order to begin the decision-making process.

The Decision-making Process
The European Commission's decision-making process renders the CHMP opinion legally binding and converts it into a Community MA. Following receipt of the opinion, the Commission has 15 days in which to prepare a draft application decision, taking Community law into account. The entire decision-making process takes 67 days.

The European Commission is not required to automatically accept the CHMP opinion (although in practice, it generally does). No real appeal mechanism exists for the applicant should the Commission disagree with the CHMP opinion. The only avenue of appeal in this instance is that offered by the treaty establishing the European Community. It has been proposed that the decision-making process be transferred to EMA, although doing so would necessitate an amendment to the treaty.

A positive European Commission decision results in the publication of an EPAR, which summarises the product's approval process. A positive Commission decision also represents product approval and results in publication of the product in the Community medicinal product register. The product is then allocated a reference number, which must appear on all packaging. An extract of the Commission decision must appear in the *Official Journal of the European Union*, and the MA decision is made available in all EU languages.

Status of a Community Authorisation
A centralised authorisation is valid for the entire Community market, with one exception: under Article 4 of Directive 2001/83/EC, as amended, Member States may prohibit the sale, supply or use of contraceptive or abortifacient medicinal products. A Community MAH currently is not required by law to market the medicinal product in all Member States, although such an authorisation confers the same rights and obligations in each Member State as one issued by that state.

Licence Maintenance
A Community MA is valid for five years and may be renewed once. The renewal application must be submitted to EMA six months before expiration. Variations to Community MAs also are made through EMA and are described in Commission Regulation (EC) No 1085/2003.

Transfer of a centralised MA to a new party is governed by Commission Regulation (EC) No 2141/96, which requires that the transfer request and all relevant documentation be submitted for EMA evaluation within 30 days.

A Community MA may be amended, suspended or withdrawn. This procedure is described in Regulation (EC) No 726/2004.

The Mutual Recognition Procedure

In contrast to the Centralised Procedure, mutual recognition applications remain under the control of each Member State's Competent Authority. As the name suggests, the procedure is based on first obtaining an MA in one Member State (the Reference Member State or RMS) and then requesting one or more others to recognise that authorisation within 90 days (see **Table 19-3**). Under the current legislation, the procedure can be used only for products that already have an MA in at least one Member State.

The legal basis for mutual recognition was Article 7a of Directive 93/39/EEC (amending Directive 65/65/EEC), which in turn has been codified into Council Directive 2001/83/EC, as amended. Starting on 1 January 1998, automatic mutual recognition has existed between Member States unless a state "considers that there are grounds for supposing that the authorisation of the medicinal product concerned may present a risk to public health."[2] In practice, other Member States often have objected to applications based on the risk to public health, even for minor issues.

Mutual recognition is an essential principle of Community law, by virtue of which one Member State recognises the equivalence of legislative, statutory and administrative provisions of others.

The key to the Mutual Recognition Procedure, which results in the granting of a national licence, is identical dossiers. Note that the national MA granted via the Mutual Recognition Procedure is not to be confused with the national authorisation route that was terminated in 1998.

Table 19-3. Mutual Recognition Procedure

Legal Basis	Article 7a of Directive 93/39/EEC
Aim	To obtain an MA in a number of Member States by the recognition of the results of the review by one Member State (Reference Member State)
Applicant options	• Select the Member States where it wants to obtain an MA • Select the Reference Member State
Mandatory for	Any product for which there is an MA in one or more Member States
Exclusions	Any product mandated to utilise the Centralised Procedure
Coordination Group for Mutual Recognition and Decentralised Procedure for Human Medicinal Products (CMDh)	• Started as informal facilitation group in 1995; formal status defined in Directive 2004/27/EC • Members are representatives of national Competent Authorities • Main task is to discuss scientific issues, consider points of disagreement, encourage dialogue between Concerned Member States, facilitate procedure in cooperation with EMA • Works under the supervision of the Heads of Medicines Agencies

Chapter 19

Table 19-4. Decentralised Procedure

Legal basis	Directive 2004/27/EC
Aim	To obtain national MAs in selected Member States
Advantage	Maximum review time of 120 days
Applicant options	• Select the Member States where it wants to obtain MA • Select the Reference member State
Coordination Group for Mutual Recognition and Decentralised Procedure for Human Medicinal Products (DMD(h))	• Started as informal facilitation group in 1995; formal status defined in Directive 2004/27/EC • Members are representatives of national Competent Authorities • Main task is to discuss scientific issues, consider points of disagreement, encourage dialogue between Concerned Member States, facilitate procedure in cooperation with EMA • Works under the supervision of the Heads of Medicines Agencies

Registration through the national route could also result in multiple MAs, but they would not necessarily be identical.

When a Member State cannot accept an RMS decision, points of disagreement are referred to the Co-ordination Group for Mutual Recognition and Decentralised Procedures—Human (CMDh) for the 60-days procedure, whether or not the application has been withdrawn from the dissenting Member State(s). If CMDh cannot reach consensus, the matter is referred to CHMP for arbitration. Therefore, CHMP is the ultimate arbitrator in the Mutual Recognition Procedure, and this process leads to a decision binding on all Member States.

For mutual recognition applications, it is recommended, whenever possible, that the same product trade name be used in all relevant Member States. This recommendation is to prevent companies from dividing the European market, which is contrary to single market/free movement of goods principles. Unlike the Centralised Procedure, the Mutual Recognition Procedure does not legally require a single trade name; therefore, the potential exists for some flexibility across Member States.

Role of the RMS
The spirit of the Mutual Recognition Procedure is based on identical dossiers and a significant degree of transparency among all EU Member States. In contrast, under the old multistate process, changes to pharmaceutical legislation resulting from Directive 93/39/EEC created many links between Member States' national MAs for the same medicinal product. The mutual recognition system is based on the applicant's obligation to provide a copy of any Member State MA and a list of those states in which the application is also under consideration to all other Member States (Concerned Member States (CMS)).

All Member States are not required to be involved in each Mutual Recognition Procedure, but the use of the Mutual Recognition Procedure is mandatory when an MA is required in more than one Member State.

The RMS plays a pivotal role in the mutual recognition process. In contrast to the Centralised Procedure, in which EMA selects the rapporteur and co-rapporteur, the applicant can choose the RMS from those Member States that already have granted national licences.

The primary role of the RMS is to produce the assessment report subsequently used by the CMS as the basis for mutual recognition. The RMS's role in the Mutual Recognition Procedure includes:
- helping the applicant prepare and plan subsequent mutual recognition activities
- discussing the need to update the file and expert report prior to mutual recognition
- holding discussions, meetings, teleconferences and other communications with the applicant and CMS in the final 30 days of the 90-day discussion and clarification period on potential serious public health issues, SmPC wording and other issues
- participating in discussions within CMDh, and participating in any CHMP arbitration on remaining serious public health issues

Mutual Recognition Application Submission and Scientific Review
The mutual recognition application must contain the following components:
- dossier with a completed European application form and all necessary fees
- applicant letter affirming that the file is identical to that submitted to the RMS (or describing any additions or deletions); it also must affirm that the proposed SmPC and dossier are identical in all CMS
- the SmPC in the applicant's national language
- copies of the label and package insert in the applicant's national language

The requirements for the number of dossier copies can be found in *The Rules Governing Medicinal Products in the European Union, Notice to Applicants.*[3]

Once all CMS have received the application, the RMS circulates the assessment report. As soon as it is received, the RMS signals the start of the 90-day clarification and dialogue period, during which the mutual recognition of the first authorisation occurs.

In stark contrast to the Centralised Procedure, the applicant's available time to respond to issues raised during the Mutual Recognition Procedure is short—a maximum of 10 days for the first set of questions at Day 50. This limited timeframe often causes applicants difficulty in generating an acceptable response, which can lead to the need to discuss the points of disagreement in the CMDh.

Acceptance of Recognition
If all issues are resolved at the end of the clarification and dialogue phase, national authorisations can be issued by all CMS. The applicant sends high-quality translations of the SmPC, package leaflet and labelling to the RMS and CMS.

Refusal of Recognition Referral to Co-ordination Group
A CMS can only refuse an application to recognise an MA granted by another Member State if it has reason to believe that authorising the medicinal product in question may present a serious risk to public health. This risk is not currently defined in the legal texts, although such concerns can relate only to the product's quality, safety or efficacy. The European Commission has, therefore, published *Commission Communication: Guideline on the definition of a potential serious risk to public health in the context of Article 29(1) and (2) of Directive 2001/83/EC.*[4] If no consensus can be reached by Day 90, the matter is referred to CMDh.

Arbitration
Arbitration is the procedure used to settle disputes arising from the mutual recognition of MAs as defined in Articles 32 and 33 of Directive 2001/83/EC, as amended. When serious public health concerns remain after discussion in the CMDh, the matter is referred to CHMP in accordance with Article 29 of Directive 2001/83/EC, as amended. The product goes to arbitration on those issues only.

In contrast to the appeal process under the Centralised Procedure, arbitration during the Mutual Recognition Procedure involves an appeal to a new committee (CHMP). In the first stage, CHMP appoints an arbitration rapporteur and holds a discussion of the points at issue. This step is followed by notifying the applicant of the issues to be addressed. The clock stops until the applicant's response is received. The rapporteur then assesses the written response and prepares a report for CHMP, which considers the report and makes its recommendations. Arbitration has three possible outcomes: positive, conditional or negative.

Following a negative or conditional decision, the applicant has 15 days to lodge a notice of appeal, followed by a 60-day period in which the written grounds for appeal must be lodged with CHMP. As with the Centralised Procedure, the appeal is made to the same body that gave the negative or conditional decision. CHMP will reexamine its opinion within 60 days of receipt of the applicant's written grounds for appeal.

The Decision-making Process
As is the case in the Centralised Procedure, the European Commission converts the CHMP opinion into a decision that is legally binding across all Member States (including those in which either the product is not marketed or an application for mutual recognition has not been made). In the event a Commission decision changes the basis of the original RMS authorisation, the MA must be amended by national variation.

Licence Maintenance
Despite the fact that the Mutual Recognition Procedure results in granting a national licence in the CMS, any MA variation application granted through mutual recognition must be submitted simultaneously in all CMS, in accordance with Council Regulation (EC) No 1084/2003. This requirement aims to preserve the licence's identical nature across all relevant Member States. Disagreements about variation applications for mutually recognised licences may result in arbitration. Arbitration is also used if a Member State considers it necessary to suspend or withdraw an authorisation. The transfer of a licence approved through mutual recognition is currently subject to local laws and regulations and thus varies across Member States.

The Decentralised Procedure
This procedure is to be used when there is no MA in any EU Member State. As in the Mutual Recognition Procedure, decentralised applications remain under the control of each Member State's Competent Authority. In case of disagreement, remaining (serious) public health issues are referred to the CHMP for arbitration. The Decentralised Procedure was introduced by Directive 2004/27/EC.

The Decentralised Procedure, like the Mutual Recognition Procedure, results in the granting of a national licence (see **Table 19-4**). Applicants can withdraw applications submitted via the Decentralised Procedure from one or more Member States at any point during the procedure's 210-day window. However, withdrawing an application in the dissenting Member State(s) during the 90-day assessment step II period will not prevent points of disagreement, if based on potential serious public health risk, from being referred to CMDh.

If CMDh cannot reach consensus, the matter is referred to CHMP for arbitration. CHMP is the ultimate arbitrator in the Decentralised Procedure, issuing a decision binding on all Member States.

It is recommended that products registered via the Decentralised Procedure have the same trade name in all CMS; however, more than one trade name may be permissible.

The requirements for the number of dossier copies can be found in *The Rules Governing Medicinal Products in the European Union, Notice to Applicants.*[5]

RMS Role
The applicant can select the RMS and list CMS. Not all Member States are required to be involved in each Decentralised Procedure. The RMS plays a pivotal role in the process.

The primary role of the RMS is to produce an assessment report, which is subsequently reviewed by the CMS. In addition, the RMS is responsible for:
- discussing the application (e.g., its suitability and likely clinical indications) with the applicant before filing
- helping the applicant prepare and plan the subsequent steps in the procedure
- holding discussions, meetings, teleconferences and other communications with the applicant and CMS, as appropriate
- participating in discussions within CMDh and any CHMP arbitration on any remaining serious public health issues

Positive Outcome of the Discussions Between the Member States
If all issues are resolved between Days 135 and 210, national authorisations can be issued in all CMS. The applicant sends high-quality translations of the SmPC, labelling and patient information leaflets to the CMS and the RMS.

Referral to Co-ordination Group
If agreement cannot be reached, the matter is referred to CMDh for resolution.

Arbitration
The arbitration procedure used to settle disputes arising from the Decentralised Procedure is defined in Articles 32 and 33 of Directive 2001/83/EC, as amended. If serious public health concerns remain on Day 270, after CMDh discussions, the matter is referred to CHMP in accordance with Article 29 of Directive 2001/83/EC, as amended. The product then is subject to arbitration on only those issues. For further arbitration procedure details, see the arbitration section under the Mutual Recognition Procedure.

The Decision-making Process
The European Commission converts the CHMP opinion into a decision that is legally binding across all Member States (even those in which the product is not marketed or no mutual recognition application has been made).

Licence Maintenance
The same rules for the Mutual Recognition Procedure apply.

Comparison of the Centralised Procedure, Mutual Recognition Procedure and Decentralised Procedure

In the EU, the chosen registration route for a given product is a critical commercial and strategic consideration. Once a product's registration route is selected, it cannot be switched at any stage following initial registration.

If a product is eligible for registration using either the centralised or decentralised route, the principal strategic considerations about the European filing route are the product's market access and commercialisation plans.

The Centralised Procedure offers pan-European access and identical products in all Member States. The timetable for this procedure is highly predictable. One drawback is the requirement for a single trade name, which may hinder co-marketing arrangements. However, this challenge can be overcome to a limited extent by submitting dual applications for the same product under differing trade names.

Regarding speed to market, the Centralised Procedure seems more predictable, with a 210-day maximum assessment time (excluding clock stops). The Decentralised Procedure can potentially be faster if there is no need for referral to CMDh and arbitration, but the procedure can be considerably longer if referrals and arbitration are necessary.

The Decentralised Procedure also allows the applicant to select the regulatory audience (i.e., RMS and CMSs) whereas, in the Centralised Procedure, the rapporteur and co-rapporteur are imposed on the applicant.

Another consideration is the appeal mechanism. In the Centralised Procedure, the appeal is made to the same body (CHMP) that issued the disputed decision in the first place, while in the Decentralised Procedure, CHMP only becomes involved if there is arbitration.

Both procedures impose the same fundamental licence maintenance requirements on MAHs. However, maintaining one pan-European licence is potentially simpler than maintaining multiple, individual licences. Note also that the submission of variations for national licences obtained through mutual recognition may trigger arbitration at the Community level. This is not the case for centralised licence variations.

A comparison of the three procedures is further summarized in **Table 19-5**.

EU Pharmaceutical Legislative Framework

The Council of the European Community can propose legal measures using several legislative instruments, including regulations, directives, decisions, recommendations, opinions and communications. The principal legislative instruments affecting medicinal products are regulations, directives and

Registration Procedures for Medicinal Products

Table 19-5. A Comparison of the Centralised, Decentralised and Mutual Recognition Procedures

Process/Issue	Centralised	Decentralised	Mutual Recognition
Product type	• Compulsory for biotech products, orphan medicinal products and new active substances in certain therapeutic areas • Optional for other new active substances, significant therapeutic, scientific or technical innovations or if the granting of a centralised MA is of interest at Community level to patients' health	• Compulsory for established medicinal products when the product is not authorised in any EU Member State (unless it falls within the scope of the Centralised Procedure) • Optional for new active substances in therapeutic areas where the Centralised Procedure is not mandatory	Compulsory for established medicinal products for which there is already an MA in at least one EU Member State
Marketing authorisation	Results in a Community/European licence	Results in identical national MAs, each valid in only one Member State	Results in identical national MAs, each valid in only one Member State
Review team	Consists of experts within the agencies of the rapporteur and co-rapporteur, both of whom are selected by EMA, not the applicant	Primary review carried out by experts within the RMS Competent Authority; the applicant can actively select the RMS	Primary review carried out by RMS Competent Authority experts; in some instances, the applicant can actively select the RMS
Application	Made to EMA	Submitted directly to the relevant Competent Authority	Submitted directly to the relevant Competent Authority
Trade name	Products registered via the Centralised Procedure can only have one trade name	It is recommended that products registered via the Decentralised Procedure have the same trade name in all CMS; however, more than one trade name may be permissible	It is recommended that products registered via the Mutual Recognition Procedure have the same trade name in all CMS; however, more than one trade name may be permissible
Documentation	Core documentation (SmPC, label and patient information leaflet) are required to be translated into all official languages of the EU (plus Norwegian and Icelandic)	Documentation is required in only the RMS/CMS relevant language(s)	Documentation is required in only the RMS/CMS relevant language(s)
Time period for applicant response to questions raised during dossier evaluation	Applicant's responses expected within three months; may be extended up to six months	In principle, three months; can be extended if justified	Initially 10 days (between Days 50 and 60); all issues should be resolved in 30 days (by Day 90)
Oral interaction with regulatory authorities	Potential for an oral explanation with CHMP at Day 181 prior to adoption of CHMP opinion	Ad hoc interactions with RMS possible during dossier review; further interactions between Days 100 and 105, and around Day 180	Interactions between Days 50 and 90
Appeal	Appeal to CHMP possible, but it is the same body that issued the disputed decision in the first place	Appeal possible via arbitration to a new body (CHMP)	Appeal possible via arbitration to a new body (CHMP)
Selective withdrawal of application in given Member States	Not possible	Possible, but application withdrawal in the dissenting Member State(s) during 90-day assessment step II will not prevent the points of disagreement, if based on potential serious risk to public health, from being referred to CMDh	Possible, but points of disagreement will be referred to CMDh for the 60-day procedure, whether the application has been withdrawn from the dissenting Member State(s) or not
Refusal to grant MA	Prohibits placing the product on the market in any EU Member State	Application withdrawal in Member State(s) refusing to grant authorisation possible; allows product to be marketed in remaining CMS, if CMDh does not consider there is a risk to public health and final procedure outcome is positive	Application withdrawal in Member State(s) refusing to grant authorisation possible; allows product to be marketed in remaining CMS, if CMDh does not consider there is a risk to public health and final procedure outcome is positive
MA granted by	European Commission	Each Member State's Competent Authority	Each Member State's Competent Authority
MA maintenance	Via EMA	Via the relevant Competent Authority	Via the relevant Competent Authority
Second applicant (generic) protection period under new legislation	8 + 2 + 1 rule (8 years until submission, normally 10 years until approval, 11 years until approval if, during the first 8, the MAH obtains an authorisation for one or more new significant therapeutic indications)	8 + 2 + 1 rule	8 + 2 + 1 rule

Regulatory Affairs Professionals Society

communications. Additional legislative mechanisms include Commission Communications; under some circumstances, they may have the force of law.

A regulation is binding on those to whom it is addressed without exception or amendment. It does not need to be translated into national law to take effect, and national law cannot override a regulation. A directive is binding on those to whom it is addressed with respect to achieving expected results under an agreed-upon timetable by translation into each Member State's existing national legislation. Directives are the minimum legal standard imposed by the Community.

The main directives and regulations establishing the current system are summarised below.

The Centralised Procedure

The Centralised Procedure is governed by three regulations that relate to human (and veterinary) medicines.

- Regulation (EC) No 726/2004 of the European Parliament and of the Council of 31 March 2004 laying down Community procedures for the authorization and supervision of medicinal products for human and veterinary use and establishing a European Medicines Agency

  The principal objectives of this regulation were to:
    o establish a centralised community procedure for the scientific evaluation of medicinal products
    o establish EMA
    o ensure close cooperation between the agency and scientists working within Member States
    o reinforce the scientific role and independence of CHMP and CVMP
    o establish a permanent technical and administrative secretariat to CHMP and CVMP
    o establish a pharmacovigilance system for monitoring adverse drug reactions
    o establish a system for coordinating Member States' supervisors' responsibilities with respect to GMP, GCP and GLP
    o establish a system for monitoring the environmental risk of products produced by conventional means and through the use of genetically modified organisms
- Commission Regulation (EC) No 540/95 of 10 March 1995 details the arrangements for reporting suspected unexpected adverse reactions
- Commission Regulation (EC) No 542/95 of 10 March 1995 relates to the examination of variations to MA terms falling within the scope of Council Regulation (EEC) 2309/93 (the regulation preceding 726/2004)

The Mutual Recognition Procedure

The Mutual Recognition Procedure is governed by two Council directives and one Commission regulation. Directives 93/39/EEC and 93/40/EEC amended previous Council texts and implemented the procedure for human and veterinary products, respectively. Principal objectives of Council Directive 93/39/EEC (amending Directives 65/65/EEC, 75/318/EEC and 75/319/EEC, which now have been codified into Directive 2001/83/EC, as amended) were as follows:

- establish a system for CHMP arbitration in cases in which applications in more than one Member State are not mutually recognised
- require Member States to systematically prepare assessment reports for exchange
- replace the previous requirement for import testing of all products from third countries (i.e., those from outside the EEC) with a waiver system that exempts the need for testing when appropriate arrangements have been made with the exporting country with respect to GMP
- establish a pharmacovigilance system to coordinate adverse-event monitoring in the Member States

Council Regulation (EC) No 1084/2003 of 3 June 2003 concerns the examination of variations to MA terms granted by a Competent Authority of a Member State.

Council Directive 93/41/EEC repealed Directive 87/22/EEC and converted any ongoing concertation applications to the Centralised Procedure. Commission Communication dated 19 April 1994 (94/C82/04) was issued to give insight into the fate of procedures pending as of 1 January 1995 and the operation of the two procedures. Commission Communication (C98/2016) was issued in July 1998 to more fully clarify the procedural and legal aspects of both new regulatory systems.

Council Regulation (EC) No 297/95 (amended by Commission Regulation (EC) No 249/2009) set fees payable by companies to EMA for its services under the Centralised, Decentralised and Mutual Recognition Procedures. Commission Regulation (EC) 1662/95 describes the decision-making process through which EMA's scientific opinion is converted into an enforceable decision in all Member States.

The Decentralised Procedure

The Decentralised Procedure was introduced by Directive 2004/27/EC.

- This procedure is to be used when there is no MA in any EU Member State.
- In the Decentralised Procedure, applicants can withdraw applications from one or more Member States at any point during the procedure's 210-day window. However, withdrawing an application in the dissenting Member(s) State(s) during the 90-day Assessment step II period will not prevent points of disagreement, if based on potential serious public health risk, from being referred to the CMDh.

Conclusion

The fundamental objectives of European pharmaceutical legislation governing registration procedures are to ensure a high level of public health protection and to support a single, pan-European market. Current registration procedures consist of mutually exclusive routes: a pan-European review administered by EMA, resulting in a Community licence; local review by national agencies and granting of a national licence; and for products already authorised in one or more EU Member States, recognition of the MA by other Member States.

The current procedures have gone a long way toward achieving the objective of protecting public health in the context of the single market; however, it is fair to say that the Centralised Procedure has contributed significantly more to this success than the Mutual Recognition Procedure. Issues relating to mutual recognition include the continuing reluctance of Member States to recognise the review of other Member States, resulting in overuse of the arbitration procedure. Experience with the Decentralised Procedure is still limited.

References

1. European Medicines Agency Guidance for Companies requesting Scientific Advice and Protocol Assistance (May 2010). EMA website. www.ema.europa.eu/docs/en_GB/document_library/Regulatory_and_procedural_guideline/2009/10/WC500004089.pdf. Accessed 13 June 2012.
2. Council Directive 65/65/EEC of 26 January 1965 on the approximation of provisions laid down by law, regulation or administrative action relating to medicinal products. EUR-Lex website. http://eur-lex.europa.eu/LexUriServ/LexUriServ.do?uri=CELEX:31965L0065:EN:HTML. Accessed 13 June 2012.
3. *The Rules Governing Medicinal Products in the European Union, Notice to Applicants: Volume 2A*, "Chapter 7—General Information," (Updated version—July 2008). EC website. http://ec.europa.eu/health/files/eudralex/vol-2/a/vol2a_chap7_rev_2008_07_en.pdf. Accessed 13 June 2012.
4. Commission Communication 2006/C 133/05: *Guideline on the definition of a potential serious risk to public health in the context of Article 29(1) and (2) of Directive 2001/83/EC*, March 2006. EC website. http://ec.europa.eu/health/files/eudralex/vol-1/com_2006_133/com_2006_133_en.pdf. Accessed 13 June 2012.
5. Op cit 3.

Chapter 20

Quality Systems and Inspectorate Process—Medicinal Products

By Robert Schiff, PhD, CQA, RAC, FRAPS and Thomas Padula

OBJECTIVES

- Understand the legal requirements of EU pharmaceutical legislation

- Understand the roles of the European Medicines Agency (EMA) and European Directorate for the Quality of Medicines & Healthcare (EDQM) relative to regulations for active pharmaceutical ingredients (APIs)

- Understand the *Guide to Good Manufacturing Practice* for finished products and active pharmaceutical ingredients, and the Mutual Recognition Agreements—Annexes for Good Manufacturing Practice

- Learn about inspection systems, the Pharmaceutical Inspection Convention (PIC) and the Pharmaceutical Inspectorate

- Understand how to apply International Conference on Harmonisation of Technical Requirements for Registration of Pharmaceuticals for Human Use (ICH)/ International Cooperation on Harmonisation of Technical Requirements for Registration of Veterinary Medicinal Products (VICH) processes

- Learn about the International Organization for Standardization (ISO) as a developer of international standards

REGULATIONS AND GUIDELINES COVERED IN THIS CHAPTER

- Directive 2001/82/EC of the European Parliament and of the Council of 6 November 2001 on the Community code relating to veterinary medicinal products, as amended

- Directive 2001/83/EC of the European Parliament and of the Council of 6 November 2001 on the Community code relating to medicinal products for human use, as amended

- Directive 2004/27/EC of the European Parliament and of the Council of 31 March 2004 amending Directive 2001/83/EC on the Community code relating to medicinal products for human use

- Directive 2004/28/EC of the European Parliament and of the Council of 31 March 2004 amending Directive 2001/82/EC on the Community code relating to veterinary medicinal products

- Regulation (EC) No 726/2004 of the European Parliament and of the Council of 31 March 2004 laying down Community procedures for the authorisation and supervision of medicinal products for human and veterinary use and establishing a European Medicines Agency, as amended

Chapter 20

❑ Directive 2011/62/EU of the European Parliament and of the Council of 8 June 2011 amending Directive 2001/83/EC

❑ Consolidated Versions of the Treaty on European Union and the Treaty on the Functioning of the European Union (March 2010)

❑ Charter of Fundamental Rights of the European Union (March 2010)

Introduction

In March 2010, the Consolidated Versions of the Treaty on European Union and the Treaty on the Functioning of the European Union and the Charter of Fundamental Rights of the European Union were published.[1] Article 168 discusses public health, and in Section 4(c) indicates that the EU will adopt "measures setting high standards of quality and safety for medicinal products and devices for medical use."

Quality guidelines are found in *The Rules Governing Medicinal Products in the European Union*.[2] Volume 4 concerns Good Manufacturing Practices (GMP), the Common Technical Document (CTD) and Marketing Authorisations (MA), which in the EU, are a basic part of quality.

The quality or GMP guidance reflects the International Conference on Harmonisation (ICH) guidances discussed later in this chapter. From 1965 through 1992, directives were promulgated that formed the foundation for EU GMPs, paralleling regulations proposed in the US. Directive 75/319/EEC defined the role of the Quality Person (QP) in the process of batch release.

In November 2001, two separate directives (2001/82/EC[3] and 2001/83/EC[4]) separated veterinary medicine from human medicine. In March 2004, Directive 2004/27/EC[5] provided methods for the Community-wide authorisation of medicinal products and established the European Medicines Agency (EMA). The directive further discussed biological medicinal products that can be matched to reference biological products, or biosimilars.

Regulation (EC) No 726/2004 of the European Parliament and of the Council of 31 March 2004[6] required Member States to ensure there was no conflict of interest on or in Competent Authorities, made the Centralised Procedure mandatory for new chemical entities, and stressed the importance of pharmacovigilance and post-market vigilance.

Active Pharmaceutical Ingredients

Although GMP involves all manufacturing, there are distinct regulations and rules for active pharmaceutical ingredients (APIs), or active substances. This is best demonstrated in ICH Q7 *Good Manufacturing Practice Guide for Active Pharmaceutical Ingredients*. Q7 was published as Annex 18 in *Notice to Applicants Volume 4* in 2000. Directive 2004/28/EC[7] required manufacturers to use APIs that were manufactured according to GMPs. In 2005, *Notice to Applicants Volume 4* was divided into Part I and Part II. Part I is devoted GMP for medicinal products and Part II to APIs.

In 2010, *Notice to Applicants Volume 4* defined manufacturing as including receipt of materials, "production, packaging, repackaging, labelling, relabeling, quality control, release, storage and distribution of active substances and the related controls."

When a manufacturer demonstrates GMP compliance to the Competent Authority, following an application for manufacturing authorisation, a GMP certificate is issued. The certificate usually is issued within 90 days after the inspection and entered into a database by EMA. As is the case in the US, inspectors can sample the drugs and APIs.

In 1996, the European Directorate for the Quality of Medicine (EDQM) was created. The following year, EMA contracted with EDQM for a sampling and testing programme for centrally authorised products. In 2003, Directive 2001/83/EC was revised and required the "mandatory character of European Pharmacopoeia Monographs when requesting MA for medicinal products for human and veterinary use." EDQM signed Memoranda of Understanding (MOUs) with the Pharmaceutical Inspection Convention Scheme (PIC/S) to exchange information and collaborate on inspections for APIs. Today, EDQM can issue a Certificate of European Pharmacopeia (CEP, Certificate of Suitability).

Notice to Applicants, Volume 4, Part II contains information detailing APIs in manufacturing:

- Quality Management: the principles, internal audits and product quality review
- Personnel: qualifications and consultants
- Buildings and Facilities: provides, among other things, information on design and construction, utilities or containment
- Process Equipment: covers design, construction, equipment, maintenance and cleaning, calibration and computerised systems
- Documentation and Records: specifications for the documentation system, equipment cleaning and use record, record of raw materials, intermediates, API labelling and packaging, master production instruction and batch production records (The sections on "generation and control of documentation" and "retention of documents" have been revised, in light of the increasing use of electronic documents within the GMP environment. These changes had a deadline of 30 June 2011 for coming into force.)
- Materials Management: general controls, purchasing, receipt and quarantine, sampling and testing of incoming production materials, storage and reevaluation

- Production and In-Process Controls: information on production operations, in-process controls, batch blending and contamination control
- Packaging and Identification Labelling of APIs and Intermediates: packaging materials, packaging and labelling operations and labelling controls
- Storage and Distribution: warehousing and distribution
- Laboratory Controls: Certificates of Analysis, testing of intermediates and APIs or expiry and retest dating
- Validation: documentation, qualification, process validation programme and cleaning validation
- Change Control: provides information on the procedures to follow
- Rejection and Reuse of Materials: reprocessing, reworking, returns and recovery of materials and solvents
- Complaints and Recalls: procedures and recordkeeping
- Contract Manufacturers (including laboratories): compliance with GMPs
- Agents, Brokers, Traders, Distributors, Repackers and Relabellers: quality management, stability and transfer of information
- Specific Guidance for APIs Manufactured by Cell Culture/Fermentation: cell bank maintenance and recordkeeping, cell culture, fermentation, harvesting, isolation and purification
- APIs for Use in Clinical Trials: guidance on quality, equipment and facilities, validation and laboratory controls

Process validation protocols now require a minimum of three consecutive production-scale batches. If not done for the MAA, the three production-scale batches must be prepared for postauthorisation and verified by the GMP inspector. The protocol must be in the MAA.

Pending Directives

On 1 July 2011, Directive 2011/62/EU[8] of the European Parliament and of the Council of 8 June 2011 amending Directive 2001/83/EC on the Community code relating to medicinal products for human use, as regards the prevention of the entry into the legal supply chain of falsified medicinal products was published. This Directive amends Directive 2001/83/EC on the Community code relating to medicinal products for human use.

Directive 2011/62/EU places an obligation on Member States to take appropriate measures to ensure that manufacturers of active substances on their territory comply with Good Manufacturing Practice (GMP) for active substances.

It also places an obligation on the Commission to adopt, by means of delegated acts, the principles and guidelines for GMP for active substances.

This concept paper is being released for public consultation with a view to preparing the delegated act. The adoption of the delegated act is planned for 2013.

Directive 2011/62/EU introduces EU-wide rules for the importation of active substances. According to Directive 2001/83/EC, Article 46b(2), active substances shall only be imported if, *inter alia*, the active substances are accompanied by a written confirmation from the Competent Authority of the exporting third country that confirms that the GMP standards and control of the plant that manufactured the exported product are equivalent to those in the EU.

The requirement of a written confirmation is waived for third countries listed by the Commission in accordance with Directive 2001/83/EC, Article 111b.

Article 111b(2) of Directive 2001/83/EC requires the Commission to adopt an implementing measure to apply these requirements.

Pharmaceutical Inspection Convention

The first body involved in mutual recognition of inspections was the Pharmaceutical Inspection Convention (PIC), begun in the 1970s as part of the European Free Trade Association (EFTA). The original PIC provisions were made obsolete by the European Economic Area legislation. Today, the legally based PIC multilateral agreement is inoperative. The PIC Scheme (PIC/S), an informal arrangement, the main focus of which is to build confidence and cooperation among its members (e.g., for training purposes), is now in place. Currently, 37 countries participate in PIC/S.

Unless replaced by a Mutual Recognition Agreement (MRA) treaty (including agreements with EU candidate countries), reference to PIC may still be acceptable in terms of mutual recognition of inspections. In those cases, reference must be made to each Member State's national legislation. Even in instances where mutual recognition of inspection results based on PIC membership is acceptable and GMP certificates are exchanged between authorities, product retesting on importation into the EU is required.

The PIC/S has revised its charter to include language promoting global harmonisation of Good Distribution Practices (GDPs) and confidentiality in data sharing. The revision, adopted 7 November 2011, took effect 1 January 2012.

Pharmaceutical Inspectorate

The Pharmaceutical Inspectorate prepares and maintains a quality manual. The format and design of the manual are decided by the individual inspectorate, but must cover the items in the European directives. At a minimum, the manual must reference the quality system procedures in the directives. References to any individual standards, such as ISO and EN, also are required.

Administrative Structure

The requirements of the administrative structure of the GMP Pharmaceutical Inspectorate include:

- "The structure, membership and operation of the GMP Pharmaceutical Inspectorate should be such as to enable it to meet the objectives of quality management and to ensure that impartiality is safeguarded.
- The personnel of the inspection service, including sub-contracted personnel and experts, should be free from any commercial, financial and other pressures which might affect their judgment and freedom to act. The Pharmaceutical Inspectorate should ensure that persons or organisations external to the inspection organisation cannot influence the result of inspections. The system for obtaining fees should not improperly influence the inspection procedure. Rules for deontology, ethics, conflict of interest and improper influence should be clearly defined.
- The relationship of the Pharmaceutical Inspectorate to other agencies and to other organisations within and outside the Inspectorate should be described where relevant.
- The Pharmaceutical Inspectorate should implement a policy which distinguishes between the process of inspection and that of issuing a manufacturing license.
- Where relevant, the Pharmaceutical Inspectorate should implement a policy which distinguishes between the process of inspection and that of providing an advisory service. This service should be of benefit to all of industry and not solely to individual organisations."[9]

Senior Management Responsibility

It is important that the senior levels of management of the Pharmaceutical Inspectorate be committed to the principles found in the PIC/S *Recommendation on Quality System Requirements for Pharmaceutical Inspectorates*. In the EU, the inspectorate is required to make certain that the quality policy is documented and implemented. Specifically, the PIC/S guidance states:

"The responsibility, authority and reporting structure of the Pharmaceutical Inspectorate should be clearly defined and documented. The structure should be defined in organisation charts and should be supported by written job descriptions for each member of staff.

There should be nominated an appropriately qualified and experienced person or persons with responsibility to carry out the quality assurance function, including implementing and maintaining the quality system. This person should have direct access to senior management.

The Pharmaceutical Inspectorate should have sufficient resources at all levels to enable it to meet its objectives effectively and efficiently. Senior management should ensure that all personnel are competent and qualified to carry out their assigned duties and that they receive appropriate training. Such training should be documented and its effectiveness assessed periodically.

There should be a system for periodic management review of the quality system. Such reviews should be documented and records should be retained for a defined period."

Inspection Procedures

PIC/S sets forth the following recommendations regarding inspections:

"The Pharmaceutical Inspectorate should conduct repeated inspections of manufacturers and/or wholesale distributors and should issue inspection reports in accordance with National or European Community requirements as appropriate.

The Pharmaceutical Inspectorate should have the documented procedures and resources to enable inspection of manufacturing and wholesale distribution operations to be carried out in accordance with the official guidelines and National legislation and in accordance with a formal inspection plan. All instructions, standards or written procedures, worksheets, check lists and reference data relevant to the work of the Pharmaceutical Inspectorate should be maintained up-to-date and be readily available to staff.

When more than one inspector is involved in an inspection, a lead inspector should be appointed to coordinate inspection activities. The inspection report should normally be prepared by the lead inspector and should be agreed by all participating inspectors.

Inspection report format should be in compliance with the PIC/S procedure or European model.

The report should follow the procedure above. The inspection report should be sent to the responsible person of the inspected company (preferably the authorised person or qualified person). The lead inspector and all concerned inspectors should participate in assessing the eventual reply or replies to determine the appropriateness of corrective actions and the GMP status of the company.

Observations and/or data obtained in the course of inspections should be recorded in a timely manner to prevent loss of relevant information."

As an example of the detail of an inspection, the PIC and PIC/S require validation of the wait time between completion of a process and cleaning of the equipment. "The period and when appropriate, conditions of storage of equipment before cleaning and the time between cleaning and equipment reuse, should form part of the validation of cleaning procedures. This is to provide confidence that routine cleaning and storage of equipment does not allow microbial proliferation."

Completed inspections should be reviewed to ensure that the requirements are met.

Joint Audit Programme

The EU Joint Audit Programme (JAP) validates and verifies that the appropriate provisions of European directives have been implemented into national laws. This covers authorisation, licensing, GMP compliance certification, administration of inspectors, complaints, recalls and internal quality assurance. All EEA GMP inspectorates for human and animal drugs fall under this umbrella. This is part of the quality system for the Compilation of Community Procedures on Inspections and Exchange of Information.[10]

The JAP harmonises inspection standards and the approach to the understanding and interpretation of the EU requirements for GMP and its mutual recognition of inspections. In addition, all EU Member States have agreed to the inspection and compliance procedures. This joint approach also satisfies the MRAs between the EU and some countries outside the community.

Compliance Group

The JAP is managed by the Compliance Group, whose function is to arrange the visits, review the conclusions, and actively follow up the corrective and preventive actions and attempt to resolve any major GMP concerns or problems. The EMA Inspection Services Group responsible for GMP nominates Compliance Group members.

The Compliance Group also ensures the JAP's documentation is "relevant and up to date."[11] It reports at GMP Inspection Services Group meetings, providing annual reports to the Heads of Medicines Agencies (HMA), monitors training courses for auditors and exchanges information with other regulatory bodies.

GMP Inspection Services Group

The JAP also interfaces with the GMP Inspection Services Group, whose primary tasks include:
- endorsing audit plans
- adopting final audit report and actions taken
- distributing audit reports to the group of HMA when deemed necessary
- releasing annual reports to HMA
- nominating members of the Compliance Group
- adopting/implementing documentation prepared by the Compliance Group
- discussing/resolving possible major problems received by the Compliance Group
- following up if corrective actions are not implemented within the agreed timeframe

EMA and Heads of Medicines Agencies

Other responsibilities are shared by HMA and EMA.

EMA provides coordinating support for the JAP, including:

- providing the secretariat for the Compliance Group
- maintaining JAP documents
- maintaining and updating the list of auditors and audit training records
- maintaining and updating the list of EEA audits conducted
- keeping an inventory of audit reports and follow-up measures
- sending out audit notifications
- drafting an annual report to HMA

HMA reviews the annual reports and provides resources for the JAP.

General Principles for Joint Audits

Every Member State's GMP Inspectorate should be audited every five or six years. Having 42 GMP Inspectorates in the EEA (excluding regional or federal ones) means seven to eight audits need to be conducted each year. Additional audits may be considered depending on previous evaluations. Any additional audits should be based on specific requests from the European Commission or Member States.

The Compliance Group sets the annual audit schedule, using the information from EMA. The schedule includes the EEA GMP Inspectorates to be audited, auditors, dates, rapporteurs, particular scope and rationale. For planning purposes, the Compliance Group liaises with PIC/S and MRA partners. The GMP Inspection Services Group reviews and agrees to the schedule. EMA officially announces the audits and asks Member States to nominate auditors for specific audits.

Auditor Training

Auditors are nominated by the Competent Authorities. Auditors must be well-trained, qualified and have relevant experience before joining the JAP.

Audits of the GMP Inspectorates and any relating units or institutions should cover:
- quality system, including implementation of Compilation of Community Procedures
- implementation of legislation related to the GMP supervision system
- authorisation/licensing system for manufacturer
- GMP guidance
- GMP compliance certification
- inspection administration (e.g., frequencies, resources, procedures)
- inspector qualifications and training
- inspections (planning, performance, reporting and follow-up system)
- complaints
- rapid alerts system
- obligations as an EU Member State

- internal audits
- observed inspections (if carried out)[12]

Final Report

It is the audit team leader's responsibility to write the final audit report. This report should include corrective and preventive actions and any comments by the auditee, and should be sent to the Compliance Group secretariat at EMA within eight weeks.

The Compliance Group monitors the audit information and, for any observations that are deemed critical, follows up with the GMP Inspection Services Group and HMA. If there are serious deficiencies, HMA may refer the results to the Commission for punitive action.

EMA prepares an annual report on all joint audits. All agency heads eventually review the report and concur when final.

The International Conference on Harmonisation (ICH)

ICH originally was founded to bring together regulatory organisations from the US, EU and Japan.[13] ICH is managed by a steering committee and supported by coordinators and a secretariat. Members of industry who have expertise in pharmaceuticals, science and technology, and product registration are contributors.

ICH's objectives focus on harmonising product approval requirements in the three regions. Previously, registration procedures such as clinical studies were duplicated because individual countries wanted efficacy and safety demonstrated in their own populations. The theory behind the testing was that indigenous peoples have metabolic differences and, therefore, should participate in the clinical programmes.

ICH has made recommendations to reduce the burden of duplication with the use of technical guidelines covering many areas of pharmaceutical product development, animal testing, quality assurance and quality control, etc.

Originally, the harmonisation was intended to reduce the economic burden of duplication and registration. However, guidance documents produced by ICH were very well accepted across the globe. In particular, the ICH quality series for GMPs and the ICH E6 guideline for GCPs have become standards around the world.

When ICH was established, most new drugs and medicines were developed in the US, Western Europe and Japan. The original intent was to limit ICH's activities to those three regions but, over the years, the organisation's guidance has been widely adopted.

ICH currently has six active participants and three observers, as well as the International Federation of Pharmaceutical Manufacturers & Associations (IFPMA). The six organisations represent the EU, US and Japan. The active participants include the EU, European Federation of Pharmaceutical Industries and Associations (EFPIA), Japan's Ministry of Health Labour & Welfare (MHLW), Japan Pharmaceutical Manufacturers Association (JPMA), US FDA and Pharmaceutical Research and Manufacturers of America (PhRMA). The three observers are nonvoting members and include the World Health Organization (WHO), European Free Trade Association (EFTA) and Health Canada.

The ICH guidances probably have done more to unify GMPs than any other individual activity. The guidances are divided into four groups: efficacy (E), quality (Q), safety (S) and multidisciplinary (M). The quality guidances range from Q1 to Q11 with secondary designations, such as A through E, and revision numbers.

The guidances move through a series of steps from draft to final status. The first were developed in 1995 and the last was released in June 2011. Although the guidances are to be applied uniformly throughout participating ICH regions, differences exist.

International Organization for Standardization (ISO)

Although ICH was primarily created for the drug industry, ISO serves the device industry. ISO is a developer of international standards. ISO brings together the public and private sectors and is a nongovernmental organisation (NGO). Several ISO participants are government entities while others are private, with strong associations with industry. Thus, ISO offers a mechanism to create a consensus between government and private industry.

ISO standards play a major role in minimising differences between cultures. ISO's 9000 and 14000 series of international standards emphasise the importance of audits as management tools. The standards discuss how to verify the implementation of an organisation's quality and/or environmental policy. Audits are a major part of conformity assessments, which deal with certification and registration as well as surveillance and supply-chain evaluation. These activities are independent of culture and ensure uniformity.

The ISO 9000 series is related to audits. Standards are written for auditors and others with an interest in compliance and quality. Standards also are used by companies and organisations that are beginning to utilise quality systems. Standards can be employed to audit training, certification processes and accreditation.

ISO 9000 is very adaptable for organisations of different sizes and activities. Auditing principles can be found in Clause 4. Clause 5 discusses how to manage audit programmes with assigning responsibility, coordinating activities and utilising team resources. Clause 6 goes into more detail on actually performing audits of quality management systems and again discusses the audit teams. Clause 7 suggests required auditor competence levels and describes the auditor evaluation process. The latter is particularly important because, too often, auditors "lack the training, experience and certification to perform quality evaluations."[14]

Harmonisation of Pharmacopeias

Under GMP, not only is there harmonisation under ICH guidance, there is also harmonisation of portions of the EU, US and Japanese Pharmacopoeias. An example is sterility testing of sterile drugs produced by aseptic fill. Product must be tested after filling into the final container; terminally sterilised product may undergo parametric release, which may not require final product testing.

Sterility testing is one of the oldest tests and first discussed in the British Pharmacopeia in 1932.[15] The *US Pharmacopeia* (USP <71>), *European Pharmacopoeia* (EP 2,6,1) and the *Japanese Pharmacopoeia* (JP 4.06) harmonised the sterility test in 2009.

Conclusion

Industry globalisation necessitates changes in inspection systems. These changes require European cooperation. With treaties and cooperative agreements such as MRAs, ICH and PIC/S, the process takes on a worldwide dimension, with ICH GMP guidelines being developed and then adopted as part of the EU regulatory framework. This global process will be encouraged and strengthened to build a fully harmonised ICH GMP Guide that can facilitate manufacturers' work and ensure patient access to innovation.

References

1. The Consolidated Versions of the Treaty on European Union and the Treaty on the Functioning of the European Union, and Charter of Fundamental Rights of the European Union (March 2010). EUR-Lex website. http://eur-lex.europa.eu/LexUriServ/LexUriServ.do?uri=OJ:C:2010:083:FULL:EN:PDF. Accessed 7 May 2012.
2. European Commission, *EudraLex: The Rules Governing Medicinal Products in the European Union*. EC website. http://ec.europa.eu/health/documents/eudralex/index_en.htm. Accessed 15 May 2012.
3. Directive 2001/82/EC of the European Parliament and of the Council of 23 October 2001 on the Community code relating to veterinary medicinal products. EUR-Lex website. http://eur-lex.europa.eu/LexUriServ/LexUriServ.do?uri=CONSLEG:2001L0082:20090807:EN:PDF. Accessed 15 May 2012.
4. Directive 2001/83/EC of the European Parliament and of the Council of 6 November 2001 on the Community code relating to medicinal products for human use. EMA website. www.emea.europa.eu/docs/en_GB/document_library/Regulatory_and_procedural_guideline/2009/10/WC500004481.pdf. Accessed 15 May 2012.
5. Directive 2004/27/EC of the European Parliament and of the Council of 31 March 2004 amending Directive 2001/83/EC on the Community code relating to medicinal products for human use. EUR-Lex website. http://eur-lex.europa.eu/Notice.do?val=343604:cs&pos=1&page=1&lang=en&pgs=10&nbl=1&list=343604:cs,&hwords=&action=GO&visu=%23texte. Accessed 15 May 2012.
6. Regulation 726/2004 of the European Parliament and of the Council of 31 March 2004 laying down Community procedures for the authorisation and supervision of medicinal products for human and veterinary use and establishing a European Medicines Agency. EUR-Lex website. http://eur-lex.europa.eu/LexUriServ/LexUriServ.do?uri=OJ:L:2004:136:0001:0033:en:PDF. Accessed 15 May 2012.
7. Directive 2004/28/EC of the European Parliament and of the Council of 31 March 2004 amending Directive 2001/82/EC on the Community code relating to veterinary medicinal products. EUR-Lex website. http://eur-lex.europa.eu/LexUriServ/LexUriServ.do?uri=CELEX:32004L0028:EN:HTML. Accessed 15 May 2012.
8. Directive 2011/62/EU of the European Parliament and of the Council of 8 June 2011 amending Directive 2001/83/EC on the Community code relating to medicinal products for human use, as regards the prevention of the entry into the legal supply chain of falsified medicinal products. EC website. http://ec.europa.eu/health/files/eudralex/vol-1/dir_2011_62/dir_2011_62_en.pdf. Accessed 15 May 2012.
9. Pharmaceutical Inspection Co-operation Scheme. Recommendation on Quality System Requirements for Pharmaceutical Inspectorates. September 2007. PIC Scheme website. www.picscheme.org/publication.php?id=17. Accessed 10 May 2012.
10. EMA. Compilation of Community Procedures on Inspections and Exchange of Information. EMA website. www.ema.europa.eu/ema/index.jsp?curl=pages/regulation/document_listing/document_listing_000156.jsp. Accessed 10 May 2012.
11. EMA. Joint Audit Programme for EEA GMP Inspectorates. EMA website. www.ema.europa.eu/docs/en_GB/document_library/Other/2009/10/WC500004862.pdf. Accessed 10 May 2012.
12. Ibid.
13. ICH. Official ICH website. http://www.ich.org/. Accessed 10 May 2012.
14. ISO 9000:2001, Quality Management Systems—Requirements.
15. Sykes G. The technique of sterility testing, . 8:573-588, 1956.

Chapter 21

Generic Medicinal Products

Updated by Jill M.E. Bunyan, PhD, MRPharmS, MTOPRA, MIOS

OBJECTIVES

- Learn about generic products and the history of the generic medicines industry

- Obtain a perspective on the current issues facing the generic product industry

- Understand Marketing Authorisation Applications for generic products in Europe

---

DIRECTIVES, REGULATIONS AND GUIDELINES COVERED IN THIS CHAPTER

- Directive 98/44/CE of the European Parliament and of the Council of 6 July 1998 concerning the legal protection of biotechnological inventions

- Directive 2001/83/EC of the European Parliament and of the Council of 6 November 2001 on the Community code relating to medicinal products for human use, as amended

- Regulation (EC) No 726/2004 of the European Parliament and of the Council of 31 March 2004 laying down Community procedures for the authorisation and supervision of medicinal products for human and veterinary use and establishing a European Medicines Agency

- Directive 2004/27/EC of the European Parliament and of the Council of 31 March 2004 amending Directive 2001/83/EC on the Community code relating to medicinal products for human use

- Commission Regulation (EC) 1234/2008 of 24 November 2008 concerning the examination of variations to the terms of marketing authorisations (MAs) for medicinal products for human use and veterinary medicinal products

- Communication from the Commission—Guideline on the operation of the procedures laid down in Chapters II, III and IV of Commission Regulation (EC) No 1234/2008, adopted December 2009.

- CPMP/EWP/QWP/1401/98 Rev. 1/Corr**, Guideline on the Investigation of Bioequivalence, Adopted January 2010

- Regulation (EC) 469/2009 of the European Parliament and of the Council concerning the Supplementary Protection Certificate for medicinal products

- Directive 2009/53/EC of the European Parliament and of the Council of 18 June 2009 amending Directive 2001/82/EC and Directive 2001/83/EC, as regards variations to the terms of MAs for medicinal products

- The Rules Governing Medicinal Products in the European Union, Volume 2A, Notice to *Applicants*, European Commission, 1998, chapters 1-7 individually updated: 2005–11

Historical Perspective

The brand-name pharmaceutical industry did not really take shape until the mid-1950s. Its rise was followed by the appearance of the generics sector when brand-name medicine patents began to expire. In the early years, the pharmaceutical industry was research-driven, and new compounds were introduced to market as soon as they were discovered. No restrictions were placed on price or profitability, and governments imposed little or no regulatory delay, so new products came to market with most of their patent life ahead of them.

Rising healthcare costs had a profound influence on the growth of the generics industry. Price controls appeared in various forms, including reimbursement schemes and linking of new product marketing approvals to pricing agreements between European governments and manufacturers. Such factors as ageing populations, medicines' accounting for an increasing percentage of healthcare expenditures and the high costs of new medicines have created an environment in which generics have an increasingly valued role in healthcare delivery. This environment, combined with patent expirations for important products, has fostered the growth of the generics industry. Generic medicines, which are priced 20%–90% lower than name brands, are currently creating €25–30 billion in savings across the Community each year for EU healthcare systems. The European market for generics is forecast to grow at more than 6% annually, a pace faster than that of the total pharmaceutical market.[1,2]

Some EU Member States have introduced measures to encourage the generics sector. Brand-name pharmaceutical companies have attempted to maintain a larger share of the off-patent market themselves, either through a generic subsidiary of their own or by entering into alliances with generics companies (e.g., licensing a generics supplier to start marketing a major product before patent expiration). In that way, the generics company gets a head start in the market while the originator continues to earn royalties from sales of the off-patent product.

The trend for major research and development companies to acquire generics subsidiaries began in the US, where the generics market was first established. US generic pharmaceutical manufacturer sales in 2007 were $58.5 billion.[3] A key reason for these high sales is that the US has long been a single market. In contrast, Europe is divided into national markets and by national laws and medical and administrative cultures. The European generics industry grew in a much more fragmented manner since companies generally limited their activities to their home countries. Now, however, European registration procedures, international mutual recognition agreements and harmonised approaches to pharmaceutical standards and registration document requirements are facilitating the development of pan-European and international generic companies.

European Generic Medicines Association

In 1993, the European Generic Medicines Association (EGA) was formed as the representative body for the European generic pharmaceutical and active pharmaceutical ingredient industries. Within the past few years, EGA has also become involved in representing the biosimilar medicines industry. EGA is the industry's official trade association or representative body, representing generic pharmaceutical companies and their subsidiaries (either directly or through national associations) throughout Europe. The accession in 2004 and 2007 of Central and Eastern European countries (whose domestic pharmaceutical markets are largely comprised of branded generics) further increased the importance and strength of the EU generic market.

EGA's policymaking, position statements and technical reviews of EU and national proposals are carried out by six committees: the Regulatory and Scientific Affairs Committee, the Health Economics Committee, the Legal Affairs (IP) Committee, the CEE & Accession Committee, the Biotechnology & Biosimilars Committee and the National Associations Committee.

EGA is regularly involved in developing pharmaceutical legislation and guidelines and maintains constant dialogue with EU institutions and various national, European and international agencies. EGA provides scientific, regulatory and legal expertise at the request of national, EU and international bodies and provides a network of information and a system of cooperative assistance with other generic pharmaceutical associations at the national, regional and international levels.[4] It liaises with other international associations and is one of the founding members of the International Generic Pharmaceutical Alliance (IGPA), established in 1997.

What Is a Generic Product?

(Article 3(3) of EC Regulation 726/2004 and Article 10(1) of Directive 2001/83/EC, as amended)

A generic medicinal product is essentially similar to an already authorised product (the "reference product"). It has the same qualitative and quantitative composition in terms of active substances as the reference product. A generic medicinal product has the same pharmaceutical form, is used at the same dose(s) to treat the same disease(s), and is equally safe and effective, which is confirmed by the appropriate bioequivalence studies.[5]

In accordance with Article 10.2(b) of Directive 2001/83/EC, as amended, different salts, esters, ethers, isomers, mixtures of isomers, complexes or derivatives of an active substance shall be considered to be the same active substance, unless they differ significantly in properties with regard to safety and/or efficacy. In such cases, additional information providing proof of the safety and/or efficacy of the various salts, esters or derivatives of an authorised active substance must be supplied by the applicant. The various immediate-release oral pharmaceutical forms (i.e., tablets and capsules) shall be considered to be one and the same pharmaceutical form for the concept of essential similarity.

When the patent for the original, brand-name product expires, the medicinal product enters the public domain. Any manufacturer may produce and market the product, provided it obtains the necessary manufacturing and MAs from the appropriate regulatory authorities. The originator's brand name, however, cannot be used. Instead, the new manufacturer/Marketing Authorisation Holder (MAH) must give the product a new brand name or generic name or supply the medicine under its recognized short chemical name, known as the International Nonproprietary Name (INN), followed by the MAH's name.

The key to a generic application is that the applicant relies on the originator's established safety and efficacy data; although they are not in fact granted actual access to this data, which remains confidential. Repetition of animal and human studies is discouraged; regulatory authorities use the originator's data to avoid the need for such studies. To protect the originator and provide an incentive for innovation, EU medicines legislation also includes data exclusivity concepts (please see Data Exclusivity below).

Bioequivalence

Directive 2001/83/EC, as amended, gives the legislative basis for bioequivalence.

A generic manufacturer must demonstrate that its product is "essentially similar" to (and therefore interchangeable with) the "reference" (i.e., original) medicinal product. It must show the same safety, quality and efficacy as the original product, which usually is accomplished by studies proving bioequivalence. Bioequivalence means that the generic and reference products have no significant differences in the rate and extent of absorption in the human body; that is, when the same dosage is administered, they produce essentially the same biological availability of the active ingredient in the body. The bioequivalence study compares the same dose under the same conditions.

The main criteria for conducting bioequivalence studies are:
- detailed study (protocol) design
- protocol approved by an Ethics Committee
- sufficient number of volunteers/patients (in specific cases)
- appropriate and thorough medical examinations of volunteers/patients (in specific cases)
- usually a cross-over study design
- randomised study design
- compliance with Good Clinical Practice (GCP) and Good Laboratory Practice (GLP)
- standardised study conditions
- sufficient wash-out periods between tests[6]

The detailed criteria for conducting bioequivalence studies (i.e., the requirements for their design, conduct and evaluation) are set forth in the *Guideline on the Investigation of Bioequivalence*.[7] This guideline specifies the requirements for immediate-release dosage forms with systemic action. However, bioequivalence study requirements for different dosage forms are specified in Appendix 2 of this guideline.

The original *Note for Guidance* (CPMP/EWP/QWP/1401/98) became outdated in many aspects; experiences with the use of the Mutual Recognition Procedure and Decentralised Procedure clearly showed that some issues were interpreted differently among Member States, and better clarity was required. In January 2010, after much discussion, a new guideline was proposed and adopted by the Committee for Medicinal Products for Human Use (CHMP).

The new *Guideline on Bioequivalence* is more transparent and should improve the general understanding of the recommendations, and, most importantly, lead to more-consistent interpretation of regulatory requirements overall, which should result in improved bioequivalence study design and success. The guideline now also clarifies cases where a bioequivalence study may not be required, the so-called "biowaiver."

For further information, refer to the EGA "Questions & Answers on the Revised EMA Bioequivalence Guideline"[8] and the European Medicines Agency's "Questions and answers on generic medicines."[9]

Data Exclusivity, Patents and Supplementary Protection Certificates

Under Directive 2001/83/EC,[10] EU data exclusivity laws guaranteed market protection for originator medicines by preventing regulatory authorities, during a given period, from accepting applications for generic products without the originator's agreement. In other words, the generic manufacturer cannot make an application for an MA during the six or 10 years (depending on the country) after the original medicinal product obtains its first authorisation in the EU. After that time, the generic medicine can be authorised by the Competent Authority, but cannot be marketed until the patents and, if relevant, the Supplementary Protection Certificates (SPCs) covering the originator product have expired.

Data Exclusivity

Exclusivity was originally introduced to compensate for a lack of patent protection, mainly for biotechnology products (which can now be patented; see Directive 98/44/CE[11]). The EU pharmaceutical legislation review (Directive 2004/27/EC[12]) resulted in a compromise period of eight years of data exclusivity, with an additional two years of market exclusivity, which is extended by a further year (8+2+1) if a new indication is added within the first eight years, for all registration procedures. In other words, generic medicines companies can apply for an MA based on bioequivalence only after the eight-year data exclusivity period has expired, and can only market their products two or three years after that. The effective period of marketing exclusivity is therefore 10 or 11 years.[13] This arrangement is only applicable to originator products submitted after 31 October 2005 and, therefore, will not impact the generics industry until after October 2013. Specific data protection may be available for the extension of the original product's indication to children (legislation under co-decision procedure ongoing).

Market exclusivity for significant clinical change (e.g., a new indication) is only available to the originator and only within the eight years of the 8+2+1 period; the one-year extension is available only once. New indications after the eight years will not be granted market exclusivity. Other product variations (such as new formulations, strengths, isomers, polymorphic forms, etc.) will not receive additional periods of protection under regulatory law.[14,15]

According to Article 89 of Regulation (EC) No. 726/2004,[16] the above-mentioned periods of protection (8+2+1) do not apply retrospectively to reference medicinal products for which the initial application for authorisation was submitted before 20 November 2005. For such products, periods of protection are:

- six-year data exclusivity periods for national authorisations granted by: Austria, Cyprus, Czech Republic, Denmark, Estonia, Finland, Greece, Hungary, Ireland, Latvia, Lithuania, Malta, Poland, Portugal, Slovak Republic, Slovenia and Spain, as well as Norway, Lichtenstein and Iceland
- 10-year exclusivity periods for national authorisations granted by: Belgium, Germany, France, Italy, Luxembourg, The Netherlands, Sweden and the UK
- 10-year period of data for all medicinal products authorised through the Centralised Procedure

Patents

Patents are awarded to inventions that fulfil the criteria of novelty (new and different), utility (useful) and non-obviousness (inventive, not previously predictive). Patents are used to protect the following four statutory classes of patentable inventions relevant to the pharmaceutical industry: a product, process, composition or use that has a practical purpose.

Patents are available for a medicinal product's active substance, compound, formulation, usage, process, mechanism of action and intermediates. Registration provides a patentee the right to prevent anyone from making, using, selling or importing the invention for 20 years. The EU now has the highest patent protection level in the world,[17] resulting in part from the following regulatory situation:

- Patents are now available for biotech products.
- Market protection periods for 20-year patents on medicinal products are extendable by a further maximum five-year period by the *Supplementary Protection Certificate Regulation* (Regulation (EC) No 469/2009[18]).
- Patents are increasingly granted for new uses, dosages and changes in formulations.

The European Patent Organisation was set up in 1977 (on the basis of the European Patent Convention (EPC) signed in Munich in 1973). It is an intergovernmental organisation consisting of two bodies: the European Patent Office (EPO) and the Administrative Council, which supervises the office's activities.[19] The EPO does not grant "international patents" or international patent protection. It provides a uniform procedure (the so-called international application), for individual inventors and companies seeking patent protection in up to 40 European countries. After 30 months from the first filing in any EU country (or, for a few countries, after 20 months) an international application must be converted into a national or regional patent application, and is then subject to a national or regional grant procedure, which gives the inventor patent protection. In other words, once the patent is granted by EPO, any Member State can give the applicant patent protection without performing its own search (on the acceptability and appropriateness of the patent application).[20]

SPCs

The SPC (Council Regulation 1768/92/EEC[21]) was a regulatory initiative introduced to give extended market protection to patented pharmaceutical products to compensate for time lost between patent filing and market authorisation. Essentially, the SPC guarantees the originator pharmaceutical company five more years of marketing exclusivity and serves as an effective delay to generic competition. After several substantial amendments, Regulation 1768/92/EEC was finally repealed by Regulation EC/469/2009, which came into effect in June 2009.

Bolar (Experimental and Testing) Provisions

The term "Bolar provision" originated in the US *Hatch-Waxman Act* (the *Drug Price Competition and Patent Term Restoration Act* of 1984 [US public law 98-417]).[22] This act extended market exclusivity to compensate originator pharmaceutical companies for the loss of patent life caused by the lengthy drug product development and registration process. At the same time, the *Roche/Bolar Amendment* to this act allowed generic companies to develop (including testing and experimental work required for registration) versions of patent-protected products while the original patent was still in force. Thus, the generics companies could be fully prepared for market entry immediately after patent expiration.

A Bolar-type provision is now largely implemented across the EU, albeit with some differences in interpretation in national territories.[23]

To harmonise the law and to bring the European pharmaceutical industry (and, in particular, the generics industry) closer to an equal footing with the US, the EU introduced a new exemption in Article 10(6) of Directive 2004/27/EC amending Directive 2001/83/EC on the Community code relating to medicinal products for human use. Under Article 10(6), a patent or SPC will not be infringed where studies and trials are conducted with a view to obtaining an EU MA for a generic medicinal product. This provision only applies to those acts, and "consequential practice requirements," which are necessary to make that application.[24]

It should be noted that this provision is not identical to the US exemption. Article 10(6) does not provide an exemption for all activities. Only studies and trials supporting abridged applications, hybrid applications and biosimilar applications are exempted from patent infringement (which is defined by Paragraphs 1, 2, 3 and 4 of Article 10).

Directive 2004/27/EC should have been implemented in national legislation by 30 October 2005, at the latest. However, most Member States did not fully complete the national implementation process by that date. Moreover, there is disparity among EU Member States with regard to interpretation. Some Member States have implemented the directive to provide just the minimum required exemption; others have provided a broader exemption than the directive requires. Some Member States appear to extend the exemption to cover studies and experiments undertaken in order to make an application for any medicinal product, not just a generic product. Germany and Italy, for example, have a broader interpretation, while the UK and the Netherlands, on the other hand, have narrower restrictions than provided for in the directive.[25]

The MA Process

In addition to the two different European MA procedures offered in the EU legislation since 1995—the Centralised Procedure and the Mutual Recognition Procedure—a Decentralised Procedure came into force with the revised law from November 2005 (see Chapter 17 Overview of Authorisation Procedures for Medicinal Products). Generic manufacturers of centrally approved reference products have the option of applying through the Centralised Procedure, Decentralised Procedure or Mutual Recognition Procedure. National procedures, of course, still exist where an MA is required in only a single country.

Currently, most generic applications are submitted through the Decentralised Procedure, but many applicants still use the Mutual Recognition Procedure. Since November 2005, the number of Decentralised Procedure applications has been growing rapidly. In 2006, only 57 Decentralised Procedures were finalised, while in 2010, 1,452 Marketing Authorisation Applications (MAAs) were approved via the Decentralised Procedure. In comparison, in 2006, 535 Mutual Recognition Procedures were finalised, while in 2010 this number was reduced to 325.[26]

The Mutual Recognition Procedure enables the national assessment done as part of the MA in one Reference Member State (RMS) to be mutually recognised by other Member States (i.e., Concerned Member States (CMS)). For any first application not previously submitted and evaluated at the national level, the Decentralised Procedure must be followed. This procedure involves the CMS at an earlier stage of the evaluation than the Mutual Recognition Procedure to minimise disagreements between the Member States and the applicant and facilitate MAAs in a number of Member States. If the product is to be marketed in only one EU Member State, an application is submitted via the national route, and a subsequent Mutual Recognition Procedure is possible at a later date, if required. In accordance with Articles 17 and 18 of Directive 2001/83/EC, as amended, the application for the same medicinal product submitted through the national route in two or more Member States at the same time shall be declined.[27] The legal text for the Mutual Recognition Procedure and Decentralised Procedure is provided in Article 27-39 of Directive 2001/83/EC, as amended, and further guidance is given in the *Notice to Applicants, Vol. 2A, Chapter 2* (February 2007).[28]

An abridged application—as opposed to a full application with preclinical and clinical data—is required for a generic product. Thus, generic applications typically include only chemical-pharmaceutical and bioequivalence data (supported by expert reports and literature). For the remaining information, the regulatory agencies may refer to the originator product's safety and efficacy data once the data exclusivity period has expired (see Data Exclusivity above).

As previously mentioned, the reference product shall mean a medicinal product authorised under Article 6 of Directive 2001/83/EC, as amended, and, in accordance with the provisions of Article 8 of the directive. This means that the reference must be made to the dossier of a reference product for which an MAA has been granted in the Community on the basis of a complete dossier. Therefore, a generic application referring to a generic dossier is not possible.[29]

European Reference Medicinal Product (ERP)

Usually, the reference is made to a medicinal product that is or has already been authorised in the Reference Member State. In some cases, a generic application can also be submitted in a Member State where the reference medicinal product has never been authorised. In this case, the applicant has to identify in the application form the name of the Member State in which the reference medicinal product has been authorised. At the request of the Competent Authority of the Member State in which the application is submitted, the Competent Authority of the other Member State shall transmit, within a period of one month, a confirmation that the reference medicinal product is or has been authorised, together with the full composition of the reference product and, if necessary, other relevant documentation.[30,31] If the European Reference Medicinal Product (ERP) is used, the period of data protection must also have expired in the Member State where the medicinal product is already authorised and/or marketed.[32]

More details of the European procedures and the legal basis for the possible applications for generic products can be found in Chapter 17 Overview of Authorisation Procedures for Medicinal Products.

Variations

Variations to existing national MAs are carried out in accordance with the *Variations Regulation* (Regulation (EC) 1234/2008)[33,34] and the guideline on variations (January 2010).[35] This regulation specifies new, more practical and workable requirements for medicinal products approved via Community and National Procedures.

The original regulation applied only to European and not National Procedures, although many Member States permitted national variations to be submitted under the same rules. This was subsequently updated by Directive 2009/53/EC,[36] which amended the rules to apply to national variations as well, with an implementation deadline of 20 January 2011.

For more details, please see Chapter 24 Pharmaceutical Postmarket Requirements and Compliance With the Marketing Authorisation.

European Initiatives and Challenges for Generic Medicines

Generic medicines promotion by EU healthcare authorities has led to a range of national initiatives. Reference price systems (that set prices in a given Member State at an average of those in a range of other Member States), generic prescription (prescribing by INN or active ingredient rather than by brand name) and generic substitution (which allows a pharmacist to replace a prescribed brand name product with a generic version) exist in at least half of the EU Member States. Currently in the UK and Germany, generic drugs account for more than half of the medicines market share (by volume) and in France, this is about 40%. In contrast, in less-mature generic markets, such as Italy and Spain, the generic portion of the market is relatively low, at approximately 25%.[37] When considered as a proportion of off-patent drugs, these figures are considerably higher.

Despite the aforementioned initiatives, generic companies face some hurdles. According to IMS data published in 2009,[37] some of the major challenges to the generic medicines industry in Europe arise from:

- increasing costs in a market undergoing constant price erosion
- unsustainable policies and an unequal playing field compared to other geographic regions with regard to taxes
- regulations and incentives

All of these limit the competitiveness and sustainability of the European generics sector.

Summary

- MAAs for generic medicines can be submitted as abridged applications mainly through European procedures: Centralised, Decentralised or Mutual Recognition; the standard National Procedure is less-often used.
- If there is no reference product authorised in the Member State where the application is made, the European Reference Product (ERP) can be used; data exclusivity must have expired at the time of submission in both the Member State where the application is made and the Member State of the ERP.
- The abridged application must demonstrate that the generic product is equally safe and effective as the originator product and must supply data proving safety and efficacy through bioequivalence studies. A full quality section of the dossier is required.
- Market protection periods for 20-year patents on medicinal products are extendable by a further maximum period of five years through the *Supplementary Protection Certificate Regulation* (EC 469/2009).
- The new EU data exclusivity laws guarantee 8+2+1 years' data protection/market exclusivity for originator products.
- A Bolar-type provision, which allows generic product development within the innovator product's patent period, was implemented in the EU in November 2005 under the revised legislation.

References

1. "The Role of Generic Medicines in Europe." European Generics Association, Brussels. September 2007. EGA website. www.egagenerics.com/gen-geneurope.htm. Accessed 2 February 2012.
2. Generic Medicines: Essential contributors to the long-term health of society. IMS Health website. www.imshealth.com/imshealth/Global/Content/Document/Market_Measurement_TL/Generic_Medicines_GA.pdf. Accessed 2 February 2012.
3. Generic Pharmaceutical Association. GPhA website. www.gphaonline.org/about-gpha/about-generics/facts. Accessed 2 February 2012.
4. European Generics Association. EGA website. www.egagenerics.com/. Accessed 2 February 2012.
5. Directive 2001/83/EC of the European Parliament and of the Council of 6 November 2001 on the Community code relating to medicinal products for human use, as amended. EUR-Lex website. http://

eur-lex.europa.eu/LexUriServ/LexUriServ.do?uri=OJ:L:2001:311:0067:0128:en:PDF. Accessed 3 May 2012.
6. "EGA Fact Sheet on Generic Medicines" Bioequivalence, European Generics Association, Brussels. EGA website. www.egagenerics.com/doc/ega_factsheet-08.pdf. Accessed 2 February 2012.
7. *Guideline on the Investigation of Bioequivalence*, Doc. Ref.: CPMP/EWP/QWP/1401/98 Rev. 1/ Corr. ** European Medicines Agency, Committee on Proprietary Medicinal Products. Adopted January 2010. EMA website. www.emea.europa.eu/docs/en_GB/document_library/Scientific_guideline/2010/01/WC500070039.pdf. Accessed 3 May 2012.
8. Questions & Answers on the Revised EMA Bioequivalence Guideline. Summary of the discussions held at the 3rd EGA Symposium on Bioequivalence June 2010 London. EGA website. www.egagenerics.com/doc/EGA_BEQ_Q&A_WEB_QA_1_32.pdf. Accessed 3 May 2012.
9. EMA/393905/2006 Rev. 1. "Questions and answers on generic medicines," EMA, London, 17 March 2011. EMA website. www.emea.europa.eu/docs/en_GB/document_library/Medicine_QA/2009/11/WC500012382.pdf - accessed 3 February 2012
10. Op cit 5.
11. Directive 98/44/EC of the European Parliament and of the Council of 6 July 1998 concerning the legal protection of biotechnological inventions. EUR-Lex website. http://eur-lex.europa.eu/smartapi/cgi/sga_doc?smartapi!celexapi!prod!CELEXnumdoc&lg=en&numdoc=31998L0044&model=guichett. Accessed 3 May 2012.
12. Directive 2004/27/EC of the European Parliament and of the Council of 31 March 2004 amending Directive 2001/83/EC on the Community code relating to medicinal products for human use. EC website. http://ec.europa.eu/health/files/eudralex/vol-1/dir_2004_27/dir_2004_27_en.pdf. Accessed 3 May 2012.
13. "EGA Fact Sheet on Generic Medicines" Generic Medicines, Data Exclusivity and Patents. European Generics Association, Brussels. EGA website. www.egagenerics.com/doc/ega_factsheet-10.pdf. Accessed 3 February 2012.
14. Regulation (EC) No 726/2004 of the European Parliament and of the Council of 31 March 2004 laying down Community procedures for the authorisation and supervision of medicinal products for human and veterinary use and establishing a European Medicines Agency. EC website. http://ec.europa.eu/health/files/eudralex/vol-1/reg_2004_726_cons/reg_2004_726_cons_en.pdf. Accessed 3 May 2012.
15. Op cit 12.
16. Op cit 14.
17. Op cit 13.
18. Regulation (EC) No 469/2009 of the European Parliament and of the Council of 6 May 2009 concerning the supplementary protection certificate for medicinal products. EUR-Lex website. http://eur-lex.europa.eu/LexUriServ/LexUriServ.do?uri=OJ:L:2009:152:0001:0010:en:PDF. Accessed 3 May 2012.
19. European Patent Organisation. EPO website. www.epo.org/about-us/organisation.html. Accessed 3 February 2012.
20. How to apply for a European patent**.** EPO website. www.epo.org/applying/basics.html. Accessed 3 February 2012.
21. Council Regulation (EEC) No 1768/92 of 18 June 1992 concerning the creation of a supplementary protection certificate for medicinal products. EUR-Lex website. http://eur-lex.europa.eu/LexUriServ/site/en/consleg/1992/R/01992R1768-20070126-en.pdf. Accessed 3 May 2012.
22. Bolar Provision: A Global History and The Future For Europe. Genericsweb website. www.genericsweb.com//index.php?object_id=238. Accessed 3 February 2012.
23. Roox K. "The Bolar Provision: A Safe Harbour in Europe for Biosimilars." Informa UK Ltd., Colchester, UK. July 2006. www.crowell.com//documents//DOCASSOCFKTYPE_ARTICLES_614.pdf.. Accessed 3 February 2012.
24. Op cit 12.
25. Op cit 23.
26. CMD(h) Annual Reports on Mutual recognition and Decentralised procedure, Heads of Medicines Agencies. HMA website. www.hma.eu/. Accessed 3 February 2012.
27. Op cit 5.
28. *Notice to Applicants, Volume 2A*, Chapter 2 (February 2007).
29. *Notice to Applicants, Volume 2A*, Chapter 1 (November 2005).
30. Ibid.
31. Op cit 12.
32. Op cit 29.
33. Commission Regulation (EC) No 1234/2008 of 24 November 2008 concerning the examination of variations. EUR-Lex website. http://eur-lex.europa.eu/LexUriServ/LexUriServ.do?uri=OJ:L:2008:334:0007:0007:EN:PDF. Accessed 3 May 2012.
34. Communication from the Commission – Guideline on the operation of the procedures laid down in Chapters II, III and IV of Commission Regulation (EC) No 1234/2008. EC website. http://ec.europa.eu/health/files/eudralex/vol-2/c323_9/c323_9_en.pdf. Accessed 3 May 2012.
35. Directive 2009/53/EC of the European Parliament and of the Council of 18 June 2009 amending Directive 2001/82/EC and Directive 2001/83/EC, as regards variations to the terms of marketing authorisations for medicinal products. EUR-Lex website. http://eur-lex.europa.eu/LexUriServ/LexUriServ.do?uri=OJ:L:2009:168:0033:0034:en:PDF. Accessed 3 May 2012.
36. Ibid.
37. Op cit 2.

Chapter 22

Nonprescription Medicinal Products

Updated by Martha Anna Bianchetto, PharmD, MBA

OBJECTIVES

- Comprehend the political background for self-medication in the EU

- Review EU pharmaceutical legislation dealing with medicinal products not subject to medical prescription

- Review the policy for changing the legal classification of medicinal products not subject to medical prescription

- Comprehend the regulatory framework for traditional herbal medicinal products in the EU

REGULATIONS, DIRECTIVES AND GUIDELINES COVERED IN THIS CHAPTER

- Directive 2004/24/EC of the European Parliament and of the Council of 31 March 2004 amending, as regards traditional herbal medicinal products, Directives 2001/83/ on the Community code relating to medicinal products for human use

- Directive 2001/83/EC of the European Parliament and the Council of 6 November 2001 on the Community code relating to medicinal products for human use

- European Commission, The Rules Governing Medicinal Products in the European Union, Notice to Applicants: Volume 2C, Guideline on Changing the Classification for the Supply of a Medicinal Product for Human Use, (revision January 2006)

- European Commission, The Rules Governing Medicinal Products in the European Union, Notice to Applicants: Volume 2C, Guideline on the Readability of Labelling and Package Leaflet of Medicinal Products for Human Use revision 1 (12 January 2009)

- European Commission, The Rules Governing Medicinal Products in the European Union, Volume 3B; Multidisciplinary Guidelines, Medicinal products for human use, Safety, environment and information, Excipients in the Label and Package Leaflet of Medicinal Products for Human Use (July 2003)

- Directive 2011/83/EC on the Community code relating to medicinal products for human use, as regards the prevention of the entry into the legal supply chain of falsified medicinal products (8 June 2011)

- "Improving the Decision Making Process for Nonprescription Drugs: A Framework for Benefit - Risk Assessment" (2 November 2011) Position Paper

Definition of Self-medication

The World Self-Medication Industry (WSMI) defines "self-medication" as:

> "…the treatment of common health problems with medicines especially designed and labeled for use without medical supervision and approved as safe and effective for such use…"[1]

"In line with a philosophy of individual participation and empowerment, the World Health Organization has stated that responsible self-medication can:

- Help prevent and treat symptoms and ailments that do not require medical consultation;
- Reduce the increasing pressure on medical services for the relief of minor ailments, especially when financial and human services are limited;
- Increase the availability of health care to populations living in rural or remote areas where access to medical advice may be difficult; and
- Enable patients to control their own chronic conditions."[2]

Political Support for Self-medication in the EU

In the EU, development of the pharmaceutical sector for nonprescription medicinal products has required strong political support. The high cost of medicinal products (based on national pricing regulations), safety profiles of certain medicinal products and the opportunity for EU citizens to self-diagnose minor ailments has led to the creation of legislation and guidelines for changing a medicinal product's classification from a prescription to nonprescription status.

In 1996, the European Parliament issued a resolution stating:

> "…responsible self-medication should be further promoted, which will foster the growing desire of the European Union's citizens to take responsibility for their own health and also help reduce health expenditure. In recent years, responsible self-medication has been identified as an important element in long-term health policy by the institutions of the European Community…"[3]

Various national and pan-European trade associations champion the use of nonprescription medicines in the EU. The Association of the European Self-Medication Council of Ministers (AESGP) has regular dialogue with the European Commission, the European Parliament, the Council of Ministers, the European Directorate for the Quality of Medicines & Healthcare (including the European Pharmacopoeia) and the European Medicines Agency (EMA) to register the interests of its members.

During 2011, a WSMI task force worked with external global experts in medicines, risk management and modeling to develop a position paper illustrating a new benefit:risk model for nonprescription medicines. The position paper arose from recognition that regulators in many parts of the world are discussing or developing benefit:risk models to provide tools for a more-structured way to frame or discuss data and knowledge regarding medicines. For nonprescription medicines, evaluating risk:benefit models is particularly challenging: risks are frequently well documented and publicised, while the benefits can be harder to quantify or define, particularly in the case of quality-of-life improvement and understanding the value of something as fundamental as convenience and accessibility. The paper, entitled "Improving the Decision-Making Process for Nonprescription Drugs: A Framework for Benefit-Risk Assessment," was published on 2 November 2011.[4]

Three core themes are discussed, including the following:
- OTC benefits:risks are incremental to the same ingredient when prescription.
- Risks are comparatively easy to define, while incremental benefits are less so.
- A more explicit framework can better draw out relevant questions before and during development, evaluation, risk management and monitoring.

Furthermore, the paper develops tools or a model that seeks to:
- comprehensively identify nonprescription drug benefit and risk characteristics
- allow early, transparent agreement among stakeholders around benefits and risk
- optimise benefit:risk assessment tools for application to nonprescription drugs while providing flexibility for regulators to adapt to unique needs
- illustrate the application of the proposed tool

EU Legislation for Nonprescription Medicines

Nonprescription medicines are formally recognised and defined in Article 72 of Directive 2001/83/EC,[5] as amended. Article 72 implies that all medicinal products should be nonprescription, unless they meet the criteria listed in Article 71 of the same directive.
- likely to present a danger, either directly or indirectly, even when used correctly, if utilised without medical supervision
- frequently and to a very wide extend used incorrectly, and as a result are likely to present a direct or indirect danger to human health
- contain substances or preparations thereof, the activity/adverse reactions of which require further investigation
- normally prescribed by a doctor to be administered parentally

This approach makes the notion of nonprescription medicines unequivocal, although some Member States still have subcategories of nonprescription medicinal products. For example, in France, not all nonprescription medicines can be advertised to the public, and in the UK, some nonprescription medicines can only be purchased in a pharmacy.

Article 74 of the same directive states:

"When new facts are brought to their attention, the competent authorities shall examine and, as appropriate, amend the classification of a medicinal product by applying the criteria listed in Article 71…"

Competent Authorities are, therefore, obliged to regularly consider the classification status of medicinal products. However, because the responsibility for legal status remains the remit of each Competent Authority, classification differences in Member States persist.

The following text is also in Article 74:

"Where a change of classification of a medicinal product has been authorised on the basis of significant preclinical tests or clinical trials, the competent authority shall not refer to the results of those tests or trials when examining an application by another applicant for or holder of marketing authorisation for a change in the classification of the same substance for one year after the initial change was authorised…"

The notion of one year of data exclusivity is a reward to applicants that generate safety (preclinical) and/or efficacy (clinical) data that successfully demonstrate the legal classification of a medicine (usually from prescription to nonprescription) should be changed.

The Centralised Procedure is available for nonprescription medicines that are of significant therapeutic value or benefit to society and/or patients. The first nonprescription medicinal product approved via the Centralised Procedure was ALLI (orlistat) 60 mg capsules, indicated for weight loss in adults aged 18 and over who are overweight.

Switching the Legal Classification of a Medicine in the European Union

In Resolution COM(93)0718-C3-0121/94, the European Parliament stated:

"As part of the process of improving the legal environment for nonprescription medicines, it will be important to establish more transparent procedures which define the method by which prescription medicines can be transferred to nonprescription status…"[6]

As mentioned above, the availability of medicines as nonprescription items varies considerably in different Member States. The disparities are largely due to previous national evaluations, the reimbursement policies of Member States and cultural differences. An issue of consideration is whether the change of legal status refers to a product or an active substance. In Germany, a switch normally refers to an active substance and not to a specific medicinal product. In other Member States, such as Italy, the switch process is based on individual products. The switch process in Member States can also differ in active substance doses, therapeutic indications and pharmaceutical forms allowed for nonprescription medicines (see **Table 22-1**).

In an attempt to harmonise basic medicinal product assessment and classification principles in the EU, the European Commission has issued the *Guideline on Changing the Classification for the Supply of a Medicinal Product for Human Use*[7] for use by applicants and Competent Authorities.

The guideline has five parts: Part 1 defines classification criteria; Part 2 describes the data (including safety/efficacy data and product information) required to support a switch; Part 3 discusses the potential for data exclusivity; Part 4 outlines principles and procedure to claim one year of data exclusivity; and Part 5 provides options for naming the medicinal product. Although the guideline is not binding, it has furthered the harmonisation process.

Most Member States have similar application dossier formats for product switching. The package includes safety evidence based on prescription use, switching experience gained from other nations and efficacy data, if the proposed indication differs from that for prescription use.

Some Member States still link switching with reimbursement considerations. For example, in Austria, Ireland, Portugal and Spain, manufacturers cannot use the same brand name for nonprescription products if one or more versions with the same ingredients remain available as a prescription-only medicine. In addition, pricing controls and negotiation policies for nonprescription medicines often have a dramatic influence on the switching climate in some Member States. In Greece, the National Authorities control the prices for nonprescription medicines, removing normal market mechanisms. This may deter some manufacturers from applying for nonprescription status.

Drug Information

Title V of Directive 2001/83/EC, as amended, states medicinal products (including those not subject to medical prescription) must be accompanied by clear instructions for use. A comprehensive list of mandatory product information is provided.

Drug information is of particular importance for nonprescription products because diagnosis of the condition, and selection and administration of the product often are the responsibility of the consumer rather than the medical practitioner. Providing legible, clear and easy to use information is crucial for the following texts: instructions for use,

Chapter 22

Table 22-1. Legal Classification Status* of Selected Ingredients in the EU

Ingredient	Austria	Belgium	France	Germany	Italy	Netherlands	Sweden	UK
ALIMENTARY TRACT AND METABOLISM								
Stomatological Preparations								
Fluoride (sodium)	OTC	OTC	OTC	OTC (1986)	OTC	OTC	OTC	OTC
Drugs for Acid-related Disorders								
Cimetidine	OTC	Rx	OTC (1997)	Rx	OTC (1993)	OTC (1996)	Rx	OTC (1994)
Ranitidine	OTC	OTC (2003)	OTC (1997)	OTC (1999)	Rx	OTC (1996)	OTC (1995)	OTC (1994)
Omeprazole	Rx	Rx	RX	Rx	Rx	OTC (2008)	OTC (1999)	OTC (2004)
Antiobesity Preparations								
Orlistat	OTC (2009)	OTC (2009)	OTC (2009)	OTC (2009)	OTC (2009)	OTC (2009)	OTC (2009)	OTC (2009)
BLOOD AND BLOOD FORMING ORGANS								
Antianemic Preparations								
Iron and folic acid preparations	OTC	OTC	OTC	OTC	Rx	OTC	OTC	OTC
CARDIOVASCULAR SYSTEM								
Cardiac Therapy								
Adenosine	Rx	OTC	OTC	OTC	Rx	Rx	Rx	OTC (2004)
DERMATOLOGICAL								
Antifungals for Dermatological Use								
Miconazole (topical)	OTC	OTC	OTC (1983)	OTC	OTC	OTC	OTC (1983)	OTC
Nystatin	Rx	OTC	Rx	OTC	Rx	Rx	Rx	Rx
Corticosteriods, Dermatological Preparations								
Hydrocortisone (topical)	Rx	OTC	OTC (1996)	OTC (1996)	OTC (1983)	Rx	OTC (1983)	OTC (1987)
GENITO-URINARY SYSTEM AND SEX HORMONES								
Sex Hormones and Modulators in the Genital System								
Levonorgestrel	Rx	OTC (2001)	OTC (1999)	Rx	Rx	OTC (2005)	OTC (2001)	OTC (2001)
ANTIINFECTIVES FOR SYSTEMIC USE								
Antimycotics for Systemic Use								
Itraconazole	Rx	Rx	Rx	Rx	Rx	Rx	Rx	Rx
MUSCULO-SKELETAL SYSTEM								
Antiinflammatory and Antirheumatic Products								
Diclofenac (topical)	Rx	Rx	Rx	OTC (2004)	OTC (1983)	OTC (1998)	OTC	Rx
Ibuprofen (oral)	OTC	OTC	OTC (1992)	OTC (1989)	OTC (1984)	OTC	OTC (1988)	OTC (1983)
NERVOUS SYSTEM								
Anaesthetics								
Cinchocaine (topical)	Rx	OTC	Rx	Rx	OTC	Rx	Rx	OTC
Lidocaine (topical/oral topical)	OTC	OTC	OTC (1958)	OTC	OTC	OTC	OTC (1987)	OTC
Analgesics								
Paracetamol	OTC	OTC	OTC	OTC	OTC (1990)	OTC	OTC	OTC
Sumatriptan	Rx	Rx	Rx	Rx	Rx	Rx	Rx	OTC (2006)
Other Nervous System Drugs								
Nicotine (gum)	OTC	OTC	OTC (1997)	OTC (1994)	OTC	OTC (1992)	OTC (1990)	OTC (1991)

Ingredient	Austria	Belgium	France	Germany	Italy	Netherlands	Sweden	UK
Antiparasitic Products, Insecticides and Repellants								
Anthelmintics								
Mebendazole	Rx	OTC	Rx	Rx	Rx	OTC	Rx	OTC (1989)
RESPIRATORY SYSTEM								
Nasal Preparations								
Beclometasone (nasal)	Rx	OTC (2008)	OTC (2002)	OTC (1997)	Rx	Rx	OTC (1999)	OTC (1994)
Oxymetazoline	OTC	OTC	Rx	OTC	OTC	OTC	OTC	OTC
Phenylephrine	OTC	OTC	OTC	OTC	OTC	Rx	Rx	OTC
Cough and Cold Preparations								
Codeine	Rx	OTC	OTC (1984)	Rx	Rx	OTC	Rx	OTC
Antihistamines for Systemic Use								
Diphenhydramine	OTC	OTC	OTC	OTC	OTC	Rx	Rx	OTC
SENSORY ORGANS								
Other Ophthalmological and Otological Preparations								
Chloramphenicol	Rx	OTC	Rx	Rx	Rx	Rx	Rx	OTC (2005)

Over-the-Counter (OTC)/Nonprescription status; (year in brackets refers to the year when the first switch took place) Rx = Prescription-only status
*WSMI should be referred to for the footnotes attached to this table, which give the specific details of the classification (source WSMI, last major update December 2008)

product label (outer packaging and/or immediate container) and the package leaflet (if required).

For consumer protection, suitable warning statements should be included in the product labelling and package leaflet as detailed in the European Commission guideline, *Excipients in the Label and Package Leaflet of Medicinal Products for Human Use*.[8] For example, if the product contains lactose (in a quantity less than 5g per dose of the medicinal product), the following statement should be added to the product label:

"Contains lactose. See leaflet for further information."

The package leaflet should contain the following statement:
"If you have been told by your doctor that you have an intolerance to some sugars, contact your doctor before taking this medicinal product."

The European Commission *Guideline on the Readability of the Label and Package Leaflet of Medicinal products for Human use*[9] provides detailed recommendations for preparing a package leaflet, e.g., font type and size, design and layout of information, writing style and consideration for blind and partially sighted patients. Quality Review of Documents (QRD) templates for labelling can be found on the EMA website.

One way to ensure key product information is conveyed to consumers in a consumer-friendly fashion is consumer testing of the package leaflet. The *Guideline on the Readability of the Label and Package leaflet of Medicinal Products for Human Use*[10] defines user testing as:

"...readability of a specimen with a group of selected test subjects. It is a development tool which is flexible and aims to identify whether or not the information as presented, conveys the correct messages to those who read it..."

Since nonprescription medicines are primarily sold directly to the consumer (user), package artwork designs tend to be more colourful and consumer-focused than those of prescription medicines. The regulatory professional will need to work closely with marketing and commercial colleagues to ensure artwork and text meet all applicable regulatory requirements, e.g., inclusion of mandatory statements discussed above and compliance with Summary of Product Characteristics (SmPC) text.

Advertising to the General Public

As stated in Directive 2001/83/EC, as amended, Title VIII, Article 88, it is permissible in the EU to advertise nonprescription medicines to the general public. It is not permissible to advertise prescription-only medicines to the general public.

Article 89 of the same directive lists conditions to be fulfilled when advertising a nonprescription medicinal product to the general public. An advertisement must:
- be set out in such a way that it is clear that the message is an advertisement and that the product is clearly identified as a medicinal product
- include the following minimum information:

- o the name of the medicinal product, as well as the common name if the medicinal product contains only one active substance
- o the information necessary for correct use of the medicinal product
- o an express, legible invitation to carefully read the instructions on the package leaflet or on the outer packaging, as the case may be

Article 90 provides clear rules detailing what should not appear in an advertisement for a medicine. The advertisement must not contain information that:

- gives the impression that a medicinal consultation or surgical operation is unnecessary, in particular by offering a diagnosis or by suggesting treatment by mail
- suggests that the effects of taking the medicine are guaranteed, are unaccompanied by adverse reactions or are better than, or equivalent to, those of another treatment or medicinal product
- suggests that the subject's health can be enhanced by taking the medicine
- suggests that the subject's health could be affected by not taking the medicine; this prohibition shall not apply to the vaccination campaigns referred to in Article 88(4)
- is directed exclusively or principally at children
- refers to a recommendation by scientists, healthcare professionals or persons who are neither of the foregoing but who, because of their celebrity, could encourage the consumption of medicinal products
- suggests that the medicinal product is a foodstuff, cosmetic or other consumer product
- suggests that the medicinal product's safety or efficacy is due to the fact that it is natural
- could, by a description or detailed representation of a case history, lead to erroneous self-diagnosis
- refers, in improper, alarming or misleading terms, to claims of recovery
- uses, in improper, alarming or misleading terms, pictorial representations of changes in the human body caused by disease or injury, or of the action of a medicinal product on the body or parts thereof

In the EU, there is a belief that advertising may increase the purchase of medicines, which could create a burden for the national reimbursement systems. Thus, Article 88 of Directive 2001/83/EC, as amended, has a provision that:

"Member States shall be entitled to ban on their territory, advertising to the general public of medicinal products, the cost of which may be reimbursed."

Use of the same brand name for both prescription and nonprescription versions of a medicinal product is not allowed in some Member States (e.g., Italy, Portugal and Spain). In addition, these Member States, do not allow immediate public advertising of switched medicinal products. In France, Ireland, Italy, Norway and Spain, nonprescription medicines automatically lose reimbursement status if the manufacturer advertises them in the general media.

Control of Advertising to the General Public

Different systems of advertising control (e.g., preapproval at a Member State level, voluntary control by self-regulatory bodies, post-publication survey) have been established in the EU in order to fulfil the requirements documented in Article 97 of Directive 2001/83/EC, as amended, which states:

"Member States shall ensure that there are adequate and effective methods to monitor the advertising of medicinal products. Such methods, which may be based on a system of prior vetting, shall in any event include legal provisions under which persons or organisations regarded under national law as having a legitimate interest in prohibiting any advertisement inconsistent with this Title, may take legal action against such advertisement, or bring such advertisement before an administrative authority competent either to decide on complaints or to initiate appropriate legal proceedings."

Methods available to Member States include stopping (by legal means, if necessary) existing or planned advertising deemed to be misleading and publishing corrective statements if necessary.

Herbal Medicinal Products

The *Traditional Herbal Medicinal Products Directive*[11] (*THMPD*), formally Directive 2004/24/EC (an amendment to Directive 2001/83/EC), and Regulation (EC) No 726/2004, established the Committee on Herbal Medicinal Products (HMPC) as part of EMA.

In accordance with *THMPD* Article 16h, HMPC's primary task is to establish a "Community list of herbal substances, preparations and combinations thereof for use in traditional herbal medicinal products" and to generate Community herbal monographs for medicinal products containing the substances in this list. The Community list is defined in Article 16f of the same directive and can be found on the EMA website.

The *THMPD* provides definitions for medicinal products, substances and preparations. Herbal medicinal products contain one or more herbal substances (whole, fragmented or cut plants, plant parts, algae, fungi and lichen) or herbal preparations (refined herbal substances). The pathway for the simplified "traditional use" registration of these products was also introduced in the *THMPD*. Previously, there was no formal EU-wide authorisation procedure, so each EU Member State regulated these products at the national level.

Under the *THMPD*, all herbal medicinal products are required to obtain an authorisation to market within the EU. For those herbal medicinal products that were not on the market before 30 April 2004, authorisation must be obtained prior to marketing.

The only herbal medicines that are exempted from the *THMPD*'s provisions are those unlicensed remedies made up for a patient following a consultation with a herbalist.

Herbal medicinal products must now be manufactured under Good Manufacturing Practices (GMPs) to ensure finished product quality and demonstrate safety.

Under the THMPD, a company needs to demonstrate that the herbal medicine has been in use within the EU for at least 30 years, or 15 years within the EU and 30 years outside the EU.

The key eligibility criteria for an herbal medicinal product to qualify under this legislation are:
- indications that are intended and designed for nonprescription use
- exclusively for administration in accordance with a specified strength and posology
- an oral, external and/or inhalation preparation
- sufficient data on the traditional use of the medicinal product; in particular, the product proves not to be harmful in the specified conditions of use and the pharmacological effects or efficacy of the medicinal product are plausible on the basis of long-standing use and experience
- vitamins and minerals may be added to the herbal medicinal product provided that their use is ancillary to the herbal ingredient(s)

The simplified registration procedure for traditional herbal medicinal products was based on evidence not supported by safety and efficacy tests and trials. Instead the applicant is asked to present bibliographic or expert evidence on the product's traditional use, as well as a bibliographic safety data review and an expert report. However, products under consideration are subject to the same pharmaceutical quality (chemistry, manufacturing and controls) requirements as other medicinal products.

A traditional herbal medicinal product complying with a Community monograph or containing substances, preparations or combinations on the Community list in one of the Member States should be recognised by other Member States. The Community list is available on the EMA website.

Furthermore, the *THMPD* mandates that product labelling for traditional herbal medicinal products contain a statement to the effect that:

"…the product is a traditional herbal medicinal product for use in specified indication (s) exclusively based upon long-standing use… the user should consult a doctor or a qualified healthcare practitioner if the symptoms persist during the use of the medicinal product or if adverse effects not mentioned in the package leaflet occur…"

Any advertising information should also contain the statement:

"…Traditional herbal medicinal product for use in specified indication(s) exclusively based upon long-standing use"

Summary

This chapter provides an overview of the EU political and regulatory environment for medicinal products not subject to medical prescription. Profiled are details regarding regulatory legislation and switch process requirements. The regulatory framework for traditional herbal medicinal products is also discussed.

References
1. World Self-Medication Industry. FAQs. WSMI website. www.wsmi.org/faqs.htm. Accessed 3 May 2012.
2. WSMI. "About self-medication—Government and health professional outlooks." WSMI website. www.wsmi.org/aboutsm2.htm. Accessed 3 May 2012.
3. COM(93)0718-C3-0121/94, *Resolution on the communication from the Commission to the Council and the European Parliament on the outlines of an industrial policy for the pharmaceutical sector in the European Community. Official Journal*, No. C 141,13 May 1996:0063. EUR-Lex website. http://eur-lex.europa.eu/LexUriServ/LexUriServ.do?uri=CELEX:51996IP0104:EN:HTML. Accessed 4 May 2012.
4. "Improving the Decision-Making Process for Nonprescription Drugs: A Framework for Benefit-Risk Assessment." Clinical Pharmacology and Therapeutics (online). 2 November 2011. Nature.com website. www.nature.com/clpt/journal/v90/n6/full/clpt2011231a.html. Accessed 3 May 2012.
5. Directive 2001/83/EC of the European Parliament and of the Council of 6 November 2001 on the Community code relating to medicinal products for human use (codifying former directives relating to medicinal products for human use). EMA website. www.emea.europa.eu/docs/en_GB/document_library/Regulatory_and_procedural_guideline/2009/10/WC500004481.pdf. Accessed 4 May 2012.
6. Op cit 3.
7. European Commission, *The Rules Governing Medicinal Products in the European Union, Notice to Applicants: Volume 2C, Guideline on Changing the Classification for the Supply of a Medicinal Product for Human Use*, (revision January 2006). EC website. http://ec.europa.eu/health/files/eudralex/vol-2/c/switchguide_160106_en.pdf. Accessed 4 May 2012.
8. European Commission, *The Rules Governing Medicinal Products in the European Union, Notice to Applicants: Volume 3B, Multidisciplinary Guidelines, Medicinal Products for human use, Safety, environment and information, Excipients in the label and package leaflet of medicinal products for human use* (July 2003). EMA website. www.ema.europa.eu/docs/en_GB/document_library/Scientific_guideline/2009/09/WC500003412.pdf. Accessed 4 May 2012.
9. European Commission, *The Rules Governing Medicinal Products on the European Union, Notice to Applicants, Volume 2C, Guideline on the Readability of the Label and the Package Leaflet of the Medicinal Products for Human Use* (January 2009). EC website. http://ec.europa.eu/health/files/eudralex/vol-2/c/2009_01_12_readability_guideline_final_en.pdf. Accessed 4 May 2012.

10. Ibid.
11. Directive 2004/24/EC of the European Parliament and of the Council of 31 March 2004 amending as regards traditional herbal medicinal products, Directives 2001/83 on the Community code relating to medicinal products for human use (*Traditional Herbal Medicinal Products Directive* (*THMPD*)). EUR-Lex website. http://eur-lex.europa.eu/LexUriServ/LexUriServ.do?uri=OJ:L:2004:136:0085:0090:en:PDF. Accessed 4 May 2012.

Chapter 23

Marketing Authorisations for Products Derived From Biotechnology

Updated by Nicole Beard, MSc, PhD

OBJECTIVES

❑ Understand the special considerations involved in developing a biotechnology-derived product for the EU market

❑ Understand the registration principles for a biotechnology-derived product for the EU market

❑ Recognise the advantages and disadvantages of obtaining an EU Marketing Authorisation through the Centralised Procedure

❑ Become familiar with sources of information about EU regulatory procedures

DIRECTIVES AND REGULATIONS COVERED IN THIS CHAPTER

❑ Regulation (EC) No 726/2004 of the European Parliament and of the Council of 31 March 2004 laying down Community procedures for the authorisation and supervision of medicinal products for human and veterinary use and establishing a European Medicines Agency, as amended (Consolidated version 20 April 2009)

❑ Regulation (EC) No 1394/2007 of the European Parliament and of the Council of 13 November 2007 on advanced therapy medicinal products and amending Directive 2001/83/EC and Regulation (EC) 726/2004

❑ Directive 2001/83/EC of the European Parliament and of the Council of 6 November 2001 on the Community code relating to medicinal products for human use, as amended (Consolidated version 5 October 2009)

❑ Directive 2004/27/EC of the European Parliament and of the Council of 31 March 2004 amending Directive 2001/83/EC on the Community code relating to medicinal products for human use

Introduction

In Europe, several marketing authorisation (MA) procedures are available to register a medicinal product. The distinction depends on the type of drug: new chemical entities, products derived from biotechnology or other innovative products.

European legislation prescribes certain procedures for specific product types. In February 1995, the European Medicines Agency (EMA) implemented the Centralised Procedure. This procedure is mandatory for biotechnology-derived products, orphan drugs and drugs designed for certain disease groups. Other products can be registered via the national route or using one of the other European procedures, namely the Mutual Recognition Procedure (MRP) or the Decentralised Procedure (DCP).

Regulation (EC) No 726/2004, as amended,[1] provides the legal basis for the Centralised Procedure and describes the marketing application and review processes specifically for biotechnology-derived products. The Centralised Procedure involves a single application; a single evaluation of the highest possible standard for these products' quality, safety and efficacy; and a single authorisation allowing direct access to the entire Community market. This regulation also established the Committee for Medicinal Products for Human Use (CHMP, previously CPMP (Committee for Proprietary Medicinal Products)) as part of EMA. Following a positive CHMP opinion, the European Commission makes the final decision about granting a MA. This regulation reinforced the need for a centralised approval process for products derived from biotechnology and for new active substances for certain therapeutic areas.

An MA granted through the Centralised Procedure is valid for the entire Community market. The Marketing Authorisation Holder (MAH) has one European licence to market the product, rather than individual national licences in EU Member States. Consequently, a medicinal product may be marketed in all EU Member States; however, it is still necessary to arrange price and reimbursement on a country-by-country basis. This is unlikely to change in the near future because financial aspects of the medicinal product supply are still regulated by national laws.

Registration Procedures of Biotechnology Products

Products Eligible for the Centralised Procedure

Community authorisation via the Centralised Procedure is compulsory for products appearing in the annex to Regulation (EC) No 726/2004, as amended. These include:

1. Medicinal products developed via one of the following biotechnological processes:
   - recombinant DNA technology
   - controlled expression of gene coding for biologically active proteins in prokaryotes and eukaryotes, including transformed mammalian cells
   - hybridoma and monoclonal antibody methods
2. Advanced therapy medicinal products:
   - gene therapy medicinal products
   - somatic cell therapy medicinal products
   - tissue-engineered products
   - combination (with medical device) advanced medicinal products
3. Medicinal products for human use containing a new active substance that, on the date of entry into force of this Regulation, was not authorised in the Community and for which the therapeutic indication is the treatment of any of the following diseases:
   - acquired immune deficiency syndrome
   - cancer
   - neurodegenerative disorder
   - diabetes
   and, with effect from 20 May 2008:
   - auto-immune diseases and other immune dysfunctions
   - viral diseases
4. Medicinal products designed as orphan medicinal products pursuant to Regulation (EC) No 141/2000[2]

Community authorisation via the Centralised Procedure is optional for certain product types detailed in Article 3 of Regulation (EC)No 726/2004:
- medicinal products containing new active substances not authorised in the Community at the date of entry into force of the regulation
- medicinal products for which a significant therapeutic, scientific or technical innovation can be demonstrated in the interest of patients' health

Similar biological ("biosimilar") medicinal products that are developed by means of biotechnological processes must be authorised via the Centralised Procedure.

Centralised Procedure

The Centralised Procedure is described in detail in *The Rules Governing Medicinal Products in the European Union, Notice to Applicants, Volume 2A*, Chapter 4.[3] A summary of the Centralised Procedure is provided in Chapter 17 Overview of Authorisation Procedures for Medicinal Products and Chapter 19 Registration Procedures for Medicinal Products of this publication.

EMA issues specific presubmission guidance for applications under the Centralised Procedure. An eligibility request must be submitted within 18 months prior to the intended submission date. An eligibility request form is available, and dates for submission of requests, linked to CHMP meeting dates, are given in the presubmission guidance.

EMA encourages applicants to request a presubmission meeting with the agency to discuss the authorisation process. This meeting should take place approximately seven months prior to submission.[4] Whether a meeting is scheduled or not, the applicant must notify EMA of its intention to submit an application seven months prior to submission.

A rapporteur and co-rapporteur, who are CHMP members, are assigned to a particular application to assess the product's quality, safety and efficacy. Applicants may indicate in a letter of intent (to submit an application) their request for appointment of a rapporteur and co-rapporteur. These requests should be received approximately seven months prior to the intended submission date and at least two weeks prior to a CHMP meeting so the appointment can take place six months prior to submission. The names of the rapporteur and co-rapporteur are communicated to the applicant before the start of the evaluation process.

Medicinal products authorised via the Centralised Procedure after implementation of the amended legislation (20 November 2005) have eight years of data protection and a 10-year market exclusivity period in all EU Member States, Liechtenstein, Norway and Iceland. Products for which the initial submission was made prior to this time continue to benefit from the previous period of protection, which is 10 years for products approved via the Centralised Procedure.

Applications in Exceptional Circumstances

Article 14(8) of Regulation (EC) No 726/2004 permits authorisations to be issued in exceptional circumstances, including a situation where the applicant is unable to provide the normal efficacy and safety data because the indication is rarely encountered. In such cases, it rarely will be possible to generate the full data; hence, the authorisation will not be converted into a "normal" MA.

The grounds for claiming exceptional circumstances are detailed in Annex I of Directive 2001/83/EC, as amended.[5] Conditions relating to the product's safety, notification of adverse events and actions taken are described in detail in the *Guideline on Procedures for the Granting of a Marketing Authorisation Under Exceptional Circumstances* (EMEA/357981/2005).[6]

The authorisation's continuation is linked to an annual assessment of these conditions.

Conditional Authorisation

Regulation (EC) No 507/2006 permits the granting of a conditional licence, valid for one year, where there is specific patient need.[7] Possible examples include products for life-threatening diseases, designated orphan medicinal products and medicinal products for use in emergency situations.

Applications should contain—unless otherwise justified—the same quality and nonclinical data as for a normal authorisation.[8] The applicant will be required to finalise ongoing clinical trials or conduct new studies to verify a presumed positive risk:benefit balance. The authorisation is subject to specific obligations that are reviewed annually. The authorisation will not remain conditional. Once the missing data are provided, the conditional MA becomes a "normal" MA. If appropriate, sponsors applying for conditional authorisations may also apply for accelerated assessment.

Accelerated Assessment Procedure

A legal provision was introduced in Regulation (EC) No 726/2004, Article 14(9) for the applicant to formally request an accelerated evaluation. This procedure applies to products that represent a therapeutic innovation and are of major interest to public health. The 210-day assessment period is reduced to 150 days.[9] (For more details about the Centralised Procedure, see Chapter 17 Overview of Authorisation Procedures for Medicinal Products and Chapter 19 Registration Procedures for Medicinal Products.)

Advantages and Disadvantages of the Centralised Procedure

While the Centralised Procedure has proven to be efficient, it is, in any case, mandatory for biotechnology products.

Important new features introduced in 2005 included an expanded scope of the procedure, establishment of a procedure for conditional MAs, formalisation of an accelerated procedure and available assistance for small and medium-sized enterprises (SMEs).[10]

It also has some disadvantages. One of the main drawbacks is the requirement that the product be made available in all 27 EU countries plus Norway, Iceland and Liechtenstein; selective filing or withdrawals are not possible, whether the MAH has a commercial interest in a particular country or not.

Among other things, this requirement involves preparing the Summary of Product Characteristics (SmPC), patient leaflet and labelling—and, subsequently, the mock-ups—in all 24 EU languages, in accordance with the Quality Review of Documents (QRD) templates.

Another potential Centralised Procedure problem is the requirement that the product have only one EU trade name.

Normally, only one invented name can be used for a product registered via the Centralised Procedure. A guideline (CPMP/328/98)[11] is available on features of proposed invented names that tend to give rise to public health concerns. The guideline describes the EMA criteria for identifying difficulties with such names:

- misleading therapeutic or pharmaceutical connotations
- misleading with respect to product composition
- likely to cause confusion in print, handwriting or speech with the trade name of an existing medicinal product

The applicant should use the request form to submit the proposed name at most 12 months, and at least four to six months, prior to the planned submission date. The (Invented) Name Review Group (NRG), a satellite group of CHMP, considers proposals, which are then presented at a subsequent CHMP meeting. Submission dates with respect to NRG/CHMP meetings are provided in the presubmission guidance. An additional form is available for justifying a previously unacceptable invented name.

In general, a minimum of three letters distinguishing the proposed trade name from an existing trade name are required. In practice, the requirement for one legally and linguistically acceptable trade name in all EU Member States has proven to be a challenge for the industry.

Another possible Centralised Procedure disadvantage is that, following the issuance of the MA, the European Public Assessment Report (EPAR) is made available via the EMA website. The sponsor has the opportunity to delete commercially sensitive, confidential information before it is published, but the EPAR still gives the competition a good idea of the basis for product approval.

Maintenance of the Marketing Authorisation
Once a product has been granted a Community MA, any postauthorisation regulatory activities, e.g., variations or renewals, must be done via the Centralised Procedure.

Variations
The MAH has an obligation to update the MA by variation applications as new data emerge. This is particularly important for new information that affects the risk:benefit balance.

A large proportion of variations relate to changes in the dossier's chemical-pharmaceutical section, i.e., Module 3 in the Common Technical Document (CTD). In January 2010, previous legislation was replaced by Regulation (EC) No 1234/2008[12] to provide a simpler and more flexible legal framework for the handling of variations.

The primary change allows annual reporting of all Type IA variations within the 12-month period following the implementation of the variations. However, for some of these minor changes, notification submitted immediately after the implementation of the variation is required (Type IA_{IN}).

Detailed dossier requirements, per variation type, are described in the regulation and guidances.

(For more details about variations, see Chapter 24 Pharmaceutical Postmarketing Requirements and Compliance.)

Renewals
An MA is valid for five years and will then be renewed based on a reevaluation of the risk:benefit balance. Once renewed, the MA is valid for an unlimited period unless there are justified grounds related to pharmacovigilance. In such a case, one additional five-year authorisation would be necessary.

The frequency of Periodic Safety Update Report (PSUR) submissions has been increased to compensate for the reduced requirements related to renewals.

Development Aspects Particular to Biotechnology Products
An MA for a biotechnology-derived product for human use will be granted following assessment of its quality, safety and efficacy. Although details of the assessment differ among the various authorities, the approval criteria are generally similar in the EU and US. Biotechnology products must fulfil the same basic quality, safety and efficacy criteria as any other pharmaceutical product. In addition, all general requirements—such as Good Laboratory Practice (GLP), Good Clinical Practice (GCP), Good Manufacturing Practice (GMP) and the need to have a manufacturing licence—also apply equally to biotechnology and conventional products.

Along with the standard regulatory requirements, however, a number of issues are specific to biotechnology products.

Quality—Chemical, Pharmaceutical and Biological Information
Development Pharmaceutics
A fair number of guidelines describe specific production and testing requirements for various biotechnology-derived product types. Many of these have been developed as International Conference on Harmonisation (ICH) guidelines and are applicable in the EU, US and Japan, as well as other countries that recognise ICH.

The section on development pharmaceutics (CTD Module 3.2.P.2, detailed in ICH guideline Q8(R2)[13]) is an important part of any EU dossier. It requires special attention for biotechnology products (ICH guidelines Q5D[14]). Underlying physicochemical differences between biological/biotechnological products and chemically synthesised products may necessitate special pharmaceutical and biopharmaceutical considerations during the research and development programme. For instance, to maintain biological activity, the active moiety's integrity must be preserved biologically and chemically during the manufacturing process and throughout the defined shelf life, requiring design of appropriate stability-indicating assays.

Rationale and experimental processes that lead to a finalised manufacturing process and established product specifications usually require a more elaborate description than is required for a conventional product. This description includes nonactive constituent selection and role, process development and optimisation, reason for cell line choice, etc. While conventional products often reference standard pharmaceutical techniques or excipients, this is not an option for biotechnology products.

Manufacturing Information
Production of biotechnological drug substances requires high-quality processes and testing, including a detailed description of source material and production strain or cell line preparation, genetic stability testing, cell bank system details, fermentation and harvesting information, purification details, a full product characterisation, analytical development of the special techniques involved, process validation and a detailed explanation of potential impurities, including batch results.

Biotechnology product quality is defined by the production and manufacturing process. Minor process changes can affect the drug product's quality. Detailed establishment of the manufacturing process is, therefore, of paramount importance. It must be known which manufacturing parameters (e.g., pH, heat, shear) can affect the drug substance's quality and stability in a formulated product to ensure consistency. This is particularly important in relation to scaling up the manufacturing process. In contrast to traditional drugs, biotechnology products typically are complex and labile proteins. For authentic *in vivo* activity, the primary amino acid sequence is essential, as are the secondary linkages and tertiary folding of the molecule to reveal the appropriate functional sites. Small changes in structure can radically alter the *in vivo* immunogenicity and pharmacokinetics of proteins.

Because of biotechnology products' physicochemical properties, it is usually not possible to terminally sterilise them in the final container by autoclaving. In most instances, they are sterilised by membrane filtration before filling. Aseptic techniques are an absolute requirement.

Compatibility with excipients and primary packaging components requires special attention. When infusion sets are used to administer the product in the clinic, compatibility studies with the infusion lines, filters and fluids are necessary.

Transmissible Spongiform Encephalopathy (TSE)
After many years of heated discussions and near bans on the use of ingredients of animal origin in medicinal products, the EU situation has stabilised. Concern about the use of animal ingredients is related to the potential for causing transmissible spongiform encephalopathy (TSE). Scrapie in sheep and goats, bovine spongiform encephalopathy (BSE) in cattle and Creutzfeldt-Jakob disease (CJD) in humans all belong to the TSE family.

TSE is believed to be caused by prion proteins and not associated genetic material. TSE agents are difficult to destroy; such conventional sterilisation methods as autoclaving at 121ºC for 15 minutes and dry heat processes such as 160ºC for one hour or irradiation at 25 kGy, do not inactivate the agents. Because TSE-associated diseases, particularly CJD, are incurable and fatal, the policy has aimed to eliminate the use of tissues at particular risk for carrying BSE.

Unfortunately, the pharmaceutical industry uses many materials from bovine, ovine or caprine sources and their derivatives. Many organs, tissues and sera, such as heparin, glucagons, lactose, foetal calf serum and bovine serum albumin, are used as raw material sources. Materials are extracted from hair and wool, and derivatives of materials of animal origin (in particular gelatine and tallow derivatives) are used in many pharmaceutical products. In addition, animal tissues are used to manufacture incubation media for the production of biotechnology products. Banning the use of bovine-derived materials in producing pharmaceuticals would have resulted in removal of a vast range of products from the European market. Instead, EU legislation has been amended to require the applicant to demonstrate that the medicinal product is manufactured in accordance with a *Note for Guidance on Minimising the Risk of TSE*.[15–17]

The ultimate goal still is to replace all ingredients of animal origin in human medicinal products with vegetable-derived or synthetic materials, using the appropriate variation procedures. Animal-derived materials may still be used, at least temporarily, provided compliance with the requirements is demonstrated by:
- submitting detailed information on animal materials used, including manufacturing procedure details, to the Competent Authorities
- submitting a European Pharmacopoeia (Ph. Eur.) certificate of TSE compliance (Certificate of Suitability)[18]

The information required in both cases is the same. The difference in the second case is that the information must be assessed only once, as the Certificate of Suitability is recognised by both the 28 signatory states of the European Pharmacopoeia Convention and the EU. The manufacturers or suppliers of any drug substance or excipient with TSE risk that is used in producing or preparing pharmaceutical products can apply to the European Directorate for the Quality of Medicines (EDQM) for a certificate evaluating TSE risk reduction according to a specific TSE monograph. A full dossier on the substance's manufacturing method and associated impurities must be sent to EDQM. The dossier is reviewed by independent experts. Once a certificate is issued, the applicant can include it in the dossier as proof the substance concerned will not pose a TSE risk.

The Certificate of Suitability can be used every time the particular substance is used in the production of any medicinal product. In contrast, when the first route is followed, each Competent Authority must make the assessment separately for every final product application. The Competent Authorities strongly encourage the use of the certification scheme. The information required is as follows:
- geographic source of the animals from which materials are derived (some countries are considered higher risk than others)
- nature of the animal tissue used in manufacture (certain tissues carry a higher risk)
- production and inactivation processes

No single approach necessarily establishes a product's safety. Therefore, these three approaches should be used in combination in assessing an ingredient's risk in pharmaceutical production.

Information regarding the raw material source and manufacturing processes must be supplemented with information regarding the material's traceability and a summary of the auditing procedures employed to demonstrate control over the material's source.

Viral Clearance
When ingredients of animal or human origin are used in producing a medicinal product, the capacity of the manufacturing process to remove all viral contamination is vitally

important. Testing and evaluating biotechnology products' viral safety are standard requirements.[19] The three complementary approaches for addressing viral safety are:
- selecting and testing cell lines and other raw materials, including media components, for the absence of undesirable viruses that may be infectious or pathogenic to humans
- assessing the capacity of the production process to clear infectious viruses by virus inactivation and virus removal
- testing the product at appropriate production steps for the absence of contaminating infectious viruses

All three approaches are necessary to establish product safety, and it is crucial to demonstrate that the purification regimen can remove and inactivate the viruses. Viral clearance requirements continue to become more stringent and—although there may be differences in implementing certain requirements—global regulatory requirements are comparable.

Release Testing in Europe
When a medicinal product is manufactured outside the EU/EEA and imported into the market, release testing must be performed on every batch in the EU/EEA. Therefore, a company should carefully consider which tests to list under release specifications and which could be considered in-process or bulk final product tests. The repeat testing requirement applies to all tests presented as final product release tests. Although this requirement is not specific to biotechnology products, the complexity of some release tests, the often small batch sizes and significant product cost may necessitate special attention to this issue.

Preclinical Information
Regulatory standards for biotechnology-derived products generally are comparable across the EU, Japan and the US. All regions have adopted a flexible, case-by-case, science-based approach to preclinical safety evaluations.[20,21]

Safety concerns may arise from the product itself and/or from the presence of impurities or contaminants. Cellular host contaminants may result in allergic reactions and other immunopathological effects. As is the case for conventional products, the product used in the pivotal pharmacology and toxicology studies should be comparable to the product proposed for clinical studies.

Toxicity studies are expected to be performed in compliance with GLP.

Conventional pharmaceutical toxicity testing may not be appropriate for biopharmaceuticals due to their unique and diverse structural and biological properties, which may include species specificity, immunogenicity and unpredicted pleiotropic activities.

In vitro studies usually play an important role in pharmacological testing of these substances to determine product properties. They also help select an appropriate animal species for further *in vivo* pharmacology and toxicology studies.

The *in vivo* safety evaluation should involve relevant animal species (i.e., species in which the test material is pharmacologically active due to the expression of the receptor or an epitope). The species commonly used for conventional products are not necessarily relevant for biotech products. Normally, safety evaluations should include two species; in justified cases, one relevant species may suffice (when only one relevant species can be determined or when the biopharmaceutical's biological activity is well understood). Toxicity studies in nonrelevant species are discouraged. If there is no relevant species, the use of transgenic animals expressing the human receptor, gene knockout animal models or homologous proteins should be considered. When these models or proteins are not available, it still may be prudent to assess some aspects of potential toxicity in limited toxicity evaluations. For instance, a repeat-dose toxicity study of a few weeks' duration that includes an evaluation of important functional endpoints (e.g., cardiovascular and respiratory) might be performed.

Many biotechnology-derived products for human use are immunogenic in animals, whether through binding antibodies, neutralising antibodies and/or allergic reactions to the intended medicinal product or one of its impurities (cell substrates, media components, fragments, aggregates). Antibody responses should be characterised (titre, number of responding animals, neutralising or non-neutralising), and their appearance should be correlated with any pharmacological or toxicological changes.

Antibody detection should not be the sole criterion for the early termination of a preclinical safety study unless the immune response neutralises the product's pharmacological and/or toxicological effects in a large proportion of animals.

Nevertheless, the usefulness of preclinical animal studies may be limited to repeat-dose studies or intermittent dosing studies of limited duration in a model as closely related to humans as possible. Immunogenicity and toxicokinetic data should be obtained after the first and nth dose in repeat-dose studies. Local tolerance must also be determined, if applicable.

A factor to consider when designing a biotechnology product's preclinical development program is the available quantity of test material. Especially in the early development phases, products of adequate quality may be available only in small quantities and at high costs.

Clinical Information
Clinical studies must be tailor-made for each medicinal product and should consider the route of administration, indication, intended treatment population, treatment duration,

etc. Several guidelines have been published by CHMP on each therapeutic area and are available on EMA's website.

Due to the nature of biotechnology products, immunogenic reactions are not unexpected and must be considered when determining the optimal posology.

In addition, the EPARs published on other biotechnology products can be useful sources of information. These EPARs also are available on EMA's website.

Comparability Guideline

Medicinal products of biotechnological origin are often subject to manufacturing process changes (drug substance, drug product or both) during the development phase or after the MA has been granted. In either case, it is necessary to compare the product derived from the modified process with the one derived from the current process to confirm that the change did not alter the product's physicochemical and biological characteristics. A change in these characteristics may lead to a different safety or efficacy profile.

The means of demonstrating comparability in either case—that is, one (or a related) manufacturer amending its own process or a product claiming similarity to a product already on the market (generic/"biosimilar")—should be identical.

Comparability must be shown for product quality, safety and efficacy in a sequential process.[22,23] Even changes classified as minor may result in relevant quality profile modifications for a biotechnology product.

As an initial approach when introducing a process change, the following parameters, on which specifications have been based, should be considered key:
- characterisation studies
- validated manufacturing process
- release data
- stability data
- in wider perspectives, preclinical and clinical experiences

Parameters should be evaluated in a step-by-step manner when discussing comparability. Of primary importance is the ability of analytical techniques to detect slight or discrete modifications to the characteristics of biotechnology-derived products. The manufacturer must provide evidence that the analytical method has the sensitivity and selectivity to discern such changes.

Products Claiming to be Similar to One Already Marketed—Biosimilars

"Biosimilar" or "follow-on biologic" are terms used to describe copies of innovator biotechnological products. At present, the term "generic" is not applied to products derived from biotechnology processes.

Biologics' specificity has created a concern that copies of products might perform differently from the original version of the drug. In the EU, a specially adapted regulatory framework has been developed for certain protein drugs, termed "similar biological medicinal products."[24–26] This framework is based on a thorough demonstration of comparability of the biosimilar product to an existing approved product. Product-specific guidelines have been published in Europe.[27–31] Some others have been released for consultation.[32,33]

Similar biological medicinal products are manufactured and controlled according to their own development, taking into account relevant and up-to-date information.

Comparison can be made against the official data, e.g., pharmacopoeial monographs, or against other published scientific data. However, such comparisons at the level of both drug substance and drug product are limited and not sufficient to establish all aspects pertinent to the evaluation. Consequently, an extensive comparability exercise will be required to demonstrate that the similar biological medicinal product has a quality, safety and efficacy profile analogous to the reference medicinal product.

It is acknowledged that the manufacturer developing similar biological medicinal products will normally not have access to all necessary information to allow an exhaustive comparison with the reference medicinal product. Nevertheless, the level of detail must be such that firm conclusions can be reached.

Based on the comparability approach and supported by sufficiently sensitive analytical systems, the comparability exercise at the quality level may allow a reduction of the nonclinical and clinical data requirements compared to a full dossier. The similar biological medicinal product may refer to the reference product's previously generated nonclinical and clinical data; however, nonclinical and clinical data will normally be required as identified in related nonclinical and clinical guidelines on similar biological medicinal products.

Summary

In the EU, medicinal products derived from biotechnology can only be registered using the Centralised Procedure, resulting in one EU licence that is valid in all EU Member States.

Biotechnology products' special and sensitive nature requires a chemical-biological-pharmaceutical and preclinical development program that is specific to the concerned product. These requirements are described in ICH and EMA guidelines.

The manufacturer should also demonstrate compliance with the *Note for Guidance on Minimising the Risk of Transmitting Animal Spongiform Encephalopathy Agents via Human and Veterinary Medicinal Products*.

References

1. Regulation (EC) No 726/2004, as amended, of the European Parliament and of the Council of 31 March 2004 laying down Community procedures for the authorisation and supervision of medicinal products for human and veterinary use and establishing a European Medicines Agency (Consolidated version 20 April 2009). EC website. http://ec.europa.eu/health/files/eudralex/vol-1/reg_2004_726_cons/reg_2004_726_cons_en.pdf. Accessed 11 May 2012.
2. Regulation (EC) No 141/2000 of the European Parliament and of the Council of 16 December 1999 on orphan medicinal products. EUR-Lex website. http://eur-lex.europa.eu/LexUriServ/LexUriServ.do?uri=OJ:L:2000:018:0001:0005:en:PDF. Accessed 11 May 2012.
3. European Commission. *The Rules Governing Medicinal Products in the European Union, Notice to Applicants: Volume 2A*, "Chapter 4 — Centralised Procedure," April 2006. EC website. http://ec.europa.eu/health/files/eudralex/vol-2/a/chap4rev200604_en.pdf. Accessed 11 May 2012.
4. European Medicines Agency. *European Medicines Agency pre-authorisation procedural advice for users of the centralised procedure*, February 2012 (EMA/339324/2007). EMA website. www.ema.europa.eu/docs/en_GB/document_library/Regulatory_and_procedural_guideline/2009/10/WC500004069.pdf. Accessed 11 May 2012.
5. Directive 2001/83/EC, as amended, of the European Parliament and of the Council of 6 November 2001 on the Community code relating to medicinal products for human use (Consolidated version: 05/10/2009). EMA website. www.emea.europa.eu/docs/en_GB/document_library/Regulatory_and_procedural_guideline/2009/10/WC500004481.pdf. Accessed 11 May 2012.
6. Guideline on procedures for the granting of a marketing authorisation under exceptional circumstances, pursuant to Article 14 (8) of Regulation (EC) 726/2004, 15 December 2005 (EMEA/357981/2005). EMA website. www.ema.europa.eu/docs/en_GB/document_library/Regulatory_and_procedural_guideline/2009/10/WC500004883.pdf. Accessed 11 May 2012.
7. Commission Regulation (EC) No 507/2006 of 29 March 2006 on the conditional marketing authorisation for medicinal products for human use falling within the scope of Regulation (EC) 726/2004 of the European Parliament and of the Council. EC website. http://ec.europa.eu/health/files/eudralex/vol-1/reg_2006_507/reg_2006_507_en.pdf. Accessed 11 May 2012.
8. Guideline on the scientific application and the practical arrangements necessary to implement Commission Regulation (EC) 507/2006 on the conditional marketing authorisation for medicinal products for human use falling within the scope of Regulation (EC) 726/2004, 5 December 2006 (EMEA/509951/2006). EMA website. www.emea.europa.eu/docs/en_GB/document_library/Scientific_guideline/2009/10/WC500004908.pdf. Accessed 11 May 2012.
9. Guideline on the procedure for accelerated assessment pursuant to article 14 (9) of Regulation (EC) 726/2004, 17 July 2006 (EMEA/419127/05). EMA website. www.ema.europa.eu/docs/en_GB/document_library/Regulatory_and_procedural_guideline/2009/10/WC500004136.pdf. Accessed 11 May 2012.
10. Commission Regulation (EC) No 2049/2005, of 15 December laying down, pursuant to regulation (EC) No 726/2004 of the European Parliament and of the Council, rules regarding the payment of fees to, and the receipt of administrative assistance from, the European Medicine Agency by micro, small and medium-sized enterprises. EC website. http://ec.europa.eu/health/files/eudralex/vol-1/reg_2005_2049/reg_2005_2049_en.pdf. Accessed 11 May 2012.
11. Guideline on the acceptability of trade names for human medicinal products processed through the centralised procedure, 11 December 2007 (CPMP/328/98, Revision 5). EMA website. www.emea.europa.eu/docs/en_GB/document_library/Regulatory_and_procedural_guideline/2009/10/WC500004142.pdf. Accessed 11 May 2012.
12. Commission Regulation (EC) No 1234/2008 of 24 November 2008 concerning the examination of variations to the terms of marketing authorisations for medicinal products for human use and veterinary medicinal products. EUR-Lex website.http://eur-lex.europa.eu/LexUriServ/LexUriServ.do?uri=OJ:L:2008:334:0007:0007:EN:PDF. Accessed 11 May 2012.
13. ICH Q8(R2) *Pharmaceutical Development*, August 2009. ICH website. www.ich.org/fileadmin/Public_Web_Site/ICH_Products/Guidelines/Quality/Q8_R1/Step4/Q8_R2_Guideline.pdf. Accessed 11 May 2012.
14. ICH Q5D *Quality of biotechnological products: derivation and characterisation of cell substrates used for production of biotechnological/biological products*, 16 July 1997. ICH website. www.ich.org/fileadmin/Public_Web_Site/ICH_Products/Guidelines/Quality/Q5D/Step4/Q5D_Guideline.pdf. Accessed 11 May 2012.
15. *Note for guidance on minimising the risk of transmitting animal spongiform encephalopathy agents via human and veterinary medicinal products*, 1 July 2011 (EMA/410/01, Revision 3). EMA website. www.ema.europa.eu/docs/en_GB/document_library/Scientific_guideline/2009/09/WC500003698.pdf. Accessed 11 May 2012.
16. *EMEA/CPMP/BWP/498/01, Joint CPMP/CVMP Note for guidance on minimising the risk of transmitting animal spongiform encephalopathy agents via human and veterinary medicinal products, explanatory note for medicinal products for human use on the scope of the guideline*, 28 February 2001 (EMEA/CPMP/BWP/498/01). EMA website. www.ema.europa.eu/docs/en_GB/document_library/Scientific_guideline/2009/09/WC500003712.pdf. Accessed 11 May 2012.
17. *Questions and Answers on Bovine Spongiform Encephalopathies (BSE) and Vaccines*, 24 April 2001 (EMEA/CPMP/BWP/819/01). EMA website. www.ema.europa.eu/docs/en_GB/document_library/Other/2009/09/WC500003715.pdf. Accessed 11 May 2012.
18. Resolution AP-CSP (99)4 of the Council of Europe, Public Health Committee, certification of suitability to the monographs of the European pharmacopoeia (revised version), 22 December 1999.
19. *Note for guidance on quality of biotechnological products: viral safety evaluation of biotechnology products derived from cell lines of human or animal origin*, October 1997 (CPMP/ICH/295/95). EMA website. www.ema.europa.eu/docs/en_GB/document_library/Scientific_guideline/2009/09/WC500002801.pdf. Accessed 11 May 2012.
20. ICH S6(R1) *Preclinical safety evaluation of biotechnology-derived pharmaceuticals*, June 2011. ICH website. www.ich.org/fileadmin/Public_Web_Site/ICH_Products/Guidelines/Safety/S6_R1/Step4/S6_R1_Guideline.pdf. Accessed 11 May 2012.
21. ICH S8 *Immunotoxicity studies for human pharmaceuticals*, May 2006. ICH website. www.ich.org/fileadmin/Public_Web_Site/ICH_Products/Guidelines/Safety/S8/Step4/S8_Guideline.pdf. Accessed 11 May 2012.
22. ICH Q5E *Note for guidance on biotechnological/biological products subject to changes in their manufacturing process*, June 2005. ICH website. www.ich.org/fileadmin/Public_Web_Site/ICH_Products/Guidelines/Quality/Q5E/Step4/Q5E_Guideline.pdf. Accessed 11 May 2012.
23. *Guideline on comparability of biotechnology-derived medicinal products after a change in the manufacturing process—non-clinical and clinical issues*, 19 July 2007 (EMEA/CHMP/BMWP/101695/2006). EMA website. www.ema.europa.eu/docs/en_GB/document_library/Scientific_guideline/2009/09/WC500003935.pdf. Accessed 11 May 2012.
24. *Guideline on similar biological medicinal products*, 30 October 2005 (CHMP/437/04). EMA website. www.emea.europa.eu/docs/en_GB/document_library/Scientific_guideline/2009/09/WC500003517.pdf. Accessed 11 May 2012.
25. *Guideline on similar biological medicinal products containing biotechnology-derived proteins as active substance: quality issues*, 22 February 2006 (EMEA/CHMP/BWP/49348/2005). EMA website. www.ema.europa.eu/docs/en_GB/document_library/Scientific_guideline/2009/09/WC500003953.pdf. Accessed 11 May 2012.
26. *Guideline on similar biological medicinal products containing biotechnology-derived proteins as active substance: non-clinical and clinical*

issues, 22 February 2006 (EMEA/CHMP/BMWP/42832/2005). EMA website. www.emea.europa.eu/docs/en_GB/document_library/Scientific_guideline/2009/09/WC500003920.pdf. Accessed 11 May 2012.
27. Reflection paper, *Non-clinical and clinical developments of similar medicinal products containing recombinant interferon alfa*, 23 April 2009 (EMEA/CHMP/BMWP/102046/2006). EMA website. www.ema.europa.eu/docs/en_GB/document_library/Scientific_guideline/2009/09/WC500003931.pdf. Accessed 11 May 2012.
28. *Guideline on non-clinical and clinical development of similar biological medicinal products containing recombinant erythropoietins (Revision)*, 18 March 2010 (EMEA/CHMP/BMWP/301636/2008 Corr.). EMA website. www.ema.europa.eu/docs/en_GB/document_library/Scientific_guideline/2010/04/WC500089474.pdf. Accessed 11 May 2012.
29. *Concept paper on the revision of the guideline on non-clinical and clinical development of similar biological medicinal products containing recombinant human insulin*, 21 July 2011 (EMEA/CHMP/BMWP/506470/2011). EMA website. www.ema.europa.eu/docs/en_GB/document_library/Scientific_guideline/2011/07/WC500109587.pdf. Accessed 11 May 2012.
30. *Annex to guideline on similar biological medicinal products containing biotechnology-derived proteins as active substance: non-clinical and clinical issues* (EMEA/CHMP/BMWP/94528/2005). EMA website. www.ema.europa.eu/docs/en_GB/document_library/Scientific_guideline/2009/09/WC500003956.pdf. Accessed 11 May 2012. *Guidance on similar medicinal products containing somatropin*, 22 February 2006.
31. *Annex to guideline on similar biological medicinal products containing biotechnology-derived proteins as active substance: non-clinical and clinical issues* (EMEA/CHMP/BMWP/31329/2005). EMA website. www.ema.europa.eu/docs/en_GB/document_library/Scientific_guideline/2009/09/WC500003955.pdf. Accessed 11 May 2012. *Guidance on similar medicinal products containing recombinant granulocyte-colony stimulating factor*, 22 February 2006.
32. *Concept paper on the development of a guideline on similar biological medicinal products containing monoclonal antibodies* (EMEA/CHMP/BMWP/632613/2009). EMA website. www.ema.europa.eu/docs/en_GB/document_library/Scientific_guideline/2009/11/WC500014438.pdf. Accessed 11 May 2012.
33. *Concept paper on immunogenicity assessment of monoclonal antibodies intended for in vivo clinical use* (EMEA/CHMP/114720/09). EMA website. www.emea.europa.eu/docs/en_GB/document_library/Scientific_guideline/2009/09/WC500003910.pdf. Accessed 11 May 2012.

Chapter 24

Pharmaceutical Postmarket Requirements and Compliance With the Marketing Authorisation

Updated by Nicole Beard, MSc, PhD

OBJECTIVES

❏ Understand the postmarket requirements of Marketing Authorisation Holders in the EU

❏ Understand regulations regarding postmarket commitments

❏ Understand the variations to Marketing Authorisation Applications

❏ Understand renewal requirements

REGULATIONS AND DIRECTIVES COVERED IN THIS CHAPTER

❏ Regulation (EC) No 726/2004 of the European Parliament and of the Council of 31 March 2004 laying down Community procedures for the authorisation and supervision of medicinal products for human and veterinary use and establishing a European Medicines Agency, as amended (Consolidated version 20 April 2009)

❏ Directive 2001/83/EC of the European Parliament and of the Council of 6 November 2001 on the Community code relating to medicinal products for human use, as amended, with further amendments (Consolidated version 5 October 2009)

❏ Commission Regulation (EC) No 1234/2008 of 24 November 2008 concerning the examination of variations to the terms of marketing authorisations for medicinal products for human use and veterinary medicinal products

❏ Communication from the Commission 2009/C 323/04, Guideline on the operation of the procedures laid down in Chapters II, III and IV of Commission Regulation (EC) No 1234/2008 concerning the examination of variations to the terms of marketing authorisations for medicinal products for human use and veterinary medicinal products

❏ Communication from the Commission, 2010/C 17/01, Guideline on the details of the various categories of variations to the terms of marketing authorisations for medicinal products for human use and veterinary medicinal products

❏ Directive 2009/53/EC of the European Parliament and of the Council of 18 June 2009 amending Directive 2001/82/EC and Directive 2001/83/EC, as regards variations to the terms of marketing authorisations for medicinal products

Introduction

In accordance with Directive 2001/83/EC, as amended,[1] a medicinal product Marketing Authorisation (MA) is granted initially for a five-year period. It is renewable upon application six months before expiration. Thus, no later than six months before the end of the five-year period, the Marketing Authorisation Holder (MAH) should apply for renewal of the MA, including all currently approved presentations. Usually, the MA will be valid indefinitely after the first renewal. In certain circumstances, the MAH has to make a commitment to gain a favourable opinion for renewal. In such cases, the MAH should provide additional data to support the product's quality, safety and efficacy profile. Outstanding issues are defined as specific obligations and follow-up measures. Such authorisations may be reviewed at more frequent intervals (on a yearly basis, for example).

The new pharmacovigilance legislation (Regulation (EU) No 1235/2010 and Directive 2010/84/EU) modifies both the submission deadline for renewals from six months to nine months as well as content requirements. Draft guidelines currently are under review.

Throughout the postmarket phase, the medicinal product must be manufactured in accordance with the Marketing Authorisation Application (MAA) submission. On the other hand, the quality of the medicinal product and its safety/efficacy information have to be continuously updated, taking into account scientific and technical progress as well as the product's safety data. In such cases, the MAH is required to make changes and variations that enable the medicinal product to be manufactured and checked by generally accepted scientific methods. If, during the postmarket phase, new safety data regarding the medicinal product become available, they must be carefully evaluated and submitted to the authorities as a variation to the MAA. Sometimes such variations result in changes to the product information (Summary of Product Characteristics (SmPC), labelling and Package Leaflet).

The MAH also is responsible for ensuring the use of the medicinal product is as safe and effective as possible. It is essential that pharmacovigilance activities be conducted throughout each drug product's lifecycle. Pharmacovigilance should include collecting and evaluating safety data from all available international sources.

Specific Obligations and Follow-up Measures

Specific Obligations

When an MA is granted under certain conditions or exceptional circumstances (Articles 14(7) and 14(8) of Regulation (EC) No 726/2004[2]), the MAH must submit postauthorisation data on a defined schedule. These additional data, known as specific obligations, are described in Annex IIC of the Committee for Medicinal Products for Human Use (CHMP) opinion and of the Commission decision with a specific deadline for each obligation. The specific obligations are to be reviewed at the intervals indicated and at least annually. The annual review includes a risk:benefit profile reassessment.

Follow-up Measures

In the case of any MA, whether granted under exceptional circumstances or not, CHMP can agree to allow the MAH to submit some outstanding data expected to ensure quality, safety or efficacy after the opinion. Outstanding issues of this type are defined as follow-up measures (FUMs). FUMs can be requested at the initial CHMP opinion or following CHMP assessment of any submitted additional data/applications.[3] FUMs should be spelled out in a work plan signed by a manufacturer's representative and annexed to the CHMP assessment report. The MAH must submit the FUMs within an agreed-upon timeframe, never exceeding five years.

Resulting Variation or Change Applications

To minimise processing and review time, MAHs are encouraged to submit any variation or change applications resulting from fulfilling specific obligations or FUMs simultaneously with that fulfilment.[3]

Non-fulfilment of Specific Obligations or FUMs

An MAH must indicate realistic target dates for the submission of the postauthorisation data in its Letter of Undertaking. If no documents are submitted or in case of non-fulfilment of the obligations, in accordance with Articles 14(7) and 14(8) of Regulation (EC) No 726/2004, CHMP will formulate an opinion recommending the "variation/suspension/revocation" of the MA.[4]

At the request of the European Medicines Agency (EMA), the Commission may impose financial penalties on MAHs under Regulation (EC) No 726/2004 if they fail to meet obligations linked to the authorisations.

Variations and Changes

MAHs are responsible for medicinal products on the marketplace throughout their lifecycle. MAHs also are required to track technical and scientific developments, and make any necessary amendments to enable the product to be manufactured and verified by generally accepted scientific methods. In addition, MAHs may wish to alter or improve the medicinal product or introduce additional safeguards. Such variations to the MA may require not only administrative data, but also more substantial information. The following section describes Centralised, Mutual Recognition and Decentralised Procedure variations. Regardless of whether the MA was approved via the Centralised, Mutual Recognition or Decentralised Procedure, Regulation (EC) No 1234/2008 applies.

Legal Basis

Before 1995, there was no consistent variation system in place for either the "Concertation Procedure" (for certain high-technology products) or the "Multi-State Procedure" (predecessor to the Mutual Recognition Procedure). In 1995, Commission Regulation (EC) No 541/95 came into force, defining a variation system for medicinal products authorised under either "ex-Concertation" Procedures or Mutual

Recognition Procedures, and for Community referral products. At the same time, Commission Regulation (EC) No 542/95 was implemented for products being authorised via the Centralised Procedure.

In 2003, a common approach to variation procedures was adopted that simplified the tasks of both industry and authorities.

Commission Regulation (EC) No 1084/2003 provided the legal basis for variation applications relating to MAs granted by Member States. It applied to products approved by the Mutual Recognition Procedure and the ex-Concertation Procedure, and to those that had been subject to a Community referral. The regulation replaced the previous requirements of Commission Regulation (EC) No 541/95, as amended by Commission Regulation (EC) No 1146/96.

Commission Regulation (EC) No 1085/2003 provided the legal basis for variation applications relating to centralised MAs. It replaced Commission Regulation (EC) No 542/95, as amended by Commission Regulation (EC) No 1069/98.

Both Regulations (EC) No 1084/2003 and (EC) No 1085/2003 took effect 1 October 2003 without any transition period.

A few years later, experiences of different stakeholders (authorities and industry) led to another revision of the legal framework to establish simpler, clearer and more flexible regulations for handling variations for all authorised medicinal products, including those authorised at a purely national level. The new *Variations Regulation*, Regulation No (EC) 1234/2008, was approved by the European Commission on 10 June 2008 and replaced both Regulations (EC) No 1084/2003 and (EC) No 1085/2003. It became mandatory on 1 January 2010 and applies to variations to MAs granted through the Decentralised, Mutual Recognition and Centralised Procedures. Currently, the new regulation is not applicable to variations for products authorised by purely National Procedures. For national approvals, a co-decision procedure has been carried out and adopted by the European Parliament and Council. However, a number of Member States have already adopted the new variations regulation and transposed it into national law.

With the new *Variations Regulation,* an update of the best practice guide in the Mutual Recognition Procedure has become available (CMDh/094/2003/Rev16).[5]

It must be remembered that the *Variations Regulation* does not apply to transfers of an MA from one MAH to another.

Classification of Variations

Variations to medicinal products can be classified in different categories, depending on the level of risk to public health and the impact on the concerned medicinal product's quality, safety and efficacy. Certain changes that have the highest potential impact on medicinal products' quality, safety or efficacy require a complete scientific assessment, the same as for the evaluation of new MAAs.[6]

The different types of MA variations (e.g., administrative, quality, safety, efficacy and pharmacovigilance) have been categorised:

- Type IA Variation: any well-defined, minor change with minimal or no impact on the concerned product's quality, safety or efficacy. The Type IA variation classification is listed in Annex II(1) of the *Variations Regulation*. These variations do not require prior approval before implementation ("Do and Tell" procedure) and are classified in two subcategories: Type IA_{IN} (requiring immediate notification) and Type IA (not requiring immediate notification). The review time is 30 calendar days following receipt of the documentation by the Competent Authority.

- Type II Variation: any major change to the MAH's proposed documentation with potentially significant impact on product quality, safety or efficacy. Type II variations require prior approval before implementation ("Prior authorisation" procedure). The standard assessment time is 60 days for the adoption of the opinion; however, the regulation includes the possibility of reducing or extending the review time (30 or 90 days, respectively).[7] Once the application is reviewed, an assessment report is written. The Type II variation classification is listed in Annex II(2) of the *Variations Regulation*.

- Minor Type IB Variations, which are neither classified as Type IA variations nor major Type II variations or extensions, are also considered notifications. Such minor variations (notifications) must be notified to the Competent Authority but do not require formal approval. However, the MAH must wait 30 days to ensure that the notification is deemed acceptable by the Competent Authority ("Tell, Wait and Do" procedure).[8]

- Line Extension Application: a major change that requires a full assessment in accordance with Article 17 of Directive 2001/83/EC (i.e., 210 days). The categories are listed in Annex I of the *Variations Regulation*.

- Urgent Safety Restriction (USR): an interim product information change resulting from new information with a bearing on the product's safe use, particularly concerning one or more of the following items in the SmPC: the indication(s), posology, contraindications, warnings, target species and withdrawal periods. This variation is used in the event of risk to public health. A USR shall be implemented within a timeframe agreed upon with the Competent Authority. The corresponding variation application must be submitted within 15 days of initiating the USR in accordance with Article 22 (3) of the *Variations Regulation*.

Detailed classification of variations together with information on the conditions to be fulfilled and documents to support the variation application are provided in the guideline on the details of the various categories of variations.[9]

Type IB by Default

If a change is not mentioned in Annex II of the *Variations Regulation* (or the classification guideline) or the conditions for a specific change could not be fulfilled and the change is not already classified as a Type II variation, this change can be submitted as a Type IB variation by default. However, if the change is supposed to have significant impact on the medicinal product's safety, efficacy or quality, it must be submitted as Type II variation.[10]

Unforeseen Variations

A variation is considered "unforeseen" when the proposed variation is not considered a minor variation of Type IB following the Commission classification guideline, or has not been classified as a Type IB variation in an Article 5 recommendation. When one or more of the conditions established in the guideline for a Type IA variation are not met, the concerned change may be submitted as a Type IB variation unless the change is specifically classified as a major variation of Type II. Prior to submission of a variation whose classification is not provided, the MAH may request the Competent Authority (Co-ordination Group for Mutual Recognition and Decentralised Procedures (CMDh) or, in the case of a centralised MA, by EMA) to provide a recommendation on the classification of the variation. This shall be delivered within 45 days following receipt of the request.

Grouping of Variations

Grouping of variations has been introduced with the new *Variations Regulation* to facilitate the review of the variations and reduce the administrative burden. Multiple variations of the same type to one or several MAs owned by the same MAH can be notified simultaneously to the same authority with a single variation application.

Groupings of variations can be used for:
- several Type IA or IA_{IN} variations affecting one medicinal product
- one Type IA or IA_{IN} variation affecting several medicinal products from the same MAH
- several Type IA and/or IA_{IN} variations affecting several medicinal products from the same MAH, provided those variations are the same for all medicinal products and are submitted to the same authority
- Type IA or IA_{IN} variations grouped with other types of variations (Type IB or II extensions)—such grouped variations will follow the review procedure of the highest variation in the group (It should be noted that when submitting Type IA/IA_{IN} variations as a part of a group, the legal deadlines for submission of each variation should be respected.[11])

Work-sharing Procedure

In order to avoid duplication of work, a work-sharing procedure was set up allowing submission of variations to be assessed by only one EU authority (Article 20 of the *Variations Regulation*). Work sharing is applicable for different medicinal products to which the same changes are expected to apply, provided that the variations are submitted by the same MAH. Work sharing is applicable for the same Type IB or Type II variations, group of the same variations and Type IA changes, if these are included in a group also containing Type IB or Type II variations. It is not applicable to line extensions.

The reference authority can be either EMA (if one of the MAs has been granted following the Centralised Procedure) or any Concerned Member State's national Competent Authority in all other cases, i.e., Mutual Recognition Procedure or Decentralised Procedure. In the latter situation, the reference authority will be chosen by CMDh, taking the recommendations from the MAH into account. The MAH is advised to announce an upcoming work-sharing procedure to CMDh at least three months in advance of the planned submission by means of a letter of intent for the submission.

It should be stressed that line extensions are excluded from work sharing. Furthermore, work sharing is not applicable to purely national MAs.

Dossier Requirements for Variations

A common application form for National, Centralised, Decentralised and Mutual Recognition Procedures, "Application for Variation to a Marketing Authorisation," should always be used. It contains the following information:
- type of procedure (Mutual Recognition, Decentralised, Centralised or National Procedure)
- type of variation (Type IA, Type IA_{IN}, Type IB unforeseen, Type IB foreseen, Type II, Type II Art. 29 (of Regulation (EC) 1901/2006), and additionally, if it is a single variation, grouping or work sharing
- for Type IB and Type II variations only, reason for change (indication, safety, safety following Urgent Safety Restriction, quality, annual variation for human influenza vaccines)
- administrative data

- products, including their invented names, active substance(s), pharmaceutical forms, strengths, MAH name, MA number and variation number
- type of change (the relevant section of the classification guideline)
- scope and background of the change and justification for grouping, work sharing and classification of unforeseen variation (if applicable)
- other related application(s), if any
- present and proposed situation/wording
- declarations of the applicant
- proposed implementation date
- applicant signature(s)

In addition to the application form, the following documents should be submitted to the Competent Authority(ies):
- cover letter
- copy of the relevant page(s) of the Commission guideline, indicating that all conditions and requirements are met
- in case the variations affect SmPC, labelling and/or package leaflet, revised product information and, if appropriate, mock-ups or specimens
- relevant data to support the proposed variation
- for unclassified variation, a detailed justification for its submission as a Type IB notification
- for variations requested by the authority following assessment of FUMs or Specific Obligations and Periodic Safety Update Reports (PSURs), or following class labelling, a copy of the request should be annexed to the cover letter
- for Type II variations, an addendum or updated Module 2 overviews or/and summaries
- proof of payment/declaration that fees have been paid (if applicable)
- if the variation is submitted via the Mutual Recognition or Decentralised Procedure, the Reference Member State (RMS) should receive from the applicant the list of dispatch dates to the Concerned Member States (CMS)

Procedures for Variations

Notification for Minor Variations of Type IA/IA$_{IN}$

For Type IA variation applications submitted through the Mutual Recognition or Decentralised Procedures, the MAH sends notification simultaneously to the RMS and CMS within 12 months (so-called "annual report") for Type IA, or immediately after implementation of a minor variation for Type IA$_{IN}$. The procedure starts at Day 0, provided that the required documentation has been submitted and the relevant fees have been paid. If all the documentation has not been provided, the notification will be deemed unacceptable and the MAH should immediately cease to apply the concerned variation(s). Alternatively, the MAH may decide to submit a new variation, which will require a new variation procedure number. The RMS only checks the notification's validity with respect to the supporting documentation. Neither the RMS nor CMS will perform a full assessment of the supporting data in detail. The CMS should not comment to the RMS or MAH about the acceptability of content; however, the CMS may comment if documentation is not received or fees are not paid. It must be stressed that for Type IA variations, there is no request by the RMS for clarification, information or documentation from the MAH and there is no clock stop or suspension of the process.[12]

The RMS will make the decision as to whether the notification is accepted or rejected within 30 days. If the notification is acceptable, the RMS will inform the MAH on behalf of the CMS that the variation is considered acceptable and issue an "Acknowledgement of an acceptable notification." If the notification is unacceptable, the MAH is also informed in writing and a reason for non-acceptance will be specified. If any amendment to the decision granting the authorisation is required, all Member States concerned will update the MA within two months following receipt of the positive outcome for the variation or within six months for minor variations of Type IA requiring immediate notification (Type IA$_{IN}$).

For Type IA variation applications submitted through the Centralised Procedure, the MAH sends notification to EMA, without involvement of the rapporteur. However, a copy of the Type IA notification will be submitted by the agency to the rapporteur for information. EMA checks the notification's validity with respect to the supporting documentation. By Day 30 after receiving the notification, EMA advises the MAH of its validity or invalidity. If the outcome is positive and the Commission decision granting the MA requires any amendments, the Commission will update the MA within two months, or within six months for minor variations of Type IA requiring immediate notification (Type IA$_{IN}$).[13]

Notification for Minor Variations of Type IB

For Type IB variation applications submitted through the Mutual Recognition or Decentralised Procedure, the MAH sends the notification simultaneously to the RMS and CMS, and sends the list of dispatch dates to the RMS. After receiving the application, the RMS and CMS will check its validity. The RMS also will check within seven calendar days whether the proposed change can be considered a Type IB minor variation, and whether the notification is correct. When the proposed variation is not considered a Type IB minor variation, and in the RMS' opinion may have a significant impact on the medicinal product's quality, safety or efficacy, the CMS and MAH are informed immediately. If the CMS do not disagree within a further seven days, the

MAH will be asked to reclassify the variation to Type II and supplement its variation application to meet the requirements for a Type II major variation application. Following receipt of the valid revised variation application, a Type II assessment procedure will be initiated. If the CMS disagree with the RMS, the RMS shall take the final decision on the classification of the proposed variation, having taken into account the comments received.

Once the classification for a Type IB notification is accepted, the RMS informs the MAH of the start date (Day 0). Until Day 20, CMS may notify RMS of their objections. If the variation can be accepted by the RMS, taking into account any CMS comments, the RMS circulates an acceptance notification to the MAH ("Acknowledgement of Approval") and informs the CMS by updating the Communication and Tracking System (CTS) record and the procedure ends (Day 30). If the variation cannot be accepted by the RMS, taking into account the CMS comments, the RMS circulates the "Notification with Grounds" to the CMS and MAH and the clock stops. Within 30 days of receipt of this notification, the MAH submits an amended notification to the RMS and CMS and a list of dispatch dates to the RMS only. The RMS restarts the clock and a New Day 0 is set up. If, after the New Day 30, the variation is accepted by the RMS and CMS, the RMS circulates an acceptance notification to the MAH and informs the CMS by updating CTS and the procedure ends. If the variation cannot be accepted by the RMS, taking into account the CMS comments, the RMS circulates a rejection notification to the CMS and MAH ("Refusal") and the procedure ends.[14]

Where necessary, the Competent Authorities will update the MA within six months following closure of the procedure by the RMS. However, accepted Type IB minor variations may be implemented without awaiting MA update.

For Type IB variation applications submitted through the Centralised Procedure, the MAH sends the notification to EMA and the rapporteur. The co-rapporteur is not involved in Type IB variations; however, a copy of the complete Type IB notification must be also submitted to the co-rapporteur. EMA checks the validity of the application within five working days and all issues identified during validation are sent to the MAH by Eudralink or fax. Once the validation phase is positively finalised, the agency sends the MAH confirmation of the positive outcome and the start day of the procedure. If, within 30 days, EMA has not informed the MAH that the notification cannot be approved, the variation shall be deemed to have been accepted. In the event of deficiencies (an unfavourable outcome), the MAH has 30 days to submit an amendment. If the MAH does not amend the notification within 30 days, as requested, the notification will be rejected. Within 30 days of receipt of the amended notification, the agency will inform the MAH of the final outcome—acceptance or rejection—and whether the Commission decision requires any amendments. If it has to be amended, the Commission will update the MA within six months following receipt of the EMA notification. However, the accepted minor variation may be implemented without awaiting the MA update.[15]

Type II Major Variations
For Type II variation applications submitted through the Mutual Recognition or Decentralised Procedure (standard 60-day timetable), the MAH sends the application simultaneously to the RMS and CMS. Additionally, the RMS should receive the list of dispatch dates indicating the Type II variation procedure number, the dates on which the applications have been sent to each CMS and confirmation that relevant fees have been paid as required by national authorities. The RMS and CMS check the application's validity, and the RMS informs the MAH of the start date (Day 0). As a general rule, a 60-day standard evaluation timetable will apply. It can be reduced to 30 days with regard to safety issues, or extended to a 90-day timetable for variations concerning changes or additions to therapeutic indications.

By Day 40, the RMS prepares the Preliminary Variation Assessment Report (PVAR) and circulates it to the MAH and CMS. In the PVAR, the RMS should clearly indicate whether it endorses the variation in its proposed form or thinks the variation should be rejected or amended. By Day 55, the CMS send their comments on the PVAR to the RMS. If there are no objections to the variation, the procedure may be finalised on Day 60. If any amendments are required, the RMS sends the request for supplementary information (RSI) to the MAH and CMS on Day 59. The procedure is suspended until the supplementary information is provided. The recommended clock-stop period is one month; however, a longer suspension is possible provided the MAH sends a justified request to the RMS. The RMS' evaluation of responses may take up to 60 days, depending on the complexity and amount of data submitted with the response. On Day 60, the RMS circulates the Final Variation Assessment Report (FVAR) to the CMS for comments and to the MAH for information. In case of disagreement between the RMS and CMS, a breakout session can be arranged (Day 75). By Day 85, the CMS send their final comments on the FVAR to the RMS. In cases where the variation is accepted, the RMS will inform the MAH and CMS that the variation is considered acceptable, together with the date of acceptance. The variation can be implemented 30 days after the MAH has been informed about its acceptance by the RMS. Competent Authorities should implement the decision nationally within two months of the end of the procedure. In cases where the variation is rejected by the RMS and CMS, the RMS will inform the MAH and CMS that the variation is considered rejected and provide a reason(s) for the rejection. If mutual recognition by one or more CMS is not possible due to a Potential Serious

Risk to Public Health (PSRPH), the matter is referred to CMDh. To avoid arbitration, the MAH may withdraw the variation application from all CMS and the RMS.[16]

For Type II variations to applications submitted through the Centralised Procedure, the MAH sends the application to EMA and the rapporteur. The co-rapporteur normally is not involved in the assessment of a Type II variation application unless it concerns a new indication. In such cases, MAHs are advised to contact EMA at least two months before the intended submission date.

EMA acknowledges receipt of a valid application and informs the MAH of the start date (Day 1) in accordance with the official start dates published on the agency's website. Under the standard 60-day timetable, the rapporteur prepares an assessment report (Day 30). Other CHMP members can send their comments until Day 50. By Day 60, CHMP formulates its opinion on the basis of the rapporteur's assessment report or makes a request for supplementary information. If supplementary information is requested, the procedure will be suspended until this information is provided. As a general rule, a standard one-month clock will apply. In justified circumstances, it can be suspended up to two months. After adoption of the CHMP opinion, the agency will inform the MAH and the Commission within 15 days about the final outcome, i.e., whether the opinion is favourable or unfavourable (including grounds for an unfavourable outcome), and whether the Commission decision granting the MA requires any amendments. Any necessary updates to the MA must be made within two months. The standard 60-day timetable may be reduced to 30 days (particularly for safety issues) or extended to 90 days (for variations concerning changes or additions to therapeutic indications).[17]

The approved Type II major variations may only be implemented after the Commission has amended the decision granting the MA and has notified the MAH. If there are no amendments to the Commission decision granting the MA, the approved variation may only be implemented once the MAH has been informed by the Commission accordingly.

Major Changes Necessitating an Extension Application

Certain changes to an MA are considered to fundamentally alter the authorisation's terms and, therefore, cannot be considered as variations. To make these changes, which are described in Annex I of the *Variations Regulation*, an extension application is necessary. Annex I of the *Variations Regulation* lists three main change categories that require an extension application:
- changes to the drug substance(s)
- changes to strength, pharmaceutical form or route of administration
- other changes specific to veterinary medicinal products to be administered to food-producing animals; change or addition of target species

These applications require a complete scientific evaluation to support the change.

Renewals

Renewals Under the Mutual Recognition and Decentralised Procedures

Legal Framework

According to Article 24 of Council Directive 2001/83/EC,[18] as amended, an MA is initially valid for five years and may be renewed on the basis of a reevaluation of the risk:benefit balance by the authorising Member State's Competent Authority. Once renewed, the MA shall be valid for an unlimited period unless the Competent Authority decides, on justified grounds relating to pharmacovigilance, to proceed with one additional five-year renewal.[19]

The MAH should agree on the common renewal date with the RMS at the completion of the initial Mutual Recognition Procedure. In practice, this agreement should take place within 30 days of Day 90. For products authorised through the Decentralised Procedure, the common renewal date should be agreed to on completion of the procedure (in practice within 30 days of the end of the procedure). This date should help in carrying out the renewal process for different product presentations and maintaining the synchronisation of PSURs, which are based on the international birth date (date of the first MA in any country in the world), the European birth date (date of the first MA in the EU) or both.

The MAH may apply for a renewal in less than five years to synchronise the renewal dates between the RMS and the CMS. It must be stressed that this is an optional procedure to be followed on a voluntary basis by the MAH and Member States.[20]

A common European renewal application form should be used for medicinal products authorised through the Centralised, Mutual Recognition or Decentralised Procedures. The European renewal application form should be completed and the MAH normally should submit one renewal application form for each MA. If any significant issues are raised by an expert that require a revised SmPC, labelling and/or package leaflet to be attached to the renewal application, the exact current and proposed wording should be specified on the application form. Alternatively, such listing may be provided as a separate attachment to the application form using a tabular format (indicating the current and proposed texts). Any proposed amendments to the SmPC should be discussed and agreed with the RMS in advance of submission.

Chapter 24

Dossier Requirement for Renewal

When applying for renewal, the MAH should submit the documents listed below,[21] presented as follows (preferably in electronic Common Technical Document (eCTD) format):

Module 1:
1.0 Cover letter
1.1 Comprehensive table of contents (not applicable for eCTD)
1.2 Renewal application form with annexes
1.3 Product Information
- revised SmPC, labelling and/or package leaflet (exact current and proposed wording should be specified), taking into account issues raised by the expert(s) (clinical, nonclinical and quality)

1.4 information about the expert(s) (quality, nonclinical and clinical, if applicable, including signature and CV)

Module 2:
2.3 Quality overview
Quality expert statement should include:
- confirmation that all changes relating to the product's quality have been made following applications for variations and that the product conforms to current CHMP quality guidelines
- confirmation of currently authorised specifications for the drug substance and the drug product (with date of latest approval and procedure number)
- qualitative and quantitative composition of the active substance(s) and the excipient(s) (with date of latest approval and procedure number)
- declaration of compliance with Directive 2001/83/EC, as amended, which obliges the MAH "...to take account of technical and scientific progress and introduce any changes..."

2.5 Clinical overview
- clinical expert statement should address the product's current risk:benefit balance based on PSUR data and safety/efficacy data accumulated since granting of the MA or its last renewal, making reference to relevant new information in the public domain
- clinical expert statement also should:
  o confirm that no new (preclinical or clinical) data are available that change or result in a new benefit:risk evaluation (Where there are new preclinical data, the MAH may submit a nonclinical expert report as appropriate.)
  o confirm that the product can be safely renewed at the end of five years for an unlimited period, or any action recommended or initiated should be specified and justified
  o confirm that the authorities have been kept informed of any additional data significant for the assessment of the benefit:risk ratio of the product concerned

Module 5:
5.3.6 Reports of postmarket experience
- PSUR data, together with any PSURs previously submitted, should cover a period of four years and four months since granting of the MA or its last renewal

Renewal Procedure

An automatic validation process begins the renewal procedure. The RMS starts the procedure based on assurance from the MAH that renewal applications have been submitted to all CMS and that the relevant national fee has been paid, where appropriate (i.e., there is no requirement for acknowledgment of receipt from CMS).

A 90-day procedure is followed and no more than 30 additional days are possible. In exceptional circumstances only, and with agreement of the RMS, the amount of time the clock is stopped may be extended. If the renewal takes longer to resolve, the product may remain on the market while the renewal application is pending.

The Member States' assessment approach focuses on a safety evaluation utilising PSUR data and any relevant new information affecting the product's benefit:risk ratio. A full reevaluation of the entire dossier normally should not take place. Module 3 quality data are not updated at renewal. The MAH is obligated to update quality data on an ongoing basis throughout the product's lifecycle using the variation procedure.

Renewal of Centrally Authorised Products

According to Regulation (EC) 726/2004, Article 14(2), an MA is valid for five years. Once renewed, the MA shall be valid for an unlimited period, unless the Commission decides, on justified pharmacovigilance grounds, to proceed with one additional five-year renewal. In accordance with Article 12(1) of the aforementioned regulation, the authorisation shall be refused when the labelling and patient leaflet do not comply with the requirements of Title V of Directive 2001/83/EC, as amended. Certain changes to the MA particulars may be made at renewal, and these changes shall not trigger a variation procedure. Further details of permitted changes are given in the *Guideline on the Processing of Renewals in the Centralised Procedure*.[22]

The renewal application should be submitted to EMA no later than six months before MA expiration. The renewal date shall take into account the international birth date as well as maintenance of synchronisation of PSURs, and should be agreed in advance with EMA and the rapporteur and co-rapporteur. A presubmission meeting with EMA (and the rapporteur) is advisable to facilitate the preparation and submission of the renewal application and should take place 10–12 months before the MA expiry date.

The dossier should be sent to EMA and should generally include:
- administrative data, i.e., renewal application form with revised SmPC, labelling and package leaflet information (Module 1)
- expert statements (quality, clinical and nonclinical, when appropriate) (Module 2)
- PSUR, with reference to the new Volume 9 of *The Rules Governing Medicinal Products in the European Union* on pharmacovigilance (Module 5)

The above data are to be submitted in EU eCTD format, similar to the previously described file for the Mutual Recognition and Decentralised Procedures. More details can be found in the *Guideline on the Processing of Renewals in the Centralised Procedure*.[23]

The application is validated by EMA. Once validated, the MAH, rapporteur, co-rapporteur and other CHMP members are informed; the timetable is adopted; and the clock starts accordingly. The assessment of the renewal application consists of a benefit:risk balance reevaluation based on a consolidated version of the submitted file, PSUR data and any relevant new information on the product's benefit:risk. A full reevaluation of the whole dossier normally should not take place.

The final CHMP opinion on the renewal application may be:
- favourable (recommending MA renewal with unlimited validity or requiring one additional five-year renewal) or,
- unfavourable (nonrenewal) if serious public health issues remain at the end of the procedure

In some cases, postauthorisation commitments are included in the renewed MA, which oblige the MAH to submit postauthorisation data (as specific obligations or FUMs). Such documentation should be reviewed in accordance with the mutually agreed timetable.[24]

If there were any amendments to product information, the MAH has to submit the relevant amended translations of the SmPC, labelling and package leaflet within five days following the CHMP opinion. Once the CHMP opinion is adopted by the European Commission, EMA updates the European Public Assessment Report (EPAR) reflecting the renewal assessment and CHMP opinion. This EPAR is made available as of the date of the Commission's MA renewal decision. If the renewal takes longer to resolve, the product may remain on the market while the renewal application is pending.

Impact of the New Pharmacovigilance Legislation on Renewals

The new pharmacovigilance legislation (Regulation (EU) No 1235/2010 and Directive 2010/84/EU) modifies the submission deadline for renewals from six months to nine months as well as content requirements. Draft guidelines are currently under review.

As of 2 July 2012, submissions of renewal applications for centrally authorised products have to comply with the data requirements provided by Article 14(2) of Regulation (EC) No 726/2004, as amended by Regulation (EU) No 1235/2010. However, the nine-month deadline should apply only to products for which the MA expires after 2 April 2013.

Likewise, submissions of renewal applications for nationally authorised products have to comply as of 21 July 2012 with the data requirements provided by Article 24(2) of Directive 2001/83/EC as amended by Directive 2010/84/EU. The nine-month deadline applies only to products for which the MA expires after 21 April 2013.

Summary

- Postmarketing activities are the most resource-intensive phase for a regulatory department and extend over the entire product lifecycle.
- Once a medicinal product is authorised, the MAH must ensure that the MA remains in compliance with the actual manufacturing process and with product information.
- MAs are subject to:
  o specific obligations
  o follow-up measures
  o variations
  o renewals
  o postmarketing pharmacovigilance activities
- Variations can be classified into different categories (Type IA, IA$_{IN}$, IB, II, Line extension, USR), depending on the level of risk to public health and the impact on the concerned medical product's quality, safety and efficacy.
- The *Variations Regulation* does not apply to transfers of an MA from one MAH to another.
- Regulation (EC) No 1234/2008 on variations gives MAHs the possibility of grouping variations and work sharing in order to avoid duplication of work for both Competent Authorities and MAHs.
- The initial MA is valid for a period of five years. At the end of this period, an application for renewal must be submitted.

- In most cases, MAs are renewed only once. Therefore, special provisions regarding pharmacovigilance activities and frequency of submission of PSURs have been reinforced. The new pharmacovigilance legislation will have a major impact on renewal procedures.

References

1. Directive 2001/83/EC of the European Parliament and of the Council of 6 November 2001 on the Community code relating to medicinal products for human use, as amended (Consolidated version: 05/10/2009). EUR-Lex website. http://eur-lex.europa.eu/LexUriServ/LexUriServ.do?uri=OJ:L:2001:311:0067:0128:en:PDF. Accessed 15 May 2012.
2. Regulation (EC) No 726/2004 of the European Parliament and of the Council of 31 March 2004 laying down Community procedures for the authorisation and supervision of medicinal products for human and veterinary use and establishing a European Medicines Agency, as amended (Consolidated version: 20/04/2009). EUR-Lex website. http://eur-lex.europa.eu/LexUriServ/LexUriServ.do?uri=OJ:L:2004:136:0001:0033:en:PDF. Accessed 15 May 2012.
3. European Commission: *The Rules Governing Medicinal Products in the European Union. Notice to Applicants, Volume 2A*, Chapter 4 "Centralised Procedure," April 2006. EC website. http://ec.europa.eu/health/files/eudralex/vol-2/a/chap4rev200604_en.pdf. Accessed 15 May 2012.
4. Ibid.
5. Commission Regulation (EU) No 1235/2010 of the European Parliament and of the Council of 15 December 2010 amending, as regards pharmacovigilance of medicinal products for human use, Regulation (EC) 726/2004 laying down Community procedures for the authorisation and supervision of medicinal products for human and veterinary use and establishing a European Medicines Agency, and Regulation (EC) No 1394/2007 on advanced therapy medicinal products (31 December 2010). EUR-Lex website. http://eur-lex.europa.eu/LexUriServ/LexUriServ.do?uri=OJ:L:2010:348:0001:0016:EN:PDF. Accessed 15 May 2012.
6. Commission Regulation (EC) No 1234/2008 of 24 November 2008 concerning the examination of variations to the terms of marketing authorisations for medicinal products for human use and veterinary medicinal products. EUR-Lex website. http://eur-lex.europa.eu/LexUriServ/LexUriServ.do?uri=OJ:L:2008:334:0007:0007:EN:PDF. Accessed 15 May 2012.
7. Ibid.
8. *European Medicines Agency post-authorisation procedural advice for users of the centralised procedure*, EMA-H-19984/03 Rev. 20, September 2011. EMA website. www.ema.europa.eu/docs/en_GB/document_library/Regulatory_and_procedural_guideline/2009/10/WC500003981.pdf. Accessed 15 May 2012.
9. *Communication from the Commission—Guideline on the details of the various categories of variations to the terms of marketing authorisations for medicinal products for human use and veterinary medicinal products (2010/C 17/01)*. EC website. http://ec.europa.eu/health/files/eudralex/vol-2/c17_1/c17_1_en.pdf. Accessed 15 May 2012.
10. *Q/A-list for the submission of variations according to Commission Regulation (EC) 1234/2008*, CMDh/132/2009/Rev12, March 2012. HMA website. www.hma.eu/fileadmin/dateien/Human_Medicines/CMD_h_/procedural_guidance/Variations/CMDh_132_2009_Rev12-Clean_2012_03.pdf. Accessed 15 May 2012.
11. Op cit 8.
12. *Best Practice Guides for the submission and processing of variations in the Mutual Recognition Procedure*, CMDh/094/2003/Rev16, March 2012. HMA website. www.hma.eu/fileadmin/dateien/Human_Medicines/CMD_h_/procedural_guidance/Variations/CMDh_094_2003_Rev16_-_clean_2012_03.pdf. Accessed 15 May 2012.
13. *Communication from the Commission—Guideline on the operation of the procedures laid down in Chapters II, III and IV of the Commission Regulation (EC) No 1234/2008 of 24 November 2008 concerning the examination of variations to the terms of marketing authorisations for medicinal products for human use and veterinary medicinal products (2009/C 323/04)*. EC website. http://ec.europa.eu/health/files/eudralex/vol-2/c323_9/c323_9_en.pdf. Accessed 15 May 2012.
14. Op cit 12.
15. Op cit 13.
16. Op cit 12.
17. Op cit 13.
18. Op cit 1.
19. *Best Practice Guide on the processing of renewals in the Mutual Recognition and Decentralised Procedures*, CMDh/004/2005/Rev6, May 2011. HMA website. www.hma.eu/fileadmin/dateien/Human_Medicines/CMD_h_/procedural_guidance/Renewal/CMDh_004_2005_Rev6_Clean_2011_06_b.pdf. Accessed 15 May 2012.
20. Ibid.
21. Ibid.
22. *Guideline on the processing of renewals in the Centralised Procedure*, EMEA/CHMP/2990/00 Rev. 3, 20 October 2005. EC website. http://ec.europa.eu/health/files/eudralex/vol-2/c/299000en_3_en.pdf. Accessed 15 May 2012.
23. Ibid.
24. Ibid.

Chapter 25

Pharmacovigilance

By Nicole Beard, MSc, PhD

OBJECTIVES

❑ Understand pharmacovigilance requirements

❑ Understand key aspects of the 2010 *Pharmacovigilance Regulation*

REGULATIONS AND DIRECTIVES COVERED IN THIS CHAPTER

❑ Regulation (EC) No 726/2004 of the European Parliament and of the Council of 31 March 2004 laying down Community procedures for the authorisation and supervision of medicinal products for human and veterinary use and establishing a European Medicines Agency, as amended (Consolidated version: 20/04/2009)

❑ Directive 2001/83/EC of the European Parliament and of the Council of 6 November 2001 on the Community code relating to medicinal products for human use, as amended (Consolidated version: 5/10/2009)

❑ Commission Regulation (EU) No 1235/2010 of the European Parliament and of the Council of 15 December 2010 amending, as regards pharmacovigilance of medicinal products for human use, Regulation (EC) 726/2004 laying down Community procedures for the authorisation and supervision of medicinal products for human and veterinary use and establishing a European Medicines Agency, and Regulation (EC) No 1394/2007 on advanced therapy medicinal products (31 December 2010)

❑ Directive 2010/84/EU of the European Parliament and of the Council of 15 December 2010 amending, as regards pharmacovigilance, Directive 2001/83/EC on the Community code relating to medicinal products for human use (31 December 2010)

Legal Framework

Pharmacovigilance is the science of the detection, collection, assessment, evaluation and prevention of adverse drug reactions (ADRs) and related activities. An ADR is a response to a medicinal product that is noxious and unintended. The limitations of clinical trials in terms of their size, duration and controlled conditions means that some ADRs will only be detected after a medicinal product has been authorised and has entered the market. The aim of pharmacovigilance is to identify new information about hazards associated with medicines and to prevent harm to patients.

The legal framework for pharmacovigilance of medicinal products for human use in the EU is given in Regulation (EC) No 726/2004[1] and Directive 2001/83/EC,[2] as amended.

In addition, detailed guidelines, definitions, standards and information regarding the precise execution of pharmacovigilance-related procedures are to be found in a number of guidance documents, principally *The Rules Governing Medicinal Products in the European Union, Volume 9A*,[3] "Pharmacovigilance" and in the pharmacovigilance-related E2 series of guidelines from the International Conference on Harmonisation (ICH).

These basic legal texts are supplemented by Commission Regulation (EC) No 540/95,[4] which regulates the procedures concerning "suspected unexpected non-serious adverse reactions."

On 31 December 2010, new pharmacovigilance legislation (Regulation (EU) No 1235/2010[5] and Directive 2010/84/EU[6]) was adopted by the European Parliament and European Council and came into force in July 2012.

This legislation is the biggest change to the regulation of human medicines in the EU since 1995. It has significant implications for Marketing Authorisation Holders (MAHs). The European Medicines Agency (EMA) is responsible for implementing the new legislation and is developing a framework for compliance and delivery of key requirements.

This legislation is the outcome of the legal proposals on pharmacovigilance that the Commission put forward in December 2008. The new legislation, which amends existing legislation, is intended to further protect public health by strengthening the current European-wide system for monitoring the safety of medicines on the EU market. The stronger legislation on pharmacovigilance will improve patient safety and public health through better prevention, detection and assessment of adverse reactions to medicines. It also will allow patients to report adverse drug reactions directly to the Competent Authorities. In addition, the legislation aims to ensure that members of the public become better informed about the benefits and risks of taking medicines.

The pharmacovigilance system in the EU operates with the management and involvement of national Competent Authorities; the European Commission, as the Competent Authority for medicinal products authorised centrally for the whole EU; and EMA. In some Member States, regional centres are in place under the coordination of the national Competent Authority. Within this system, EMA's role is to coordinate the EU pharmacovigilance system.

To ensure the provision of advice for the safe and effective use of medicines, several major measures will be implemented:
- a Pharmacovigilance Risk Assessment Committee (PRAC), as a new scientific committee created within EMA, to ensure the availability of the necessary expertise and resources for pharmacovigilance assessments at the EU level
- request for postauthorisation safety and efficacy studies (PASS/PAES) from the pharmaceutical industry
- risk-management systems for all newly authorised medicines
- all pharmacovigilance referrals will be discussed by the new PRAC and the Committee for Medicinal Products for Human Use (CHMP) or the Co-ordination Group for Mutual Recognition and Decentralised Procedures—Human (CMDh); opinions will be adopted as a result

- MAH required to maintain a Pharmacovigilance System Master File (PSMF), permanently available for submission or inspection by the national Competent Authority (The PSMF replaces the current Detailed Description of the Pharmacovigilance System (DDPS).
- MAH must submit information to EMA on medicinal products for human use authorised or registered in the EU using an electronic format provided by the agency; MAH is also responsible for maintaining this information once submitted
- modification to the submission deadline for renewals from six months to nine months as well as changes in content requirements

Periodic Safety Update Reports

Once a medicinal product is authorised in the EU or a Member State, the MAH is required to submit Periodic Safety Update Reports (PSURs). Adverse reaction report sources include spontaneous reports from healthcare professionals, data from postauthorisation studies and the published literature. The MAH may receive reports directly or indirectly from a Competent Authority.

The PSUR is an update on a medicinal product's worldwide safety experience available to a Competent Authority at defined times:
- immediately upon request
- every six months after authorisation and before marketing
- every six months during the first two years of marketing
- annually for the subsequent two years
- every three years thereafter

Each PSUR should cover the time period since the previous report was issued and should be submitted within 60 days of the last data lock point. The data lock point (DLP) is defined as the cut-off date for data to be included in a PSUR. It may be set according to the medicinal product's European birth date (EBD) or international birth date (IBD).

A medicinal product's birth date is used as the basis for defining the time points for submission of the PSURs after authorisation. The EBD is defined as the date of the first Marketing Authorisation (MA) for a medicinal product granted to the MAH in the EU. The IBD is defined as the date of the first MA for a medicinal product granted to the MAH in any country in the world. In the case the medicinal product is first authorised in Europe, the EBD and the IBD are the same.

PSURs for medicinal products authorised under the Centralised Procedure should be submitted to all Member States' Competent Authorities and EMA in accordance with Regulation (EC) No 726/2004, as amended. PSURs for medicinal products authorised nationally should be submitted to the Competent Authorities in accordance with Directive 2001/83/EC, as amended.

MAHs are expected to provide summary information and a critical evaluation of the product's risk:benefit balance in light of new or changing postauthorisation information. This evaluation should ascertain whether further investigations are required and whether changes should be made to the MA, the Summary of Product Characteristics (SmPC), the patient information leaflet or product advertising.

Ordinarily, a single PSUR can cover all dosage forms, formulations and indications for a medicinal product authorised to one MAH. Within the PSUR, separate presentations of data for different dosage forms, indications or populations (e.g., paediatric population versus adults) may be appropriate.

If an MAH is granted a subsequent MA for a product containing the same drug substance as one previously authorised, the first product's PSUR data lock points usually should be used for all products. However, the submission cycle normally will be restarted when the subsequent MA is granted, unless other conditions are imposed. In such cases, the joint PSURs submitted according to the latest MA's cycle cover data for all previous products. Preferably, generic products should have the same PSUR submission periods as those agreed for the corresponding originator product.

For combinations of substances that are also authorised individually, safety information may be reported either for the fixed combination in a separate PSUR or as separate presentations in the report on one of the components, depending on the circumstances. It is essential to cross-reference all relevant PSURs.

Where a product is authorised to more than one MAH, joint PSURs may be submitted provided the products remain identical and the PSURs are submitted independently by or on behalf of the respective MAH for its product. The data lock point should be based on the birth date of the first authorised product.

Requirements for PSURs have been significantly amended in the new legislation:
- Routine PSUR reporting is no longer necessary for products with low risk or for old or established products, i.e., for many generic and traditional herbal medicinal products. However, Competent Authorities can request PSURs for these products on the basis of pharmacovigilance concerns.
- MAHs shall submit PSURs to EMA containing
  o summaries of data relevant to the product's benefits and risks
  o a scientific evaluation of the medicinal product's risk:benefit balance
  o all data relating to the volume of sales and any data in the MAH's possession relating to the volume of prescriptions, including an estimate of the population exposure
- PSUR reporting will be electronic following the establishment of an EU repository. PSURs will be sent directly to EMA.
- PSURs will have a single assessment for the same active substance or a combination of active substances.

Development Safety Update Report

The Development Safety Update Report (DSUR) ICH E2F[7] guidance has reached ICH Step 4 for periodic reporting on the safety of investigational drugs. The guidance was adopted by CHMP in September 2010 and was implemented in the EU 1 September 2011. This means that as of 1 September 2011, all MAHs are required to submit DSURs instead of Annual Safety Reports (ASRs).

At present, some ICH countries and regions accept submission of a PSUR to fulfil national and regional requirements for periodic reporting on the safety of approved drugs. Although the focus of the DSUR is on investigational drugs, there can be overlap between the content of the DSUR and PSUR, and some repetition is expected.

Reference Safety Information

One PSUR objective is to establish whether information recorded during the reporting period is in accordance with previous knowledge about the medicinal product's safety, and to indicate whether product information changes should be made. Reference information is needed to perform this comparison. A single information reference source facilitates a practical, efficient and consistent safety evaluation approach and makes the PSUR a unique report accepted in all areas.

It is common for the MAH to prepare its own company core data sheet covering safety, indications, dosing, pharmacology and other product information. A practical approach for the MAH to use in periodic reporting is referencing the safety information from its central document. This information is the company core safety information (CCSI).

For periodic safety reporting, the CCSI is the basis for determining whether an adverse drug reaction is listed or unlisted. The SmPC or locally approved product information is the reference document upon which expectancy is based for local expedited postauthorisation safety reporting.

Electronic Transmission of Individual Case Safety Reports

Transmission of adverse reaction reports previously relied on paper-based formats. National reporting forms were used for Member State adverse reaction reports, and Council for International Organisation of Medical Sciences II (CIOMS) forms were used for adverse reactions in a third country. Paper reporting has been replaced by electronic transmission through the EudraVigilance system among EMA, Member State Competent Authorities and MAHs.

EudraVigilance is a data processing network and database management system for exchanging, processing and evaluating Individual Case Safety Reports (ICSRs) on serious adverse reactions.

Data structuring, as required for electronic transmission, implies the use of controlled vocabularies. The Medical Dictionary for Regulatory Activities (MedDRA)—the internationally agreed-upon medical terminology designed to support medical information classification, retrieval, presentation and communication—has made an important contribution to standardising medical information. In January 2003, it became mandatory to use MedDRA terminology in all electronically transmitted adverse drug reaction reports.

The new legislation makes substantial amendments to the reporting requirements. MAHs shall record all suspected adverse reactions that are brought to their attention and shall ensure that those reports are accessible at a single point within the Community (including reports from postauthorisation studies). The MAH shall not refuse to consider reports of suspected adverse reactions received electronically or by any other appropriate means from patients and healthcare professionals, and all expedited reports have to be submitted electronically by EudraVigilance.

All serious reports must be submitted within 15 days following the day on which the MAH gained knowledge of the event. Non-serious suspected adverse reactions that occur in the Community must be submitted within 90 days following the day on which the MAH concerned gained knowledge of the event.

Good Pharmacovigilance Practice

Good Pharmacovigilance Practices (GVPs) are a set of measures drawn up to facilitate the performance of pharmacovigilance in the EU. They cover medicinal products authorised centrally via EMA as well as those authorised at the national level.

The GVP guidelines are divided into 16 modules, each of which covers one major pharmacovigilance process. Each module is developed by a team of experts from EMA and from EU Member States.

The GVP modules will replace *Volume 9A* and will set out detailed, practical guidance on how MAHs and Member States should meet the requirements.

GVPs have been released for consultation in two phases, with the first phase in February 2012 and the second phase in May/June 2012. The modules released in Phase I are:
- Module I—Pharmacovigilance Systems and their Quality Systems
- Module II—Pharmacovigilance System Master File
- Module V—Risk Management Systems
- Module VI—Management and Reporting of Adverse Reactions
- Module VII—Periodic Safety Update Report
- Module VIII—Postauthorisation Safety Studies
- Module IX—Signal Management

Summary

This new EU pharmacovigilance legislation represents the most impressive change to the EU pharmacovigilance requirements for more than a decade and the biggest changes to human medicines since the establishment of EMA in 1995.

MAHs will be impacted by the legislation in a number of key areas, since the legislation aims to make roles and responsibilities clear, minimise duplication of effort, free up resources by rationalising and simplifying reporting of adverse drug reactions and PSURs, and establish a clear legal framework for postauthorisation monitoring.

This will have a major impact on existing regulatory processes and, as a consequence, numerous new processes will have to be put in place. New legislation will have major implications on the well-trained pharmacovigilance, IT and regulatory departments and on financial resources.

References

1. Regulation (EC) No 726/2004 of the European Parliament and of the Council of 31 March 2004 laying down Community procedures for the authorisation and supervision of medicinal products for human and veterinary use and establishing a European Medicines Agency, as amended (Consolidated version: 20/04/2009). EC website. http://ec.europa.eu/health/files/eudralex/vol-1/reg_2004_726_cons/reg_2004_726_cons_en.pdf. Accessed 15 May 2012.
2. Directive 2001/83/EC of the European Parliament and of the Council of 6 November 2001 on the Community code relating to medicinal products for human use, as amended (Consolidated version: 5/10/2009). EUR-Lex website. http://eur-lex.europa.eu/LexUriServ/LexUriServ.do?uri=OJ:L:2001:311:0067:0128:en:PDF. Accessed 15 May 2012.
3. *EudraLex: The Rules Governing Medicinal Products in the European Union, Volume 9A*, "Guidelines on pharmacovigilance for medicinal products for human use" (September 2008). EC website. http://ec.europa.eu/health/files/eudralex/vol-9/pdf/vol9a_09-2008_en.pdf. Accessed 15 May 2012.
4. Commission Regulation (EC) No 540/95 of 10 March 1995 laying down the arrangements for reporting suspected unexpected adverse reactions that are not serious, whether arising in the community or in a third country, to medicinal products for human or veterinary use authorised in accordance with the provisions of Council Regulation (EEC) 2309/93. EUR-Lex website. http://eur-lex.europa.eu/LexUriServ/LexUriServ.do?uri=CELEX:31995R0540:en:HTML. Accessed 15 May 2012.
5. Commission Regulation (EU) No 1235/2010 of the European Parliament and of the Council of 15 December 2010 amending, as regards pharmacovigilance of medicinal products for human use, Regulation (EC) 726/2004 laying down Community procedures for the authorisation and supervision of medicinal products for human and veterinary use and establishing a European Medicines Agency, and Regulation (EC) No 1394/2007 on advanced therapy medicinal products (31 December 2010). EUR-Lex website. http://eur-lex.europa.eu/LexUriServ/LexUriServ.do?uri=OJ:L:2010:348:0001:0016:EN:PDF. Accessed 15 May 2012.

6. Directive 2010/84/EU of the European Parliament and of the Council of 15 December 2010 amending, as regards pharmacovigilance, Directive 2001/83/EC on the Community code relating to medicinal products for human use (31 December 2010). EUR-Lex website. http://eur-lex.europa.eu/LexUriServ/LexUriServ.do?uri=OJ:L:2010:348:0074:0099:EN:PDF. Accessed 15 May 2012.

7. ICH *Development Safety Update Report E2F* (17 August 2010). ICH website. www.ich.org/fileadmin/Public_Web_Site/ICH_Products/Guidelines/Efficacy/E2F/Step4/E2F_Step_4.pdf. Accessed 15 May 2012.

Chapter 26

Products Manufactured From Human Blood or Plasma

Updated by Gudrun Busch, MSc, PhD, MTOPRA, RAC

OBJECTIVES

❑ Learn why blood and plasma products are necessary for therapeutic treatment

❑ Understand the requirements for human medicinal products derived from human blood or plasma

❑ Understand how human blood and plasma products are classified and regulated

❑ Get an overview of which accessory products are on the market

DIRECTIVES, REGULATIONS AND GUIDANCES COVERED IN THIS CHAPTER

❑ Directive 2001/83/EC of the European Parliament and of the Council of 6 November 2001 on the Community code relating to medicinal products for human use, amended by Directives 2003/63/EC and 2004/27/EC

❑ Directive 2002/98/EC of the European Parliament and of the Council of 27 January 2003 setting standards of quality and safety for the collection, testing, processing, storage and distribution of human blood and blood components and amending Directive 2001/83/EC

❑ Commission Directive 2005/62/EC of 30 September 2005 implementing Directive 2002/98/EC of the European Parliament and of the Council as regards Community standards and specifications relating to a quality system for blood establishments

❑ Commission Directive 2005/61/EC of 30 September 2005 implementing Directive 2002/98/EC of the European Parliament and of the Council as regards traceability requirements and notification of serious adverse reactions and events

❑ Commission Directive 2004/33/EC of 22 March 2004 implementing Directive 2002/98/EC of the European Parliament and of the Council as regards certain technical requirements for blood and blood plasma

❑ Guideline on plasma-derived medicinal products of 21 July 2011 (EMA/CHMP/BWP/706271/2010)

❑ Scientific data requirements for a Plasma Master File (CHMP/BWP/3794/03, Rev. 1)

❑ Epidemiological data on blood transmissible infections (CHMP/BWP/125/04 Rev. 1)

❑ Validation of immunoassay for the detection of antibody to Human Immunodeficiency Virus (Anti-HIV) in plasma pools (CHMP/BWP/298388/05)

❑ Validation of immunoassay for the detection of hepatitis B virus surface antigen (HBSAG) in plasma pools (CHMP/BWP/298390/2005)

❑ Documents regarding official control authority batch release published by the European Directorate for the Quality of Medicines and Healthcare

❑ Directive 2000/70/EC of the European Parliament and of the Council of 16 November 2000 amending Council Directive 93/42/EEC as regards medical devices incorporating stable derivatives of human blood or human plasma

What Is Plasma?

Plasma is the fluid portion of blood that functions as a carrier for red and white blood cells, proteins and metabolic products. Blood is 55% plasma. Plasma remains after separation of all cells from blood when clotting is prevented by an anticoagulant. Plasma contains 7%–8% proteins, primarily albumin, immunoglobulins and fibrinogen.

Plasma used to manufacture plasma-derived medicinal products is obtained from healthy donors—mainly by plasmapheresis (source plasma)—in specialised plasmapheresis centres. In addition, plasma derived from whole blood donations (recovered plasma) is available as a remnant of transfusion product production.

Plasma-derived Medicinal Products and Their Indications

Plasma-derived proteins are extracted from pools of source plasma using either alcohol precipitation and subsequent biochemical separation techniques (fractionation) or chromatographic capture techniques. Manufacturing occurs on an industrial scale, starting with approximately 500–2,500 litres of pooled plasma.

The quality and safety of plasma-derived products are based on qualified measures in two major areas:
- control of starting material: includes donor selection, testing of individual plasma units, quarantine periods for plasma and testing of plasma pools for viral markers
- control of manufacturing: emphasises validated and controlled protein purification, including the choice of manufacturing process steps that inactivate or remove microbial contaminants

Both measures ensure the safety of therapies derived from human plasma.

Plasma-derived medicinal products can be divided into seven therapeutic groups:

1. coagulation factors
2. immunoglobulins
3. albumin
4. inhibitors (antiproteases)
5. fibrin sealants
6. fibrinogen
7. thrombin

Today, 26 families of blood- and plasma-derived medicinal products are available for treating about 40 indications. Life-saving treatments for conditions such as Factor VIII deficiency and immunoglobulin deficiency are among the best-known uses of plasma-derived products. **Table 26-1** summarises the seven different groups and their fields of indications.

Regulatory Environment

Political Institutions

Within the European Commission, the Directorate-General for Enterprise is responsible for the regulatory framework and market authorisations for pharmaceuticals, including those derived from human blood and plasma. In that function, this division ratifies Committee for Medicinal Products for Human Use (CHMP) opinions on all pharmaceutical products. The Commission publishes the legal framework for licensing pharmaceuticals—*The Rules Governing Medicinal Products in the European Union*.[1] The publishing organ is the *Official Journal of the European Union*.

The Directorate-General for Health and Consumers (DG SANCO) is responsible for the control and framework for blood and plasma collection.

Committee for Medicinal Products for Human Use (CHMP)

CHMP is responsible for scientific guidelines for marketing applications for all pharmaceuticals, including plasma-derived medicinal products. Draft and final guidelines released by European Medicines Agency (EMA) committees for consultation are available on EMA's website.

CHMP has established several working parties. Those with crucial impact on plasma-derived medicinal products are the Blood Products Working Group (BPWG) and the Biotechnology Working Party (BWP).

BPWG

BPWG has adopted several Notes for Guidance (NfGs) on clinical investigations of blood products (see **Table 26-1**). In addition, BPWG issues a core Summary of Product Characteristics (SmPC) that provides common ground for a product's characteristics in the EU.

Table 26-1. Medicinal Products Derived From Human Plasma and Their Indications

	Medicinal Products Derived From Human Plasma	Indications (Examples)
Coagulation Factors	Prothrombin complex concentrate (Coagulation Factors II, VII, IX, X)	Prophylaxis and therapy of haemorrhages caused by a congenital or acquired deficiency
	Coagulation Factor VII	Prophylaxis and treatment of bleeding in patients with antibodies against Factor XIII and Factor IX
	Coagulation Factor VIII	• Prophylaxis and treatment of bleeding in haemophilia A (congenital Factor VIII deficiency) • Acquired Factor VIII deficiency
	von Willebrand Factor	Prophylaxis and treatment of bleeding in von Willebrand disease
	Coagulation Factor IX	• Prophylaxis and treatment of bleeding in haemophilia B (congenital Factor IX deficiency) • Acquired Factor IX deficiency
	Coagulation Factor XI	Treatment of bleeding in congenital deficiency
	Coagulation Factor XIII	• Congenital deficiency • Haemorrhagic diatheses caused by acquired Factor XIII deficiency
Immunoglobulins	Nonspecific normal immunoglobulins (i.m./s.c.)	• Substitution in primary and secondary antibody deficiency • Prophylaxis (passive immunisation) of hepatitis A and measles • Therapy of radiogenic mucositis
	Nonspecific normal immunoglobulins (i.v.)	• Substitution and replacement therapy in primary and secondary antibody deficient disorders such as agammaglobulinaemia and hypogammaglobulinaemia • Secondary immunodeficiency syndrome due to underlying diseases (e.g., chronic lymphocytic leukaemia) • Idiopathic thrombocytopenic purpura (ITP)
	Anti-D immunoglobulin	Treatment and prevention of haemolytic disease of foetus and newborn due to Rh-incompatible blood transfusions
	Cytomegalovirus immunoglobulin	Passive immunisation
	Hepatitis A immunoglobulin	Passive immunisation
	Hepatitis B immunoglobulin	Passive immunisation
	Measles immunoglobulin	Passive immunisation
	Rabies immunoglobulin	Passive immunisation
	Rubella immunoglobulin	Passive immunisation
	Tetanus immunoglobulin	Passive immunisation
	Tick-borne encephalitis immunoglobulin	Passive immunisation
	Varicella-zoster immunoglobulin	Passive immunisation
Critical Care Products	Albumin solutions 5%, 20%, 25%	Restoration and maintenance of blood volume in volume deficiency where use of a colloid is inappropriate
Fibrin Sealants	Fibrinogen concentrates with various combinations of thrombin, Factor XIII and inhibitors	• Tissue adhesion • Suture support • Homeostasis • Wound care • Sealing of body cavities and subarachnoid space
Inhibitors	Antithrombin III	Congenital (prophylaxis and prevention of progression of deep vein thrombosis) and acquired deficiency of Antithrombin III
	C1-Inactivator (C1 Esterase Inhibitor)	Congenital angio-edema (HAE) caused by deficiency, absence or defective synthesis of C1 Esterase Inhibitor
	Alpha-1-Antitrypsin	Treatment of emphysema caused by genetic deficiency
Others	Fibrinogen	Treatment of bleeding: • Replacement therapy or • Complementary therapy in cases of acquired hypofibrinogenaemia
	Thrombin	Wound care, sealing of body vessels and cavities

Chapter 26

BWP
BWP covers the field of plasma-derived medicinal products, vaccines and all biotechnology-derived medicinal products, including gene therapy. A key manufacturing and quality control document for the plasma industry is *Guideline on plasma-derived medicinal products (*EMA/CHMP/BWP/706271/2010).[2]

One focus of BWP is virus safety and risk assessment of transmissible spongiform encephalopathy/Creutzfeldt-Jakob disease (TSE/CJD).

TSEs are a family of diseases in humans and animals characterised by spongy degeneration of the brain with severe and fatal neurological signs and symptoms.[3] In humans, the most common TSE is CJD.

European Directorate for the Quality of Medicines and Healthcare

European Pharmacopoeia
The European Pharmacopoeia (Ph.Eur.) publishes pharmacopoeial monographs, which are quality specifications for pharmaceutical preparations and their ingredients. Monograph 01/2007/0853 on human plasma for fractionation is particularly important to manufacturers: it describes general collection and storage conditions and serves as the basis for all other related monographs on plasma-derived medicinal products.

Ph.Eur. provides reference standards for tests described in the monographs. Coagulation factor standards and nucleic acid amplification technology (NAT) virus testing standards are important in plasma product testing.

Official Control Authority Batch Release
The European Directorate for the Quality of Medicine (EDQM) publishes regulatory procedures for Official Control Authority Batch Release (OCABR) for medicinal products derived from human blood or plasma. The Commission of the European Union and the Council of Europe decided on 26 May 1994 to create a network of official medicines control laboratories (OMCLs).[4] Independent from manufacturers, such OMCLs support regulatory authorities in controlling the quality of medicinal products for human and veterinary use available on the market. Within the EU, OMCLs such as the National Institute for Biological Standards and Control in the UK and the Paul-Ehrlich-Institut in Germany are nominated by the national authority responsible for the quality control of medicines in their country. The expertise of each OMCL may differ, and a manufacturer may opt to use the OMCL of its choice.

Such laboratories are responsible for batch release testing of plasma-derived medicinal products. If a Member State's Competent Authority informs the Marketing Authorisation Holder (MAH) that its authorised human biological medicinal product is subject to OCABR, samples of the batch to be released are sent to an OMCL within the EU/European Economic Area (EEA), which issues an Official Control Authority Batch Release Certificate to the MAH.[5]

Legal Framework
The legal framework for EU licensing consists of three major types of documents: regulations, directives and guidelines, which are published by the European Commission in *The Rules Governing Medicinal Products in the European Union.*[6] The following volumes are relevant for medicinal products for human use, manufactured from human blood or plasma:
- *Volume 1: Pharmaceutical Legislation: Medicinal Products for Human Use*
- *Volume 2: Pharmaceutical Legislation: Notice to Applicants*
  - *Volume 2A: Procedures for Marketing Authorisation*
  - *Volume 2B: Presentation and Content of the Dossier Volume*, 1998 edition and CTD 2001 edition
  - *Volume 2C: Regulatory Guidelines*
- *Volume 3: Medicinal Products for Human Use: Guidelines*
- *Volume 4: Medicinal Products for Humans and Veterinary Use: Good Manufacturing Practice*, Annex 14: Manufacture of Products Derived from Human Blood or Human Plasma
- *Volume 9: Pharmacovigilance*
- *Volume 10: Clinical Trials*

Regulations
Regulations are directly effective as supranational law and apply to the citizens of all EU Member States. All regulations for human pharmaceutical medicinal products naturally apply to blood- and plasma-derived products.

Directives
Directives apply to the Member States and must be implemented into national law by Member State legislation. Placing medicinal products for human use onto the EU market is governed by Directive 2001/83/EC and its amendments, which represent the codification of key directives (such as Directive 65/65/EEC, Directive 75/318/EEC, Directive 75/319/EEC and, notably, Directive 89/381/EEC, which extended the scope of Directives 65/65/EEC and 75/319/EEC to plasma-derived products).

Quality and safety standards for collecting, testing, processing, storing and distributing human blood and blood components, also pertinent to the collection phase in manufacturing medicinal products derived from human blood or plasma, are found in Directive 2002/98/EC. They apply directly to collecting such products as starting materials for human medicinal products.

Additional Commission directives implement the technical annexes of Directive 2002/98/EC:
- Commission Directive 2005/62/EC of 30 September 2005 implementing Directive 2002/98/EC of the European Parliament and of the Council as regards Community standards and specifications relating to a quality system for blood establishments
- Commission Directive 2005/61/EC of 30 September 2005 implementing Directive 2002/98/EC of the European Parliament and of the Council as regards traceability requirements and notification of serious adverse reactions and events
- Commission Directive 2004/33/EC of 22 March 2004 implementing Directive 2002/98/EC of the European Parliament and of the Council as regards certain technical requirements for blood and blood plasma

Registration Procedures
The EU offers three main authorisation routes for medicinal products, including plasma-derived products:
- National Procedure
- Noncentralised Procedure (Mutual Recognition Procedure and Decentralised Procedure), as described in Directive 2001/83/EC as amended
- Centralised Procedure, as described in Council Regulation (EEC) No 726/2004

Medicinal products manufactured from human blood or plasma do not normally fall within the scope of the annex to Council Regulation (EEC) No 726/2004; thus, the use of the Centralised Procedure is not mandatory for such products, which more often are regulated under Directive 2001/83/EC, as amended, alone or by National Procedures.

If a medical condition does not affect more than five in 10,000 people in the Community (i.e., 188,800 as of 1 January 2001), it is possible to apply for orphan medicinal product designation. Plasma-derived products are eligible for designation as orphan medicinal products under Regulation (EC) No 141/2000 and Regulation (EC) No 847/2000.

Council of Europe Publications
Prior to the establishment of Directive 2002/98/EC, the standards for collection and use of blood and its components were described in publications from the Council of Europe. Directive 2002/98/EC and its annexes establish the minimum requirements at a legislative level, but these two publications provide additional detail.
- Council Recommendation R (95) 15—*Guide to the preparation, use and quality assurance of blood components* (9th edition, published January 2003)
- Council Recommendation 98/463/EC—*Guide on the Suitability of Blood and Plasma Donors and the Screening of Donated Blood in the European Community*

General Documents and Guidelines
Guidelines issued by Ph.Eur. and the International Conference on Harmonisation (ICH) are not legally binding. If an applicant chooses not to apply a guideline, however, that decision must be explained and justified. Important examples of guidelines for blood and plasma products include:
- From CHMP and its working groups
  - *Guideline on plasma-derived medicinal products* (EMA/CHMP/BWP/706271/2010)[2] covers source material, manufacture, quality control and process validation studies, including virus inactivation/removal validation; refers to Ph.Eur. monographs; and lists more guidance documents in the annex (also revised by CHMP/BWP/1595/00). It includes an explanatory note on the use of albumin as a stabiliser (i.e., the shelf life of the albumin shall not expire earlier than the shelf life of the stabilised medicinal product).
  - Core SmPCs are released by BPWG.
  - Clinical trial guidelines are released by BPWG.
- From EDQM
  - Monographs issued by Ph.Eur. for plasma for fractionation and most plasma products.
  - Control authority batch release procedures necessitated by Directive 2001/83/EC are described in a group of documents published by EDQM that include the *EC Administrative Procedure for Official Control Authority Batch Release* (PA/PH/OMCL [2002] 68) and the *Procedure for Official Control Authority Batch Release of Centrally Authorised Immunological Medicinal Products for Human Use and Medicinal Products Derived From Human Blood and Plasma* (PA/PH/OMCL [2000] 83).

Control of Sourcing and Manufacture
In general, sourcing and manufacturing control requirements for medicinal products derived from human blood or plasma are the same as those for other biological and biotechnology products, with some key focus areas.

Testing of Donations
Directive 2002/98/EC and Ph.Eur. monograph 01/2007/0853 prescribe the basic testing requirements for whole blood and plasma donations. For starting materials for medicinal products—namely plasma for fractionation—testing for hepatitis B (HBs-Ag), hepatitis C (anti-HCV)

and HIV 1 and 2 (anti-HIV 1.2) are the minimum requirements.

Plasma pool testing for viral markers for HIV 1 and 2, hepatitis C virus (HCV) and hepatitis B virus (HBV) was introduced for medicinal product starting materials 1 November 1994 by Guidance III/5193/94 (renamed 3ab13a). Since July 1999, NAT for detecting HCV in plasma pools has been mandatory in the EU (CHMP/BWP/390/97).[8] Validation requirements for viral marker assays have been revised and are set out in CHMP/BWP/298388/05 and 298390/2005.

Some Member States conduct plasma pool testing during batch release procedures. Appropriate samples of starting material pools and intermediate plasma pools must be provided to the OMCLs.

Virus Safety Evaluation

Note for Guidance on virus validation studies (CPMP/BWP/268/95), describes the design, contribution and interpretation of studies validating virus inactivation and removal. For plasma-derived products, the manufacturing process should bear independent and validated inactivation and removal steps with a significant reduction factor. (Although Guidance III/5512/93 on the contribution of Part II of the dossier for the Marketing Authorisation Application (MAA), which describes the required virological documentation, has not been formally retracted, it became defunct with the introduction of the Common Technical Document (CTD), compulsory from 1 July 2003.)

TSE Safety Evaluation

A CHMP expert group is assessing the impact of TSE (variant CJD) on the safety evaluation for medicinal products derived from human plasma or human urine. Although cumulative epidemiological evidence and other considerations do not support transmission of sporadic, familial or iatrogenic CJD by plasma-derived products, donor residence in a high-risk country such as the UK is recognised as a risk factor to be taken into account with regard to donor exclusion criteria. The following guidance documents[9] in this field are produced as meeting reports or position statements that reflect the field's developmental nature:

- Expert workshop on human TSEs and plasma-derived medicinal products, 15–16 May 2000 (CHMP/BWP/1244/00 EMEA)
- Expert meeting on human TSEs and medicinal products derived from human blood and plasma, 1 December 2000 (EMEA/CHMP/BWP/450/01 EMEA)
- Position statement on CJD and plasma- and urine-derived medicinal products (EMEA/CHMP/BWP/2870/02 CHMP)

The Marketing Authorisation Dossier

In general, the marketing authorisation (MA) process for plasma-derived medicinal products is the same as that for other pharmaceutical products. The current legally binding requirements for the dossier content for an EU MAA are described in *The Rules Governing Medicinal Products in the European Union, Notice to Applicants, Volume 2B*. Effective 1 July 2003, all dossiers, whether for new submissions or variations, are required to conform to the five-module CTD structure released by ICH. The EU-CTD format is published in the *Notice to Applicants, Volume 2B*.

Dossier Contents

The MAA dossier table of contents was originally designed for pharmaceuticals in general and did not take into account the specific needs for plasma product documentation. The table of contents was integrated into the new CTD of the ICH dossier, but it still does not fully match the needs of plasma products. Module 3.2.S.2.3 requires extended information on blood or plasma sourcing.

The Plasma Master File

Information on plasma starting material collection and control must be documented either as part of the dossier or, preferably, as a Plasma Master File (PMF). The original *Note for Guidance on the Contribution to Part II of the Structure of the Dossier for Application for Marketing Authorisation—Control of Starting Materials for the Production of Blood Derivatives* (III/5272/94) was revised as CHMP/BWP/2053/01 and has been superseded by *Guideline on the Scientific Data Requirements for a Plasma Master Filed (PMF)* (CHMP/BWP/3794/03) to take the new CTD structure into account and provide further detail on the PMF concept. A PMF contains information on plasma used for manufacturing all intermediates and plasma products used as active substances or excipients of one company. If another manufacturer uses human albumin as a stabiliser for an active ingredient, the excipient manufacturer's PMF may be referenced. The structure and content of the PMF are set out in CPMP/BWP/3794/03 Rev. 1 and the *Guideline on Epidemiological Data on Blood Transmissible Infections* (CPMP/BWP/125/04 Rev. 1).

Currently, the PMF can be introduced either directly as part of the dossier of each single licence for a medicinal product or cross-referenced as a PMF master file, authorised centrally. The standalone PMF allows PMF management and approval through EMA.

Batch Release (OCABR)

Batch-release requirements for plasma-derived medicinal products were set forth in Directive 89/381/EEC, which was incorporated into the codified Directive 2001/83/EC.

Article 114 thereof allows, but does not require, a Member State laboratory to test a batch of a medicinal product derived from human blood or plasma before it can be marketed. The procedure is described in detail in EDQM documents, namely PA/PH/OMCL (2002) 68 and PA/PH/OMCL (2000) 83 in the case of blood products.[10]

Guidance originally available on control authority batch release of blood products (III/3008/93 for coagulation factors, III/3010/93 for immunoglobulins and III/3009/93 for albumin) was overhauled during a review of OCABR procedures in 2002 and has been replaced and extended by several documents produced by the EDQM.

Labelled samples of each batch shall be delivered for testing to the OMCLs. Thereafter, OMCLs issue an EU batch release certificate that is valid in all EU Member States.

Postmarket Requirements: Renewal and Pharmacovigilance

All licences for medicinal products, including plasma-derived medicinal products, approved through the Centralised Procedure, Mutual Recognition Procedure or Decentralised Procedure must be renewed after the first five years. Thereafter, the MA usually is unlimited.

Drug safety surveillance of licensed medicinal products (pharmacovigilance) is regulated by Council Regulation (EEC) No 2309/93 and Directive 2001/83/EC. Commission Regulation (EC) No 540/95 sets forth specific requirements for reporting non-serious, unexpected adverse reactions. Since December 2001, all guidance documents have been summarised in *The Rules Governing Medicinal Products in the European Union, Volume 9*.[11]

Companies provide individual adverse reaction case reports, Periodic Safety Update Reports (biannually and annually during the first five years of an MA) and—depending upon licencing conditions—postauthorisation safety studies.

Outlook

- Directive 2002/98/EC: This directive covers all blood components for transfusion (e.g., red blood cells, platelets) and plasma for fractionation. It sets high standards of quality and safety for blood and blood derivatives across the EU. The directive was adopted 27 January 2003 and was required to be transformed into national law by 8 February 2005. A number of Commission directives implement the technical annexes of Directive 2002/98/EC.

- Structure of the dossier: With the introduction of the CTD format for all dossiers from 1 July 2003, information on starting materials, such as those for human blood and plasma, was placed in Module 3.2.S.2.3. To facilitate submission, applicants may refer to the PMF, which is intended to be distinct from the submission dossier. This guidance can help develop a more suitable MAA dossier table of contents for plasma-derived products.

- Medical devices incorporating blood products: As of 13 June 2002, the *Medical Devices Directive* (Directive 93/42/EEC) was amended by Directive 2000/70/EC to include devices that incorporate a medicinal product derived from human blood or plasma. A Notified Body shall seek a scientific opinion from EMA as part of the approval process. The transition phase for this directive ended 15 November 2005.

Summary

Medicinal products for human use derived from human blood or plasma are regulated in the EU as medicinal products under Directive 2001/83/EC, as amended. Due to quality and safety concerns about such products, extensive rules and guidance are provided. These publications focus on two areas—starting material source and medicinal product manufacture, including virus and TSE risk assessments.

References

1. European Commission, *Eudralex: The Rules Governing Medicinal Products in the European Union* (European Commission, April 1998). EC website. http://ec.europa.eu/health/documents/eudralex/index_en.htm. Accessed 18 May 2012.
2. *Guideline on plasma-derived medicinal products of 21 July 2011, EMA/CHMP/BWP/706271/2010* Rev. 2 of 25 January 2001. EMA website. www.ema.europa.eu/docs/en_GB/document_library/Scientific_guideline/2011/07/WC500109627.pdf Accessed 2 June 2012.
3. World Health Organization. Bovine Spongiform Encephalopathy (BSE). www.who.int/zoonoses/diseases/bse/en/. Accessed 18 May 2012.
4. European Directorate for the Quality of Medicines and HealthCare. General European OMCL Network. www.edqm.eu/en/General-European-OMCL-Network-46.html. Accessed 18 May 2012.
5. Ibid.
6. Op cit 1.
7. Op cit 2.
8. Ibid.
9. Ibid.
10. Op cit 1.
11. Ibid.

Chapter 27

Human Tissue Regulation

Updated by Isabel Zwart, PhD

OBJECTIVES

- Understand regulatory issues related to human tissues and cells
- Detail key aspects of EU directives for human tissues and cells
- Learn about issues associated with tissue donation
- Discuss tissue engineering and stem cell research
- Discuss existing regional and national regulations applicable to various countries
- Understand major topics regarding tissue- and cell-derived medicinal products

DIRECTIVES AND REGULATIONS CITED IN THIS CHAPTER

- Directive 2004/23/EC of the European Parliament and of the Council of 31 March 2004 on setting standards of quality and safety for the donation, procurement, testing, processing, preservation, storage and distribution of human tissues and cells
- Directive 2006/17/EC of 8 February 2006 implementing Directive 2004/23/EC of the European Parliament and of the Council as regards certain technical requirements for the donation, procurement and testing of human tissues and cells
- Commission Directive 2006/86/EC of 24 October 2006 implementing Directive 2004/23/EC of the European Parliament and of the Council as regards traceability requirements, notification of serious adverse reactions and events and certain technical requirements for the coding, processing, preservation, storage and distribution of human tissues and cells
- Directive 2001/83/EC of The European Parliament and of the Council of 6 November 2001 on the Community code relating to medicinal products for human use
- Regulation (EC) No 1394/2007 of the European Parliament and of the Council of 13 November 2007 on Advanced Therapy Medicinal Products and amending Directive 2001/83/EC and Regulation (EC) No 726/2004
- Commission Directive 2009/120/EC of 14 September 2009 amending Directive 2001/83/EC of the European Parliament and of the Council on the Community code relating to medicinal products for human use as regards advanced therapy medicinal products
- Draft guideline on the risk-based approach according to Annex I, part IV of Directive 2001/83/EC applied to Advanced

Chapter 27

  Therapy Medicinal Products, EMA/CAT/
  CPWP/686637/2011

- Guideline On Human Cell-Based Medicinal Products, EMEA/CHMP/410869/2006

- Reflection paper on stem cell-based medicinal products, EMA/CAT/571134/2009

- Guideline On Xenogenoic Cell Based Medicinal Products, EMEA/CHMP/CPWP/83508/2009

- CHMP/CAT position statement on Creutzfeldt-Jakob disease and advanced therapy medicinal products, EMA/CHMP/BWP/353632/2010

- Guideline on Safety and Efficacy Follow-up—Risk Management of Advanced Therapy Medicinal Products, EMEA/149995/2008

Introduction

Regulation of products comprising human tissue or cells has been a much-debated topic among industry, public health and regulatory groups in Europe over the past decade. Industry seeks to market cell-based products through a central or single approval system that will instil confidence in the public, operate under standardised requirements for all players (manufacturers, universities, hospitals, tissue banks, etc.), and promote innovation with intellectual property protection. Public health groups want to ensure patient safety, while regulatory groups want to standardise product quality requirements and establish a risk:benefit balance. In order to fully understand the current situation in the EU, the evolution of human tissue-based products and their regulation must be considered.

In the late 1990s, when many tissue-based products were becoming commercially available, most personnel at manufacturing companies involved had medical device backgrounds. This new genre of biological materials was developed primarily for orthopaedic or wound-care cases (such as cartilage or skin repair), so in many ways this was a natural progression. Although the EU *Medical Devices Directive* (*MDD*, Directive 93/42/EEC) had been implemented, it was widely recognised that many tissue-engineered products did not fall within the scope of the *MDD*'s structure or definitions.[1] In this regard, the *MDD* specifically states that it does not apply to "transplants or tissues or cells of human origin nor to products incorporating or derived from tissues or cells of human origin." However, Directive 2001/83/EC of the European Parliament and of the Council on the Community code relating to medicinal products for human use, which classified cell-based products as medicinal products, was also considered inappropriate to the specific requirements of human tissue-engineered products. Recognising the need for some form of regulation, companies approached the regulatory authorities for advice. This process led to a plethora of different national regulations regarding the development and use of such products, which was further complicated by national requirements for obtaining and storing human tissues and cells.

To safeguard public health, which could be compromised by the existence of a diverse set of national regulations (or lack of regulation), the Commission put forward a framework legislative proposal in 2002 to ensure the safe collection and use of human tissues in Europe.[2] The resulting Directive 2004/23/EC of the European Parliament and of the Council of 31 March 2004 on setting standards of quality and safety for the donation, procurement, testing, processing, preservation, storage and distribution of human tissues and cells, was published in 2004 and is commonly known as the *European Union Tissues and Cell Directive* (*EUTCD*). This directive laid down requirements for the safety and quality of human tissues and cells, with a further mandate for the Commission to provide legislation on setting technical standards for cell and tissue donation, procurement and storage. A set of implementing directives was adopted in 2006 to fulfil this mandate, with Directive 2006/17/EC providing standards for donation, procurement and testing, while Directive 2006/86/EC covers processing, preservation, storage and distribution. These directives are outlined in further detail in this chapter.

However, while these directives aimed to facilitate the exchange of tissues or cells among Member States, and ensure patients receiving such materials would be protected from transmissible disease, they did not intend to harmonise how such products were authorised for clinical use and distribution. Until 2007, there was no agreement on the definition of tissue engineering and no EU-wide regulatory framework for tissue-based products (i.e., each country still had the ability to define its own requirements). Furthermore, many products did not fit into the existing categories of transplant, medicinal product or medical device legislation, contributing to the confusion. As a result, various human tissue-derived products that were being successfully used in the clinic during this period were developed without coverage by any specific pan-European regulation. Undoubtedly, this situation was frustrating from the prospect of commercialisation, with companies finding it extremely labour-intensive and time-consuming to navigate the regulatory maze across Europe, often without reward.

The debate on responsibility for tissue regulation continued until 2007, when European legislation was introduced in the form of Regulation (EC) No 1394/2007. This regulation defined a new category of medicinal products called advanced therapy medicinal products (ATMPs) that fall under the overarching medicinal product legislation through amendments to Directive 2001/83/EC and Regulation (EC) No 726/2004. Understandably, this proposal initially caused great debate within industry, particularly among companies manufacturing tissue- or cell-based products that were licensed under less stringent requirements than are in place for pharmaceuticals, or were approved as medical devices or transplants. These products were now to be regarded in a new light, as a consequence of the important concepts that arose from this new regulation:

- ATMPs are to be regarded as medicinal products. However, the regulation does acknowledge that specific testing and control parameters are required that may differ from more conventional biologics.
- A new Committee for Advanced Therapies (CAT) was formed under the auspices of the European Medicines Agency (EMA) to provide scientific opinions to the Committee for Medicinal Products for Human Use (CHMP) on applications for ATMPs and to give companies scientific advice when requested.
- Product approval requires submission to EMA according to traditional pharmaceutical principles and using recognised formats.
- Postmarketing activities, such as pharmacovigilance, are required to demonstrate continued efficacy and risk management.
- Product/patient traceability and specific labelling requirements also apply.

This chapter aims to outline how this legislation on ATMPs, as well as the directives on tissues and cells, have been implemented, and considers the current requirements for human tissue- and cell-based products, along with developments that may affect future regulation of these products.

Human Tissue Regulation in Europe

The overarching *EUTCD* is applicable to all somatic cells, stem cells (including haematopoietic and bone marrow-derived stem cells), reproductive cells and embryonic and foetal tissue. The directive excludes blood and blood products, which are regulated by other directives, as discussed in Chapter 26 in this book, and organs, which are regulated under local transplant law, as well as the new Directive 2010/53/EU of the European Parliament and of the Council of 7 July 2010 on standards of quality and safety of human organs intended for transplantation, that is to be implemented in August 2012. It also excludes organs, tissues and cells of animal origin.

Important concepts for the donation, procurement, testing and distribution of human tissues and cells, as well as traceability, are provided in the *EUTCD*, with the aim of facilitating pan-European trade and use of tissues. The directive also outlines the role of various establishments in such activities, and requires the accreditation of tissue establishments,—i.e., the facility where the activities of processing, preservation, storage or distribution of the human tissues and cells are undertaken—by the relevant national Competent Authorities. Any licensed tissue establishment within the EU must, therefore, conform to the directive, as well as any additional national legislation, before any human tissue can be banked or used in the clinic. These tissue establishments are also responsible for the import and export of tissues to and from countries outside the EU, and must ensure that all imported and exported material meets EU legislation with regard to the standards for the quality and safety of human tissues and cells.

Following on from this basic framework, two further directives were then published that provide details with regard to the implementation of Directive 2004/23/EC:

- Directive 2006/17/EC of the European Parliament and of the Council of 8 February 2006 implementing Directive 2004/23/EC of the European Parliament and of the Council as regards certain technical requirements for the donation, procurement and testing of human tissues and cells
- Directive 2006/86/EC of the European Parliament and of the Council of 24 October 2006 implementing Directive 2004/23/EC of the European Parliament and of the Council as regards traceability requirements, notification of serious adverse reactions and events and certain technical requirements for the coding, processing, preservation, storage and distribution of human tissues and cells

These two implementing directives provide detailed requirements for the donation, procurement and testing of human tissues and cells, as well as traceability, as described below.

Requirements of the *EUTCD*

Donation

The EU legislation on tissues and cells covers the donation of such material from both living and deceased donors, and also specifies requirements for autologous or allogeneic tissue donation. Article 13 of the *EUTCD* requires that all donors give informed consent; in this regard, the information to be provided to donors at the time of consent is specified in the annex to this directive. Further details of the actual procedure for obtaining consent and donor identification are set out in Annex IV of the implementing Directive 2006/17/EC. This directive states that consent should be obtained by persons appropriately qualified, provided with timely and relevant training and, where appropriate, be registered in accordance with the appropriate professional and/or statutory bodies. This information should be documented in training records that are updated regularly.

In addition to outlining the donor identification and consent procedures, the *EUTCD* specifies whether financial incentives may be provided to donors. Since the aim of the directive is to promote the altruistic donation of tissue and cells to help ensure the safety of such material, donors may only receive compensation to cover the expenses and inconveniences related to the donation, and not for the donation itself. The directive allows each Member State to individually define the conditions under which compensation may be granted.

Donor Selection and Testing

To select appropriate consenting donors of human tissue, donor identification procedures should comply with the requirements set out in Annexes I and III to Directive 2006/17/EC. Procedures and standards employed for the selection of appropriate donor(s) and the exclusion of high-risk or otherwise unsuitable candidates should be clearly delineated and justified. A review of a donor's medical and behavioural history should be performed to highlight potential risk factors, such as a previous transplantation with a xenograft that would render the donor unsuitable.

In addition to a medical history assessment, the donor should be tested for transmissible diseases using a range of laboratory tests. The laboratory tests for infectious disease are specified in Annex II of Directive 2006/17/EC, and are summarised in **Table 27-1**. It should be noted that these tests must be carried out by a qualified laboratory, authorised as a testing centre by the Member State's Competent Authority, using CE-marked testing kits where appropriate. It is recommended that nucleic acid amplification techniques be used where possible because, otherwise, repeat donor testing is required for some diseases after 180 days.

In the case of donor embryos for the derivation of human Embryonic Stem (hES) cell lines, both the oocyte and the sperm donor should be tested as defined in Annex III of Directive 2006/17/EC. Where tissue is taken from neonates, for example in the derivation of fibroblasts, the biological testing defined in Annex II of Directive 2006/17/EC can be carried out on the mother to avoid medically unnecessary interventions on the infant.

In certain circumstances, additional testing may be required, depending on the donor's history and the characteristics of the tissue or cells donated (e.g., RhD, HLA, malaria, CMV, toxoplasma, EBV, Trypanosoma cruzi). Furthermore, as the *EUTCD* only sets the minimum standards of quality and safety for donation, procurement and testing, each Member State can introduce more stringent donor testing requirements. In its three-year report issued in June 2010[3] on the application of the *EUTCD* by the 27 Member States, the European Commission noted that 14 Member States "apply additional testing requirements to take into account their specific national epidemiological situation." The meaning of this statement is not described, but it is inferred that a higher risk exists from donors originating from a nation that adds more testing requirements. For further details of additional national requirements, please see **Table 27-1**.

Procurement

In addition to specifying the donor identification requirements to ensure the tissue's quality and safety, Annex IV to Directive 2006/17/EC also sets regulatory requirements for the procurement procedure itself. The intent is to ensure the safety of the donor during the procurement procedure, as well as the collection of the material under aseptic conditions to minimise the risk of microbial contamination of the tissue. In this regard, Annex IV requires the establishment performing the procurement to produce a procurement report that is then passed on to the tissue establishment.

Traceability

A system allowing complete traceability of the patient as well as of the product and its starting materials is required to monitor the safety of human tissues and cells. The *EUTCD* lays down the requirements for traceability, and notes that systems should be put in place to ensure that all tissues and cells can be traced from donor to recipient, and vice versa. In this regard, Directive 2006/17/EC Annex IV requires that donor records be maintained by the tissue establishment for a minimum of 30 years after clinical use of the tissue. In addition, appropriate labelling systems should be put in place, including a donor identification code, as well as identification of the intended recipient. The full requirements for tissue traceability and notification of adverse events associated with its use are further provided in implementing Directive 2006/86/EC.

Implementation of the *EUTCD*—What It Means in Practice

It is important to note that all three directives have to be transposed into national law in order for the requirements listed above to be enforced. As a result, Member States have the option to impose additional country-specific requirements to those set out in the directives, leading to subtle differences in legislation across the EU. Furthermore, the European Commission allowed a transitional period for the implementation of the *EUTCD* into national law, with 7 April 2006 being the deadline. It would appear that all 27 Member States have implemented most of the requirements of the *EUTCD*, particularly with regard to the minimum testing requirements.[4,5] However, not all Member States have implemented some of the requirements regarding the accreditation of tissue establishments, inspections, importation and exportation of tissues and reporting of adverse events. These issues are compounded by the fact that the bodies responsible for policing these transpositions are different for each country. As a result, a patchwork of different regulations is still found across the EU. This poses a challenge for industry and regulatory professionals, and hinders not only distribution to Member States from third parties (countries) but also sharing of tissues among Member

Table 27-1. Donor Testing for Infectious Diseases

Disease *	Test	Additional National Requirements
HIV 1 and 2	Anti-HIV-1,2	HIV-antigen: Czech Republic, France, Malta, Romania HIV-1 NAT: Denmark, Estonia, Hungary, Italy, Portugal, Slovakia
Hepatitis B	HBsAg Anti-HBc	HBV NAT: Denmark, Hungary, Italy, Portugal, Spain
Hepatitis C	Anti-HCV-Ab	HCV NAT: Denmark, Germany, Hungary, Italy, Portugal, Spain
Syphilis	validated testing algorithm	-
T-Lymphotropic virus (donor living in or originating from a high incidence area)	Anti-HTLV-1: HTLV-I antibody testing must be performed for donors living in, or originating from, high-incidence areas or with sexual partners originating from those areas or where the donor's parents originate from those areas	This test is required without regard to the donor's risk for HTLV in the following countries: Bulgaria, Germany, Greece, Spain, France, Italy, Hungary, Romania
Chlamydia (Sperm donor only)	NAT	-
NAT = Nucleic acid amplification technique * In certain circumstances, additional testing may be required depending on the donor's history and the characteristics of the tissue or cells donated (e.g., RhD, HLA, malaria, CMV, toxoplasma, EBV, Trypanosoma cruzi)		

States. Furthermore, the subsequent application of tissues that have not been substantially manipulated or engineered (i.e., those that are exempt from the ATMP legislation) is regulated differently in each Member State; these differences in national legislation are briefly outlined below.

Current National Regulation of Human Tissues for Clinical Application

France

The situation in France allows latitude for interpretation. The legislative system dictates that a law is enforced by a decree, which in turn is enacted by a set of rules known as an *arrêté*. Several laws and decrees (the *Bioethics Law*, the Law of 98-535 and decrees relating to L.1211, L.1241 to L.1245) give the background for controlling tissue products, including the *Décret n° 2008-968 du 16 Septembre 2008*. As a result, tissues must be screened through the Microbiological Safety Committee prior to use. Human tissue products are distributed under the jurisdiction of *Agence nationale de sécurité du médicament et des produits de santé* (ANSM), and tissue banks are licensed and inspected by the agency. In the case of cell-based products that are not manufactured industrially and so are not considered medicinal products, these products must receive authorisation from ANSM prior to distribution and clinical use; this authorisation procedure takes into account the opinion of the Biomedicines Agency, *Agence de la Biomédecine*, in France. Furthermore, ANSM is also responsible for pharmacovigilance of these products.

Germany

Human tissues in Germany are ostensibly controlled by the *Arzneimittelgesetz* (*AMG*) or *German Drug Law*. Again, the regulations are not straightforward because the level of control differs by product and is therefore determined on a product-by-product basis. For example, autologous tissues used in orthopaedic reconstructions within the same institution are classified as unfinished drugs; although the *AMG* applies, no approval or submission processes exist. A non-centralised approval system in Germany leads to assessment of product data in individual *Lander* (states within Germany), which adds complexity because individual methods differ.

The fact that the *AMG* applies to tissues implies that guidelines and principles of pharmaceutical development are relevant. This includes manufacturing, which must comply with Good Manufacturing Practice (GMP) guidelines. In general, therefore, any tissue-based product intended for importation into Germany must comply with the *AMG* and is authorised by the Paul-Ehrlich-Institut (Division of Medical Biotechnology).

Italy

In Italy, the control of human tissue has passed to the *Centro Nazionale Trapianti* or the National Transplant Centre (CNT). This organisation prepares a list of approved tissue processors from which hospitals or tissue banks can purchase tissue. A network of six regional tissue banks within this organisation controls the sourcing and distribution of human tissue products, giving priority to tissues procured and processed in Italy and using the list of approved processors to permit distribution of tissues from outside the country.

Spain

Spain has had tissue product regulations in place for several years. All activities concerning the use of human tissue are regulated by Royal Decree 411/1996, which includes ethical considerations and technical details. The decree allows the introduction of tissue products to the Spanish market, provided they originate from a Spanish tissue bank or tissue services foundation (TSF). TSFs service several hospitals in a district, provided the hospitals are certified to perform specific implantation or transplant procedures by the autonomous regional government. For tissue product companies based outside Spain, the regulations inevitably lead to contracts and distribution via the TSFs, which act in many ways as third-party quality brokers. The TSFs must be notified of each product batch used in Spain. They maintain batch records and the name of the destination hospital.

It should be noted that products derived from human tissue containing lyophilised, crushed demineralised bone in powder form and subsequently embedded in a gel or paste were previously authorised by the *Agencia Española de Medicamentos y Productos Sanitarios* (AEMPS). As of March 2010, they fall under the remit of the *Organización Nacional de Trasplantes* (ONT, National Transplant Organization) and must meet the standards for cells and tissues set in the Royal Decree of 1301/2006.

Sweden

Sweden, like Germany, has indicated that human tissues are regulated as pharmaceuticals. The *Medicinal Products Act* (SFS 1992:859) states that any product that contains substances or combinations of substances with a pharmacologic, immunologic or metabolic effect is classified as a medicinal product. This classification brings with it the rules and regulations attached to pharmaceuticals, including manufacturing and quality requirements and demonstrated product safety and efficacy. Although Sweden takes a pragmatic approach to regulation, the application of pharmaceutical rules and guidelines can complicate assessment. For example, the definition of batch size, identification of active substances, product composition and safety profiles are challenges for regulators and industry.

UK

The UK government has a particularly pragmatic approach to regulating human tissue products. Products that are not classified as ATMPs currently have no official Marketing Authorisation (MA) approval routes, although interaction with the Medicines and Healthcare products Regulatory Authority (MHRA) is recommended as part of any marketing activity.

In 2004, the UK issued the *Human Tissue Act*, which provides wide-ranging legislation and a specific regulatory framework to cover the handling, storage, use, research and "human application" of any and all human tissues and cells. In short, any testing, research, display, processing or distribution for transplant is covered. The act also provided for the establishment of the regulatory and licensing authority, the Human Tissue Authority (HTA). HTA came into being in April 2005 and assumed full statutory responsibility and authority on 1 April 2006. All activities covered by this legislation are subject to licensing by this authority, with HTA providing licences to organisations/centres where human application of tissues is being performed. In addition, HTA routinely inspects all licensed establishments. In this regard, HTA announced recently (March 2012) that it is seeking to work with the Care Quality Commission and Human Fertilisation and Embryology Authority to deliver regulation more effectively while ensuring that safety and quality of service are maintained.

The UK has also issued two publications that are pertinent to sourcing control of human tissues and cells and that should be referred to by tissue establishments:
- *Guidance on the Microbiological Safety of Human Organs, Tissues and Cells used in Transplantation* (August 2000)
- *A Code of Practice for Tissue Banks*

These were revised and came into force on 15 September 2009.

Regulation of Stem Cells

Stem cells are another complex and rapidly evolving technology considered to hold great promise for tissue repair and replacement. Stem cells can be categorised into three groups: embryonic, adult and foetal (e.g., umbilical cord blood).[6] All groups must follow the requirement for procurement, testing, storage and traceability, as outlined above. However, in the case of embryonic stem (ES) cells, an additional layer of regulatory complexity exists.

ES cell regulations are the most highly debated among scientific and sociological groups. Since these stem cells originate from live human embryos, generally obtained as surplus embryos from IVF clinics, ethical issues are of particularly great concern. Currently, European legislation regarding ES cell research varies greatly from country to country.

Both the EU 6th Research Framework Programme (FP6 2003–06) and current 7th Research Framework Programme (FP7 2007–13) allow funding of human ES cell research to fight major diseases. However, to deter the creation of more embryos and satisfy country-specific ethical requirements, the Commission included a restriction to the scope of the funding to exclude "proposals for projects which include research activities intended to destroy human embryos, including the procurement of stem cells. The exclusion of funding of this step of research will not prevent Community funding of subsequent steps involving human embryonic stem cells."[7] This compromise was reached following objection to the initial FP7 proposal by Germany and Italy. In both these countries, research and importation is strictly limited, and the procurement of ES cells from the embryo is banned. It should be noted that five other countries also voted against the agreement and did not accept the compromised text due to ethical reasons, but could not block it due to a lack of majority vote: these countries are Lithuania, Austria, Malta, Slovakia and Poland. In these countries, with the exception of Austria, any research involving ES cell lines is explicitly prohibited. This is in stark contrast to the most liberal countries in Europe (such as the UK, Belgium, Spain and Sweden), which not only allow the procurement and generation of new ES cell lines, but also allow the funding and creation of human embryos for the procurement of ES cells under particular circumstances. In other cases, countries have no clear stance on the use of ES cells, with several countries (including Bulgaria, Cyprus, Ireland, Luxembourg and Romania) having no specific legislation on research using these cells. However, the regulatory landscape is still changing in this area, and certain countries have relaxed the laws somewhat, with Germany now allowing research using ES cells derived before a later cut-off date than what was originally in place (1 May 2007 versus 1 January 2002), giving researchers access to a wider range of ES cell lines.

More detailed information on national requirements for ES cell research is provided by the European Consortium for Stem Cell Research (also called EuroStemCell), which is funded by the FP7, and the European Human Embryonic Stem Cell Registry.

It should be noted that in cases where ES cells are used as starting materials for cell therapies classified as medicinal products (discussed below), Regulation (EC) No. 1394/2007 has provided a caveat that allows Member States to create their own policies on the development and authorisation of such medicinal products. As a result, although all ES cell therapies that fall under the ATMP legislation must receive a pan-European MA (as discussed below), marketing of the product may still be prohibited in certain Member States that express conservative views towards the use of ES cells.

Advanced Therapy Medicinal Products Legislation

The regulation of medicinal products for human use in the EU is codified in Directive 2001/83/EC, as amended. In recent years, this directive has been amended by Regulation (EC) No 1394/2007 on Advanced Therapy Medicinal Products (*ATMP Regulation*) and Commission Directive 2009/120/EC on the Community code relating to medicinal products for human use as regards Advanced Therapy Medicinal Products. The *ATMP Regulation* defines ATMPs in Article 2.1 as gene therapy medicinal products, somatic cell medicinal products and tissue-engineered products.

Any material that is classed as an ATMP is subject to an MA granted by the European Commission, as defined in Paragraph (9) of the *ATMP Regulation*. Therefore, any somatic cell therapy or tissue-engineered product, including those containing genetically-modified stem cells, must enter the market through the Centralised Procedure.

The Centralised Procedure to obtain an MA involves an evaluation of the data package by the Competent Authorities. In this regard, the implementation of the *ATMP Regulation* has led to the formation of a new review body under the auspices of EMA; the aforementioned Committee for Advanced Therapies (CAT). This committee provides advice on the approvability of all advanced therapies, from tissue-engineered products to gene therapies. During the centralised review process, the CAT is responsible for the scientific review of the dossier, though progress and issues are also discussed at CHMP meetings. CAT prepares the draft opinion for final approval by CHMP. It is anticipated that both committees usually will reach a consensus decision, however this may not always be the case (as has already been seen with the Amsterdam Molecular Therapeutics submission for Glybera).[8] Where a consensus is not seen, an annex to the scientific opinion sent to the European Commission will be appended detailing the scientific grounds for the differences, which will be considered by the Commission, resulting in the application's approval or rejection.

In the context of human tissue regulation, it is important to distinguish between products that are defined as medicinal products and fall under the ATMP legislation, for which a centralised approval is mandatory; and those that are not defined as medicinal products, and are instead regulated at the national level. In both cases, therapies derived from human cells or tissues must comply with the "donation, procurement and testing" aspects of the *EUTCD* (and the implementing Directive 2006/17/EC). However, once these tissues or cells are classified as medicinal products, the aspects of processing, preservation, storage and distribution outlined in the *EUTCD* and implementing directives are no longer applicable.

In order to distinguish ATMPs containing human tissues and cells from other materials that are fully covered by the *EUTCD* through to clinical application, the definitions of an ATMP must be clarified.

Directive 2001/83/EC Annex I, Part IV, has been updated in accordance with the *ATMP Regulation*, and defines somatic cell therapies:

"Somatic cell therapy medicinal product means a biological medicinal product which has the following characteristics:
(a) contains or consists of cells or tissues that have been subject to substantial manipulation so that biological characteristics, physiological functions or structural properties relevant for the intended clinical use have been altered, or of cells or tissues that are not intended to be used for the same essential function(s) in the recipient and the donor;
(b) is presented as having properties for, or is used in or administered to human beings with a view to treating, preventing or diagnosing a disease through the pharmacological, immunological or metabolic action of its cells or tissues."

The definition of a tissue-engineered product is provided in the *ATMP Regulation*:

"A Tissue engineered product means a product that:
– Contains or consists of engineered cells or tissues, and
– Is presented as having properties for, or is used in or administered to human beings with a view to regenerating, repairing or replacing a human tissue.

A tissue engineered product may contain cells or tissues of human or animal origin, or both. The cells or tissues may be viable or nonviable. It may also contain additional substances, such as cellular products, biomolecules, bio-materials, chemical substances, scaffolds or matrices."

Furthermore, part (c) of Article 2, states that:
"Cells or tissues shall be considered 'engineered' if they fulfil at least one of the following conditions:
– the cells or tissues have been subject to substantial manipulation, so that biological characteristics, physiological functions or structural properties relevant for the intended regeneration, repair or replacement are achieved. The manipulations listed in Annex I, in particular, shall not be considered as substantial manipulations,

– the cells or tissues are not intended to be used for the same essential function or functions in the recipient as in the donor."

An important factor in these definitions is that in order for cell-based or tissue-derived products to be classified as medicinal products, the cells or tissues have to have undergone substantial manipulation. The definition of substantial manipulation is provided in *ATMP Regulation* Annex I. This annex lists the following activities that are not considered to be substantial manipulations:
- cutting
- grinding
- shaping
- centrifugation
- soaking in antibiotic or antimicrobial solutions
- sterilisation
- irradiation
- cell separation, concentration or purification
- filtering
- lyophilisation
- freezing
- cryopreservation
- vitrification

Based on this definition, peripheral blood stem cells isolated through apheresis, for example, would not fall under the definition of an ATMP. Neither would the isolation of cells from human tissue through means such as enzymatic dissociation be classified as substantial manipulation. However, any expansion of cells *ex vivo* is considered as substantial manipulation, and would then automatically lead to classification as an ATMP. It should be noted that whether the cells are to be used in an autologous or allogeneic situation is irrelevant for classification as a medicinal product, with the main defining factor for cell-based medicinal products being that they are not to be used for the same function they served in the donor when administered to the recipient. For example, isolated pancreatic islet cells administered to patients to improve pancreatic function are not considered as ATMPs. In cases of doubt, a sponsor may request a formal classification from CAT with regard to whether a tissue-based product meets the criteria that define an ATMP. This ATMP classification is a 60-day procedure that is normally performed early on in product development. The outcome of the classification procedure is a scientific recommendation in which CAT will also state whether the product falls under the definition of a gene therapy medicinal product, a somatic cell therapy medicinal product or a tissue-engineered product.

Once a tissue-derived product has been classified as an ATMP (either as a somatic cell therapy or a tissue-engineered product), it must meet the requirements of the *ATMP Regulation*, as well as the overarching Directive 2001/83/

EC, which covers the regulation of medicinal products for human use in the EU. Since all ATMPs are considered "medicines," they are subject to the rigours of pharmaceutical registration and approval processes. As a result, ATMPs, like other medicinal products, require proof of quality, safety and efficacy. However, unlike more traditional medicines, the demonstration of continued efficacy postapproval is required, particularly if the treatment is expected to result in long-term correction of a genetic disorder, for example. Manufacturers need to develop data to satisfy these criteria and present them in a format traditionally recognised by the regulatory agencies. In this regard, Directive 2009/120/EC of 14 September 2009, provides specific information as to the data that are required on the quality, nonclinical and clinical testing of such products in order to support an MA. As a result, the development programme for an ATMP largely follows that for conventional medicinal products, with data on the manufacturing process, product quality, pharmacodynamics, pharmacokinetics, safety and efficacy required. However Directive 2009/120/EC also introduces the concept of a "risk-based approach," which can be applied to determine the extent of quality, nonclinical and clinical data to be included in the Marketing Authorisation Application (MAA). At the time of updating this chapter, draft guidance has been published to describe the methodology for applying a risk-based approach, and how this information should be presented in the CTD format: *Draft guideline on the risk-based approach according to Annex I, Part IV of Directive 2001/83/EC applied to ATMPs* (EMA/CAT/CPWP/686637/2011).

The pharmaceutical categorisation of these products also requires that other rules and guidelines are followed, such as GMP and the conduct of clinical investigations in accordance with Directive 2001/20/EC (Good Clinical Practice). With regard to GMP, a second consultative review of Annex 2 to *Volume 4 of the EU Guidelines for Good Manufacturing Practice for Medicinal Products for Human and Veterinary Use* was completed in July 2010. The original Annex 2 was published to address GMP requirements for biologics. In light of Article 5 of the *ATMP Regulation*, the Commission has since proposed revisions to Annex 2 to increase the breadth of biological products covered to include several new product types, such as transgenic-derived products and ATMPs. Part B of the draft Annex 2 discusses GMP concerns specific to cell therapies and tissue-engineered products, including segregation of source materials, and contamination during processing and storage (e.g., at cryopreservation). The finalised version of the revised document had yet to be published at the time this chapter was updated.

It should be noted that although ATMP manufacturing must be GMP-compliant, the processes to obtain the starting materials are not covered by the GMP guidance. As previously noted, the donation, procurement and testing processes are regulated by the *EUTCD*. In this regard it is important to reiterate that the *EUTCD* and implementing directives do not have any role in placing products on the market, but do address public safety issues. As a consequence, the manufacturer of a cell-based ATMP is required to:

- Obtain tissues and cells that have been released by a designated "responsible person" at an accredited tissue establishment. There are specific qualification requirements and reporting responsibilities (adverse reaction, activity) for the Responsible Person, and this person may be legally responsible for the product itself (similar to the role of the Qualified Person in the pharmaceutical industry).
- Ensure there is a contract in place between the manufacturer and the tissue establishment that defines the responsibilities of the Responsible Person and the Qualified Person.
- Ensure that the tissue establishment from which the material was received provides the manufacturer with the donor/material test results for adventitious agents. Where the manufacturer acts as the tissue establishment, it must conduct all relevant safety testing on donated tissue, as defined by national transpositions of the *EUTCD* (as noted previously, this can be inconsistent among Member States).
- Control product traceability and conformity aspects from donor to patient, right through the manufacturing process. Guidance on the individual roles of the tissue establishment, manufacturer, sponsor and investigator/institution in ensuring traceability are provided in the *Detailed guidelines on good clinical practice specific to advanced therapy medicinal Products* (ENTR/F/2/SF/dn D(2009) 35810).

Therefore, while the *ATMP Regulation* is applicable for defining the regulatory route to market, the cells and tissues will be regulated at the national level with regard to donation and procurement. As a consequence, sourcing the cells will require the involvement of national Ethics Committees and Competent Authorities; the extent of their involvement will depend on the source of material used to manufacture the ATMP, and differs in degree in each Member State. As previously noted, for any tissues or cells imported from outside the EU, the tissue establishments are responsible for ensuring that all imported and exported material meets EU legislation with regard to the quality and safety standards for human tissues and cells. These factors should be taken into consideration when determining the source of cells for the development of a cell-based medicinal product. In the UK, for example, any stem cell-based products that involve the destruction of a human embryo in their formulation are initially licensed by the Human Fertilisation and Embryo Authority (HFEA). At the point where the embryo has been destroyed and the cells are harvested, these human cells would then fall under HTA's remit. The development of a product using these cells is under the remit of HTA until such time as the national Competent Authority, MHRA, classifies the product as an Investigational Medicinal Product (IMP)/ATMP. Once this classification has been confirmed, the clinical trial authorisation falls under MHRA's remit, while the MA procedure is centralised and coordinated by EMA.

Guidance

To aid applicants developing ATMPs intended for use in the EU, the European Commission has published various guidance documents. The guidelines cover quality, nonclinical, clinical and other issues. While guidance published by the European Commission and EMA is not legally-binding, it represents the harmonised view of the Community and its agencies on a particular issue, and any deviation from the guidelines during product development will need to be justified by the applicant when seeking an MA.

The most important guidelines for the development of an ATMP containing human cells or tissue are:
- *Draft guideline on the risk-based approach according to Annex I, part IV of Directive 2001/83/EC applied to Advanced Therapy Medicinal Products* (EMA/CAT/CPWP/686637/2011)
- *Guideline on Human Cell-Based Medicinal Products* (EMEA/CHMP/410869/2006)
- *Reflection paper on stem cell-based medicinal products* (EMA/CAT/571134/2009)
- *Guideline on Xenogeneic Cell-Based Medicinal Products* (EMEA/CHMP/CPWP/83508/2009)
- *CHMP/CAT position statement on Creutzfeldt-Jakob disease and advanced therapy medicinal products* (EMA/CHMP/BWP/353632/2010)

These documents provide guidance on manufacturing and quality aspects, including:
- starting material safety and control
- cell-culturing procedures
- product characterisation
- final product specifications
- handling procedure validation
- batch identification
- product-release testing and quality control prior to patient administration

These ATMP guidelines also provide recommendations for nonclinical and clinical studies; however, it should be noted that clinical development should also follow indication-specific guidance, in addition to any requirements laid down for cell-based products. There is also one specific guideline in relation to the follow-up of safety and efficacy for ATMPs:

- *Guideline on Safety and Efficacy Follow-up—Risk Management of Advanced Therapy Medicinal Products* (EMEA/149995/2008)

It should be noted that much of the guidance provided concerns the data requirements specific to an MAA for a cell-based product. However, due to the perceived higher risk of cell-based products and the novelty of any such product, in particular those containing stem cells, similar requirements may be required for a clinical trial application (CTA), although these are regulated by national Competent Authorities.

Hospital Exemption

Under the *ATMP Regulation* and as laid down in Article 3 (7) of Directive 2001/83/EC, there is an exemption from central authorisation for ATMPs that are "prepared on a non routine basis according to specific quality standards, and used within the same Member State in a hospital under the professional responsibility of a practitioner, in order to comply with an individual medicinal prescription for a custom-made product for an individual patient." The exemption was created in recognition of the small-scale and developmental nature of activity carried out in some hospitals, which would benefit from a degree of flexibility over the nature of regulatory requirements. The main issue with this exemption is the definition of "non-routine," and how this and the terminology used in the exemption have been interpreted by national Competent Authorities. This greatly influences the extent to which national agencies "regulate" these exempt products.

For ATMPs that fall under the hospital exemption rule, the manufacture of these products will be authorised by the national Competent Authorities and must still be GMP compliant. These products also must comply with the same requirements for traceability, quality and pharmacovigilance that are applicable for ATMPs that are authorised centrally by the Commission. In addition, such use of human tissue through hospital tissue banks still will be subject to the *EUTCD* with respect to donation, procurement and testing, as described above.

Devices

ATMPs can incorporate, as an integral part of the product, one or more medical devices, in which case they are referred to as "combined ATMPs" as defined in Article 2(d) of the *ATMP Regulation*. A combined ATMP is defined as follows:

'Combined advanced therapy medicinal product' means an advanced therapy medicinal product that fulfils the following conditions:
- it must incorporate, as an integral part of the product, one or more medical devices within the meaning of Article 1(2)(a) of Directive 93/42/EEC or one or more active implantable medical devices

within the meaning of Article 1(2)(c) of Directive 90/385/EEC, and
- its cellular or tissue part must contain viable cells or tissues, or
- its cellular or tissue part containing nonviable cells or tissues must be liable to act upon the human body with action that can be considered as primary to that of the devices referred to."

Therefore, the definition of combined ATMPs will be of particular relevance to the field of tissue-engineering, which is rapidly developing technologies that focus on producing viable and nonviable biomaterials. It should be emphasised that the applicability of EU ATMP legislation to any therapeutic product is determined by its primary intent and the mode of action. Products containing a device that are used in or administered to human beings with a view to regenerating, repairing or replacing a human tissue, even though they contain nonviable cells, will be classified as combined ATMPs if the primary mode of action is dependent on the cells. It should be noted that any product containing a device and viable cells will automatically be classified as an ATMP (combined), regardless of the role of the device. In contrast, products containing nonviable human tissues and cells with an ancillary action to that of the device are excluded from the *ATMP Regulation*. Normally, a combined product containing a medicinal product with ancillary action to that of the device would be assessed in accordance with the *Medical Devices Directive* (*MDD*, Directive 93/42/EEC). However, the *MDD* explicitly states that it does not apply to products containing human tissues and cells, with the exception of "human blood derivatives." This creates an interesting conundrum, as tissue engineering can potentially straddle both the ATMP and device camps, with true "borderline" characteristics. Furthermore, this has led to a group of products that are non-regulated devices, in which the nonviable materials do not have a medicinal claim (i.e., as standalone products, these would not meet the definition of a medicinal product as defined in Directive 2001/83/EC), and so are considered exempt from the *ATMP Regulation*. Examples of such products include human skin substitutes containing nonviable fibroblasts, and human bone void fillers containing human bone tissue. These products are excluded from both the ATMP and the devices legislation and are subject to national legislation, which may vary from country to country.

To attempt to address these gaps and simplify the devices legislation, while ensuring as high a level of protection of public health as possible, the European Commission launched a public consultation with a commitment to "recast" Directives 90/385/EEC and 93/42/EEC, and the results were published in December 2008.[9] The overall outcome of this consultation was that stakeholders confirmed that medical devices consisting exclusively of nonviable human cells, tissues or their derivatives, and medical devices incorporating such cells/tissues/derivatives with an action ancillary to that of the medical device, are currently not regulated at the EU level. In this regard, the majority of respondents took the view that medical devices consisting of or incorporating nonviable human tissue or cells should be regulated under the *MDD*, through revision of the provisions of Directive 2003/32/EC regarding nonviable animal tissues or cells. In contrast, a minority of respondents considered that such products should fall under the *ATMP Regulation*. In addition, tissue banks highlighted concerns about how the *EUTCD* fits into the possible future regulation of nonviable human tissues and cells.

So far, there has been no amendment to the scope of the *MDD* and the *Active Implantable Medical Devices Directive* (*AIMDD*, Directive 90/385/EEC) to include certain human tissue derivatives, based on the outcome of the consultation. However, the European Commission has released a roadmap for 2012, which contains the *Proposal for a Regulation of the European Parliament and of the Council concerning medical devices and repealing Directives 90/385/EEC and 93/42/EEC*.[10] This proposal includes a possibility for an extension of the scope of the EU legislation on medical devices to cover products manufactured utilising nonviable tissues and cells of human origin. No defined timelines for such revisions have been put forward at this time.

In any case, for products that clearly fall under the definition of a combined ATMP, manufacturers will still need to consider the requirements of the *MDD* (including the requirements of CE marking) for the device element of the product. Although the MAA for such a product will be reviewed by CAT, as for other ATMPs, the application should include evidence to show that the device meets the requirements of the medical devices legislation, as well as evidence of compatibility of the cells with the device. Medical devices are usually assessed by an appropriate Notified Body (NB). In the case of a combined ATMP, the applicant can provide the results of a previous assessment performed by an NB in the MAA dossier. If this is not the case, then CAT will seek additional assessment by an NB as part of the MAA procedure prior to affixing the CE Mark and approving the product, unless it deems that the involvement of an NB is not required. The exact relationship between the CAT, the manufacturer and the NB has been clarified, with EMA publishing a document entitled, *Procedural advice on the evaluation of combined advanced therapy medicinal products and the consultation of Notified Bodies in accordance with Article 9 of Regulation (EC) No 1394/2007*. This guidance provides information on how the assessment procedure for a combined ATMP will be coordinated and the associated timelines.

Standards and Coding

The main purpose of the *EUTCD* was to set standards for the quality and safety of human-derived material. In addition to the quality testing set out in the *EUTCD*, Article 25 of the directive also specified the creation of a European-wide coding system, since it was considered that adoption of a universal coding, nomenclature and labelling system would enhance tissue sharing (exchange and importation) among nations and additionally improve traceability. The *EUTCD* states that Member States should "establish a system for the identification of human tissues and cells, in order to ensure the traceability of all human tissues and cells" and that "the Commission, in cooperation with the Member States, shall design a single European coding system to provide information on the main characteristics and properties of tissues and cells." This coding system was intended to complement coding/traceability systems already in place at the national level, rather than replace them.

The European Commission requested that the European Standards Committee (CEN) set out the specifications of this European coding system for human tissues and cells, as well as provide guidance on how to implement the system. This was based on previous work performed by the Tissue and Cells Regulatory Committee Expert Working Group that was established in accordance with Article 29 of the *EUTCD*. During a workshop in 2008, the working group analysed three candidate coding systems proposed by Member State representatives, and, together with a panel including DG SANCO representatives and lawyers, recommended use of ISBT 128 as the basis for the EU coding scheme. The outcome of this workshop was published in a recommendation in June 2008.[11] This is seen to be the first step toward a worldwide standard in tissue and cell therapy.

In addition to the use of ISBT 128, due to the pre-existence of coding schemes defined at the national or organisational level, it was proposed at the workshop that an additional component be created to support both use of ISBT 128 and the existing coding schemes; this would involve unique identification by means of a "key code." The task of further defining the "key code" was assigned to the Tissue and Cells Regulatory Committee Expert Working Group. In a more recent meeting of the working group, it was proposed that this key code could be used with existing coding systems to provide unique identification and allow EU traceability of all materials from one donation event. Therefore, the coding system would serve to link the existing national traceability systems. Specifically, it is proposed that the code will include a national identification number and an EU-identification number.[12] The EU-identification number will consist of a donor identification code that is unique to the country (ISO 3166-1) and tissue establishment, and contains a local donation number. In addition, a product identification code will be included; both ISBT-28 and EUROCODE are under consideration as suitable systems to identify product characteristics. The classification and coding system is still under development at the time of this update.

In addition to this EU-wide coding system, other standards work is ongoing in Europe, with release of a revised draft version of the publicly available specification *(PAS) 83: Guidance on codes of practice, standardised methods and regulations for cell-based therapeutics.*[13] This document provides recommendations on the standards necessary for cell-based therapies to be used in clinical trials in the UK, and describes the accompanying legislation, codes of practice, guidance documents and standards for this process. This document was developed by the Department of Trade and Industry (DTI) with the British Standards Institution (BSI) in 2006 and is being revised to incorporate the *ATMP Regulation*. It is anticipated that this updated version will be ready sometime in 2012–13. Additional standards recently published include *PAS 93:Characterization of human cells for clinical applications.*[14] This document is a best practice guide for organisations that develop products for clinical applications, using human cells as their building blocks, and provides details on the characterisation of such products and associated methods. While these documents do not constitute a formal British Standard, they still serve to create management systems, product benchmarks and codes of practice that will aid the development of cell- and tissue-derived products.

Summary

Since this chapter was last updated, significant regulatory progress has been made, and there has been a gradual transposition into national law by Member States of the *EU Tissues and Cells Directive* (*EUTCD*, Directive 2004/23/EC), as well as its implementing directives, 2006/17/EC and 2006/86/EC. Industry no longer has to speculate about minimum EU requirements for human tissue products or to guess which guidelines and requirements to implement. Member States, however, are permitted to augment or supplement the requirements of the directives, based on national legislation determined by the Member State to be necessary to ensure public health within its jurisdiction. In this regard, several countries with pre-existing legislation have transposed the directive into national law, but elected to maintain it as a minimum requirement that is supplemented by national requirements.

In addition to the implementation of the *EUTCD*, the regulation of human tissue- and cell-based products has been further harmonised across the EU through the advent of the *ATMP Regulation* (Regulation (EC) No 1394/2007), which defines how somatic cell therapy and tissue-engineered medical products are authorised for marketing and distribution. This regulation serves to remove the disparity in how such products were previously regulated in different countries, which was not conducive to product commercialisation or exchange among Member States.

The *ATMP Regulation* became applicable in all Member States on 30 December 2008; however, a transitional period was provided for cell therapy and tissue-engineered products that were legally marketed prior to that date. In the case of cell therapies, the transitional period ended in December 2011, while tissue-engineered products have until 30 December 2012 to comply with the regulation. At the time of this update, only one cell-/tissue-based product has received marketing approval under the *ATMP Regulation* framework. In response to industry feedback, CAT has proposed a five-year Work Programme to 2015,[15] with the aim of making the new framework more accessible to small companies and academia that are at the forefront of developing ATMPs, and eventually increasing the number of ATMPs that make it from the bench onto the market. Furthermore, the Commission has promised to publish a general report on the application of the *ATMP Regulation* by 30 December 2012, which shall include comprehensive information on the different types of ATMPs authorised pursuant to this regulation.

References

1. European Commission "Consultation Document," *Need for a legislative framework for human tissue engineering and tissue-engineered products,* (June 2002). EC website. http://ec.europa.eu/health/files/advtherapies/docs/st09756_en.pdf. Accessed 24 May 2012.
2. "Proposal for a Directive of the European Parliament and of the Council on setting standards of quality and safety for the donation, procurement, testing, processing, storage, and distribution of human tissues and cells." COM(2002) 0319 final; 2002/0128(COD), 19 June 2002. EUR-Lex website. http://eur-lex.europa.eu/smartapi/cgi/sga_doc?smartapi!celexplus!prod!DocNumber&type_doc=COMfinal&an_doc=2002&nu_doc=0319&lg=en. Accessed 24 May 2012.
3. Communication from the Commission to the Council, the European Parliament, the European Economic and Social Committee and the Committee of the Regions on the application of Directive 2004/23/EC on setting standards of quality and safety for the donation, procurement, testing, processing, preservation, storage and distribution of human tissues and cells, COM (2009) 0708 January 2010. EUR-Lex website. http://eur-lex.europa.eu/LexUriServ/LexUriServ.do?uri=COM:2009:0708:FIN:EN:HTML. Accessed 24 May 2012.
4. Ibid.
5. Summary Table of Responses from Competent Authorities for Tissues and Cells: Questionnaire on the transposition and implementation of the European Tissues and Cells regulatory framework, December 2009 (SANCO C6 /PL/hp/D(2010)360016). EC website. http://ec.europa.eu/health/blood_tissues_organs/docs/tissues_responses_2008_en.pdf. Accessed 24 May 2012.
6. The European Association for Bioindustries (EuropaBio). *Biotech Fact Sheet: Human Cell and Tissue Based Products*.Brussels, Belgium. May 2003.
7. Statements by the Commission—Re Article 6. Official Journal of the European Union L 412/42, December 2006. EUR-Lex website. http://eur-lex.europa.eu/LexUriServ/LexUriServ.do?uri=OJ:L:2006:412:0042:0043:EN:PDF. Accessed 24 May 2012.
8. EMA/CHMP/845661/2011,Questions and answers: Refusal of the marketing authorisation for Glybera (alipogene tiparvovec): Outcome of re-examination. EMA website. www.ema.europa.eu/docs/en_GB/document_library/Summary_of_opinion_-_Initial_authorisation/human/002145/WC500116926.pdf. Accessed 24 May 2012.
9. Recast Of The Medical Devices Directives Summary Of Responses To The Public Consultation, December 2008 (ENTR/F/3/D(2008) 39582).
10. Roadmap: Proposal for a Regulation of the European Parliament and of the Council concerning medical devices and repealing Directives 90/385/EEC and 93/42/EEC; November 2011. SANCO/B2. EC website. http://ec.europa.eu/governance/impact/planned_ia/docs/2008_sanco_081_proposal_medical_devices_en.pdf. Accessed 24 May 2012.
11. CEN Workshop Agreement: CWA 15849 - Coding of Information and Traceability of Human Tissues and Cells, June 2008. CEN website. ftp://cenftp1.cenorm.be/PUBLIC/CWAs/e-Europe/Tissues_cells/CWA15849-2008-publishedtext.pdf. Accessed 24 May 2012.
12. Meeting of the Competent Authorities for Tissues and Cells—Summary Report, June 2011 (SANCO D4/IS/hp ARES(2011). EC website. http://ec.europa.eu/health/blood_tissues_organs/docs/tissues_mi_20110623_en.pdf. 24 May 2012.
13. PAS 83:2006 Guidance on codes of practice, standardised methods and regulations for cell-based therapeutics—from basic research to clinical application. BSI website. http://shop.bsigroup.com/en/Browse-by-Sector/Healthcare/PAS-832006/. Accessed 24 May 2012.
14. PAS 93:2011 Characterization of human cells for clinical applications. Guide. Available from BSI. http://shop.bsigroup.com/en/ProductDetail/?pid=000000000030213318.
15. Committee for Advanced Therapies (CAT) Work Programme 2010–2015, 30 June 2010. EMA/CAT/235374/2010. EMA website. www.ema.europa.eu/docs/en_GB/document_library/Work_programme/2010/11/WC500099029.pdf. Accessed 24 May 2012.

Chapter 28

Vaccines

By Shailesh S. Dewasthaly

OBJECTIVES

- Understand pre- and post-licensure development of vaccines in Europe
- Understand regulation of vaccines in Europe
- Understand lot release requirements for vaccines
- Understand special topics in vaccines such as adjuvants, lot release, influenza vaccines, etc.

DIRECTIVES, REGULATIONS AND GUIDELINES COVERED IN THIS CHAPTER

- Commission Directive 2003/94/EC of 8 October 2003 laying down the principles and guidelines of good manufacturing practice in respect of medicinal products for human use and investigational medicinal products for human use
- Commission Directive 2005/28/EC of 8 April 2005 laying down principles and detailed guidelines for good clinical practice as regards investigational medicinal products for human use, as well as the requirements for authorisation of the manufacturing or importation of such products
- Directive 2001/83/EC of the European Parliament and of the Council of 6 November 2001 on the Community code relating to medicinal products for human use
- Directive 2001/20/EC of the European Parliament and of the Council of 4 April 2001 on the approximation of the laws, regulations and administrative provisions of the Member States relating to the implementation of good clinical practice in the conduct of clinical trials on medicinal products for human use
- Directive 2001/18/EC of the European Parliament and of the Council of 12 March 2001 on the deliberate release into the environment of genetically modified organisms and repealing Council Directive 90/220/EEC
- Directive 2008/27/EC of the European Parliament and of the Council of 11 March 2008 amending Directive 2001/18/EC on the deliberate release into the environment of genetically modified organisms, as regards the implementing powers conferred on the Commission
- Council Directive 89/105/EEC of 21 December 1988 relating to the transparency of measures regulating the prices of medicinal products for human use and their inclusion in the scope of national health insurance systems
- Regulation (EC) No 726/2004 of the European Parliament and of the Council of 31 March 2004 laying down Community procedures for the authorisation and supervision of medicinal products for human and veterinary use and establishing a European Medicines Agency

Chapter 28

- Proposal for a Directive of the European Parliament and of the Council relating to the transparency of measures regulating the prices of medicinal products for human use and their inclusion in the scope of public health insurance systems

- The Rules Governing Medicinal Products in the European Union, Volume 1, EU pharmaceutical legislation for medicinal products for human use

- The Rules Governing Medicinal Products in the European Union, Volume 5, EU pharmaceutical legislation for medicinal products for veterinary use

- Guideline on quality, non-clinical and clinical aspects of live recombinant viral vectored vaccines, January 2011 (EMA/CHMP/VWP/141697/2009)

- Concept Paper on guidance for DNA vaccines, October 2007 (EMEA/CHMP/308136/2007)

- Note for Guidance on the Clinical Evaluation of Vaccines, February 2007 (EMEA/CHMP/VWP/164653/05)

- Guideline on Clinical Evaluation of New Vaccines Annex: SPC Requirements, February 2007 (EMEA/CHMP/VWP/382702/2006)

- CHMP Position Paper on Thiomersal: Implementation of the Warning Statement Relating to Sensitisation, January 2007 (EMEA/CHMP/VWP/19541/2007)

- Explanatory Note on Immunomodulators for the Guideline on Adjuvants in Vaccines for Human Use, July 2006 (CHMP/VWP/244894/2006)

- Guideline on Adjuvants in Vaccines for Human Use, July 2005 (CHMP/VEG/134716/04)

- EMEA Public Statement on Thiomersal in Vaccines for Human Use—Recent Evidence Supports Safety of Thiomersal-containing Vaccines, March 2004 (EMEA/CPMP/VEG/1194/04)

- Guideline on the Scientific Data Requirements for a Vaccine Antigen Master File (VAMF), March 2004 (CPMP/BWP/3734/03)

- Guideline on Requirements for Vaccine Antigen Master File (VAMF) Certification, February 2004 (CPMP/4548/03/Final/ Rev 1)

- CPMP Position Statement on the Quality of Water used in the production of Vaccines for parenteral use, October 2003 (CPMP/BWP/1571/02 Rev 1)

- Note for Guidance on the Development of Vaccinia Virus Based Vaccines Against Smallpox, July 2002 (CPMP/1100/02)

- Points to Consider on the Reduction, Elimination or Substitution of Thiomersal in Vaccines, May 2001 (CPMP/BWP/2517/00)

- Public Statement on the Evaluation of Bovine Spongiform Encephalopathies (BSE)—risk via the use of materials of bovine origin in or during the manufacture of vaccines, February 2001 (CPMP/BWP/476/01)

- Concept Paper on the Development of a Committee for Proprietary Medicinal Products (CPMP) Points to Consider on Stability and Traceability Requirements for Vaccine Intermediates, 2000 (CPMP/BWP/4310/00)

- Note for Guidance on Pharmaceutical and Biological Aspects of Combined Vaccines, January 1999 (CPMP/BWP/477/97)

- Note for Guidance on Preclinical Pharmacological and Toxicological Testing of Vaccines, December 1997 (CPMP/SWP/465/95)

- Concept paper for a guideline on the quality of porcine trypsin used in the manufacture of human biological medicinal products, September 2011 (EMA/CHMP/BWP/367751/2011)

- Concept paper on a revision of the guideline on pharmaceutical aspects of the product information for human vaccines, July 2009 (EMEA/CHMP/BWP/290688/09)

- Guideline on Virus Safety Evaluation of Biotechnological Investigational Medicinal Products, February 2009 (EMEA/CHMP/BWP/398498/05)

- Guideline on Environmental Risk Assessments for Medicinal Products Consisting of, or Containing, Genetically Modified Organisms (GMOs) (Module 1.6.2), July 2007 (EMEA/CHMP/473191/06 Corr)

- Guideline on Pharmaceutical Aspects of the Product Information for Human Vaccines, November 2003 (CPMP/BWP/2758/02)

- Note for Guidance on the Use of Bovine Serum in the Manufacture of Human Biological Medicinal Products, October 2003 (CPMP/BWP/1793/02)

- Testing for SV40 in poliovirus vaccines, April 2002 (CPMP/BWP/1412/02)

- Development Pharmaceutics for Biotechnological and Biological Products—Annex to Note for Guidance on Development Pharmaceutics, October 1999 (CPMP/BWP/328/99)

- Position Paper on Viral Safety of Oral Poliovirus Vaccine (OPV), May 1998 (CPMP/BWP/972/98)

- Note for Guidance on Virus Validation Studies: The Design, Contribution and Interpretation of Studies Validating the Inactivation and Removal of Viruses, August 1996 (CPMP/BWP/268/95 3AB8A)

European Institutions Involved With Vaccines

European Commission

The European Commission is a pan-European organisation based in Brussels and is responsible for drafting proposals for new European laws. It is the body that issues licenses for medicinal products authorised through the Centralised Procedure.

European Medicines Agency

The European Medicines Agency (EMA), based in London, is responsible for scientific evaluations for applications (including licence applications) through the Centralised Procedure. EMA's Committee for Medicinal Products for Human Use (CHMP) is responsible for human medicines. It, in turn, has several working parties that make recommendations on specific product types, one of which is the Vaccine Working Party (VWP).

VWP's tasks include providing scientific advice on general and specific aspects of vaccines at the request of CHMP, supporting dossier evaluation for vaccines, issuing vaccine guidelines, working with other organisations like the World Health Organization on vaccine-related matters, and many other functions related to vaccines. The detailed mandate description is provided on the EMA website.

Vaccines

Vaccines and vaccinations are considered one of the 10 great public health achievements of the 20th century.[1] Although vaccines are medicinal products (and, therefore, follow the same development pathways as drugs), vaccines are different from other medicinal products in many respects. Vaccines are produced in biological systems that are more complex than "chemical reactions." In terms of manufacturing, they use biological systems that make vaccine quality control very complex. In a way, they are unique with short exposure and long-term response. They generally are provided as a preventive (prophylactic) measure to healthy individuals, the majority of whom are children at a vulnerable age; hence, very high levels of safety are required during development. Additionally, as there is no immediate health benefit for an individual who is vaccinated, there is a limited acceptance of risks. Therefore, vaccines are assessed through a different risk:benefit profile than therapeutic drugs.

Development of Vaccines

Vaccine development follows the same path as other drugs for human use. In general, during development, there is a short- to medium-term goal of ensuring activities for clinical trial authorisation, and a long-term goal of fulfilling requirements for product licensure. Given the nature of vaccines, some aspects of the product require special attention even during development.

Many guidelines for the development of medicinal products are also applicable to vaccines. Other guidelines that may apply to vaccines fall under the "Biologics/Biotechnological Products" category. Some general guidelines apply to all vaccines (see **Table 28-1**), while others deal with specific vaccines like Influenza vaccines (mentioned later) and the development of Vaccinia virus-based vaccines (second generation) against smallpox (CPMP/1100/02). Although smallpox has been eradicated, smallpox vaccines are part of certain national stockpiles. Many of these vaccines now are produced by tissue culture process, not from live animals, as was previously the case.

Important European vaccine guidelines for the development of vaccines are discussed in the following sections.

Manufacturing and Quality Control

Vaccines are biological/biotechnological products that involve biological processes. Compared to a chemical (drug) or mechanical (device) process, a biological process is complicated by the involvement of live organisms. As a

Chapter 28

Table 28-1. Vaccine Guidelines

Title	Date	Number
Guideline on quality, non-clinical and clinical aspects of live recombinant viral vectored vaccines	January 2011	EMA/CHMP/VWP/141697/2009
Concept Paper on guidance for DNA vaccines	October 2007	EMEA/CHMP/308136/2007
Note for Guidance on the Clinical Evaluation of Vaccines	February 2007	EMEA/CHMP/VWP/164653/05
Guideline on Clinical Evaluation of New Vaccines Annex: SPC Requirements	February 2007	EMEA/CHMP/VWP/382702/2006
CHMP Position Paper on Thiomersal: Implementation of the Warning Statement Relating to Sensitisation	January 2007	EMEA/CHMP/VWP/19541/2007
Explanatory Note on Immunomodulators for the Guideline on Adjuvants in Vaccines for Human Use	July 2006	CHMP/VWP/244894/2006
Guideline on Adjuvants in Vaccines for Human Use	July 2005	CHMP/VEG/134716/04
EMEA Public Statement on Thiomersal in Vaccines for Human Use—Recent Evidence Supports Safety of Thiomersal-containing Vaccines	March 2004	EMEA/CPMP/VEG/1194/04
Guideline on the Scientific Data Requirements for a Vaccine Antigen Master File (VAMF)	March 2004	CPMP/BWP/3734/03
Guideline on Requirements for Vaccine Antigen Master File (VAMF) Certification	February 2004	CPMP/4548/03/Final/ Rev 1
CPMP Position Statement on the Quality of Water used in the production of Vaccines for parenteral use	October 2003	CPMP/BWP/1571/02 Rev 1
Note for Guidance on the Development of Vaccinia Virus Based Vaccines Against Smallpox	July 2002	CPMP/1100/02
Points to Consider on the Reduction, Elimination or Substitution of Thiomersal in Vaccines	May 2001	CPMP/BWP/2517/00
Public Statement on the Evaluation of Bovine Spongiform Encephalopathies (BSE)—risk via the use of materials of bovine origin in or during the manufacture of vaccines	February 2001	CPMP/BWP/476/01
Concept Paper on the Development of a Committee for Proprietary Medicinal Products (CPMP) Points to Consider on Stability and Traceability Requirements for Vaccine Intermediates	January 2001	CPMP/BWP/4310/00
Note for Guidance on Pharmaceutical and Biological Aspects of Combined Vaccines	January 1999	CPMP/BWP/477/97
Note for Guidance on Preclinical Pharmacological and Toxicological Testing of Vaccines	December 1997	CPMP/SWP/465/95

result, every manufactured "lot" is slightly different from the previous one, complicating the process of assuring the quality and consistency of biotechnological/biological products. The assurance of quality also impacts the risks and benefits to trial subjects and to vaccinees once the product is licensed. It must be remembered that trial subjects for vaccines are drawn from a "healthy population," thus the level of acceptable risks is significantly lower than for therapeutic products, e.g., cancer treatments.

EU directives and EMA guidances for medicinal products provide the basic principles of vaccine production and control. A recent draft guideline based on the International Conference on Harmonisation (ICH) Q11 document, *Development and manufacture of drug substances* (EMA/CHMP/ICH/425213/2011) has completed the consultation phase. This guideline discusses both chemical entities and biotechnological products. For biotechnological products (like vaccines), certain principles should be considered during the development stage because the manufacturing process defines the product.

Another new guideline not yet adopted discusses *Requirements for quality documentation concerning biological investigational medicinal products in clinical trials* (EMEA/CHMP/BWP/534898/08). This guidance is specifically aimed at harmonising requirements and the assessment of quality information for biological/biotechnological investigational medicinal product or clinical trial material throughout the EU. Similar guidance already exists that covers all investigational medicinal products (IMPs) in clinical trials (CHMP/QWP/185401/2004). In terms of quality documentation for a clinical trial, manufacturers need to submit an Investigational Medicinal Product Dossier (IMPD).

Vaccines, like other medicinal products, must be manufactured in compliance with GMP regulations, found in *The Rules Governing Medicinal Products in the European Union, Volume 4*, and Directive 2003/94/EC (the *GMP Directive*), for both clinical trial materials and approved products. In 2010, the EC released draft guidance for biologics' CGMPs, *Manufacture of Biological Medicinal Substances and Products for Human Use* (ENTR/C/8/SF D(2010) 380334) for public consultation. The guidance was revised to include advanced therapy medicinal products (ATMPs). Although the guidance has not been finalised, it does indicate the current thinking of EU experts on this topic.

In the EU, all firms manufacturing medicinal products, even investigational products, are required to obtain manufacturing authorisation issued by the respective national or regional authority of the Member State (Directive 2005/28/EC). Another specific EU requirement for both drug and biological manufacturers is that a Qualified Person (QP) must certify that every lot/batch is in compliance with the approved product specification for use in clinical trials and on the market. The QP's role in lot certification throughout the development process became mandatory in the EU under Directive 2001/83/EC. Previously, the QP was involved only in approved products in most EU Member States, while in some there was no requirement for a QP; since 2004, a QP also must be involved with IMPs. The QP is bound by the law to ensure the suitability of every lot before it is released for human use in any EU Member State. Details of the QP role can be found in EMA's CGMP guidelines and are applicable for all medicinal products, including vaccines and drugs. Lots manufactured outside the EU are also subject to QP certification and release.

Interestingly, there is a specific CHMP position paper on quality of water used for parenteral vaccines in the EU (CPMP/BWP/1571/02 Rev 1). This guideline clarifies that Water for Injection (WI) must be used for final formulation of vaccines; lesser quality water may be used for other manufacturing steps.

Local requirements for clinical trials vary to some extent among the EU Member States. For example, for the authority lot/batch release of vaccines or biologics for IMPs, some authorities do not require an official release of lot/batch for clinical trials as long as the Clinical Trial Application (CTA) is in place and the company's QP has certified the lot. However, other Members States require lot release before the IMP can be used in humans; usually this is a "paper release," i.e., only lot relevant documents like CoA documentation must be submitted and approved, while other Member States specify certain Official Medicines Control Laboratory (OMCL) tests, including vaccine potency. Austria and the Netherlands require lot release of vaccine IMPs; while Germany, the UK and other Member States do not require specific lot release by the authorities; clinical trial approval and the release of the lot by the company QP is sufficient for administering the medicine in clinical trials provided other required approvals (e.g., Ethics Committees) are in place. Due to these differing requirements, manufacturers are always advised to contact the respective clinical trial authority for vaccine IMP lot release requirements. Manufacturers should remember that all lots of marketed vaccines are subject to authority lot release, which is discussed later in this chapter.

Vaccines contain certain typical additives apart from the impurities resulting from the manufacturing process (e.g., host cell proteins). Thiomersal is one such additive (preservative) used historically in vaccines (especially in multidose vials). In 2004, EMA issued a public statement on the safety of vaccines containing thiomersal (EMEA/CPMP/VEG/1194/04). EMA also encourages vaccine manufacturers to produce vaccines with very low to no thiomersal. Specific guidance exists on how to implement the warning statement to sensitisation in the Summary of Product Characteristics (SmPC) (EMEA/CHMP/VWP/19541/2007). Process impurities like host cell proteins are inevitable and the levels must meet the specifications in the 1998 WHO guideline on the use of animal cells for the production of biological products.[2] Some additives used in vaccines are adjuvants and stabilisers. Adjuvants are discussed later in the chapter and stabilisers generally are covered in vaccine (CMC) guidelines.

Vaccine Antigen Master File

Vaccines are continuously being developed that will be part of combination vaccines. A combination vaccine offers obvious advantages such as convenient administration and protection against multiple diseases. If an antigen used in one component of a combination vaccine is also part of the other vaccine, then this antigen can be subject to Vaccine Antigen Master File (VAMF) certification, whereby the Competent Authority reviews and issues a VAMF. Information on the scientific requirements and evaluation of the VAMF can be found in *Guideline on the Scientific Data Requirements for a Vaccine Antigen Master File* (EMEA/CPMP/BWP/3734/03). The guideline also clarifies the number of certificates required for certain vaccines, e.g., Polio (3); 23-valent Pneumococcal polysaccharide (23), etc. A VAMF is designed to help both manufacturers and Competent Authorities reduce the number of submissions and assessments, and ensure vaccine consistency throughout the EU. A manufacturer may choose to apply for VAMF certification at the Community level through EMA. A positive assessment of the submission results in the issuance of a VAMF certificate that can be used in all vaccines containing the same antigen. The certificate is also valid in all European countries. The procedural guidance is mentioned in *Guideline on requirements for Vaccine Antigen Master File (VAMF) certification* (EMEA/CPMP/BWP/4548/03).

The content of the VAMF application is identical to the 3.2.S section of the Common Technical Document (CTD), in addition to the relevant CTD 3.2.A sections on equipment and facilities and adventitious safety evaluation.

Nonclinical

Nonclinical aspects of vaccine development are discussed by EMA in *Note for guidance on preclinical pharmacological and toxicological testing of vaccines* (CPMP/SWP/465/95). According to this guidance, many typical toxicological studies for "drugs" are generally not necessary for vaccines, e.g., genotoxicity, etc. The guidance also suggests that the omission of certain toxicology tests should be properly justified.

A few years ago, due to an industry initiative,[3] the need for a dedicated acute toxicology test was re-assessed and, as a result, the guideline was withdrawn. According to *Questions and answers on the withdrawal of the 'Note for guidance on single dose toxicity'* (EMA/CHMP/SWP/81714/2010), EMA recognises that traditional single-dose toxicity studies are of limited value and that eliminating them also will help reduce the number of animals used for testing. Data about acute toxicity can be obtained from other toxicology studies. Similar changes have also been made to the ICH M3(R2) guideline.

Clinical

Clinical trials performed in the EU are required to be conducted in accordance with the EU *Clinical Trials Directive* (Directive 2001/20/EC) and must be in compliance with Good Clinical Practices (GCPs). Almost all the elements in the EU directive have been incorporated into Member States' legislation. Although this has ensured similar standards and requirements across Member States, there are also additional local requirements. Similar to those for drugs, vaccine clinical trials are regulated at the national level. Therefore, in addition to following the EU directives, trial sponsors should expect minor local differences at the national level during the review of the CTA. This can be especially true for such complex products as vaccines and biotechnological products. As mentioned previously, since vaccines are administered to healthy individuals, the safety review of the vaccine is particularly critical. It might be prudent to consider clinical trials in countries with "experienced" Competent Authorities in a specific disease/product area. It also may be pointed out that the healthcare locations generally used for clinical trials with specific "patients" and clinical research organisations often are clustered in the same regions.

Requirements for conducting a clinical trial are defined in *The Rules Governing Medicinal Products in the European Union, Volume 10*, Clinical trial guidelines (http://ec.europa.eu/health/documents/eudralex/vol-10/). *Volume 10* is a collection of information on clinical trials in the EU, ranging from legislation to inspections. A CTA is set of documents submitted to a national Competent Authority for approval of a clinical trial. It contains administrative documentation, quality documentation, the clinical trial protocol, etc. The quality documentation is the IMPD mentioned above. The IMPD follows CTD granularity, which has no specific requirements for vaccines. IMPD structure and content can be found in the *Guideline on requirements to the chemical and pharmaceutical quality documentation concerning investigational medicinal products in clinical trials* (CHMP/QWP/185401/2004 final).

Requirements for the clinical development of vaccines are described in *Guideline on clinical evaluation of new vaccines* (EMEA/CHMP/VWP/164653/2005). This guideline outlines requirements for vaccine clinical studies. It also discusses situations where efficacy studies for vaccines are not possible. In general, all vaccine developers are encouraged to establish immunological correlates of protection during the development process. The annex to this main guidance (EMEA/CHMP/VWP/382702/2006) deals with SmPC requirements for vaccines and provides details on some sections (4 and 5, i.e., clinical particulars and pharmacological properties) of the standard SmPC template provided by the Quality Review of Documents (QRD) convention that are unique to vaccines.

Vaccine Licensure in the EU

Vaccine licensure in the EU (Marketing Authorisation (MA)) follows the same route as other medicinal products,

Table 28-2. Adjuvants Licensed in the EU

Adjuvant	Contains Mainly	Manufacturer	Vaccines
Alum	Aluminium hydroxide/phosphate	*many*	Hep A,B, DTaP, Tdap, Hib, HPV, Anthrax, Rabies, Pneumococcal conjugate vaccine etc.
MF59	Oil in water emulsion	Novartis	Influenza (Fluad/pandemic influenza)
AS03	Oil in water emulsion+tocopherol	GSK	Pandemic influenza
AS04	MPL+alum	GSK	HPV (Cervarix), HBV (Fendrix)
Liposomes	Oil in water emulsion	Crucell	HAV, Influenza

(Modified from Mbow et al 2010 New Adjuvants for human vaccines. Curr Opinion Immunol. 22: 411-16)

Figure 28-1. OCABR Decision Flowchart

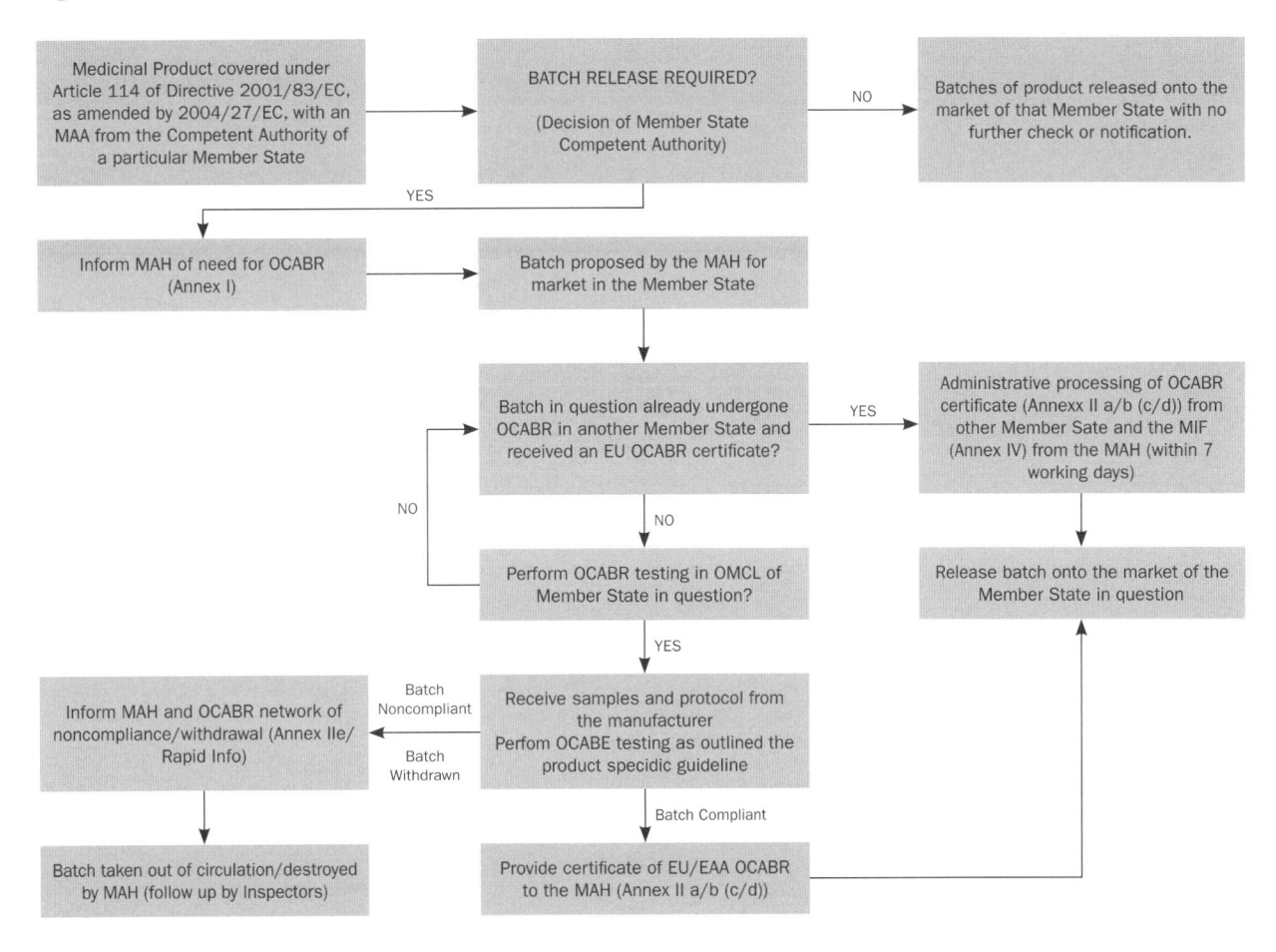

(from: http://www.edqm.eu accessed Jan 2012)

i.e., Centralised, Decentralised, Mutual Recognition or National Procedure. The Centralised Procedure is mandatory for certain types of products, e.g., orphan drugs, etc., and offers the advantage of having a single Marketing Authorisation Application (MAA), single process and MAs in all EU Member States and the EEA states of Iceland, Liechtenstein and Norway. It is interesting to note that the company may choose not to simultaneously market the product in all countries. The MAA should be in CTD format. The electronic CTD (eCTD) is now the standard for submitting MAAs in the EU, and there are no special requirements for vaccines.

If the MAA contains a VAMF, the appropriate documents must be included in the application (in CTD section 3.2 S). A summary of the section is also included in section 2.3.S, Quality Overall Summary (QOS).

For more information on the licensure procedure in the EU, please refer to Chapter 17.

Other Aspects of Vaccines

Many vaccines are incomplete without adjuvants. This section discusses some aspects unique to vaccines like adjuvants and DNA vaccines.

Adjuvants

Charles Janeway called adjuvants "immunologists' dirty secrets." Adjuvants are components that help enhance or modulate the immune response either by higher titres, long-lived titres or both, or by influencing the immune response in a particular direction (e.g., cellular rather than humoral). Although adjuvants have been used for a long time, their complete and precise mechanism of action still is unknown.

Universally, alum (either aluminium hydroxide or aluminium phosphate) is the most commonly used adjuvant in vaccines licensed for human use. In the EU, the requirements for adjuvants are defined in *Guideline on adjuvants in vaccines for human use* (EMEA/CHMP/VEG/134716/2004). This guidance discusses almost all aspects of adjuvant

Regulatory Affairs Professionals Society

Table 28-3. European Guidelines for Influenza Vaccines

Title	Date	Number
Seasonal Vaccines		
Guideline on quality aspects on the isolation of candidate influenza vaccine viruses in cell culture	February 2012	CHMP/BWP/368186/2011
Procedural advice on the submission of variations for annual update of human influenza inactivated vaccines applications in the centralised procedure	February 2011	EMA/CHMP/BWP/99698/2007
Points to Consider on the Development of Live Attenuated Influenza Vaccines	August 2003	CPMP/BWP/2289/01
Cell Culture Inactivated Influenza Vaccines—Annex to Note for Guidance on Harmonisation of Requirements for Influenza Vaccines (CPMP/BWP/214/96)	August 2002	CPMP/BWP/2490/00
Note for Guidance on Harmonisation of Requirements for Influenza Vaccines	April 1997	CPMP/BWP/214/96
Pandemic Vaccines		
Concept paper on the revision of guidelines for influenza vaccines	October 2011	EMA/CHMP/VWP/734330/2011
Annex I variation application(s) content for live attenuated influenza vaccines	October 2011	EMA/CHMP/BWP/577998/2010
Core SPC for Pandemic Influenza Vaccines	July 2010	EMEA/CHMP/VWP/193031/2004 Rev-1
Standard Paediatric Investigation Plan for non-adjuvanted or adjuvanted pandemic influenza vaccines during a pandemic	March 2010	EMA/185099/2010
CHMP Recommendations for the Pharmacovigilance Plan as part of the Risk Management Plan to be submitted with the Marketing Authorisation Application for a Pandemic Influenza Vaccine	September 2009	EMEA/359381/2009
Guideline on Dossier Structure and Content for Pandemic Influenza Vaccine Marketing Authorisation Application	January 2009	CHMP/VEG/4717/03 Rev 1
Guideline on Dossier Structure and Content of Marketing Authorisation Applications for Influenza Vaccines Derived from Strains with a Pandemic Potential for Use Outside the Core Dossier Context	January 2007	CHMP/VWP/263499/06
Guideline on Submission of Marketing Authorisation Applications for Pandemic Influenza Vaccines through the Centralised Procedure	April 2004	CPMP/4986/03

development, including manufacturing, characterisation, etc. Adjuvants are not licensed independently in the EU, but are licensed as a part of the vaccine product. One aspect worth mentioning is that the EU does not employ a Drug Master File (DMF) system. Consequently, all EU licence applications are expected to provide full information of the adjuvant (even if it is proprietary information held by a different party). It is interesting to note that more novel adjuvants are licensed in the EU than in the US. **Table 28-2** lists the adjuvants and their vaccines licensed in the EU.

Based on the previously mentioned guideline, all novel adjuvants are expected to be thoroughly characterised through physicochemical-biological methods. In addition, microbiological and chemical purity should be ascertained. Studies to show adjuvant-antigen mechanism of action, stability and other routine studies generally are recommended. Preclinical studies are required both with and without antigens. Preclinical studies for a novel adjuvant are determined based on the current guidance and the adjuvant-antigen combination and, in general, the strategy is decided on a case-by-case basis. Clinical studies should include, at a minimum, studies to show the adjuvant's benefit. If the adjuvant is intended to replace a licensed adjuvant-antigen (vaccine), immune response non-inferiority studies generally are expected.

The field of adjuvants has now expanded with immunomodulators included in certain products. EMA clarified through its *Explanatory note on immunomodulators for the guideline on adjuvants in vaccines for human use* (EMEA/CHMP/VWP/244894/2006) that if compounds are given separately from the vaccine antigen, these will be considered not adjuvants, but immunomodulators.

GMOs and DNA vaccines

Newer vaccines are being developed that contain genetically modified organisms (GMOs), bacteria and viruses, as vaccine candidates. Usually, these vaccine candidates contain a vector that could be an attenuated virus or bacteria that contains a heterologous antigen or gene. These vaccine candidates are treated as GMOs that require environmental risk assessment in addition to the quality, safety and efficacy assessment for both MA and clinical trial approval. Special regulations and guidelines are in place for medicinal products using GMOs like Regulation (EC) No 726/2004, Directive 2001/18/EC and Directive 2008/27/EC (amending the previously mentioned directive) and guidelines like *Environmental Risk Assessments for Medicinal Products Consisting of, or Containing, Genetically Modified Organisms (GMOs)* (EMEA/CHMP/BWP/473191/2006). Readers are also advised to refer to the guideline on quality, nonclinical and clinical aspects of live recombinant viral vectored vaccines (EMA/CHMP/VWP/141697/2009).

Usually a GMO vaccine product requires more time for clinical trial assessment and includes additional reviews during licence approval, e.g., the Paul-Erlich-Institut, Germany, suggests a 90-day assessment of the CTA for a product containing a GMO in contrast to only 30 days for other medicinal products like simple vaccines. As every country has different regulations and pathways, manufacturers are advised to check with their respective Competent Authority for more details on GMOs.

Assessing the environmental risks posed by a GMO product due to its release and/or excretion is an important aspect of the application. Live attenuated vaccines (not always GMOs) are subject to critical environmental assessment as they may find their way into the environment (*Environmental risk assessment of medicinal products for human use*, CHMP/SWP/4447/00).

There has been a lot of interest in DNA vaccines at the research level and, lately, some of the vaccines also have been the subject of human development. Although a concept paper was released by EMA on guidance for DNA vaccines, there is no specific guidance on the subject yet. Until such specific guidance is available, the note for guidance on the quality, preclinical and clinical aspects of gene transfer medicinal products (CPMP/BWP/3088/99) should be followed.

Therapeutic Vaccines

There is a great deal of ongoing research on therapeutic vaccines. Most of the research focusses on cancer and other life-threatening indications. Some of the products involve genetically modified cells as therapeutic vaccines. These generally are classified as ATMPs in the EU. Therapeutic vaccines are relatively new, and there are not many regulations in this field at this time. In the EU, there is no specific EMA guideline on this subject. However, applicable guidelines on ATMPs, biologicals, cell-based products, etc., are used. As all cancer therapies have access to the Centralised Procedure, any cancer vaccine also will be regulated through the Centralised Procedure. Under circumstances where specific guidelines are not available, guidelines for similar products or indications should be followed, e.g., in this particular case, *Guideline on evaluation of anticancer medicinal products in men*. Until such a specific guideline is available in the EU, manufacturers are advised to adhere to the US guideline, *Guidance for Industry: Clinical Considerations for Therapeutic Cancer Vaccines* (October 2011).

Lot Release of Licensed Vaccines

Vaccines, as biological/immunological products, are subject to special lot release requirements in almost all EU Member States. In addition to a company's QP release, vaccines also are tested by laboratories assigned by the Competent Authorities, OMCLs.

OMCLs

OMCLs in each Member State support the Competent Authorities in quality control of both human and veterinary medicines. Independent from manufacturers, OMCLs test products (or at least check their release documentation) before they can be released onto the market. A product certified by one OMCL is recognised by all other laboratories in the network. Within this OMCL organisation, the Official Control Authority Batch Release (OCABR) network is responsible for human biologicals (vaccine) testing.

EMA recommends that contact with potential OMCLs to exchange information should begin, ideally, approximately one year prior to submission of the MAA. This is important because it is possible not all agencies will have the resources and the technical capabilities for a particular assay or product. The OMCL decides which tests to perform as part of the lot release. Often, technology transfer may be required from the manufacturer to the OMCL for vaccine testing, which may be time consuming if special

> "Legal framework of OCABR is a part of the regulation of biological medicinal products, Article 114 of Directive 2001/83/EC relating to medicinal products for human use, as amended by Directive 2004/27/EC, of the European Parliament and of the Council provides that a Member State laboratory may, but is not required to, test a batch of an immunological medicinal product or a medicinal product derived from human blood or plasma before it is placed on the market. OCABR performed by any given Member State must be mutually recognised by all other member states requiring OCABR for that product."
>
> *From OCABR, EDQM (EDQM definition)*

Chapter 28

Figure 28-2. Process for Production and Licensing of Seasonal Influenza Vaccines in Europe

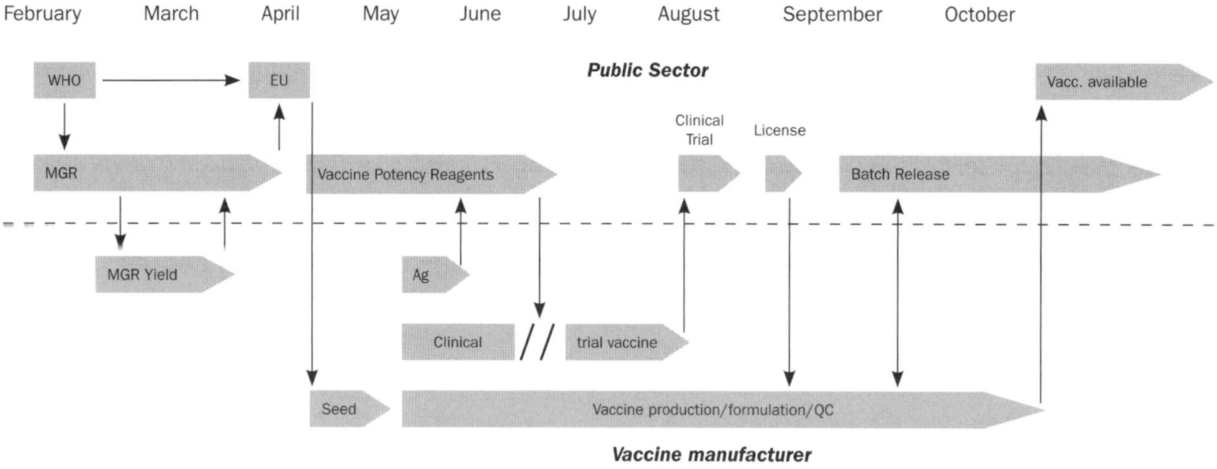

(from: Minor P D Clin Infect Dis. 2010;50:560-565)

tests are required. It is interesting to note that in some countries, OMCLs are different organisations than the Competent Authorities, e.g., the UK, where the Medicines and Healthcare products Regulatory Agency (MHRA) is the regulatory authority while the National Institute of Biological Standards and Control (NIBSC) is the OMCL. Information on the OMCL is discussed during the presubmission meeting with the Competent Authority. There are some advantages if the OMCL and rapporteur are from the same country and/or institution.

The Marketing Authorisation Holder (MAH) is expected to send the designated OMCL samples of each batch to be released onto the market along with the required documentation. The OMCL reviews the documentation and also tests the lot with specific test(s). If the test results are satisfactory, the OMCL issues an "Official Control Authority Batch Release Certificate," which essentially confirms that the batch has been tested and found to be compliant with the OCABR-defined guidelines, specifications in the MA and relevant European Pharmacopoeia monographs. This certificate is recognised by all OMCL network countries. **Figure 28-1** describes the algorithm for OMCL lot release of medicinal products.

A list of contacts for all OCABRs can be downloaded from www.edqm.eu/site/annex_iii_human_ocabr_contact_list_updated_2802201zip-en-30773-2.html

Risk Management Plans and Pharmacovigilance of Vaccines

Serious adverse events that are clinically relevant usually are rare and therefore are unlikely to be seen during vaccine development because exposure to vaccines is limited. Additionally, since vaccines are biological products and generally safe (as compared to drugs), related serious adverse events are usually very rare during development. Hence post-licensure monitoring of vaccines through Risk Management Plans (RMPs) and pharmacovigilance (PV) are very important. Although RMPs and PV plans are required for all medicinal products, PV plans and RMPs for vaccines are unique in some ways:

- Vaccines are given to healthy people, including children; consequently there is low tolerance for risks.
- There is no immediate benefit as diseases can be very rare, sometimes nonexistent (e.g., polio in Europe).
- Vaccines are provided to large populations.
- The population is very sensitive to a vaccine scare.

Vaccine dossiers, like those for other medicinal products, need to contain RMPs according to the *Guideline on Risk management systems for medicinal products for human use* (EMEA/CHMP/96268/2005). The RMP template is also provided by EMA.

In the EU, there is no specific equivalent of the US Vaccine Adverse Event Reporting System (VAERS). Like any other medicinal products, vaccines are also subject to various postmarketing reporting requirements and studies. All adverse events, including those involving vaccines, are reported to either Member State Competent Authorities or centrally to Eudravigilance (http://eudravigilance.ema.europa.eu/human/index.asp). It is important to note that vaccine failures are considered adverse reactions.

The Rules Governing Medicinal Products in the European Union, Volume 9, contains EU pharmacovigilance requirements (*Volume 9A* for human products and *Volume 9B* for veterinary products). *Volume 9A* describes overarching rules for pharmacovigilance procedures, documentation, etc. This will be updated sometime during 2012 to reflect the new requirements under the *Pharmacovigilance Regulation*

(Regulation (EU) No 1235/2010). The regulation was adopted in December 2010 to overhaul the PV system and is effective from July 2012. The regulation is applicable to all medicinal products, including vaccines. Guidance issued by EMA provides additional information about vaccine pharmacovigilance (*Guideline on the conduct of pharmacovigilance for vaccines for pre- and post-exposure prophylaxis against infectious diseases* (EMEA/CHMP/PhVWP/503449/2007)). This guidance also discusses adjuvants, preservatives, etc., that are normally inherent in vaccines, as these components may be responsible for adverse events.

PV reporting in Europe is slightly complicated due to the licensure pathway; not all Member States have electronic reporting at this time and some need to be informed specifically apart from the central Eudravigilance reporting. These reporting requirements are similar to those for other medicinal products, and there are no special requirements for vaccines. With the new pharmacovigilance legislation, all MAHs will submit the reports directly to Eudravigilance instead of using the current procedures. Additionally, this legislation is considered to be the biggest change in human medicine regulations in the EU since 1995, so it is important for manufacturers to ensure they are familiar with the updated requirements. For more information on risk management and pharmacovigilance in the EU, please refer to Chapter 25.

A Qualified Person for Pharmacovigilance (QPPV) is essential for companies marketing their products in the EU. The requirements for this key role are described in detail in *Volume 9A*. The QPPV is tasked with establishing and maintaining the MAH's pharmacovigilance system, overseeing product safety profiles, preparing periodic and other safety reports and acting as a central point of contact with authorities on a 24-hour basis. There are no special QPPV requirements for vaccines.

Influenza Vaccines

Although influenza vaccines are like any other vaccines, from a regulatory perspective, they follow a unique pathway. Influenza vaccines can be classified as seasonal and pandemic. Seasonal vaccines are produced every year for the strains that are most predominant. Pandemic influenza vaccines, on the other hand, are produced only when there is an influenza pandemic, as in 2009. Some influenza vaccine guidelines (both seasonal and pandemic) in the EU are listed in **Table 28-3**.

Seasonal influenza vaccine manufacture and approval is well-organised and standardised for regulators and manufacturers at every step (**Figure 28-2**), starting with a review of the WHO epidemiology data in mid-February every year.[4] This is followed by the EU recommendation on the use of reassortants for influenza vaccine manufacture through the EU Ad hoc Influenza Working Party, which takes place at EMA every March. Following the recommendation, manufacturers start vaccine production and submit chemistry, manufacturing and control (CMC) information. The submission is a "Type II Variation" to EMA (Centralised Procedure) and is essentially a two-step procedure, i.e., submission of quality documentation followed by clinical documentation. EMA has published guidance on the specific variation procedure for the annual update of the influenza vaccines, *Procedural advice on the submission of variations for annual update of human influenza inactivated vaccine applications in the centralised procedure* (EMA/CHMP/BWP/99698/2007 Rev. 1).

Note that some manufacturers have moved to a quadrivalent seasonal influenza vaccine.

For pandemic influenza vaccines, EMA and the European Commission have developed an innovative Core Pandemic Dossier approach, where a company submits a licence application with a "mock" strain of influenza. The strain used in the core pandemic dossier is a strain for which the population is naïve but could cause a pandemic. This way, the core dossier would mimic the future pandemic vaccine in quality, nonclinical and clinical aspects. Naturally, the safety and immunogenicity data in the core dossier are based on the premise that subjects will respond similarly to the actual pandemic strain. As soon as the pandemic starts, the strain is replaced, specific predefined development steps are performed and resulting data are submitted and evaluated as a variation to the MA. This process significantly accelerates the licensure and availability of such vaccines within a reduced pandemic response time.

Several guidelines are in place for influenza vaccines. Due to pandemic scares and the lessons learned from them, CHMP has decided to develop a single comprehensive influenza vaccine guideline that deals with quality, nonclinical and clinical requirements for all kinds of influenza vaccines. The *Concept paper on the revision of guidelines for influenza Vaccines* was published and released in September 2011, and consultation ended in December 2011. The first draft of the guidance is expected in 2012. This new guideline is expected to streamline development of all kinds of influenza vaccines.

Pricing, Reimbursement and Policy Making in the EU

Most medicines in the EU are under price controls, and almost all vaccines are reimbursed. Hence, pricing and reimbursement of vaccines are important elements of EU regulatory activities. Reimbursement and pricing are determined at a national level, regardless of the authorisation pathway used. Often, Member States use different schemes and policies due to their own medical and economic pricing and reimbursement needs. Each Member State has its own reimbursement assessment authority based on health technology assessment (HTA). Almost all childhood vaccines are provided free of cost in the EU and costs are borne

Table 28-4. Some Organisations Involved in Vaccine Recommendations in the EU

Country	Committee	Acronym
Germany	Standing Vaccination Committee at the Robert Koch Institut (*Staendige Impfkommission*)	STIKO
UK	Joint Committee on Vaccination and Immunisation	JCVI
France	Advisory Board on Immunisation	CTV
Spain	Technical Working Group on Vaccines of The Commission on Public Health	
Czech Republic	Ministry of Health	
Ireland	National Immunisation Advisory Committee of Royal College of Physicians	

completely or in part by either social health insurance systems or the national health service. Pricing and reimbursement are discussed in the recently revised *Transparency Directive* (http://ec.europa.eu/enterprise/sectors/healthcare/files/docs/transpadir_finalprop01032012_en.pdf). This directive covers the speed of pricing, transparency and reimbursement decisions. Under this directive, Member States must make a reimbursement decision within 120 days of approval of an innovative drug and 30 days for a generic product. This is a significant reduction from the previously required 180 days. A public consultation on the *Transparency Directive* (Directive 89/105/EEC) was completed in 2011 and is slated to be implemented in 2014.

Some institutions involved in reimbursement include:
- Sweden: The Dental and Pharmaceutical Benefits Agency (TLV (www.tlv.se/in-english/)
- Denmark: Danish Medicines Agency (www.medicinpriser.dk/)

The EU Policy-making Process

Although not a direct regulatory activity, vaccination policy or recommendation is an important part of post-licensure activity. For vaccines, there is no single official Pan-European policy body. Recommendations are made at the Member State level (for examples, see **Table 28-4**). Sometimes, a national recommendation is also modified at the local level, primarily based on reimbursement arrangements and general practitioners' recommendations, e.g., Germany. In countries like France and Austria, reimbursement schedules are set at the national level and are not modified locally. There also are minor differences in vaccination schedules among EU Member States. More information on EU vaccination schedules is available from the EUVAC network (www.euvac.net/graphics/euvac/vaccination/vaccination.html).

Summary

- Vaccines are regulated at the Community level through several EU directives and regulations, and at the national level by laws and legislation.
- Guidelines are issued centrally by EMA and by national Competent Authorities, making marketing in the EU complex due to the number of organisations involved in regulation of and drafting guidelines for medicinal products.
- General guidelines that are applicable to medicinal products also apply to vaccines.
- Biological and biotechnological product guidelines and those specifically for vaccines are more relevant than some medicinal product guidelines. Guidelines also are available for different disciplines such as the quality, nonclinical and clinical aspects of vaccine development.
- Since vaccines are produced from biotechnological processes, many licensure considerations must be implemented during the development process.
- Unique EU manufacturing requirements include site manufacturing authorisations (even for IMPs) and QP certification.
- Vaccines are subject to lot release by OMCLs that are involved in vaccine lot testing and certification.
- EU adjuvant requirements are clearly defined and a number of adjuvants are licensed.
- Nonclinical activities for vaccines may be limited, with proper justification.
- Vaccines that contain live virus vectors also are regulated as GMOs. Both licensure and clinical assessments of these products add complexity due to environmental assessments.
- Seasonal influenza vaccines follow a well-defined path; pandemic influenza vaccines follow a core pandemic dossier approach.
- PV activities are centrally organised through Eudravigilance. The EU PV system currently is being revised.
- Every EU Member State makes policies on vaccinations and reimbursement.

References

1. US Centers for Disease Control. Ten great public health achievements—United States, 1900–1999. MMWR 1999;48:241–3. CDC website. www.cdc.gov/mmwr/preview/mmwrhtml/00056796.htm. Accessed 28 May 2012.
2. WHO: Requirements for the use of animal cells as in vitro substrates for the production of biologicals (Requirements for Biological

Substances No. 50). WHO Technical Report Series, No. 878. 1998; Annex 1. WHO website, www.who.int/biologicals/publications/trs/areas/vaccines/cells/WHO_TRS_878_A1Animalcells.pdf. Accessed 28 May 2012.
3. Robinson S. et al. A European pharmaceutical company initiative challenging the regulatory requirement for acute toxicity studies in pharmaceutical drug development, *Regul. Toxicol. Pharmacol.* (2008), 50 (3): 345-52. NCBI website. www.ncbi.nlm.nih.gov/pubmed/18295384. Accessed 12 May 2012.
4. Minor PD. Vaccines against seasonal and pandemic influenza and the implications of changes in substrates for virus production. *Clin Infect Dis* 2010; 50: 560-565. Oxford Journals website. http://cid.oxfordjournals.org/content/50/4/560.full. Accessed 28 May 2012.

Chapter 29

Orphan Medicinal Products

Updated by Gautam Maitra

OBJECTIVES

- Examine the special regulations for rare indications involving small patient populations.

- Obtain a basic understanding of the considerations for developing orphan medicinal products for the European market.

- Learn how to apply for orphan medicinal product designation.

- Understand that orphan medicinal products include only medicinal products, not devices.

- Understand the two basic approaches to support an orphan medicinal product designation application.

REGULATIONS AND GUIDELINES COVERED IN THIS CHAPTER

- The Rules Governing Medicinal Products in the European Union (European Commission, April 1998)

- Directive 2001/83/EC of the European Parliament and of the Council of 6 November 2001 on the Community code relating to medicinal products for human use

- Directive 2004/27/EC of the European Parliament and of the Council of 31 March 2004 amending Directive 2001/83/EC on the Community code relating to medicinal products for human use

- Regulation (EC) No 141/2000 of the European Parliament and of the Council of 16 December 1999 on orphan medicinal products

- Commission Regulation (EC) No 847/2000 of 27 April 2000 laying down the provisions for implementation of the criteria for designation of a medicinal product as an orphan medicinal product and definitions of the concepts similar medicinal product and clinical superiority

- Regulation (EC) No 726/2004 of the European Parliament and of the Council of 31 March 2004 laying down Community Procedures for the authorisation and supervision of medicinal products for human and veterinary use and establishing a European Medicines Agency

- Regulation (EC) No 1901/2006 on medicinal products for paediatric use and amending Regulation (EEC) No 1768/92, Directive 2001/20/EC, Directive 2001/83/EC and Regulation (EC) No 726/2004

- Regulation (EC) No 1394/2007 of the European Parliament and of the Council of 13 November 2007 on advanced therapy medicinal products and amending Directive 2001/83/EC and Regulation (EC) No 726/2004

Introduction

Orphan medicinal products (OMPs) are intended for diagnosis, prevention or treatment of life-threatening or very serious conditions affecting fewer than five in 10,000 people. These products are called "orphans" because the pharmaceutical industry has little interest, under normal market conditions, in developing and marketing products intended for only a small number of patients suffering from very rare conditions. For the drug companies, the cost of bringing a medicinal product for a rare disease to the market would not be covered by the expected sales of the product. For this reason, governments and organisations representing patients suffering from these rare diseases have emphasised the need for economic and regulatory incentives to encourage drug companies to develop and market medicines for patients who have the many neglected rare conditions.

The *Orphan Medicinal Product Regulation* (Regulation (EC) No 141/2000)[1] was proposed by the European Commission in July 1998 and has been in force since 2000. It sets up the criteria for orphan designation in the EU and describes the incentives (e.g., 10-year market exclusivity, protocol assistance and access to the Centralised Procedure for Marketing Authorisation (MA)) to encourage the research, development and marketing of medicines to treat, prevent or diagnose rare diseases. The regulation does not concentrate on access or research.

In 2000, the Committee for Orphan Medicinal Products (COMP) was established to review designation applications from persons or companies intending to develop medicines for rare diseases. This committee is responsible for studying the applications for orphan designation, for giving opinions on the designation as orphan medicinal products and for advising and assisting the Commission in discussions on orphan drugs.

Drugs with the orphan designation are entered in the Community Register for Orphan Medicinal Products.

Orphan Medicinal Product Legislation and Guidelines

On 16 December 1999, the European Parliament approved Regulation (EC) No 141/2000 of the European Parliament and the Council on orphan medicinal products. This regulation set forth implementation rules and definitions essential for the regulation of orphan medicinal products.

Other regulations and guidelines clarify specific concepts or provide procedural guidelines following Commission Regulation (EC) No 847/2000[2] of 27 April 2000 laying down the implementation provisions of criteria for designating a medicinal product an orphan medicinal product and defining the concepts of "similar medicinal product" and "clinical superiority."

Orphan Designation Application

- *Guideline on the format and content of applications for designation as orphan medicinal products and on the transfer of designations from one sponsor to another,* October 2002 (ENTR/6283/00 Rev. 2)
- Annex to *Guideline on the Format and Content of Applications for Designation as Orphan Medicinal Products,* July 2004
- *Final Points to Consider on the Calculation and Reporting of the Prevalence of a Condition for Orphan Designation,* Adopted March 2002 (EMEA/COMP/436/01)
- *Draft guideline on elements required to support the medical plausibility and the assumption of significant benefit for an orphan designation,* released for consultation September 2004 (EMEA/COMP/66972/04 COMP)
- *Overview of comments received in draft guideline on elements to support the medical plausibility and the assumption of significant benefit for an orphan designation* (EMEA/337053/2005)

Orphan Procedures

- *Procedures for Orphan Medicinal Product Designation–General Principles,* 19 July 2007 (EMEA/14222/00/Rev 3)
- *General Information for Sponsors of Orphan Medicinal Products,* 18 July 2007 (EMEA/4795/00/Rev 3)
- *Note for Sponsors of Orphan Medicinal Products regarding Enlargement of the European Union,* October 2006 (EMEA/422264/06)
- *Appeal Procedure for Orphan Product Designation,* 9 February 2001 (EMEA/COMP/50/01)
- *Practical information for sponsors during the early phase of an orphan drug application,* 18 July 2007 (EMEA/114593/07 Rev 1)
- *Members' interaction with sponsors of applications for orphan designation,* 12 July 2006 (EMEA/COMP/150409/06)
- European Medicines Agency (EMA) Orphan Designation webpage[3]
- *Recommendation on elements required to support the medical plausibility and the assumption of significant benefit for an orphan designation*[4] (EMA/COMP15893/2009)
- *Practical information for sponsors during the early phase of an orphan drug application*[5] (EMA/710916/2009/Rev 5)

Protocol Assistance

- *EMEA Guidance for Companies Requesting Scientific Advice (SA) or Protocol Assistance (PA),* Updated 19 January 2007 (EMEA/H/4260/01 Rev. 4)

Transfer of Orphan Designation
- *Checklist for sponsors applying for the transfer of orphan medicinal product designation,* April 2007 (EMEA/41277/07 Rev. 1)

Annual Report
- *Final Note for Guidance on the Format and Content of the Annual Report on the State of Development of an Orphan Medicinal Product,* April 2002 (EMEA/COMP/189/01)

It should be noted that there is significant emphasis on trans-Atlantic simplification in the orphan designation area. For example, the US Food and Drug Administration (FDA) Office of Orphan Products Development now accepts the Annual Report for EMA. Additionally, there is a harmonised application form for orphan designation accepted by both FDA and EMA.

As of January 2012, 977 applications for orphan medicinal product designation had obtained a positive opinion from COMP. Of these, the European Commission granted designation to 945. It should be noted that 346 applications were withdrawn, and 18 applications received a final negative COMP opinion. Almost all designations were granted on the basis of prevalence and only a very limited number on the basis of the financial clause. Several MAs have been granted for orphan medicinal products. These numbers are higher than expected and suggest that the legislation is a great success. Interestingly, the Committee for Medicinal Products for Human Use (CHMP) has adopted negative opinions for orphan medicinal products (e.g., somatropin for the treatment of AIDS-related wasting and trabectedin for the treatment of ovarian cancer).

Background

Starting in the mid-1980s, individual EU Member States began to adopt specific measures to improve the knowledge of rare conditions. These measures also were intended to improve the detection, prevention and treatment of those diseases. Following the example of the US and Japan, where orphan drug legislation was enacted in 1983 and 1993, respectively, legislators aimed to provide incentives for research and development of medicinal products for rare diseases.

These early national initiatives, however, did not lead to significant progress in research, and only rarely were medicinal products for rare diseases developed. Interestingly, in those cases, it is unlikely that national incentives played an important role.

The *OMP Regulation* was the outcome of a resolution adopted by the Council of Ministers on 20 December 1995 asking the European Commission to investigate the need for a European orphan drug policy.

One of the guiding principles of the European OMP legislation is the rights of people affected by orphan diseases. At the time the legislation was implemented, nearly 5,000 rare conditions affecting approximately 25–30 million people in the 15 Member States were known. Today, it is estimated that between 5,000 and 8,000 distinct rare diseases exist, affecting 6%–8% of the EU population (27–36 million people in total). It is estimated that 80% of rare diseases have identified genetic origins. The *OMP Regulation* states that patients suffering from rare conditions should be entitled to the same quality of treatment as other patients. This concept is based on principles of social justice and equality, and the fact that patients affected by rare disorders have the same desire for effective treatments as those affected by common diseases. Therefore, it was considered important to stimulate the research, development and marketing of medicinal products for rare conditions.

As stated earlier, the aim of the OMP legislation is to stimulate research and development of medicinal products for rare conditions by providing incentives to the pharmaceutical industry, including:
- development input through protocol assistance
- eligibility for Community and Member State initiatives
- access to the Centralised Procedure
- fee reductions from EMA
- 10-year market exclusivity once authorised

The last incentive of 10 years' market exclusivity can be extended to 12 years under Article 37 of the *Paediatric Regulation* (1901/2006/EC):

"Where an application for a marketing authorization is submitted in respect of a medicinal product designated as an orphan product pursuant to Regulation (EC) No 141/2000 and that application includes the results of all studies conducted in compliance with an agreed paediatric investigation plan, and the statement referred to in Article 28(3) of this Regulation is subsequently included in the MA granted, the ten-year period referred to in Article 8(1) of Regulation (EC) No 141/2000 shall be extended to twelve years."[6]

This extension is dependent only on completion of the agreed-upon studies and not on the outcomes of those studies.

The market exclusivity incentive is tempered by Article 8(2) of the *OMP Regulation*, which states, "This period may…be reduced to six years if, at the end of the fifth year, it is established, in respect of the medicinal product concerned, that the criteria laid down in Article 3 are no longer met."[7]

This procedure is not intended to be applied systematically according to Article 8(2), but only where a Member

Table 29-1. Comparison of the EU and US Orphan Programmes

	European Orphan Programme	US Orphan Programme
Date of implementation	Directive 141/2000/EC (2000)	*Orphan Drug Act* (1983)
Prevalence	< 5/10,000 (approx. 246,000 people in EU Member States)	< 200,000 patients in the US (approx. <7.5/10,000)
Products	Medicinal products as defined in 2001/83/EC as amended by Directive 2004/27/EC	Medicinal products
Designation criteria	Epidemiological or financial, with the requirement that no other authorised method exists; or if one does exist, that the product has significant benefit to patients	Epidemiological or financial
Market exclusivity	• 10 years (six if criteria are no longer met or 12 if paediatric development completed) • Clinical superiority clause for second applicant	• Seven years (no reduction even if prevalence changes) • Clinical superiority clause for second applicant
Supervising bodies	• European Commission: grants legal decision on orphan medicinal product designation • European Medicines Agency (EMA): administrative body supporting Committee for Orphan Medicinal Products (COMP) • COMP: advisory body providing opinion on the application to the European Commission	• US Food and Drug Administration (FDA): grants legal decision on orphan drug designation • Office of Orphan Products Development: advisory body providing opinion on the application to FDA
Other incentives	• Possible financial incentives on a national basis • Access to protocol assistance • Fee waiver upon request • Use of Centralised Procedure	• Tax credits • Government grants • Assistance for clinical research • Fee reduction
	• Programme does not include devices	• Programme includes drugs and devices

State indicates to EMA that it believes a product no longer fulfils the designation criteria.

Article 8(5) requires the European Commission to draw up guidelines on the application of this process. A draft for public consultation was issued in March 2007 with a deadline of early May 2007. The final guideline, *Guideline on aspects of the application of Article 8(2) of Regulation (EC) No. 141/2000 of the European Parliament and of the Council: Review of the period of market exclusivity of orphan medicinal products,* was published in September 2008.

Orphan Drugs Legislation: EU versus US

As noted previously, OMP designation procedures exist in several other countries, including, Japan, Australia, Singapore, South Korea and Switzerland. Many of these procedures are based on principles similar to those of the US system. **Table 29-1** compares the EU system with the US system.

OMP Designation

Criteria for Orphan Designation

To obtain an EU OMP designation, an applicant must establish that the product meets two criteria described in Article 3 of Regulation (EC) No 141/2000:

1. Rarity of the condition—The medicinal product is intended for the diagnosis, prevention or treatment of a life-threatening or chronically debilitating condition that affects not more than five in 10,000 persons in the European Community at the time of the submission (Article 3.1(a)i of Regulation (EC) No 141/2000). Or, the medicinal product is intended for the diagnosis, prevention or treatment of a life-threatening, seriously debilitating, or serious and chronic condition in the EU, and without incentives, it is unlikely that marketing this product in the European Community would generate sufficient financial return to justify the investment (Article 3.1(a)i of Regulation (EC) No 141/2000).

2. Approved methods of diagnosis, prevention or treatment—Applicants should demonstrate that, at the time of submission, no satisfactory method of diagnosis, prevention or treatment of the condition in question has been authorised in the European Community. If such a method has been approved, the applicant should demonstrate that its medicinal product will be of significant benefit to those affected by that condition.

Figure 29-1 presents a simplified view of the designation criteria.

Committee for Orphan Medicinal Products

Article 4 of Regulation (EC) No 141/2000 established COMP. The tasks of this committee are:
- to examine any application submitted for designation of a medicinal product as an OMP in accordance with Regulation (EC) No 141/2000
- to advise the European Commission on the establishment and development of a policy on OMPs for the EU
- to assist the European Commission in liaising internationally on matters relating to OMPs and in liaising with patient support groups

COMP consists of:
- one member nominated by each of the 27 Member States
- three members nominated by the European Commission to represent patients' organisations
- three members nominated by the European Commission on the basis of an EMA recommendation
- one member nominated by each EEA-EFTA state (Iceland, Liechtenstein and Norway)
- one European Commission representative
- general observers

Members are appointed for a renewable, three-year term. COMP members elect the chair and vice chair for a three-year term that can be renewed once. EMA provides the COMP secretariat.

COMP is supported by two working parties:
- EMA's Human Scientific Committees' Working Party with Patients' and Consumers' Organisations (more commonly known as the Patients' and Consumers' Working Party, or PCWP) was established to provide recommendations to EMA and its human scientific committees on all matters of interest to patients in relation to medicinal products.
- In the interest of public health, and with a view toward improving access to medicinal products for patients affected by orphan diseases, the COMP Working Group with Interested Parties (COMP-WGIP) prepares proposals for COMP concerning:
  o transparency of EMA/COMP activities relating to the orphan designation procedure
  o optimisation of the orphan designation procedure
  o COMP policy recommendations on orphan medicinal products
  o any other topic of interest at the request of COMP

OMP Designation Procedure

Submission of an Application

Note that the European *OMP Regulation* clearly states that only medicinal products for human use, as defined in Article 2 of Directive 2001/83/EC[8] and as amended by Directive 2004/27/EC,[9] are eligible for OMP designation. The scope includes drugs, biological and biotechnological products, and cell and gene therapy products; it excludes medical devices and certain tissue products.

A sponsor can submit an application to obtain OMP designation at any medicinal product development stage before the Marketing Authorisation Application (MAA) is submitted. Once an MAA for a medicinal product is submitted by that sponsor in any EU Member State or centrally through EMA, regardless of the outcome, it is no longer eligible for orphan product designation if the MAA is for the same therapeutic orphan indication. However, a sponsor may apply for an OMP medicinal product designation for an already approved product provided the proposed orphan indication concerns an unapproved therapeutic indication. In this context, please note that a MA for an OMP covers only therapeutic indications that fulfil the criteria for designation according Article 7 of Regulation (EC) No 141/2000.[10]

EMA requests that sponsors send notification of their intent to submit an application, preferably two months in advance and in writing. This notification should include the following information (see ENTR/6283/00):
- medicinal product name
- proposed orphan indication
- sponsor name and address
- planned submission date

This notification permits EMA to appoint two coordinators (one COMP and one EMA staff member). COMP also may identify experts to be involved in evaluating an application. EMA encourages sponsors to request a presubmission meeting prior to filing. In general, presubmission meetings are important to fine-tune the submission.

Sponsors are asked to submit the application in triplicate and include an additional copy in electronic format. A separate application should be submitted for each orphan indication. Documentation for an OMP designation application includes an application form and a core dossier containing the rationale for orphan designation; the documentation requirements are detailed in Commission Guideline ENTR/6283/00.

Validation and Assessment

After application submission, EMA will validate the dossier. If the application is incomplete, the sponsor will be asked to supplement it before the coordinators start the review. The 90-day assessment starts after successful validation. Usually, the timetable is set in such a way that Day 0 (clock start), Day 60 and Day 90 of the procedure coincide with COMP meetings. Note that no clock stops are possible under this procedure.

During the assessment phase, the EMA coordinator, in close cooperation with the COMP coordinator and, if appropriate, experts in the field, prepares a summary report on the application. This summary report is circulated among all COMP members and is discussed at Day 60 during the COMP meeting, where members may raise questions about the application. Questions are sent to the sponsor for response, or COMP may invite the sponsor to an oral explanation session at procedure Day 90. No opinions are discussed in the sponsor's presence.

Opinion and Commission Decision

According to *OMP Regulation* Article 5, COMP should provide an opinion within 90 days. Usually, an opinion is adopted between Day 60 and Day 90, just after the COMP meeting. Whenever possible, opinions are adopted by consensus. In the absence of consensus, opinions are deemed adopted if supported by a two-thirds majority.

EMA then forwards the opinion, accompanied by the COMP assessment report, to the European Commission and to the sponsor.

In the event of a negative opinion, the sponsor is permitted one appeal. The sponsor should notify EMA in writing of its intent to appeal within 15 days of receiving the negative opinion. The reasoning for the appeal should be submitted to EMA within 90 days of receiving the opinion. EMA then forwards the grounds for appeal to COMP, which considers them at its next meeting. The appeal should be based only upon data provided in the application.

The sponsor may decide at any time during the normal procedure to withdraw an application. After a withdrawal, the sponsor may resubmit the application. COMP will issue a negative opinion following a withdrawal.

The European Commission decides on the designation within 30 days of receiving the opinion. Upon a favourable Commission decision, designated OMPs are published in the Community Register of Orphan Medicinal Products, available on the European Commission website.

Since March 2002, EMA has published the Public Summary of the COMP Opinion after adopting any European Commission opinion. This document is available on EMA's website and provides summary information on the following topics:
- orphan indication
- available treatment methods
- estimated prevalence or financial aspects (depending upon which criterion is used for the application)
- mode of action
- stage of development
- sponsor's contact details

Before publishing the Public Summary, EMA consults patients' organisations to ensure readability. EMA also consults with the sponsor to ensure that any information considered proprietary or commercially confidential is removed.

OMP Designation Dossier

The following documentation must be supplied in any OMP designation application:

1. Application form, which requests the following information:
   - active substance name
   - proposed indication and ATC code (if available)
   - proposed medicinal product details (if available)
   - name and permanent address of sponsor or corporate contact person
   - name and manufacturer of active substance
2. Additional data (i.e., the core dossier), which consists of the following information:
   - description of the condition
   - details of the condition
   - proposed orphan indication
   - medical plausibility
   - justification of the condition's life-threatening or debilitating nature
   - prevalence of the condition
     - orphan disease or condition's prevalence in the Community (to be completed if the application follows Article 3.1(a)i of the *OMP Regulation* (i.e., is based upon prevalence))
     - orphan disease or condition's prevalence and incidence in the Community (to be completed if the application follows Article 3.1(a)ii of the regulation (i.e., is based upon insufficient return on investment))
     - participation information on other Community projects
   - potential for return on investment (to be completed if the application follows Article 3.1(a)ii of the *OMP Regulation* (i.e., is based upon insufficient return on investment))
     - grants and tax incentives
     - past and future development costs
     - production and marketing costs
     - expected revenues
     - certification by a registered accountant
   - existence of other diagnostic, prevention or treatment methods
     - details of existing diagnostic, prevention or treatment methods
     - justification why existing methods are not satisfactory (to be completed if no medicinal product is authorised in the Community for the indication)

Figure 29-1. Orphan Designation Criteria

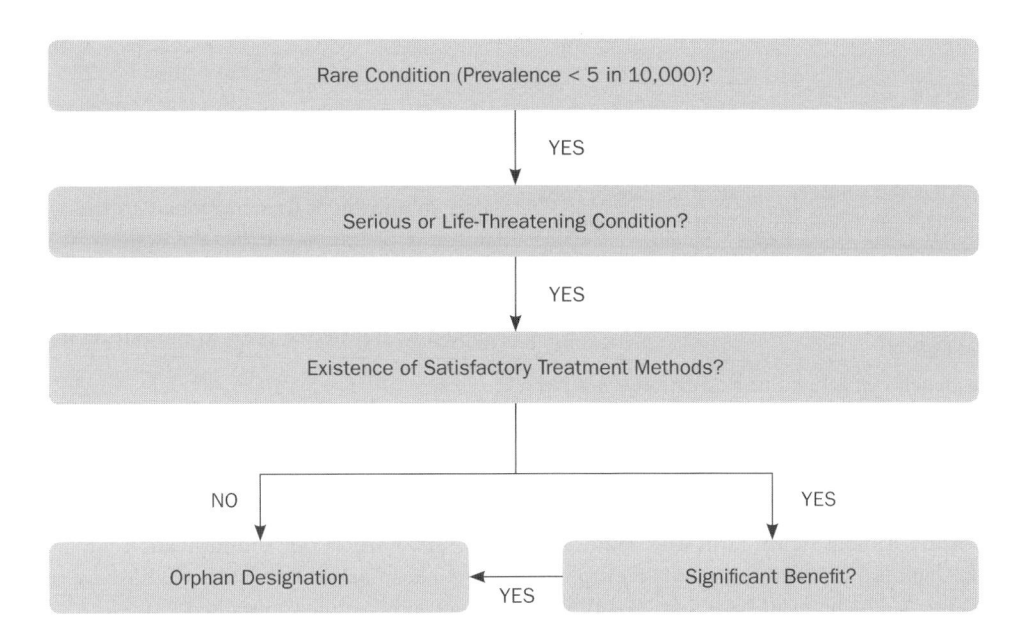

```
Rare Condition (Prevalence < 5 in 10,000)?
                    │
                   YES
                    ▼
      Serious or Life-Threatening Condition?
                    │
                   YES
                    ▼
      Existence of Satisfactory Treatment Methods?
              │                  │
             NO                 YES
              ▼                  ▼
      Orphan Designation ◄──── Significant Benefit?
                          YES
```

- o justification of significant benefit (to be completed if medicinal products are authorised in the Community for the indication)
- description of the development stage
  - o summary of product development
  - o current regulatory status and marketing history details
- bibliography

Unified EU-US Application

Due to their relatively small numbers, patients with orphan diseases may be distributed around the world, requiring a global regulatory strategy. The introduction of a joint US-EU orphan drug application is the first step in simplifying the procedure. FDA and EMA are working together on other orphan development initiatives, possibly one for therapeutics for tropical diseases.[11]

Medical Plausibility

Experience has shown that a large proportion of unsuccessful orphan designation applications were due to so-called "salami slicing." This refers to applying for artificial subsets of conditions that, as a whole, have a prevalence greater than five in 10,000 people.

It is important to distinguish between the proposed orphan indication, which is the designation application's subject, and the proposed therapeutic indication, which is the subject of an MAA. The proposed therapeutic indication in the MAA should reflect the results of clinical development and usually describes a specific population in whom benefit has been demonstrated. The proposed orphan indication, however, should be described as broadly as possible. Distinct medical entities that can be defined according to specific clinical, pathophysiological or histopathological characteristics are generally acceptable. A subset of a frequent disease could be considered a valid condition for orphan status if patients in the subset show distinct and unique quantitative characteristics with a plausible link to the condition. In addition, the following must apply:

- The characteristics in patients are essential for the medicinal product to carry out its action.
- The absence of these characteristics in patients will render the product ineffective in the rest of the population.

Prevalence

In March 2002, COMP issued *Points to Consider on Calculation and Reporting of the Prevalence of a Condition for Orphan Designation* (EMEA/COMP/436/01). "Prevalence" is defined as the number of people in the European Community affected by the condition at the time of submission. Prevalence should not be confused with incidence—the number of new cases of a condition in a specified time period. Only in the case of conditions with a very short duration (less than one year) has COMP adopted positive opinions on the basis of annual incidence rather than prevalence.

The sponsor should present precise evidence (including published literature and data from reference databases) demonstrating that prevalence is lower than five in 10,000 in the

Community. A justification for using selected references or databases in the calculating prevalence should be provided.

Significant Benefit

When seeking orphan designation for an authorised medicinal product, the sponsor should provide justification for the assumption that the product will significantly benefit those affected by the condition. In general, any medicinal product already authorised in an EU Member State for the proposed orphan indication will be viewed as a "satisfactory method," and the sponsor will be required to argue "significant benefit."

"Significant benefit" is defined in Regulation (EC) No 847/2000[12] as a clinically relevant advantage or a major contribution to patient care. Because sponsors can submit an application at any stage of development, COMP will be looking for a justification for an assumption of potential benefit rather than a demonstration of it. The significant benefit should be demonstrated later to maintain the orphan designation prior to MAA approval. Note that COMP has taken the position that a new mode of action (i.e., improved efficacy) or a new method of administration (e.g., from intravenous administration to oral) could be acceptable as a justification for significant benefit.

Finally, sponsors should be aware that during the development phase, other diagnostic, prevention or treatment methods for the same condition may be approved in the European Community or one of its Member States. In such cases, it may be necessary to change the basis of the OMP designation from "no authorised treatment available" to "significant benefit." This change can be made at the time of the annual report on the OMP development.

In this context, applicants should provide the justification for significant benefit and/or why the chemical or molecular entity is not a similar active ingredient (as defined in the orphan legislation) in Module 1.7 when submitting an MAA for an orphan designated product.

Incentives

To stimulate research and development of medicinal products for rare conditions, the OMP legislation provides incentives. Member States can add further stimulus by providing such inducements as tax incentives, grants and free scientific input on a national level.

Fee Reductions

OMPs are eligible for reductions of all fees payable under Community rules pursuant to Regulation (EC) No 726/2004,[13] including:
- preauthorisation activities—scientific advice and consultation on ancillary medicinal products or blood derivatives in medical devices
- new applications, referrals and inspection
- postauthorisation activities—variations, transfers, extensions, minimum risk levels, renewals, annual fees

On an annual basis, the European Parliament allocates a budget for granting OMP fee exemptions. EMA manages the budget, and the sponsor can obtain fee reductions only after submitting a written request to the agency. For this reason, it is important that the designated OMP sponsor and proposed Marketing Authorisation Holder (MAH) are the same legal entity. If that is not the case, sponsorship should be transferred prior to submitting the request.

Access to the Centralised Procedure

The Centralised Procedure is obligatory for medicinal products included in the Annex of Council Regulation (EEC) No 726/2004.[14] In accordance with Regulation (EC) No 141/2000 Article 7(1) and Regulation (EEC) No 726/2004, as stated in annex point (4), OMPs have unreserved and direct access to the Centralised Procedure.

Protocol Assistance

General Information

There are many challenges in developing medicinal products for rare conditions. Often, animal models of the disease are not available for studies assessing the product's pharmacological activity. In addition, in many cases the conditions are heterogeneous; therefore, it is difficult to recruit patients for clinical studies and, more specifically, it is sometimes challenging to perform adequately powered clinical studies to show statistically significant effects. This situation often results in long multinational and multicentre studies with few patients per centre.

To guide OMP sponsors toward a successful application, EMA considers it important to provide development advice as well as regulatory assistance on the content of a future MAA (so-called Protocol Assistance). Protocol Assistance can be requested at all stages of OMP development. EMA is responsible for providing Protocol Assistance in consultation with CHMP and its Scientific Advice Working Party (SAWP). The procedure for Protocol Assistance is similar to that for Scientific Advice. The main differences between OMP Protocol Assistance and Scientific Advice, which reflect the main purpose of the OMP legislation, are:
- Two COMP members and specific experts from the field (e.g., researchers in the field of an orphan indication, methodologists, statisticians and patient representatives) participate in the process to provide an extended and collaborative forum that takes broad views and new ideas into consideration.
- An interactive dialogue is sought. In general, sponsors are invited to present an oral explanation during the Protocol Assistance procedure.

- Fee reductions can be requested approximately two months prior to the protocol assistance request. In the last few years, the fee reduction has been 100%.

EMA Protocol Assistance is not binding on EMA, CHMP or the sponsor with regard to any future OMP MAA.

Content of Request and Procedure

On 27 February 2002, EMA issued a guidance document for companies requesting Protocol Assistance on scientific issues (EMEA/H/238/02). This document describes the procedure's legal background, requested content and the procedure itself. In general, the request should contain prospective questions concerning quality and preclinical and clinical aspects of the proposed future development.

The two main types of questions concern:
1. MA quality, safety and efficacy criteria:
   - development of medicinal products for rare conditions
     o pharmaceutical development (e.g., new technologies)
     o preclinical and clinical development (e.g., methodologies for small populations or new methodological approaches)
   - study design to demonstrate clinical superiority over similar orphan products authorised for the same indication
2. orphan drug status designation criteria

Annual Report

After OMP designation has been granted, sponsors are required, under Regulation (EC) No 141/2000 Article 5.10, to provide annual reports on the state of development within two months of the anniversary date. This information includes the following components:
- Administrative update—Provided as an updated application form (annex to Guideline ENTR/6238).
- Summary of product development—A concise summary of development plan advances compared with the original application or previous annual report. A tabulated overview that includes initiated, ongoing and completed preclinical and clinical studies, as well as a short summary of the results, should be provided. This information can be provided in Investigator Brochure style; full reports should only be provided when requested. The summary also should include a brief description of the upcoming year's development plan and follow-up information on Protocol Assistance received. Of particular interest are difficulties encountered in implementing such advice.
- Update on the product's current regulatory status—An update on the OMP's regulatory status in EU and non-EU countries, including active compassionate use programs and the status of the orphan designation request and MAA (including those requested, rejected, granted and planned for each country, with submission dates).
- Incentives received—Estimates of total financial incentives directly related to the orphan designation received during the reporting year; the incentive source(s) (Member States, European Commission, EMA) should be provided.

Transfer of Sponsorship

An OMP designation can be transferred from one sponsor to another in accordance with Regulation (EC) No 141/2000 Article 5(11).[15] The sponsor holding the designation should submit an application to EMA that includes:
- a copy of the Commission decision on the designation
- a comprehensive document (Template 1, available on the EMA website) signed by both the current and new sponsor, including:
  o identification of the sponsor of the designation to be transferred ("current sponsor") and of the sponsor to whom the transfer is to be granted ("new sponsor") including contact details
  o a statement certifying that a copy of the complete and up-to-date designation application has been made available or has been transferred to the new sponsor
  o a statement as to the date on which the new sponsor can actually assume responsibility for and the rights of the designation for the medicinal product concerned from the current sponsor (i.e., the date of implementation of the transfer)
- identification (i.e., name and address) for both the existing and proposed sponsors
- proof that the proposed sponsor is established in the EEA
- depending on the approval date of the orphan designation, translation of either the name of the active ingredient or subset in all EU languages plus Icelandic and Norwegian are required

EMA should adopt an opinion within 30 days of receiving this application. The opinion, signed by the EMA executive director, will be forwarded to the existing sponsor, the proposed sponsor and the European Commission. If it agrees, the Commission will amend the decision granting the designation. The transfer is accepted from the date of notification of the amended European Commission decision.

Humanitarian Medical Devices

In 2008, the European Organisation for Rare Diseases (EURODIS) proposed the creation of a Humanitarian

Medical Device (HMD) category at the EU-level, similar to the programme in the US, which would allow for fee waivers for the registration of specified devices. This would provide a class for medical devices similar to the orphan designation for medicinal products, while recognising the specificities of the two different products.

Summary

The European *OMP Regulation* has been successfully implemented in the EU. Many companies have used or are using this regulation, as demonstrated by the large number of applications to COMP. Several products with OMP designation have reached the market. It will be interesting to follow their availability to patients (e.g., by examining reimbursement processes). There are a few orphan disorders, such as pulmonary arterial hypertension and hereditary angioedema, for which various companies are developing or have developed treatments. It remains to be seen what will happen when competitors seek MA (clinical superiority, similarity, market exclusivity, etc.). Such analyses, and experience with other products, will create an even better understanding of the EU *OMP Regulation's* true impact.

References

1. Regulation (EC) No 141/2000 of the European Parliament and of the Council of 16 December 1999 on orphan medicinal products. EUR-Lex website. http://eur-lex.europa.eu/LexUriServ/LexUriServ.do?uri=OJ:L:2000:018:0001:0005:en:PDF. Accessed 29 May 2012.
2. Commission Regulation (EC) No 847/2000 of 27 April 2000 laying down the provisions for implementation of the criteria for designation of a medicinal product as an orphan medicinal product and definitions of the concepts similar medicinal product and clinical superiority. EC website. http://ec.europa.eu/health/files/eudralex/vol-1/reg_2000_847/reg_2000_847_en.pdf. Accessed 29 May 2012.
3. EMA Orphan Designation webpage. www.ema.europa.eu/ema/index.jsp?curl=pages/regulation/general/general_content_000029.jsp&mid=WC0b01ac05800240ce. Accessed 29 May 2012.
4. EMA/COMP15893/2009 *Recommendation on elements required to support the medical plausibility and the assumption of significant benefit for an orphan designation*. EMA website. www.ema.europa.eu/docs/en_GB/document_library/Regulatory_and_procedural_guideline/2010/07/WC500095341.pdf. Accessed 29 May 2012.
5. EMA/710916/2009/Rev 5 Practical information for sponsors during the early phase of an orphan drug application. EMA website. www.ema.europa.eu/docs/en_GB/document_library/Regulatory_and_procedural_guideline/2009/09/WC500003771.pdf. Accessed 29 May 2012.
6. Regulation (EC) No 1901/2006 of 12 December 2006 on medicinal products for paediatric use and amending Regulation (EEC) 1768/92, Directive 2001/20/EC, Directive 2001/83/EC and Regulation (EC) No 726/2004. EUR-Lex website. http://eur-lex.europa.eu/LexUriServ/LexUriServ.do?uri=OJ:L:2006:378:0001:0019:en:PDF. Accessed 29 May 2012.
7. Op cit 1.
8. Directive 2001/83/EC of the European Parliament and of the Council of 6 November 2001 on the Community code relating to medicinal products for human use. EMA website. www.emea.europa.eu/docs/en_GB/document_library/Regulatory_and_procedural_guideline/2009/10/WC500004481.pdf. Accessed 29 May 2012.
9. Directive 2004/27/EC of the European Parliament and of the Council of 31 March 2004 amending Directive 2001/83/EC on the Community code relating to medicinal products for human use. EC website. http://ec.europa.eu/health/files/eudralex/vol-1/dir_2004_27/dir_2004_27_en.pdf. Accessed 29 May 2012.
10. Op cit 1.
11. *SCRIP*, "Drug Market Developments." 2008; 19(5). Taylor Wessing website. www.taylorwessing.com/uploads/tx_siruplawyermanagement/scrip_rehmann_morgan.pdf. Accessed 29 May 2012.
12. Op cit 2.
13. Regulation (EC) No 726/2004 of the European Parliament and of the Council of 31 March 2004 laying down Community Procedures for the authorisation and supervision of medicinal products for human and veterinary use and establishing a European Medicines Agency. EC website. http://ec.europa.eu/health/files/eudralex/vol-1/reg_2004_726_cons/reg_2004_726_cons_en.pdf. Accessed 29 May 2012.
14. Ibid.
15. Op cit 1.

Chapter 30

Combination Products

Updated by Gudrun Busch, MSc, PhD, MTOPRA, RAC

OBJECTIVES

❑ Understand the prerequisites for the proper classification of combination products in the European market

❑ Obtain an overview of the regulatory pathways towards CE-marking of drug-device combination products

❑ Understand the pharmaceutical consultation procedure and the role of the European Medicines Agency in it

❑ Obtain a general insight into appeal procedures against an assigned classification that is disputed by the manufacturer

---

REGULATIONS AND GUIDELINES COVERED IN THIS CHAPTER

❑ Council Directive 93/42/EEC of 14 June 1993 concerning medical devices, as amended

❑ Directive 2001/83/EC of the European Parliament and of the Council on the Community code relating to medicinal products for human use, as amended

❑ MEDDEV 2.1/3 Rev. 3 Borderline Products, drug-delivery products and medical devices incorporating as an integral part, an ancillary medicinal substance or an ancillary human blood derivative (December 2009)

❑ MEDDEV 2.4/1 Rev. 9 Classification of Medical Devices

❑ Manual on Borderline and Classification in the Community Regulatory Framework for Medical Devices (document periodically updated by the European Commission)

❑ GHTF SG1 N11: 2008 Summary Technical Documentation for Demonstrating Conformity to the Essential Principles of Safety and Performance of Medical Devices (STED)

NOTE: For the effective use and comprehension of this chapter it is helpful to be familiar with the Medical Devices Directive *93/42/EEC as amended, and the* Medicinal Products Directive *2001/83/EC (MPD) as amended.*

Introduction

The demarcation between medicinal products and devices becomes increasingly important. Novel technologies lead to more drug/device combination products and medical devices incorporating a medicinal substance. Also, cell therapy and tissue-engineered products are being combined with both medicinal products and medical devices. Statistical evaluations estimate a market potential with up to 15% annual growth.

This chapter provides practical guidance on the borderline issues concerning these combination products and advice on the regulatory strategy to follow.

What are combination products? Combination products, as the name implies, are products that share the attributes of two product categories. Many combination products, such as device-blood products, device-nutritionals or device-cosmetics, are feasible or imaginable. In this chapter we will only discuss combinations of medical devices and medicinal products. They are by far the most common and the most disputed in terms of the regulatory framework and the market potential.

In the EU, a combination product is regulated by either the *Medical Devices Directive* (*MDD*, Directive 93/42/EEC), as amended, or Directive 2001/83/EC on medicinal products. In general, the primary mode of action (or function) of the product determines how it is classified and regulated. In contrast to US regulations, in the EU, the same product can never be both a pharmaceutical product and a medical device. To make it even more complicated, there is no clear definition or specific regulation for combination products. A complex framework of regulations has to be considered to come to a decision and implement a regulatory strategy.

The decision whether a drug-device combination must lead to a pharmaceutical dossier review by a national Competent Authority or by the European Medicines Agency (EMA) is one with major repercussions on time to market and money. The lack of a sole regulatory body with which a manufacturer can communicate and get a reasonably fast response that is legally binding in the EU is one of the more glaring deficiencies in the current European healthcare product classification system. It is likely one area where the recast of the *MDD*—a major update tentatively scheduled for 2015—should bring improvement.

As a result, it is not uncommon for combination products to be submitted for adjudication to the manufacturer's Notified Body (NB). Because the manufacturer expects to be able to rely on the NB's statement in case of a future dispute with a national Competent Authority, most NBs will get a binding opinion from the national Competent Authority under which they operate. The design and development of a combination product invariably are more demanding than those of a "pure" medical device. This should be reflected in the manufacturer's business plan.

Once the manufacturer has established that a pharmaceutical consultation is required, this procedure may begin. It is reasonably well defined, but may differ substantially from country to country, depending on the national Competent Authority involved and, in the case of advanced therapies, EMA's recommendation.

Definitions

Although medical devices and medicinal products in Europe have been defined in the respective directives covering these products, their use in combination is only described in a medical devices guidance document, MEDDEV 2.1/3 Rev. 3. However, MEDDEV documents are non-binding on the authorities and, therefore, not enforceable in court. That makes them comparable to harmonised standards; they describe the current state of science.

The legally valid definition of a "medical device" can be found in Article 1, Section 2 of the *MDD*. To be classified as a medical device, the product must among other preconditions: "….not achieve its principal intended action in or on the human body by pharmacological, immunological or metabolic means, but which may be assisted in its function by such means."

So, the medical device function is achieved principally by mechanical means, including, but not limited to, mechanical action, physical barrier or replacement of or support to organs or body functions (MEDDEV 2.1/3 rev. 3 (A2.1.1.1)). In the vast majority of combination products, the principal mode of action is self-evident. Admittedly, there is no binding legal definition available. For a combination of a device and drug, the classification is essentially driven by the principal mode of action and the product's auxiliary component(s), how they interface, the nature of the non-device component and, finally, how they are labelled and marketed.

The legal definition of a "medicinal product" in Article 1(2) of Directive 2001/83.EC is:

"(a) any substance or combination of substances presented as having properties for treating or preventing diseases in human beings; or

(b) Any substance or combination of substances which may be used in or administered to human beings either with a view to restoring, correcting or modifying physiological functions by exerting a pharmacological, immunological or metabolic action, or making a medical diagnosis."

Overview of Directives, Guidance Documents and National Practices and Their Implications

Directives

There are key references to combination products included in the current *MDD*, which are summarised here:

- Article 1, paragraph 3 states, "Where a device is intended to administer a medicinal product within the meaning of Article 1 of Directive 2001/83/EC, that device shall be governed by this Directive, without prejudice to the provisions of Directive 2001/83/EC with regard to the medicinal product."

  An example is an insulin pump or a syringe intended for parenteral administration of pharmaceuticals. These medical devices will be governed exclusively by the *MDD*.

- Paragraph 3 further states, "If, however, such a device is placed on the market in such a way that the device and the medicinal product form a single integral product which is intended exclusively for use in the given combination and which is not reusable, that single product shall be governed by Directive

2001/83/EC. The relevant essential requirements of Annex I to this Directive (i.e., the *MDD*) shall apply as far as safety and performance-related device features are concerned."

An example is a disposable syringe prefilled with insulin or another drug, or a disposable, pre-filled drug delivery device. This product is classified as a pharmaceutical product, but has to meet additional requirements.

- Article 1, paragraph 4 of the *MDD* states, "Where a device incorporates, as an integral part, a substance which, if used separately may be considered to be a medicinal product within the meaning of Article 1 of Directive 2001/83/EC and which is liable to act upon the body with action ancillary to that of the body, that device shall be assessed and authorized in accordance with this directive."

These products constitute the major thrust of this chapter because of their enormous diversity and, at times, complexity. Examples are heparin-coated catheters, platelet irradiation solutions for the reduction of pathogen load, joint replacements coated with bone growth factor, in vitro fertilisation media and many others.

- Article 1, paragraph 4a states, "Where a device incorporates, as an integral part, a substance which if used separately, may be considered to be a medicinal product constituent or a medicinal product derived from human blood or human plasma within the meaning of Article 1 of Directive 2001/83/EC and which is liable to act upon the human body with action ancillary to that of the device, hereinafter referred to as a "human blood derivative," that device shall be assessed and authorized in accordance with this Directive."

A company that wants to market a combination device should follow a cascade of regulatory questions to determine which legal framework is applicable:

Question 1: Is a medicinal product included?
The manufacturer should assess whether the product contains, as an integral part, a medicinal product. This is the case not only, for example, for a coating, but must also be considered if a medicinal product is included in the packaging that will be placed on the market. If the pharmaceutical component is sold separately (i.e., not included within the device packaging), it is a medicinal product and not a medical device (only one can apply). This has given rise to many disputes and will likely continue to do so until the next major overhaul of the device legislation.

Question 2: Is the substance a medicinal product?
It has to be evaluated whether a "substance, if used separately is considered ....a medicinal product." Many substances may be used in different ways and indications. Examples include:
- surface tension-reducing substances used to reduce foaming in bubble oxygenators, but also to the same purpose in certain stomach conditions
- vitamin E (alpha-tocopherol) used as an oxygenation enhancer in certain pathogen reduction processes
- heparin solutions to rinse laboratory glassware in order to prevent clotting when used with blood in the laboratory
- human growth hormone in combination with a mechanical scaffold to promote bone growth in large bone defects that will not heal completely by themselves
- nano-sized silver particles or silver derivatives either imbedded or eluted from wound dressings

National Competent Authorities and, consequently, NBs and courts of justice tend to consider any substance or chemical that may have any pharmacological, metabolic, immunological and, at times, even nutritional (as a precursor to metabolic) property as fitting within the medicinal products aspect. Therefore, a manufacturer wishing to consider the design of any combination product should seek to establish with certainty the planned product's proper classification.

Question 3: Does the substance act on the human body?
The final consideration is "...and which is liable to act upon the body with action ancillary to that of the body..." This statement is more contentious than it may first appear and will be explained by an example: A wound dressing contains solidly embedded silver particles. It has been demonstrated that the silver is not released in the wound. The manufacturer claims that the silver is used only to reduce microbial colonization inside the dressing to extend the dressing's duration of use (and not to enhance the reduction of the pathogen load in the wound), so this is not considered a combination product. However, if any of these conditions is not met, a consensus published by the European Commission (the *Manual on Borderline and Classification in the Community Regulatory Framework for Medical Devices* vs.1.6 02-2010, section 8.15) unequivocally classifies the product as Class III under Rule 13 of the *MDD*, Annex IX dealing with classification of medical devices: "All devices incorporating, as an integral part, a substance which, if used separately can be considered to be a medicinal product as defined in Article 1 of Directive 2001/83/EC and which is liable to act upon the body with action ancillary to that of the devices, are in Class III."

However, Article 1, Section 4 of the *MDD* states: "Where a device incorporates, as an integral part, a substance which, if used separately may be considered to be a medicinal product within the meaning of Article 1 of

Directive 2001/83/EC and which is liable to act upon the body with action ancillary to that of the device, that device shall be assessed and authorised in accordance with this directive."

There are subtle but important differences between these two statements, the main one being the interpretation of what is a medicinal product "defined in" or "within the meaning of." There is a growing tendency to use an all-encompassing interpretation of what constitutes a medicinal product. As a result, a conformity assessment consistent with Class III is performed in the vast majority of drug-device combination products. The resulting pharmaceutical consultation is discussed later in this chapter.

Question 4: What is the principal component?
What is the product's principal component and what is its auxiliary component? The principal mode of action can be determined by theoretically deleting one component, then assessing whether the intended use is still possible. If the intended use is no longer possible, then the hypothetically deleted component provides the principal mode of action. For instance, in a dressing that releases an antibiotic substance into the wound to combat an infection, the principal mode of action is clearly a pharmacological intervention. But a dressing with paraffin to soothe and mechanically protect a burn wound is a device with paraffin as an auxiliary pharmaceutical. If considered separately, the paraffin may be used as a drug.

Question 5: Intended product claims
The configuration of the product is a vital factor in determining the pathway to CE marking. Individually placing different components of a segregated drug-device combination intended to be used together is likely to have major repercussions, primarily for the pharmaceutical component, which probably will require a full pharmaceutical registration.

European Guidelines

The classification rules for medical devices are codified in *MDD* Annex IX. Medical devices cover a vast spectrum of products and in the early years of the directive, the need for further guidance became obvious. Two guidance documents have been formulated: MEDDEV 2.4/1 Rev. 9 describing the risk classification system and MEDDEV 2.1/3 Rev.3. MEDDEV 2.1/3 Part A explores the various borderline areas between pharmaceuticals and devices; Part B contains an extensive interpretative description of the various parameters and permutations for drug-device combination products; and Part C covers the consultation procedure, which is described later in this chapter.

Because MEDDEV 2.1/3 Part B is a consensus document, it could only contain examples and rulings that are not contentious. Unfortunately, it leaves many manufacturers of products that do not fit the "common mold" with major uncertainty on how to determine the correct pathway to CE marking their products. To overcome these problems, the European Commission implemented the Medical Devices Expert Group (MDEG) to compile cases that defy the normal classification rules in the *Manual on Borderline and Classification in the Community Regulatory Framework for Medical Devices*.[1] The manual is updated two or three times per year and is intended to reflect the consensus between the national Competent Authorities of the Member States, the medical devices industry and the NB. To be included in the manual, unanimity is not required, but a "qualified" majority is required. That means that none of the national Competent Authorities can disagree. It is a helpful and pragmatic approach and should be considered by manufacturers for further advice.

Neither the MEDDEVs nor the manual has the force of law. Dissenting Member States may legally block a product from their national markets even if the manufacturer complies with the guidance and the opinion of its NB. That opens the door to national guidelines, the main vehicle for re-nationalisation of the medical devices regulatory framework.

National Regulations and Guidance

Most Member States have some dissenting opinions on specific product categories. A whole set of well-defined and elaborate rulings on both borderline and combination products is not available. Few national approaches have been made in this direction. Bulletin No. 17, entitled "Medical Devices and Medicinal Products," from the UK's Medicines and Healthcare products Regulatory Agency (MHRA) is one of them.[2] The document presents MHRA's current views on the interpretation of the *Medical Devices Regulations* and the *Medicines Act* as they relate to drug/device demarcation issues. It is intended as general guidance and should not be regarded as an authoritative statement of the law or as having any legal consequence.

Therefore, manufacturers should not rely on national guidances if they want to market their products EU-wide. They should consult the legislation and make their own decisions in conjunction with their lawyers and other professional advisers.

It is important for a manufacturer to be aware that although a CE Mark is valid in all of the jurisdictional territories of the EAA and Switzerland, the NB and its rulings are governed by the Member State in which it is located. In other words, a British NB is governed by its national Competent Authority, MHRA, but the resulting CE Mark is valid throughout Europe. If, for instance, France or the Netherlands disagrees with the classification as a combination product, it may invoke the Safeguard Clause of the

MDD to protect its citizens' health and well-being. Such a procedure may end in a number of ways, but that is outside the scope of this chapter.

The Pharmaceutical Consultation Procedure

A product that has been classified as a "device incorporating, as an integral part, an ancillary medicinal substance or an ancillary human blood derivative" combination product must be reviewed by a national Competent Authority located in any Member State. The choice of such a reviewing agency is the NB's prerogative, but in practice, it is limited by two factors:
- manufacturer preference
- national Competent Authority availability

This essentially reduces the choice to either the authorities in the Netherlands, UK, Germany or France. Other agencies either refuse to perform the review or have extremely lengthy waiting periods. Both the Dutch and the British agencies have descriptors of what they expect regarding data, format and documentation. Dossier criteria focus on product safety and "usefulness," with other aspects such as pharmacodynamics and pharmacokinetics less pronounced. According MEDDEV2.1/3 Rev. 3, "safety" is defined as the potential inherent risks assessed against the benefit to be obtained, and "usefulness" as the suitability of the medicinal substance to achieve its intended ancillary action. As it is important to limit the scope of the dossier to those data relevant to this assessment, the agencies mentioned here actually encourage the manufacturer to meet with them prior to submission. The results of such discussions are binding, regardless of how they were formulated. To prevent misunderstandings, the manufacturer should always summarise these discussions in writing.

The format of the submission is described in some detail in section C3 of MEDDEV 2.1/3 Rev. 3. The guidance reflects specified parts of a drug submission in the Common Technical Dossier (CTD) format.

The manufacturer has to submit the documentation to the NB, which pre-assesses it for the device aspects. Subsequently, the national Competent Authority checks it for completeness and format. If the submission is rejected, the manufacturer usually has one more chance but, obviously, the review clock stops. If the submission is accepted, the review may lead to one or two question-and-answer cycles. The overall review process takes about 12 months in the UK and somewhat less in the Netherlands, but both agencies also significantly deviate from this practice. In France and Germany, the timeline is not predictable.

Ancillary blood derivatives and certain new pharmaceuticals, or existing products with a new use (e.g., drug eluting stents) are subject to submission to and review by EMA and its Committee for Advanced Therapies (CAT).[3] It is expected that the evidence of conformity with the Essential Requirements of the medical device directives is documented in the STED format,[4] including an Essential Requirements checklist and a description of the interaction and compatibility between genes, cells and/or tissues and the structural components.

The steps of the consultation procedure and the timelines are summarised in **Figure 30-1**. Eighty days after the NB assessment has been provided, CAT identifies questions for the NB, which generally should be answered by Day 120 of the procedure. The second consultation cycle results in a Letter of Questions on Day 170. On Day 200, CAT adopts an opinion, and discussion with CHMP takes place on Day 210. Either the draft opinion will become final, or an oral explanation will be provided. Assuming the NB needs four months for the assessment, and a scientific evaluation by CAT takes about seven months, the time before the manufacturer gets a reliable decision is close to one year. This is a comparably long period for the development of a medical device. On the other hand, it is a rather reliable timeline that a manufacturer can use for planning purposes.

Once the results of the national Competent Authority or EMA review are final, a "recommendation" will be issued that must be followed by the NB. A negative opinion of the national Competent Authority means a combination product cannot be placed on the market.

Several aspects will impact the review:
- data submitted to other agencies (e.g., the US Food and Drug Administration (FDA))
- the use of an Active Substance Master File (ASMF) for pharmaceuticals as a "fast track" approach)
- careful crafting of the labelling to avoid "drug" type claims

Pathways for Appeals and Remedial Actions

Given the complexity and sometimes unclear formulated definitions and regulations, there is only a small proportion of classifications that may take some time to obtain a clear-cut outcome.

The vast majority of cases in which a classification is disputed by the NB and the manufacturer end with the NB requesting a ruling from the national Competent Authority under whose jurisdiction it falls. If the manufacturer tries a "don't ask, don't tell" approach, the national Competent Authorities can reinforce their market vigilance. This could mean high costs and loss of reputation for the manufacturer.

The manufacturer can file a formal complaint with the national Competent Authority, which then has to review the case. The manufacturer can also ask the national Competent Authority to initiate an enquiry among the Member States in a standardised format (the Helsinki Enquiry and the Dublin form). If such an enquiry yields a strong majority, the result usually is announced in the MDEG's Committee

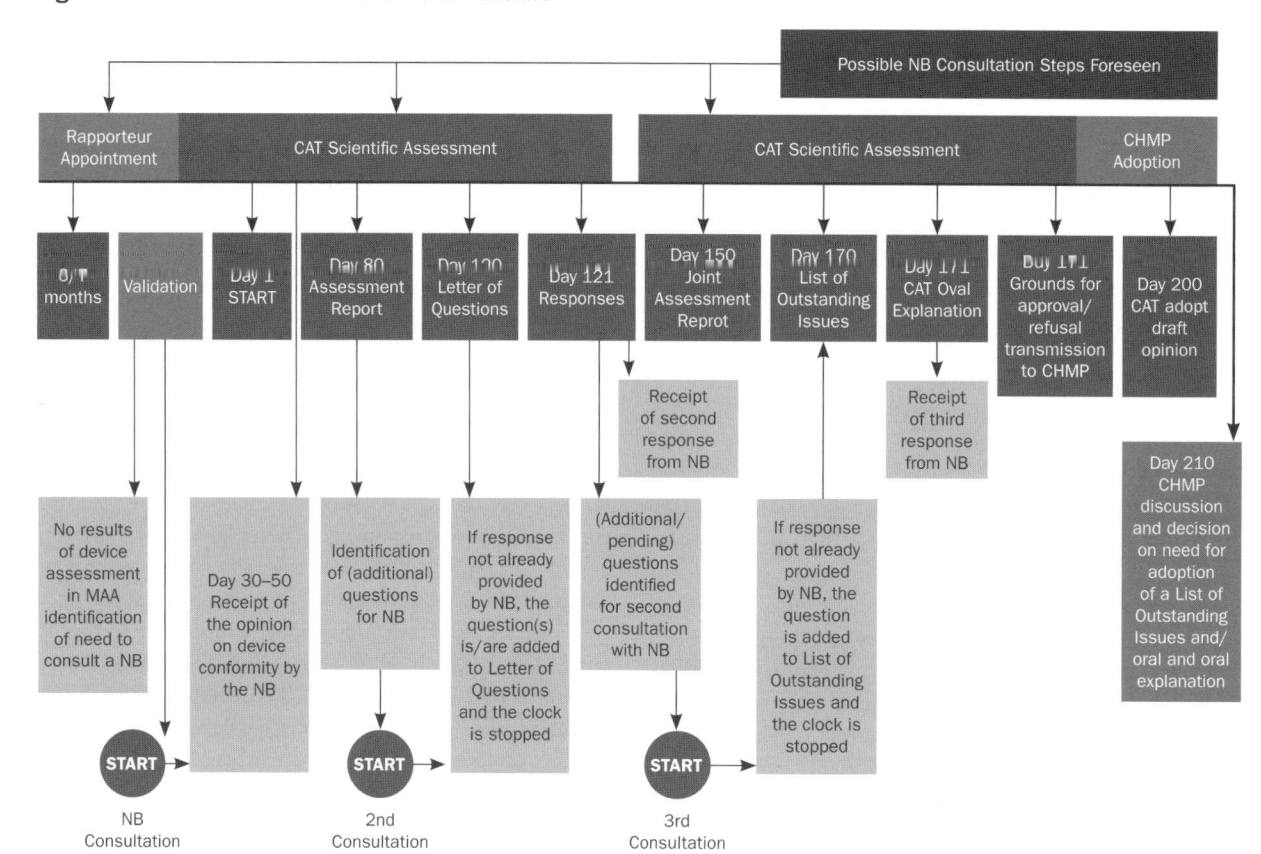

Figure 30-1. Consultation Procedure and Timeline

Rapporteur Appointment	CAT Scientific Assessment					CAT Scientific Assessment				CHMP Adoption
0/T months / Validation	Day 1 START	Day 80 Assessment Report	Day 120 Letter of Questions	Day 121 Responses		Day 150 Joint Assessment Report	Day 170 List of Outstanding Issues	Day 171 CAT Oral Explanation	Day 171 Grounds for approval/refusal transmission to CHMP	Day 200 CAT adopt draft opinion

Possible NB Consultation Steps Foreseen

- Receipt of second response from NB (after Day 150)
- Receipt of third response from NB (after Day 171)
- Day 210 CHMP discussion and decision on need for adoption of a List of Outstanding Issues and/oral and oral explanation

NB Consultation (START): No results of device assessment in MAA identification of need to consult a NB → Day 30–50 Receipt of the opinion on device conformity by the NB

2nd Consultation (START): Identification of (additional) questions for NB → If response not already provided by NB, the question(s) is/are added to Letter of Questions and the clock is stopped

3rd Consultation (START): (Additional/pending) questions identified for second consultation with NB → If response not already provided by NB, the question is added to List of Outstanding Issues and the clock is stopped

---

for Classification of Borderline and Combination Products, and in case of a consensus, is entered into the manual. These enquiries have three major drawbacks:

- The manufacturer has no way to obtain intermediate status information, whether the enquiries were launched, or learn the result before the enquiry has been finished.
- There is no mandatory participation or limit on response time.
- Because there is no mechanism for managing enquiries, they can last indefinitely (some have lasted as long as five years). In the meantime, the manufacturer is left with uncertainty at a minimum, or the impossibility of proceeding at worst. There is no procedure to appeal against an unreasonably slow or incomplete enquiry.

The manufacturer can also lodge a formal complaint against a national Competent Authority with the European Commission. If its result is not acceptable, the manufacturer can go to the ultimate arbiter of appeals, the European Court of Justice in Luxembourg. Although the procedure itself is not prohibitively expensive, by this time most small and mid-sized manufacturers have exhausted their funds and abandoned the effort in view of the lost time and sales opportunities. However, it is possible to win. The important consequence is that such adjudications not only are binding law in all EEA countries and Switzerland, but also represent precedents and "predicates" to subsequent cases. In addition, for most Class I and IIa and some IIb products, the verdict has repercussions for submissions in Canada and Australia, countries with similar device classification systems.

In conclusion, the best way to resolve any contentious classification issues is to reach a negotiated outcome that satisfies all parties, even if the national Competent Authority would like to escalate the matter along the pathway described.

Case Studies

A. Heparin coating of an active implantable medical device (artificial heart) intended for auxiliary heart pump function in severe cardiac deficiency

This combination product contains a tiny quantity of heparin (1/20,000[th] of the daily dosage to achieve systemic anticoagulation) and was solidly bound to the pump material. However, its mere presence necessitated a pharmaceutical consultation procedure under Annex IX, Rule 13, Class III procedures. The resulting pharmaceutical consultation increased the lead time by about 12 months.

This example is quoted in MEDDEV2.1/3 Rev. 3, section B.4.1 (first example).

B. In vitro fertilisation solutions and solutions to transport transplant organs or tissue (simulated environment)

These fairly complex and largely empirically formulated products have been used in Europe and the US in millions of patients in the past 25 years. Even so, a sudden whistleblower action by a competitor almost resulted in an (unintended) classification as a drug, because several national Competent Authorities maintained that there was a metabolic action of the media on the spermatocytes and the fertilised oocyte. After about three years of tough negotiations, the European Commission successfully forged a compromise, which has been published in the manual under 4.3, p. 23. The gist is that products will be treated in principle as Class IIb medical devices if no medicinal substance, no blood derivative and no animal-based derivative is used. If the product contains one or more of these components, the applicable route will apply. For example, the use of human serum albumin (HSA) necessitates a review by EMA, which easily adds 18 months to the review process and a sizeable fee. In addition, the HSA is subject to batch release.

C. Bone substitute with bone growth hormone (BGH)

Bone additives have long been a huge point of contention, depending on whether the manufacturer added an osteoconductive, an osteoinductive, an antibiotic or a human BGH. Again, reference is made to MEDDEV 2.1/3 for the respective examples.

The bone substitute with BGH has been regulated as a "classic" Rule 13 product because the primary mode of action is considered the substitute, with the BGH as an ancillary action. In case of a matrix (scaffold) where the BGH plays the primary role, the combination product is considered a medicinal product.

D. Set for local anesthesia with lidocaine

In this example, the packaging configuration plays a major role. Unlike FDA, under which such a product may be subject to a straightforward 510(k) notification process, in Europe it really depends on whether:

- the lidocaine has been approved as a generic or branded drug and is added as an approved, labeled entity to the set, or
- it is sold separately as a drug, but may be used with the device set, or
- it is "imbedded" in the device set, and has not been labelled as an approved separate drug entity

In the latter case only, the combination will be classified as Class III under Rule 13 and subject to a pharmaceutical consultation procedure. This is an excellent exercise to test whether the omission or modification of a packaging configuration would result in a different primary mode of action.

E. Sunblock cream with imbedded titanium oxide for vitiligo (barrier)

Even though the product would qualify as a straightforward medical device because of the mechanical action, the titanium oxide may be considered a medicinal substance and, consequently, subject the product to Rule 13. The primary mode of action, though, is physical and consequently, the *MDD* applies.

Conclusion

Products that combine a medical device and a medicinal product are regulated by a complex framework of legislation. The primary mode of action, the kind of pharmaceutical active substance and its interaction with the human body are important for the product's classification according to device or drug law. For manufacturers, it is difficult to find a regulatory pathway with predictable timelines. Due to the large number of different medical devices, the implementation of a centralised authority would not resolve the current problems, as novel products are developed continuously.

References

1. Manual on Borderline and Classification in the Community: Regulatory Framework for Medical Devices. European Commission website. http://ec.europa.eu/health/medical-devices/files/wg_minutes_member_lists/borderline_manual_ol_en.pdf. Accessed 30 May 2012.
2. Bulletin No. 17, Medical Devices and Medicinal Products. Medicines and Healthcare products Regulatory Agency website. www.mhra.gov.uk/home/groups/es-era/documents/publication/con007498.pdf. Accessed 30 May 2012.
3. Procedural advice on the evaluation of combined advanced therapy medicinal products and the consultation of Notified Bodies in accordance with Article 9 of Regulation (EC) No. 1394/2007.
4. Summary Technical Documentation for Demonstrating Conformity to the Essential Principles of Safety and Performance of Medical Devices (STED). February 2008. GHTF website. www.ghtf.org/documents/sg1/sg1final-n11.pdf. Accessed 30 May 2012.

Chapter 31

Cosmetic Products

Updated by Andrea Martter, RAC

OBJECTIVES

❏ Understand what a cosmetic product is in the EU

❏ Understand how cosmetics are regulated

❏ Learn the critical requirements for placing a cosmetic on the market

❏ Learn how changes are made to EU regulations

❏ Understand the major differences between cosmetics regulations in the EU and US

REGULATIONS AND GUIDELINES COVERED IN THIS CHAPTER

❏ Council Directive 76/768/EEC of 27 July 1976 on the approximation of the laws of the Member States relating to cosmetic products[1]

❏ On 30 November 2009, this directive was amended for the eighth time. It is now Regulation (EC) No 1223/2009 of the European Parliament and of the Council on cosmetic products.[2] The Cosmetics Regulation takes full effect 11 July 2013 with a few exceptions.

Implementation of the Cosmetics Regulation

❏ 1 December 2010: The provisions in the Cosmetics Regulation regarding carcinogenic, mutagenic or toxic for reproduction (CMR) substances came into force, repealing corresponding sections of the Cosmetics Directive.

❏ 11 January 2012: The Cosmetic Products Notification Portal (CPNP) was made available and can be used for centralised electronic cosmetic notifications.

❏ 11 January 2013: Notification of nanomaterials used in cosmetic products commences.

❏ 11 July 2013: The Cosmetics Regulation enters into force, replacing the Cosmetics Directive. Compliance with the new product information file (PIF) requirements, nanomaterials notifications and labelling and CPNP are mandatory.

Note: cosmetic products placed on the market before 11 July 2013 may comply with the new provisions of the *Cosmetics Regulation* to ensure a smooth transition between the directive and regulation. Cosmetic products that were on the market prior to 11 July 2013 must be in compliance with the *Cosmetics Regulation* as of 11 July 2013. Information provided in this chapter will refer to the *Cosmetics Regulation* unless otherwise noted.

Cosmetic Products Legislation

Cosmetic products are regulated by Regulation (EC) No 1223/2009 relating to cosmetic products, the *Cosmetics Regulation*.[2] This regulation consists of forty articles and ten annexes.

A "cosmetic product" is defined in Article 1 of the regulation as:

"any substance or mixture intended to be placed in contact with the external parts of the human body (epidermis, hair system, nails, lips and external genital organs) or with the teeth and mucous membranes of the oral cavity with a view exclusively or mainly to cleaning them, perfuming them, changing their appearance, protecting them, keeping them in good condition or correcting body odours."

and furthermore:

"a substance or mixture intended to be ingested, inhaled, injected or implanted into the human body shall not be considered to be a cosmetic product."

Cosmetic products may include the following product types:
- creams, emulsions, lotions, gels and oils for the skin
- face masks
- tinted bases (liquids, pastes, powders)
- make-up powders
- after-bath powders, hygienic powders
- toilet soaps, deodorant soaps
- perfumes, toilet waters and eau de cologne
- bath and shower preparations (salts, foams, oils, gels)
- depilatories
- deodorants and anti-perspirants
- hair colorants
- products for waving, straightening and fixing hair
- hair-setting products
- hair-cleansing products (lotions, powders, shampoos)
- hair-conditioning products (lotions, creams, oils)
- hairdressing products (lotions, lacquers, brilliantines)
- shaving products (creams, foams, lotions)
- make-up and products removing make-up
- products intended for application to the lips
- products for care of the teeth and the mouth
- products for nail care and make-up
- products for external intimate hygiene
- sunbathing products
- products for tanning without sun
- skin-whitening products
- anti-wrinkle products

It may be confusing sometimes whether a product is a cosmetic or falls under different legislation, e.g., a biocide, medicinal product or medical device. A product is either a cosmetic or another type of product (e.g., medicinal product) but cannot be both ("principle of non-cumulation"). Questions may be raised about the classification of a product that is on the borderline between the definition of a cosmetic product and that of other product types.

For borderline situations, the European Court of Justice has repeatedly stated that, in seeking to classify products, not only the legal definition but all product characteristics (i.e., the product's composition, its properties, the way in which it is used, the extent to which it is sold, consumer familiarity with it and the risks its use may entail) must be taken into account on a case-by-case basis. To clarify borderline situations and facilitate interpretation, the Commission has published a number of guidance documents on its website (http://ec.europa.eu/consumers/sectors/cosmetics/cosmetic-products/borderline-products/index_en.htm), including a "manual"[3] on the scope of the *Cosmetics Directive* and on the demarcation between, respectively, the *Cosmetic Products Directive* and the *Medicinal Products Directive*, *Biocidal Products Directive* and *General Products Safety Directive*. Borderline products discussed in the "manual" include:

Borderline with Toys
- make-up to be used on dolls
- make-up to be used on children
- bath products for children with a play value

Borderline with Biocides
- antiseptic or antibacterial leave-on products presented as "antiseptic" or "antibacterial"
- antiseptic or anti-bacterial mouthwash

Borderline with Medicinal Products
- products intended to exclusively or mainly relieve joint pain
- products intended to address itching
- product containing substances that restore, correct or modify physiological functions by exerting a pharmacological, immunological or metabolic action
- products to stimulate hair growth or reduce hair loss
- products that make eyelashes grow
- products for in-grown hairs
- products that make the lips swell
- products reducing cellulite
- substances applied with skin-patches
- products to treat dry mouth
- products for superficial moisturizing of female genital organ in cases of extreme mucosal dryness
- topical breast augmentation products
- products for atopic skin
- products to reduce dark circles under the eyes

Borderline with Medical Devices
- products that, according to their presentation, are intended to peel the skin
- products against head lice

Borderline with Other Legislations
- products to detect plaque on teeth
- products to remove glue used to fix articles on the skin or nails
- products to stimulate sexual activity

Marketing Requirements for a Cosmetic Product

Cosmetics must not cause damage or harm to humans when applied or used under normal or reasonable conditions, taking into account the product's presentation, labelling, instructions for use and disposal and any other information provided by the manufacturer or distributor. Further, products must be properly labelled and have a Product Information File (PIF), which must be made available to the Competent Authorities upon request (within 72 hours). They cannot contain or use ingredients prohibited or restricted outside the scope of the constraints.

Responsible Person and Distributor

The Responsible Person (RP) is the legal or natural person designated within the EU who is ultimately responsible for ensuring compliance with the *Cosmetics Regulation*. The RP is responsible for holding the PIFs and making them available upon request to the Competent Authority; employing corrective measures to bring products into conformity or withdrawing and recalling products if necessary; and completing product notifications.

The selection of the RP is extremely important. For products manufactured within the EU, the RP is generally the manufacturer. For imported cosmetics, the importer placing the product on the market shall be the RP. Importers may use outside services to respond if they do not want their sensitive information available to distributors.

Distributors are responsible for ensuring that the products they place on the market have compliant labelling (including the appropriate language requirements), products have not passed their date of minimum durability, appropriate product storage and transport conditions are employed and corrective actions are taken as needed (including product withdrawal and recall). Distributors are also responsible for a limited product notification if they are placing a product on the market (that is already available in another Member State) and they have translated any element of the label on their own initiative to comply with national law. See information on premarket notification below.

Premarket Notification

One of the major changes in the *Cosmetics Regulation* is a new single, centralised notification process. Under the *Cosmetics Directive*, premarket approval is not required, although in practice, some Member States (e.g., Denmark and Spain) might require premarket approval or notification to their Poison Centres. Therefore, in essence, the *Cosmetics Regulation* replaces multiple Member State notifications with one centralised notification.

The Cosmetic Products Notification Portal (CPNP) is now available, although the use of this electronic filing method is not mandatory until 11 July 2013. Notification to the European Commission of cosmetic products must be made prior to placing them on the market. The Commission will then submit relevant information to the Member States' Poison Centres.

The following information should be included in the notification:
- product name and category
- name and address of the RP
- country of origin, if imported
- Member State where the product is to be placed on the market
- contact details of a physical person in case of necessity
- presence of nanomaterials
- name and CAS number of any CMR (carcinogen, mutagen and reprotoxic) substances
- frame formulation (ingredient names and concentrations, ranges are optional)
- labelling and packaging

The RP and the Poison Centres will have access to all information. Competent Authorities will not have access to the formulation information.

Distributors selling a cosmetic product in a Member State that is already available in another Member State are responsible for the electronic filing of the following information:
- product name and category
- Member State in which the product is made available
- distributor's name and address
- name and address of the RP where the PIF is made readily accessible

Labelling

Cosmetics must have the following labelling information in indelible, easily legible and visible lettering on the container and packaging (however, the list of ingredients may be indicated on the packaging alone):

1. name and address of the RP (If there are multiple EU addresses on the label, the address where the PIF can be consulted shall be underlined.)
2. package contents, either by weight or volume, except for packaging of less than 5 g or ml, free samples and single-application packs
3. date of minimum durability or Period After Opening (PAO)

Chapter 31

- If there are fewer than 30 months of stability, the label must bear the phrase "Best used by" or the hourglass pictogram (found in Annex VII 3) followed by the date (month+year or day+month+year).
- For products with more than 30 months of stability, the label must include the PAO, which is the period after the product has been opened by the consumer during which it will cause no harm to the consumer. The PAO symbol is an open jar (found in Annex VII 2) followed by months and/or years.
- European Commission guidelines on the practical implementation of Article 6(1)(c)[4] of the *Cosmetics Directive* state that "months" are to be expressed by "M" (for menses), and that no PAO is needed for aerosol dispensers, single-application packs or products for which there is no deterioration risk. The manufacturer may decide which method is relevant to substantiate its product's date of durability or PAO.

4. precautions for use, especially those related to the presence of certain ingredients found in Annexes III to VI
5. batch or lot number
6. product's function, unless it is obvious from its presentation
7. ingredient list, using the International Nomenclature of Cosmetic Ingredients (INCI)
    - The ingredient list shall be preceded by the word "Ingredients," and listed in descending order by weight. Ingredients comprising less than 1% can be listed in any order after the ingredients of more than 1%. Impurities in the raw materials and trace materials not present in the final product are not considered ingredients.
    - Colorants (other than hair dyes) may be listed in any order after the other cosmetic ingredients. For decorative cosmetics (other than hair dyes) that vary only in shades, all colouring agents (listed on Annex IV) may be listed if preceded by the phrase "may contain" or the symbol [+/-].
    - Perfume and aromatic compositions shall be referred to by the word "parfum" or "aroma." However, if the formulation contains more than 10 ppm for leave-on products or 100 ppm for rinse-off products of any of the 26 fragrance allergens listed in Annex III, from any source (fragrances, essential oils, plant extracts, etc.), each of these allergens must be listed in the ingredient declaration.
    - All ingredients in the form of nanomaterials shall be indicated by the word "nano" in brackets (NANO) appearing after the ingredient name.

Nominal content, date of minimum durability or PAO, precautions for use and product function have to be translated into the official national language(s) of any EU Member States where the product is marketed. If the package size or shape makes it impossible for the required information to be mentioned on the label, marketers are permitted to put the symbol of a hand pointing to an open book (found in Annex VII 1) on the label, mentioning the list of ingredients and precautions for use on an affixed label, tag, tape or card or in an enclosed leaflet. This symbol directs the consumer to look elsewhere for specific label information.

For small products, it is possible to mention the list of ingredients on a notice in immediate proximity to the cosmetic product displayed for sale.

Animal Testing of Cosmetics and Their Ingredients

Based on Article 18 of the *Cosmetics Regulation* (commonly known as the 7th Amendment to the *Cosmetics Directive*):

1. No testing of cosmetic products has been permitted to be performed on animals since 11 September 2004.
2. No testing of any cosmetic ingredient has been permitted to be performed on animals to establish its safety for use in cosmetics since 11 March 2009, with the exception of repeated-dose toxicity, carcinogenicity, reproductive toxicity and toxicokinetics.
3. No repeated-dose toxicity, carcinogenicity, reproductive toxicity or toxicokinetics testing on animals of cosmetic ingredients will be permitted to be performed as of 11 March 2013. However, it is unlikely that science will develop alternative test methods by 2013 and the date of this ban may be extended.
4. Beyond those deadlines, Member States may request the European Commission to grant a derogation to carry out animal testing, but only for an existing ingredient in wide use, which cannot be replaced by another ingredient with a similar function, and if there is a substantiated human health problem.

The Annexes

Table 31-1 shows the annex numbers, some of which have changed, for the *Cosmetics Directive* and the *Cosmetics Regulation*. References to the annexes in the following sections use the *Cosmetic Regulation* annex number unless otherwise noted.

Annex II Prohibited Substances

Annex II lists substances that are prohibited from use in cosmetics. Currently, there are more than 1,300 prohibited substances. Included in this annex are human derivatives as well as several animal-derived products because of Bovine Spongiform Encephalopathy (BSE) risk, nitrosamines,

Table 31-1. Annexes to the *Cosmetics Directive* and *Cosmetic Regulation*

Topic	Cosmetic Directive	Cosmetic Regulation
Prohibited Substances	Annex II	Annex II
Restricted Substances	Annex III	Annex III
Colorants	Annex IV	Annex IV
Preservatives	Annex VI	Annex V
UV Filters	Annex VII	Annex VI
Symbols on Packaging/Containers	Annex VIII	Annex VII
Animal Testing	Annex IX	Annex VIII

secondary alkanolamines, *o*-phenylenediamines and their salts, dimethyl sulfoxide, Vitamins D2 and D3, trichloroacetic acid and coal tar. Since September 2004, many new substances have been added to Annex II because of the systematic ban of CMRs. The latest additions are chemicals that were used in hair dyes. These were added, not because of safety issues, but because the use was so small that industry did not support the testing to include these as permitted hair dyes.

As this list is updated periodically, manufacturers should always refer to the latest annex. Until the *Cosmetics Regulation* comes into full force, the annex of the *Cosmetics Directive* should be consulted because it has been updated with more than 40 additional substances since the *Cosmetics Regulation* was published.

Traces of forbidden substances are tolerated provided their presence is technically unavoidable under Good Manufacturing Practice (GMP) and they do not present a risk to human health.

Restricted Substances

The *Cosmetics Regulation* further contains lists of substances that are prohibited except under conditions stated in Annex III. There are also three positive lists consisting of permitted cosmetic colouring agents (Annex IV), preservatives (Annex V) and UV filters (Annex VI) for skin protection (filters designed to protect only the product are not covered).

The *Cosmetics Regulation* reflects the situation of science at the time of the Commission's adoption of the proposal on 5 February 2008. The *Cosmetics Directive* annexes have been updated since then and these changes are in the process of being amended to the *Cosmetics Regulation*. In this interim period, both the directive and regulation need to be considered. Changes to the annexes of the *Cosmetics Directive* are technically considered part of Article 3 of the *Cosmetics Regulation*, which ensures the safety of cosmetic products. Therefore, until these changes have been amended to the *Cosmetics Regulation*, compliance with the directive's annexes ensures compliance with the regulation.

Note that in the *Cosmetics Directive*, each annex has a Part I for definitively allowed substances and a Part II for provisionally accepted substances. The deadlines in Part II are the dates by which a decision (such as definitively accepting the substance, banning it or maintaining it as provisionally accepted) should have been reached. The substances listed provisionally have been reviewed and moved to other annexes or are no longer permitted for use in cosmetics.

Annex III Restricted Substances

Annex III contains a list of more than 200 restricted substances that can be used only under specified conditions and restrictions. This annex includes many active ingredients used in hair waves, relaxers, dyes and bleaches as well as antidandruff agents, antiperspirant agents, fluoride compounds for oral hygiene and many other restricted ingredients. The usual conditions include field of application and/or use, maximum use levels, other limitations and requirements, conditions of use and mandatory warnings on labels. This is also where the 26 fragrance allergens are found.

Annex IV Colorants

Annex IV contains a list of more than 150 permitted cosmetic colours, including an indication of the cosmetic products in which they may be used:

1. all cosmetics
2. all cosmetics except eye care products
3. cosmetics not intended to come into contact with mucous membranes
4. cosmetics intended to be used as rinse-off products

Other colour restrictions include certain maximum levels of impurities, mainly for food colorants.

Colorants used only for hair dye are not included in this annex, though they may be included in the future, after further review.

Remember that all colours must be included in the label ingredients list using their Colour Index (CI) number, except for the last few colours that are listed by their chemical name.

Chapter 31

Annex V Preservatives
Annex V contains a list of more than 50 permitted preservatives, noting the maximum permitted levels and other limitations. Some preservatives require warnings.

Cosmetics containing formaldehyde, or preservatives that may release formaldehyde, are required to have the warning "contains formaldehyde" if the total formaldehyde concentration in the product exceeds 0.05% as determined by the approved COLIPA (now known as Cosmetics Europe) method.[5]

Annex VI UV Filters
Annex VI of the *Cosmetics Regulation* contains a list of more than 25 filters permitted in the EU to protect skin from solar UV rays. There is a maximum level for each filter. According to the *Cosmetics Regulation*, products containing more than 0.5% benzophenone-3 are required to have a warning label that says "contains benzophenone-3" (this is updated from the *Cosmetics Directive* warning "contains oxybenzone" that referred to the common name rather than the INCI name).

Other Annexes
Annex VII Symbols
Annex VII contains symbols for use on packaging or containers. The first is a hand pointing to an open book, which is used on small packaging to direct consumers to look elsewhere for information on composition and warnings. The second is the symbol representing the PAO. The third symbol is an hourglass indicating the date of minimum durability.

Annex VIII Animal Testing Alternatives
Annex VIII lists validated alternatives to animal testing that have been approved and can be used to determine the cosmetic product's safety. As of publication, no alternative test methods have been added to this annex. However, approved alternative test methods can be obtained from the European Centre for the Validation of Alternative Methods (ECVAM) website (http://ecvam.jrc.it/).

Other Ingredient Information
Nanomaterials
To ensure the protection of human health, companies must notify the Commission of any cosmetic products containing nanomaterials (except for nanomaterials used as colorants, UV filters or preservatives, which are regulated by other sections of the *Cosmetics Regulation*). Nanomaterials are defined in the *Cosmetics Regulation* as "an insoluble or biopersistant and intentionally manufactured material with one or more external dimensions, or an internal structure, on the scale from 1 to 100 nm." As the science in this field progresses, this definition may be amended in the future to be consistent with definitions at the international level.

Notifications must be made at least six months prior to being placed on the market. Notifications commence as of 11 January 2013 and are mandatory as of 11 July 2013.

Carcinogenic, Mutagenic or Toxic for Reproduction Substances (CMRs)
Category 1A, 1B, and 2 CMRs in the *Classification, Labelling and Packaging Regulation* (Regulation (EC) No 1272/2008) are prohibited. However, the *Cosmetics Regulation* allows for the use of some CMR 2 substances if they have been evaluated by the Scientific Committee on Consumer Safety (SCCS) and found safe for use in cosmetics based on their exposure and concentration.

CMR 1A or 1B substances may be used in cosmetics if the following conditions are met:
- they comply with food safety requirements
- there are no suitable alternative substances available
- the product has a particular use and known exposure
- they have been found safe by the SCCS for use in cosmetic products regarding exposure and vulnerable population groups

REACH
Cosmetic ingredients also must comply with the environmental concerns in Regulation (EC) No 1907/2006 on the Registration, Evaluation, Authorisation and Restriction of Chemicals (REACH).

Product Information File
The PIF must be accessible at the EU address of the RP and kept on file for 10 years after the final product batch date on the EU market. The information should be available in electronic or other format to the Competent Authority of the Member State where the file is kept. The file should be in a language easily understood by the respective Competent Authority. The PIF consists of five parts:

1. description of the cosmetic product in which the information is clearly attributed to the cosmetic product
2. Cosmetic Product Safety Report (CPSR), which must contain at a minimum:
   - Cosmetic Product Safety Information:
     o qualitative and quantitative composition
     o physical/chemical characteristics and stability
     o microbiological quality
     o impurities, traces and information about the packaging material*
     o normal and reasonably foreseeable use*
     o information on exposure to the product and substances
     o toxicological profile of the substances

- o undesirable effects
- o serious undesirable effects*
- o other relevant information on the product
- complete Product Safety Assessment consisting of:
  - o conclusion on the cosmetic product's safety
  - o labelled warnings and instructions for use*
  - o scientific reasoning on the conclusion, possible interactions of the substances, justification of toxicological profiles and impact of the stability*
  - o assessor's credentials (The assessor must be a person with formal qualifications in theoretical and practical study in pharmacy, toxicology, medicine or a similar discipline recognised by a Member State.)
3. description of the manufacturing method and a statement on compliance with GMPs (The required GMPs are those applicable in the manufacturing country. Generally, these must be equal to or better than the ISO 22716 international standard.)
4. proof of effect claimed (if applicable)
5. data on any animal testing

*These items are new requirements in the *Cosmetics Regulation*.

Parts That Must be Made Available to the Public

The following information must be made available to the public upon request:
- qualitative formulation and concentrations of hazardous substances
- fragrance supplier names and codes for any fragrances in the product
- adverse health effects resulting from cosmetic product use (To ensure consistent information, companies generally should compute a value for the number of undesirable effects per million marketed units, except when the actual volume placed on the market is small.)

This information may be made available electronically or by any other means (mail, etc.).

Changes to the European Commission Cosmetics Regulations

Changes to these regulations can be made by amendment. Annexes may be amended as described in Article 31 of the *Cosmetic Regulation*. These are long-term changes to the annexes including:
- changes to Annexes II to VI that address potential risks to human health arising from the use of ingredients in cosmetic products, after consulting the SCCS
- changes to Annexes III, IV, V, VI and VII for the purpose of adapting technical and scientific progress, after consulting the SCCS
- changes to Annex I to ensure the safety of cosmetic products, after consulting the SCCS

Amendment is a long process involving the European Commission, which prepares the proposals before discussion by the European Parliament and the Council of Ministers. All amendments must be passed by both the Parliament and the Council of Ministers (co-decision procedure).

If the amendment is a matter of urgency, the Commission may use the urgency procedure to review the changes.

Differences Between the US and the EU

There are several important differences between US and EU regulations. Basically, the US cosmetic regulation is static and has not changed very much since its publication, while the EU version is constantly evolving.

Definition of Cosmetic Products

One major difference is cosmetic product definition; many products regulated as cosmetics in the EU are considered over-the-counter (OTC) or nonprescription drugs in the US. The primary reason for this difference is that in the US a cosmetic product is not supposed to have any action on a physiological bodily function. Also, the US does not accept the functions of "protecting" and "maintaining in good condition" for cosmetics. OTC products include sun protection products, antiperspirants, antimicrobial cleansers, antidandruff products, skin whiteners and skin protectants. Those products are subject to the more stringent obligations described in specific US Food and Drug Administration (FDA) monographs.

Because of these differences, it is impossible to sell the same product on both markets with the same labelling. It is illegal to label a product that is considered a drug in the US as a drug in the EU if it is considered a cosmetic there. For example, drugs list their active ingredients separately and cosmetic products (like foods) have only one list of ingredients.

Composition Labelling

For products considered cosmetics in both the US and the EU, an agreement has been reached to permit single, full ingredient labelling. The INCI is used as a harmonised standard. This nomenclature is nearly the same on both sides of the Atlantic, except for cosmetic colours, botanical ingredients and some ingredients with trivial names. Canada has adopted ingredient labelling, but to satisfy Quebec, some unique changes were made. Canada accepts any name in the INCI dictionary with 57 exceptions, although the Latin names are acceptable. However, English

Chapter 31

Table 31-2. Ingredient Nomenclature for Labels

Old US Name	Old EU Name	Current Harmonised Name for EU and US	Harmonised Names for US, EU and Canada
Alcohol*	Alcohol denat.	*	same
Egg	Ovum	Egg (Ovum)	Egg/Ovum/Œuf
Flavor	Aroma	Flavour (Aroma)	Aroma/Flavor
Fragrance	Partum	Fragrance (Partum)	Parfum/Fragrance
Honey	Mel	Honey (Mel)	Mel/Honey/Miel
Microcrystalline Wax	Cera Microcistallina	Microcrystalline Wax (Cera Microcistallina)	Cera Microcistallina/ Microcrystalline Wax/Cire microcristalline
Milk	Lac	Milk (Lac)	Milk/Lac/Lait
Milk Lipids	Lactus Lipidia	Milk Lipids (Lactus Lipidia)	Milk Lipids/Lactus Lipidia/Lipides du lait
Mineral Oil	Parraffinum Liquidum	Mineral Oil (Paraffinum Liquidum)	Paraffinum Liquidum/Mineral Oil/Huile minérale
Rosin	Colophonium	Rosin (Colophonium)	Rosin/Colophonium/Colophane
Sea Salt	Maris Sal	Sea Salt (Maris Sal)	Sea Salt/Maris Sal/Sel Marin
Silk Powder	Serica	Silk Powder (Serica)	Silk Powder/Serica/Poudre de soie
Tallow	Adeps Bovis	Tallow (Adeps Bovis)	Tallow/Adeps Bovis/Suif
Water	Aqua	Water (Aqua)	Water/Aqua/Eau

* In the US, denatured alcohol is listed by its US Department of the Treasury designation (27 CFR 21). In the EU, the term is "alcohol denat." and then, in the appropriate descending order, location and the INCI designation of the denaturant. Source: *International Cosmetic Ingredient Dictionary and Handbook*. 12th ed. Labelling the product as Alcohol indicates that undenatured alcohol is the ingredient.

or combined English/Latin names must also be in French. **Table 31-2** lists some of these examples. For a complete list see: www.gazette.gc.ca/archives/p2/2004/2004-12-01/html/sor-dors244-eng.html.

Colours

The EU requires all colours to be listed by their CI number. The US requires certified organic colours and their like to be listed using FDA nomenclature:
- EU: CI 42090
- US: Blue 1 (note this format replaced the old nomenclature of FD&C Blue # 1)
- If the predominant market is the EU, the harmonised label will look like this:
  o CI 42090 (Blue 1)
- If the predominant market is the US, the label will look like this:
  o Blue 1 (CI 42090)
- The US uses INCI nomenclature for noncertified but permitted colours. Labelling would be similar:
  o EU: CI 77289
  o US: Chromium Hydroxide Green
  o Dual label: CI 77289 (Chromium Hydroxide Green) or Chromium Hydroxide Green (CI 77289)

The major difference with inorganic colours concerns iron oxides. The US lists any of the four grades of iron oxide as Iron Oxides, while the EU lists the specific CI number (i.e., CI 77489, CI 77491, CI 77492 or CI 77499). As a result, the dual label is much longer than necessary.

Botanical Ingredients

The US and the EU have now harmonised the nomenclature for botanical ingredients. Previously, the US used common names while the EU used the Linné (Latin) system used by botanists worldwide. This applied to whole oils or extracts. Any chemical modification would require INCI names. For example, in the US, "Chamomile Oil" would have been used, while in the EU, this would have been listed as "Anthemis Nobilis." There is now a common name for both markets. The resulting label is "Anthemis Nobilis (Chamomile) Flower Oil." These rules are applicable to all vegetable oils and waxes, plant extracts and oils and plant-derived gums.

Trivial Names

Table 31-2 lists the trivial names, i.e., names that can be easily understood by a consumer. The EU uses the Latin names that appear in the *EU Pharmacopoeia*.

It is important to note that the only correct name for water in the US is "Water" and in the EU is "Aqua." The use of other words such as "purified," "distilled," "natural," etc. is prohibited. (In the US, the use of the term "Purified Water" is only permitted in drugs that make no cosmetic claims. FDA views the use of this term in a cosmetic ingredient label to be a drug claim and hence it would be considered an unapproved new drug.)

Warning Labelling

FDA requires warnings on products based on types and uses, such as feminine deodorant sprays, bubble bath products for children's use, hair dye products, etc. The EU requires warnings based on the inclusion of certain ingredients (such as benzophenone-3, thioglycollic acid, ammonia, etc.) and for some substances, depending on their concentration (such as ammonia, formaldehyde, IPBC).

Claims

Therapeutic claims are not accepted in the EU or the US. There is no EU official list of unaccepted claims for cosmetics. Any claim listed in an OTC monograph is totally unacceptable for cosmetics in the US.

Regulated Ingredients

The number of substances banned or restricted in cosmetics in the US is very small (14) while, as noted previously, there are many banned and restricted substances for cosmetics in the EU, and these lists are evolving constantly. It must be noted that very few of the banned substances in the EU have ever been used in cosmetics. The huge increase was due to the EU ban on Category 1 and 2 CMRs.

The US list of positive cosmetic colorants is much shorter than the EU list. Another major difference is that only FDA-certified colorant batches can be used in the US. Such a procedure is not required in the EU.

The US has no positive list of preservatives.

On the other hand, in the US, only active ingredients listed in the OTC monographs can be used for products that would be considered cosmetics in the EU. It is extremely difficult to add a new active ingredient to the monographs.

Controls

Controls on cosmetics in the US mainly concern labelling (particularly, claims) and composition. If FDA is unhappy with claims the agency considers to be therapeutic, it usually will send a Warning Letter to the manufacturer(s).

Competent Authorities in the EU, when controlling cosmetic products, verify the presence of banned substances, restricted substance(s) concentration, labelling composition (are all ingredients included on the label?), warnings (are all compulsory warnings present on the label and translated into the national language?), claims (are they cosmetic? are they substantiated?), substantiation of durability date or PAO, etc.

Summary

The *Cosmetics Regulation* requires one centralised, electronic premarket notification for products marketed in conformance with the regulations. Cosmetics are required to have proper labels, including mandatory warnings where applicable, a disclosure of all ingredients and the address where product information is available. The EU has positive lists of permitted colours, preservatives and UV filters, as well as lists of restricted substances and banned substances.

References

1. Council Directive 76/768/EEC of 27 July 1976 on the approximation of the laws of the Member States relating to cosmetic products. EUR-Lex website. http://eur-lex.europa.eu/LexUriServ/LexUriServ.do?uri=CONSLEG:1976L0768:20080424:en:PDF. Accessed 31 May 2012.
2. Regulation (EC) No 1223/2009 of the European Parliament and of the Council of 30 November 2009 on cosmetic products. EUR-Lex website. http://eur-lex.europa.eu/LexUriServ/LexUriServ.do?uri=OJ:L:2009:342:0059:0209:EN:PDF. Accessed 31 May 2012.
3. European Commission, "Manual on the scope of application of the *Cosmetics Directive* 76/768/EEC (art. 1(1) *Cosmetics Directive*," Version 8.0 (June 2011). EC website. http://ec.europa.eu/consumers/sectors/cosmetics/files/doc/manual_borderlines_ol_en.pdf. Accessed 31 May 2012.
4. European Commission, 04/ENTR/COS/28, "Practical implementation of Article 6(1)(c) of the *Cosmetics Directive* (76/768/EEC), Labelling of product durability: 'Period of time after opening'." EC website. http://ec.europa.eu/consumers/sectors/cosmetics/files/doc/wd-04-entrcos_28_rev_version_adoptee20040419_en.pdf. Accessed 31 May 2012.
5. *Colipa Method* (Brussels, Belgium: The European Cosmetic Toiletry and Perfumery Association, 2002).

Chapter 32

Food Supplements, Health Claims and Borderline Issues

Updated by Gudrun Busch, MSc, PhD, MTOPRA, RAC

OBJECTIVES

❑ Understand EU legislation on food supplements and related national legislation

❑ Understand the requirements for food supplement labelling

❑ Learn what types of health claims may be made about food supplements

❑ Learn general safety and notification requirements relating to food supplements

❑ Learn about the *Foods for Special Medical Purposes (FSMP) Regulation*

REGULATIONS AND GUIDELINES COVERED IN THIS CHAPTER

❑ Directive 2002/46/EC of the European Parliament and of the Council of 10 June 2002 on the approximation of the laws of the Member States relating to food supplements[1]

❑ Regulation (EC) No 178/2002 of the European Parliament and of the Council of 28 January 2002 laying down the general principles and requirements of food law, establishing the European Food Safety Authority and laying down procedures in matters of food safety[2]

❑ Directive 2000/13/EC of the European Parliament and of the Council of 20 March 2000 on the approximation of the laws of the Member States relating to the labelling, presentation and advertising of foodstuffs[3]

❑ Council Directive 90/496/EEC of 24 September 1990 on nutrition labelling for foodstuffs[4]

❑ Commission Directive 2008/100/EC of 28 October 2008 amending Council Directive 90/496/EEC on nutrition labelling for foodstuffs as regards recommended daily allowances, energy conversion factors and definitions[5]

❑ Directive 2001/83/EC of the European Parliament and of the Council of 6 November 2001 on the Community code relating to medicinal products for human use, as amended by Directive 2004/24/EC and Directive 2004/27/EC[6,7,8]

❑ Regulation (EC) No 1924/2006 of the European Parliament and of the Council of 20 December 2006 on nutrition and health claims made on foods[9]

❑ Regulation (EC) No 1925/2006 of the European Parliament and of the Council of 20 December 2006 on the addition of vitamins and minerals and of certain other substances to foods[10]

❑ Regulation (EC) No 258/97 of the European Parliament and of the Council of 27 January 1997 concerning novel foods and novel food ingredients[11]

❑ Commission Directive 1999/21/EC of 25 March 1999 on dietary foods for special medical purposes[12]

❑ Directive 2009/39/EC of the European Parliament and of the Council of 6 May 2009 on foodstuffs intended for particular nutritional uses (recast)[13]

Introduction

Healthy development and life maintenance of human beings depends on several parameters: sufficient sleep and exercise, exposition to sunlight and prevention of environmental impact and distress. While an adequate and varied diet is the prominent factor for the intake of nutrients and other substances, the broad spectrum of these other parameters might affect the nutritional balance and lead to a lack of vitamins or minerals.

In fact, scientific data show that not all EU population groups are meeting these guidelines. Some consumers, due to their lifestyles or for other reasons, therefore choose to supplement their intake of dietary nutrients or other beneficial substances by using food supplements.

The increased marketing of food supplements in the EU has led Member States to develop national rules that have interfered with the free movement of goods, thus creating unequal competition and barriers to trade. As a result, the European Commission undertook a harmonisation exercise that resulted in the *Food Supplements Directive* (*FSD*) (Directive 2002/46/EC). Harmonisation of rules for all substances used in food supplements, including such essential nutrients as vitamins, minerals, amino acids and essential fatty acids, fibres, other substances with a nutritional or physiological effect (e.g., glucosamine, coenzyme Q10, various carotenoids, etc.) and various plant and herbal extracts is a huge endeavour. For practical reasons, it was decided as a first step to harmonise vitamins and minerals and to conduct a study on the need or usefulness of harmonising other substances at a later time. The *FSD* has been updated four times, most recently in 2011, to align the legal framework with current developments in the markets.

Purpose of the *Food Supplements Directive*

The *FSD* lays down specific rules for vitamins and minerals that are used as food supplement ingredients. The directive aims to harmonise Member States' national legislation based on the following elements:
- establish the category name of food supplements (previously also called diet integrators, dietary supplements, etc.) and give a precise definition, regulating them under food law
- establish positive lists of vitamins and minerals and their chemical forms that may be used in food supplements
- determine derogation and amendment procedures for the aforementioned lists
- agree on appropriate standards for labelling, presentation and advertising
- introduce safeguards in the event of a risk to public health

Scope and Definition

Directive 2002/46/EC defines "food supplements" as "foodstuffs, the purpose of which is to supplement the normal diet and which are concentrated sources of nutrients or other substances with a nutritional or physiological effect, alone or in combination, marketed in dose form." (Article 2a).

"Dose form" means "forms such as capsules, pastilles, tablets, pills and other similar forms, sachets of powder, ampoules of liquids, drop dispensing bottles, and other similar forms of liquids and powders designed to be taken in measured small unit quantities." "Nutrients" means (as a first stage) only vitamins and minerals (Article 2b), as indicated in positive lists. Only the vitamins and minerals listed are allowed in food supplements.

The *FSD* also requires food supplements to be supplied to the final consumer in pre-packaged form. *FSD* Article 1, paragraph 2, does not apply to medicinal products, including traditional herbal medicinal products (Directives 2001/83/EC and 2004/24/EC).

Given national regulations and the overlap of the definitions, some products may fall into a grey area between food and drug regulations (e.g., products with botanicals such as ginseng). In line with European Court of Justice (ECJ) case law, in cases of doubt, if, when taking into account all its characteristics, a product may fall within the definition of a "medicinal product" and within the definition of a product covered by other Community legislation, medicinal product directives prevail.

To keep up with scientific and technological developments, it is important to have a mechanism to promptly revise the lists whenever necessary. Because such revisions are often highly technical and based on scientific risk assessment by the European Food Safety Authority (EFSA), to simplify and expedite the procedure, their development and adoption are entrusted to the European Commission without much involvement of the Council or European Parliament. This is called the "comitology procedure" (regulatory procedure with scrutiny), in which the Commission is assisted by the Standing Committee on the Food Chain and Animal Health (SCFCAH), composed of experts from the Member States.

The *FSD* does not contain specific provisions relating to substances other than vitamins and minerals with a nutritional or physiological effect used as food supplement ingredients (e.g., amino acids, essential fatty acids, fibre and various plants and herbal extracts such as ginseng). Until the *FSD* is amended further, national rules remain applicable subject to *European Treaty* Articles 32 and 34 on the free movement of goods and mutual recognition.[14] Basically, this means food supplements lawfully manufactured or marketed in one Member State also should be allowed to be marketed in all other Member States. In practice, this often is difficult to achieve, and the ECJ has successfully condemned many Member States for not applying mutual recognition.[15]

One current European Commission-level focus is harmonisation of botanical food supplements and ingredients, which still are subject to divergent, case-by-case assessments by Member States.[16] Defining the product's intended use and other characteristics is paramount to assessing applicable legislative requirements.[17] The applicable legal framework for individual products or ingredients depends on these criteria. The *General Food Law Regulation* (Regulation (EC) No 178/2002) (*GFLR*) or the *Medicinal and Traditional Herbal Medicinal Product Directives* (Directives 2001/83/EC and 2004/24/EC) (*THMPD*) may apply, as well as specific ECJ case law. In principle, the EU framework allows the coexistence of botanical food supplements and herbal medicinal products.

Quality Requirements

Substance purity criteria are not yet established in the *FSD*. It is anticipated that these will be adopted in accordance with the comitology procedure. In general, however, purity criteria specified by European Commission legislation for nutritional substances used in foodstuffs apply. If purity criteria are not specified by European Commission legislation, generally acceptable international purity criteria shall be applicable and national rules setting stricter purity criteria may be maintained.

Food Supplement Labelling

Information relating to food supplements' nutrient content is essential to allow consumers to make informed choices and use supplements properly and safely. As food supplements are legally considered foodstuffs, the requirements of the EU *Labelling Directive* (Directive 2000/13/EC) relating to foodstuffs' labelling, presentation and advertising are applicable.

However, given the specific nature of food supplements, the *Nutrition Labelling Directive* (Directive 90/496/EEC, amended through Directive 2008/100/EC) for foodstuffs does not apply. Indeed, food supplements' energy, protein, fat, carbohydrate and fibre content is usually negligible, and the products are consumed in relation to the daily amount specified on the label. Specific rules are therefore detailed in the *FSD*:

Table 32-1. Vitamins and Minerals That May Be Declared and Their Recommended Daily Allowances (RDAs)

Vitamin/Mineral	Amount (RDA)	Unit
Vitamin A	800	µg
Vitamin D	5	µg
Vitamin E	12	mg
Vitamin K	75	µg
Vitamin C	80	mg
Thiamin	1.1	mg
Riboflavin	1.4	mg
Niacin	16	mg
Vitamin B6	1.4	mg
Folic acid	200	µg
Vitamin B12	2.5	µg
Biotin	0.05	mg
Pantothenic acid	6	mg
Potassium	2000	mg
Chloride	800	mg
Calcium	800	mg
Phosphorus	700	mg
Magnesium	375	mg
Iron	14	mg
Zinc	10	mg
Copper	1	mg
Manganese	2	mg
Fluoride	3.5	mg
Selenium	55	µg
Chromium	40	µg
Molybdenum	50	µg
Iodine	150	µg

Source: Annex to Directive 2008/100/EC

"As a rule, 15 % of the recommended allowance specified in this Annex supplied by 100 g or 100 ml or per package if the package contains only a single portion should be taken into consideration in deciding what constitutes a significant amount."

- The sales denomination is "food supplement" (Article 6 paragraph 1).
- Specific labelling requirements (Article 6 paragraph 3) include the indication of:
  a. the nutrient or substance category that characterises the product or an indication of those nutrients' or substances' nature
  b. the portion of the product recommended for daily consumption
  c. a warning not to exceed the stated recommended daily dose

d. a statement that food supplements should not be used as a substitute for a varied diet
e. a statement that the products should be stored out of the reach of young children
- Food supplement labelling, presentation and advertising must not include any statement or implication that a balanced and varied diet cannot provide appropriate quantities of nutrients in general (Article 7).
- The amount of the nutrients or substances with a nutritional or physiological effect present in the product must be declared per portion of the product as recommended for daily consumption (Article 8).
- The vitamin and mineral information must be expressed as a percentage of the reference values mentioned in the annex to Directive 2008/100/EC per daily recommended amount (see **Table 32-1**).

Minimum and Maximum Amounts Based on Safety

The *FSD* does not yet specify minimum and maximum amounts of vitamins and minerals in food supplements. This work is currently underway. These levels will be established by the European Commission by the comitology procedure, but it is proving to be a difficult exercise given the Member States' diverging approaches.

The *FSD*, however already specifies the principles that should be observed for setting maximum levels: the maximum amounts of vitamins and minerals present in food supplements per daily portion of consumption, as recommended by the manufacturer, shall be set based on the following:
- upper safe levels of vitamins and minerals established by scientific risk assessment based on generally accepted scientific data, taking into account, as appropriate, the varying degrees of sensitivity of different consumer groups
- intake of vitamins and minerals from other dietary sources

In addition, when the maximum levels are set, "due account" should also be taken of reference intakes of vitamins and minerals for the population.

Safeguard Measures (Public Health)

As with most European Commission regulations, the *FSD* leaves room for national measures in case new information shows that a product may endanger human health (Article 12). Even when a product complies with the directive, a Member State may then temporarily restrict the provisions' application within its territory. The Member State should immediately inform other Member States and the European Commission, providing justification. If justified, an amendment to the directive will be considered by the comitology procedure, where relevant, after EFSA renders an opinion. The Member State that has adopted the safeguard measure may, in that event, retain it until the amendment has been adopted.

Notification

To facilitate efficient monitoring of food supplements, the *FSD* also allows Member States to require manufacturers or distributors to notify Competent Authorities when food supplements are placed on the market by submitting a copy of the product label (Article 10). Most Member States have exercised this option. In some cases, Competent Authorities request additional information.

Safety Assessment of Food Supplement Ingredients

In general, food supplement substances and ingredients not used in the EU before 15 May 1997 are subject to the *Novel Foods Regulation* (*NFR*) (Regulation (EC) No 258/97). The *NFR* foresees explicit European Commission premarketing approval after the assessment of an application (submitted by an interested party) by EFSA. This approval procedure can take two to three years.

For other ingredients, the *FSD* does not include a standard safety assessment requirement. The products and production processes should be in conformity with GFLR safety requirements. However, the *Addition of Vitamins and Minerals and of Certain Other Substances to Food Regulation* (*ADMOSFR*) (Regulation (EC) No 1925/2006), which came into force 1 July 2007, covers safety assessment of other substances to some extent. Chapter III anticipates an EFSA risk assessment procedure for substances other than vitamins or minerals added to foods or used in their manufacture, resulting in the ingestion of these substances in amounts far greater than reasonably expected under normal consumption of a balanced and varied diet and/or otherwise representing a potential risk to consumers. This may also apply to ingredients used in food supplements.

Based on the EFSA opinion, the substance is then included in one of three lists:
- List A—Addition to foods or use in the manufacture of foods is prohibited.
- List B—Addition to foods or use in the manufacture of foods is allowed only under the conditions specified.
- List C—If the possibility of harmful effects on health is identified but scientific uncertainty persists, it is up to interested parties to submit a file to EFSA containing scientific data demonstrating safety for evaluation. Within four years, a decision will be made via comitology, taking into account EFSA's

opinion to generally allow the use of the substance or include it on list A or B.

To bring improvements on a number of important issues such as nanomaterials definition and labelling, a centralised and quicker authorisation procedure for novel foods and specific measures for traditional foods from third countries, a proposal for the revision of *Novel Food Regulation* (Regulation (EC) No 258/97) is being discussed and is under assessment by the European bodies. Details are available on the European Commission website.

Health Claims

The *FSD* gives no specific rules for health claims on food supplements. It only specifies that food supplement labelling, presentation and advertising must not attribute to the product the property of preventing, treating or curing a human disease or refer to such properties (Article 6, paragraph 2; Article 2).

As of 1 July 2007, Nutrition and Health Claims have been covered by the *Nutrition and Health Claims Regulation* (*NHCR*) (Regulation (EC) No 1924/2006).

The primary goal of this regulation is to ensure adequate and appropriate labelling to protect and inform consumers. It harmonises the many differences that existed between national legislative provisions relating to claims and their conditions of use that impede the free movement of goods. By involving EFSA, uniform review and approval procedures are included for the different types of claims, based on adequate scientific substantiation.

The *NHCR* covers all foods, including food supplements, where no specific provisions relating to claims have been described in the relevant regulatory texts. It covers not only labelling but also all commercial communications, including claims in advertising, in publicity and on websites. The four main types of claims for which specific procedures are in place are:

- Nutrition Claims (NCs)—These claims state, suggest or imply that a food has particular beneficial nutritional properties due to its energy content or level of nutrients or other substances it does or does not contain or contains in reduced or increased proportions. The only permissible NCs are those listed in the *NHCR* annex.
- Health Claims (HCs)—These claims state, suggest or imply that a relationship exists between a food category, a food or one of its constituents and health. There are HC provisions based on generally accepted scientific evidence and well understood by the average consumer that will, in future, only be allowed when they are included in a positive list (Article 13). HCs based on newly developed scientific evidence and/or including a request for the protection of proprietary data will only be allowed after a decision by the European Commission following the submission of a dossier and an EFSA opinion (Articles 13.5 and 18).
- Reduction of Disease Risk Claims (RDRCs)—These are any health claims that state, suggest or imply that the consumption of a food category, a food or one of its constituents significantly reduces a risk factor in the development of a human disease. RDRCs will be permissible if specifically allowed by the European Commission by comitology after the submission of a dossier and an EFSA opinion (Articles 14, 15, 16, 17 and 19).
- Claims referring to Children's Development and Health (CDHCs)—These claims will have to follow the same procedure as RDRCs.

Health claims that make reference to general, nonspecific benefits of the nutrient or food for overall good health or health-related well-being may only be made if they are accompanied by a specific, approved health claim.

The *NHCR* foresees many transition periods. In practice, due to thousands of claims submissions received,[18] the original date of January 2010 for an EFSA review has been delayed at least until January 2013. At the time this chapter was updated, several HCs had received positive opinions by EFSA (mostly vitamins and minerals), although a majority had received negative reviews (mainly probiotics, fatty acids and botanical substances), often justified by EFSA for insufficient characterisation, lack of demonstrating a beneficial health effect in a given target population or lack of demonstrating a cause-effect relationship by randomised controlled trials (RCTs). For instance, EFSA did not consider "antioxidant activity" a beneficial physiological effect. NCs not included in the annex and HCs not included in the Article 13 list will be prohibited.

Borderline Issues: Foods and Medicinal Products

The definitions of "food," "health claim" and "medicinal product" are complex and legally difficult and seem to overlap. Therefore, it is little wonder that the dispute concerning so-called "borderline products," in particular the dividing line between medicinal products and food supplements, has been a central point of ECJ proceedings for years.

Medicinal products, in accordance with the *Medicinal Product Directive* (*MPD*) (Directive 2001/83/EC), are excluded from the field of food law. Since no similar exclusion of food is included in the medicinal product definition specified in the *MPD*, the *MPD* provisions overrule those of the *GFLD* in case of challenge. How such assessment is performed is further specified in *MPD* Article 2.2, which states that the *MPD*'s provisions shall apply only in cases of doubt, i.e., taking into account all its characteristics, when a product falls within both the definition of a medicinal product and the definition of a product covered by other Community legislation.

Article 1.2.1 defines "medicinal product" in two ways:
- by virtue of its presentation—any substance or combination of substances presented as having properties for treating or preventing disease in human beings
- by virtue of its function—any substance or combination of substances that may be used in or administered to human beings either with a view to restoring, correcting or modifying physiological functions by exerting a pharmacological, immunological or metabolic action or to making a medical diagnosis

According to this definition, a product can be classified as a medicinal product either because it is presented for the prevention or therapy of a disease or because it has inherent therapeutic or diagnostic functions. However, this is not absolute because—if taken literally—many components contained in foods could be considered medicinal based on this definition. That this should not be the case stems from a number of legal arguments:
- *MPD* Article 2.2 gives conditions for the superiority of medicinal law to be applied (only to individual products, in cases of doubt, while taking into consideration all the product's characteristics).
- Directive 2004/27/EC "whereas" 7 states that, "Where a product comes clearly under the definition of other product categories, in particular food, food supplements, medical devices, biocides or cosmetics," the *MPD* should not apply.
- "Whereas" 12 of the *Traditional Herbal Medicinal Product Directive* (*THMPD*) (Directive 2004/24/EC) states that it "allows non-medicinal herbal products, fulfilling the criteria of food legislation, to be regulated under food legislation in the Community."
- The *FSD* defines food supplements as concentrated sources of nutrients or other substances with a nutritional or physiological effect, and acknowledges in "whereas" 6 that, "There is a wide range of nutrients and other ingredients that might be present in food supplements including, but not limited to, vitamins, minerals, amino acids, essential fatty acids, fibre, and various plants and herbal extracts."
- The *NHCR* explicitly covers "other substances," which are defined as substances other than nutrients that have nutritional or physiological effects.

The most explicit support for the fact that there is a limit to the superiority of medicinal law when applied to individual products comes from numerous ECJ judgements. In the judgement on "the garlic case" (Case 319/05), where the European Commission brought charges against the Federal Republic of Germany for classifying a garlic preparation in capsule form as a medicinal product although it did not satisfy the statutory definition, the ECJ spelled out once again the basic rules for distinguishing between a product's medicinal and food status.[19]

- Case-by-case approach—The ECJ has consistently held that it is up to the national authorities to determine on a case-by-case basis whether a product falls within the definition of a medicinal product, taking into account all the product's characteristics, particularly its composition; its pharmacological properties, to the extent to which they can be established in the present state of scientific knowledge; the manner in which it is used; the extent of its distribution; its familiarity to consumers; and the risks its use may entail.
- Therapeutic effect—The ECJ holds that the definition of "by virtue of its function" is broad enough to include products that, although capable of having an effect on bodily functions, have in fact another purpose. However, that criterion must not lead to classification as medicinal products by function of substances that, while having an effect on the human body, do not significantly affect metabolism and thus do not strictly modify the way in which it functions. The definition of medicinal product by function is designed to cover products whose pharmacological properties have been scientifically observed and are genuinely designed to make a medical diagnosis or to restore, correct or modify physiological functions. A physiological effect is not specific to medicinal products but is also among the criteria used for the definition of food supplements. Therefore, for a product to fall within medicinal law, it is not sufficient that it possess properties beneficial to health in general; it must, strictly speaking, have the function of treating or preventing disease. The fact that many products generally recognised as foodstuffs may also serve therapeutic purposes is not sufficient to confer on them the status of medicinal product.

This illustrates clearly that the EU legal framework intends that food supplements and medicinal products co-exist, each category in conformity with the rules of its legal framework.

Foods for Special Medical Purposes

Dietary foods for Special Medical Purposes (FSMPs), often also referred to as Medical Foods, are an important resource that healthcare professionals use to help ensure patients receive the nutrients they need. FSMPs can be either the only source of nourishment or part of the diet for acute or chronic conditions, sometimes for the rest of a patient's life. They are used under medical supervision and in quantities recommended by healthcare professionals, forming an integral part of patient management. Relevant usages of FSMPs include disease-related conditions (stroke, cancer, malnutrition, etc.), infants suffering from severe cow's milk allergy and patients with rare inborn metabolic disorders.

FSMPs are regulated by Directive 1999/21/EC covering product composition and labelling. They must comply with all other relevant food legislation including food hygiene, food safety and additives. The *Parnuts Directive* (Directive 2009/39/EC), which lists FSMPs as one of its categories, includes some further key provisions for FSMPs, such as communication to HCPs.

Enterals Versus Parenterals

FSMPs are for enteral usage (including oral nutritional supplementation) and regulated as foods. FSMPs should not be confused with parenteral nutrition (infusion of nutrients directly in the blood circulation), which is regulated under drug law.

FSMPs are consumed across all healthcare settings such as hospitals, clinics and nursing homes and at home. They have been shown to result in lower healthcare costs by reducing hospital stays and maintaining patients independently longer. In most EU Member States, many products notified or registered as FSMPs are reimbursable as part of local healthcare systems.

Summary

- In spite of current harmonisation, food supplements are still subject to largely divergent country-by-country legislation.
- The *FSD* provides, for the first time, a common EU food supplement definition. However, it currently covers only certain aspects of vitamins and minerals across the EU and, for those, minimum and maximum amounts still have to be agreed.
- Nutrition and health claims are now regulated by the *NHCR*, which provides for premarketing approval of all claims.
- Food supplements need to be in conformity with the general food safety requirements laid down in the *GFLR* and *NFR*.
- The *MPD* may overrule a given product's food status, but only in cases where there is doubt about the applicable framework and when all of the product's characteristics are considered. ECJ court rulings confirm this should essentially be a product-by-product assessment, and the fact that the product may exhibit effects beneficial to health is not in itself sufficient to classify the product as medicinal.
- FSMPs follow food law and can be either the only source of nourishment or part of the diet of patients. They are used under medical supervision and in quantities recommended by healthcare professionals.

References

1. Directive 2002/46/EC of the European Parliament and of the Council of 10 June 2002 on the approximation of the laws of the Member States relating to food supplements. EUR-Lex website. http://eur-lex.europa.eu/LexUriServ/LexUriServ.do?uri=OJ:L:2002:183:0051:0057:EN:PDF. Accessed 31 May 2012.
2. Regulation (EC) No 178/2002 of the European Parliament and of the Council of 28 January 2002 laying down the general principles and requirements of food law, establishing the European Food Safety Authority and laying down procedures in matters of food safety. EUR-Lex website. http://eur-lex.europa.eu/LexUriServ/LexUriServ.do?uri=OJ:L:2002:031:0001:0024:EN:PDF. Accessed 31 May 2012.
3. Directive 2000/13/EC of the European Parliament and of the Council of 20 March 2000 on the approximation of the laws of the Member States relating to the labelling, presentation and advertising of foodstuffs. EUR-Lex website. http://eur-lex.europa.eu/LexUriServ/LexUriServ.do?uri=OJ:L:2000:109:0029:0042:EN:PDF. Accessed 31 May 2012.
4. Council Directive 90/496/EEC of 24 September 1990 on Nutrition labelling for foodstuffs. EUR-Lex website. http://eur-lex.europa.eu/LexUriServ/LexUriServ.do?uri=CELEX:31990L0496:EN:HTML. Accessed 31 May 2012.
5. Commission Directive 2008/100/EC of 28 October 2008 amending Council Directive 90/496/EEC on nutrition labelling for foodstuffs as regards recommended daily allowances, energy conversion factors and definitions. EUR-Lex website. http://eur-lex.europa.eu/LexUriServ/LexUriServ.do?uri=OJ:L:2008:285:0009:0012:EN:PDF. Accessed 31 May 2012.
6. Directive 2001/83/EC of the European Parliament and of the Council of 6 November 2001 on the Community code relating to medicinal products for human use. EUR-Lex website. http://eur-lex.europa.eu/LexUriServ/LexUriServ.do?uri=OJ:L:2001:311:0067:0128:en:PDF. Accessed 31 May 2012.
7. Directive 2004/27/EC of the European Parliament and of the Council of 31 March 2004 amending Directive 2001/83/EC on the Community code relating to medicinal products for human use. EUR-Lex website. http://eur-lex.europa.eu/Notice.do?val=343604:cs&pos=1&page=1&lang=en&pgs=10&nbl=1&list=343604:cs,&hwords=&action=GO&visu=%23texte. Accessed 31 May 2012.
8. Directive 2004/24/EC of the European Parliament and of the Council of 31 March 2004 amending, as regards traditional herbal medicinal products, Directive 2001/83/EC on the Community code relating to medicinal products for human use. EUR-Lex website. http://eur-lex.europa.eu/LexUriServ/LexUriServ.do?uri=OJ:L:2004:136:0085:0090:en:PDF. 31 May 2012.
9. Corrigendum to Regulation (EC) No 1924/2006 of the European Parliament and of the Council of 20 December 2006 on nutrition and health claims made on foods. EUR-Lex website. http://eur-lex.europa.eu/LexUriServ/LexUriServ.do?uri=OJ:L:2007:012:0003:0018:EN:PDF. Accessed 31 May 2012.
10. Regulation (EC) No 1925/2006 of the European Parliament and of the Council of 20 December 2006 on the addition of vitamins and minerals and of certain other substances to foods. EUR-Lex website. http://eur-lex.europa.eu/LexUriServ/LexUriServ.do?uri=OJ:L:2006:404:0026:0038:EN:PDF. Accessed 31 May 2012.
11. Regulation (EC) No 258/97 of the European Parliament and of the Council of 27 January 1997 concerning novel foods and novel food ingredients. EUR-Lex website. http://eur-lex.europa.eu/smartapi/cgi/sga_doc?smartapi!celexapi!prod!CELEXnumdoc&lg=EN&numdoc=31997R0258&model=guichett. Accessed 31 May 2012.

12. Commission Directive 1999/21/EC of 25 March 1999 on dietary foods for special medical purposes. EUR-Lex website. http://eur-lex.europa.eu/LexUriServ/LexUriServ.do?uri=CONSLEG:1999L0021:20070119:EN:PDF. Accessed 31 May 2012.
13. Directive 2009/39/EC of the European Parliament and of the Council of 6 May 2009 on foodstuffs intended for particular nutritional uses (recast). EUR-Lex website. http://eur-lex.europa.eu/LexUriServ/LexUriServ.do?uri=OJ:L:2009:124:0021:0029:EN:PDF. Accessed 31 May 2012.
14. Consolidated version of the treaty on the functioning of the European Union. EUR-Lex website. http://eur-lex.europa.eu/LexUriServ/LexUriServ.do?uri=OJ.C.2010.003.0017.0200.en.PDF. Accessed 31 May 2012.
15. European Court of Justice. Case 387/99 (*Commission vs. Germany*); Case 24/00 (*Commission vs. France*); Case 150/00 (*Commission vs. Austria*); Case 192/01 (*Commission vs. Denmark*); Case 41/02 (*Commission vs. The Netherlands*).
16. European Advisory Services (2008). Marketing Food Supplements, Fortified and Functional Foods in Europe. Report. Fifth edition. ISBN 9789080699533. www.eas.eu.
17. Coppens P, Delmulle L, Gulati O, Richardson D, Ruthsatz M, Sievers S and Sidani S. "Use of Botanicals in Food Supplements. Regulatory Scope, Scientific Risk Assessment and Claim Substantiation." *Ann NutrMetab*. 2006; 50:538–554.
18. European Food Safety Authority. Register of Questions. European Food Safety Authority website. http://registerofquestions.efsa.europa.eu/roqFrontend/questionsListLoader/panel/NDA/btnSearch/1/ Accessed 6 April 2012.
19. European Court of Justice. Case 319/05 (*Commission vs. Germany*).

Chapter 33

Veterinary Medicinal Products

By Rick Clayton, DipM, MTOPRA

OBJECTIVES

- Gain a basic understanding of the types of veterinary products considered to be medicines in the EU

- Identify the main differences between the registration of human and veterinary medicinal products in the EU

- Gain an understanding of the legislation covering the registration of veterinary medicinal products in the EU

- Identify the relevant legal texts and guidelines relating to EU registration for veterinary medicinal products

- Understand the types of procedures that may be used to obtain Marketing Authorisations for veterinary medicinal products in the EU

- Understand the procedures required to maintain and extend Marketing Authorisations in the EU—Renewals and Variations

- Gain a basic understanding of associated issues: Maximum Residue Limits, pharmacovigilance, the cascade and Good Manufacturing Practice

SOURCES OF DIRECTIVE, REGULATIONS AND GUIDELINES COVERED IN THIS CHAPTER

The legislation covered in this chapter is listed in **Table 33-1**. The sources of this legislation and of the guidelines covered in this chapter are listed below (and described more fully later in the chapter).

The legislation governing medicinal products is published by the European Commission on the DG Health & Consumers Eudralex webpage (http://ec.europa.ue/health/documents/eudralex/index_en.htm) in a series of volumes of The Rules Governing Medicinal Products in the European Union. The legislation relevant to veterinary medicinal products is compiled in Volume 5. Any new legislation also will be published on this website.

The guidelines covered by this chapter are published on several websites:

1. The Eudralex webpage (above) also contains Volumes 4 to 9 of The Rules Governing Medicinal Products in the European Union, containing guidelines relevant to veterinary medicinal products.
2. Other scientific guidelines, and guidelines relevant to the Centralised Procedure, are published on the European Medicines Agency's veterinary sector webpages (www.ema.europa.eu).
4. Guidelines relevant to the Decentralised and Mutual Recognition Procedures are published on the Heads of Medicines Agencies website, in the CMDv section (www.ham.eu/cmdv.html).

Chapter 33

Introduction

Role of Veterinary Medicinal Products in 21st Century Europe

Within the last century, the availability of safe and effective medicines for human use has transformed human life expectancy and quality of life. It is impossible to imagine an existence without the benefits of vaccines or antimicrobials or access to a range of highly specialised surgical procedures and treatments specifically targeting diseases that were once incurable.

The development of veterinary medicines has had a similar impact on animal health. It has improved quality of life and life expectancy for companion animals, e.g., by preventing serious diseases such as canine distemper and feline leukaemia, and controlling a host of parasitic diseases. It also has brought considerable improvements to public health and the control of zoonotic disease, such as avian flu, rabies and bovine brucellosis. It has supported the drive toward greater agricultural efficiency in the livestock sector and prevented serious economic loss from devastating diseases (e.g., Aujezkey disease in pigs, foot-and-mouth and bluetongue in ruminants). Veterinary medicines and vaccines prevent the spread of disease in modern meat and dairy product production, without which the European livestock industry could not compete in global markets. Consumers also benefit—healthy animals mean safer food, and efficient production means more-affordable food.

However, in the future, veterinary medicines must continue to be used prudently and should always be an adjunct to, not a replacement for, good livestock management practices.

Differences Between the Animal Health and Human Health Markets

There are significant differences between the animal health and human health markets.

- Animal health sales in the EU are, by value, only a fraction (3–5%) of the human pharmaceutical market. The veterinary market is divided into many animal species and separated by geographic differences. The importance of certain species to specific communities and differences in disease prevalence across EU Member States lead to further fragmentation of the market.
- The animal health sector has no price reimbursement or national healthcare scheme; the entire cost of treatment must be borne by the animal's owner. While this may not be a problem for pet owners with recourse to insurance, livestock treatment is primarily driven by economics, as each animal has a distinct and limited monetary value.
- In the animal health market, the "patient" may end up in the human food chain. Consumers of animal products must be protected from contact with potentially harmful drug residues.
- The veterinary medicinal product user—defined as any person who may come into contact with: the product; the product components before, during or after administration to the animal; and/or animals immediately after treatment—must be safeguarded from any possible harmful effects of the product.
- The environment also must be protected; consequently, every veterinary medicine must undergo an environmental risk assessment as part of the registration procedure. However, the potential for adverse environmental effects must be balanced against the product's potential benefits. The enhancement of livestock productivity can be associated with a decrease in livestock numbers and a concomitant reduction in quantities of feed consumed and waste produced, thereby reducing the overall pressure on the environment.

Due to the veterinary sector's unique operating environment, the European animal health market is highly sensitive to any factors impacting cost. Therefore, considerable importance is attached to ensuring that legislation is appropriate and proportionate. The continuous tightening of registration requirements during the last two decades has led to a marked decline in the availability of veterinary medicinal products in the marketplace. This has become particularly acute for the *equidae* and animals classed as a "minor" species. Under the European Commission's "Better Regulation" initiative, a review of the legislation governing veterinary medicinal products began in 2010 with a view to simplification, reduction in administrative burdens and stimulating innovation. Revised legislation is expected in 2014–15.[1,2]

Definitions of Veterinary Medicinal Products in the EU

Veterinary Medicinal Products

The definition of a "veterinary medicinal product" is given in Article 1 of Directive 2001/82/EC,[3] as amended by Directive 2004/28/EC[4] and Directive 2009/9/EC,[5] on the Community code relating to medicinal products for veterinary use. It encompasses any substance or combination of substances administered to animals for the following purposes:

- treating disease in animals
- preventing disease in animals
- making a medical diagnosis
- restoring, correcting or modifying physiological functions in animals by exerting a pharmacological, immunological or metabolic action

Table 33-1. Legislative Framework for Registration of Veterinary Medicinal Products Within the EEA

Legal Text	Description	Notes
The Community Code Directive 2001/82/EC on the Community code relating to veterinary medicinal products, as amended by Directive 2004/28/EC, Directive 2009/9/EC and Directive 2009/53/EC	Harmonised procedures and requirements for MAs including mutual recognition among Member States, manufacture, import, labelling, possession, distribution, market surveillance and supervision for veterinary medicinal products; covers: • pharmaceutical products • immunological products • homeopathic products	**Supersedes**: Council Directive 81/851/EEC as amended by Council Directives 90/676/EEC, 90/677/EEC, 92/74/EEC, 93/40/EEC and 2000/37/EEC
Annex containing the data requirements Commission Directive 2009/9/EC	Describes the tests required to meet quality, safety and efficacy requirements	**Supersedes**: Annex to Directive 81/851/EC **Amending**: Directive 2001/82/EC
EMA Regulation Regulation (EC) No 726/2004	Community procedures for the centralised authorisation and supervision of human and veterinary medicinal products and establishing the European Medicines Agency (EMA)	**Supersedes**: Council Regulation (EC) No 2309/93
MRL Regulations Regulation (EC) No 470/2009	Community procedures for the establishment of residue limits of pharmacologically active substances in foodstuffs of animal origin	**Supersedes**: Regulation (EC) No 2377/90 **Amending**: Directive 2001/82/EC and Regulation (EC) No 726/2004
Commission Regulation (EC) No 37/2010	Pharmacologically active substances and their classification regarding maximum residue limits in foodstuffs of animal origin	Alphabetical listing of all substances registered as pharmacologically active and information on their MRL status
Variations Regulations Commission Regulation (EC) No 1234/2008	Procedures for variations to national and centralised MAs	**Supersedes**: Commission Regulations (EC) No 1084/2003 and No 1085/2003
Directive 2009/53/EC	Amends Directive 2001/82/EC by including an article mandating the Commission to adopt an implementing regulation on variations to the terms of MAs	**Amending**: Directive 2001/82/EC
Good Manufacturing Practice Commission Directive 91/412/EC	Principles and guideline for Good Manufacturing Practice for veterinary medicinal products	Annexes regularly updated
Pharmacovigilance Commission Regulation EC No 540/95 Directive 2001/82/EC as amended	Arrangements for reporting suspected unexpected adverse reactions in accordance with the provisions of Regulation (EC) No 726/2004 and Directive 2001/82/EC	
Genetically modified organisms Council Directive 90/219/EEC as amended	The contained use of genetically modified micro-organisms (GMOs)	Amended by Directive 98/81/EC
Directive 2001/18/EC	The deliberate release into the environment of GMOs	**Repealing**: Council Directive 90/220/EEC
Transfers Commission Regulation (EC) No 2141/96	Transfer of a MA for a medicinal product falling within the scope of Regulation (EC) No 726/2004	
Decision making Commission Regulation (EC) No 1662/95 and Regulation (EC) No 219/2009	Detailed arrangements for implementing the Community decision-making procedures in respect of MAs for products for human or veterinary use	
Sanctions Commission Regulation (EC) No 658/2007	Financial penalties for infringement of certain obligations in connection with MAs	
Miscellaneous Commission Regulation (EC) No 1950/2006	Establishing a list of substances essential for the treatment of *equidae*	
Commission Directive 2006/130/EC	Establishment of criteria for exempting certain veterinary medicinal products for food-producing animals from the requirement of a veterinary prescription	
Council Directive 78/25/EEC	Colouring matters which may be added to medicinal products	

N.B. Unless otherwise stated, all Directives and Regulations are "of the European Parliament and the Council".

This definition covers therapeutics, immunologicals (vaccines, antigens), biological substances (blood products, microorganisms, toxins), products indicated for reproductive management (oestrus synchronisation), premixes used to prepare medicated feed (see below) and certain dietary supplements.

A product may also be defined as a veterinary medicinal product if it is judged to be "medicinal." Some substances sit on the "borderline" of this definition (see Borderline Substances below), but as a rule, a product may be considered medicinal:

- by presentation (i.e., if therapeutic claims are made on the label)
- by function (i.e., if the product contains active substances above a certain level, even if no therapeutic claim is made for substances with pharmacological activity).

Borderline Substances

There is a range of animal treatment products defined as "borderline" substances, where the pattern of use or label claims will determine whether registration under veterinary medicines legislation is required. The following borderline substances are generally considered to be medicinal within the EU:

- Vitamin and mineral supplements, which by their recommended rate of use cause an overall level of any vitamin or mineral administered to an animal to exceed what is generally considered to be the normal dietary requirement, are medicinal by function.
- Insecticides applied to animals, whether as sprays, spot-on products, shampoos or collars[6] are medicinal by function.
- Non-insecticidal shampoos may be considered medicinal by presentation if reference to skin conditions such as seborrhoea and dermatitis are made.
- Teat dips applied after milking used as aids for the prevention of mastitis are considered to be medicinal by presentation by a number of EU Member States, e.g., the UK, Netherlands, Ireland and Norway.
- Products containing more than 0.3% iodine or chlorhexidine gluconate and applied to teats and udders may be considered medicinal by function in some Members States; other Member States regard these products as disinfectants, provided no therapeutic claim is made.[7]
- Antiseptic products that claim to treat or prevent disease are regarded as medicinal by presentation.
- Herbal products are considered to be medicinal if claims are made or if the active substance derived from plants has undergone processing to concentrate particular components (most herbal products containing dried or unrefined parts of plants are not medicinal).
- Colostrum products are considered medicinal when they are administered to provide passive immunity.[8]

Insect repellents without any demonstrable insecticidal activity, such as diethyltoluamide (DEET) or ethylhexanediol, are not regarded as medicinal provided the claim is only to repel insects. However, these products are classified as biocides and, as such, require registration under the *Biocidal Products Directive* (Directive 98/8/EC).[9] Similarly, a disinfectant product that makes no claims to treat or prevent disease is not considered medicinal but requires registration as a biocide.

Each EU Member State interprets the medicinal product definition slightly differently, and each has its own list of borderline substances and its own National Procedures for the registration of such products. Sponsors should always confirm the status of individual products with the relevant national Competent Authorities.

Premixes, Feed Additives and Medicated Feed

A premix used to prepare medicated feed is considered a medicinal product and falls within the scope of Directive 2001/82/EC. However, medicated feed and feed additives are covered by the following separate pieces of European legislation (and will not be covered later in this chapter except under the section 'Manufacturing and Product Control Requirements'):

- Council Directive 90/167/EC of 26 March 1990 laying down conditions governing the preparation, placing on the market and use of medicated feedstuffs in the Community—This directive is currently under review, and revised legislation is expected in 2014-15.
- Regulation (EC) No 1831/2003 of the European Parliament and of the Council of 22 September 2003 on additives for use in animal nutrition—This regulation is implemented with the following supplementary legislation:
  - Commission Regulation (EC) No 429/2008 of 25 April 2008 on detailed rules for the implementation of Regulation (EC) No 1831/2003 of the European Parliament and of the Council as regards the preparation and the presentation of applications and the assessment and the authorisation of feed additives
  - Commission Regulation (EC) No 124/2009 of 10 February 2009 setting maximum levels for the presence of coccidiostats or histomonostats in food resulting from the unavoidable carry-over of these substances in non-target feed

o Commission Directive 2009/8/EC of 10 February 2009 amending Annex I to Directive 2002/32/EC of the European Parliament and of the Council as regards maximum levels of unavoidable carry-over of coccidiostats or histomonostats in non-target feed.

This regulation is to be revised; new legislation is expected in 2014–15.

Key Sources of Legislation and Guidance

The Rules Governing Medicinal Products in the European Union

Pharmaceutical legislation and guidance on the interpretation and fulfilment of regulatory requirements are published by the European Commission in a series of 10 volumes, entitled, *The Rules Governing Medicinal Products in the European Union*. Volumes 5–8 deal exclusively with veterinary legislation and guidance; the information presented in *Volumes 4* and *9* concerns both veterinary and human products:

- *Volume 4*: Guideline for Good Manufacturing Practices for Medicinal Products for Human and Veterinary Use
- *Volume 5*: EU Pharmaceutical Legislation for Medicinal Products for Veterinary Use
- *Volume 6*: Notice to Applicants and Regulatory Guidelines for Medicinal Products for Veterinary Use
    o *Volume 6A*: Procedures for Marketing Authorisations
    o *Volume 6B*: Presentation and Content of the Dossier
    o *Volume 6C*: Regulatory Guidelines
    o *Volume 6*: Electronic Submission
- *Volume 7*: Scientific Guidelines for Medicinal Products for Veterinary Use
    o *Volume 7A*: General, Efficacy, Environmental Risk Assessment
    o *Volume 7B*: Immunologicals, Quality
- *Volume 8*: Maximum Residue Limits
- *Volume 9*: Pharmacovigilance Guidelines (Medicinal Products for Human and Veterinary Use)

These volumes are updated regularly; *Volume 6*, in particular, is subject to frequent revision and amendment. *The Rules Governing Medicinal Products in the European Union* can be found on the European Commission, DG Health & Consumers' Eudralex webpage.[10]

Guidelines from the Regulatory Bodies

There are two primary European regulatory bodies concerned with the authorisation of veterinary medicinal products in the EU: the European Medicines Agency (EMA) and the Coordination group for Mutual Recognition and Decentralised Procedures–veterinary (CMDv). These bodies are established by law, and their websites should be consulted for the latest guidelines and regulatory developments. In addition, the Heads of Veterinary Medicines Agencies group (HMA) was created by the national agencies as an informal high-level organisation to provide a forum for discussion of issues of mutual interest and to promote harmonisation and cooperation.

The EMA website[11] provides detailed scientific guidelines on specific aspects of quality, safety and efficacy studies as published by the Committee for Veterinary Medicinal Products (CVMP). EMA is also the body that provides guidance on the general procedures and regulatory issues for the Centralised Procedure for Marketing Authorisation Applications (MAAs). EMA publishes a list of new guidelines to be developed during a particular year; this can be found in the EMA Work Programme (published annually in January).

The HMAvet website[12] provides procedural guidelines developed by CMDv relevant to the Mutual Recognition and Decentralised Procedures. CMDv does not provide scientific advice or scientific guidelines.

Internationally Harmonised Guidelines

A number of veterinary guidelines (approximately 50 by 2012) have undergone international harmonisation through the International Cooperation on Harmonisation of Technical Requirements for Registration of Veterinary Medicinal Products (VICH).[13] VICH is a trilateral (EU, Japan, US) programme aimed at harmonising technical requirements for veterinary product registration. This process is also closely followed by Canada, Australia and New Zealand, which are official observers at VICH. Once adopted, these guidelines replace those in the VICH regions. In the EU, they are published on the EMA website as CVMP guidelines. The process is continual, with new guidelines undergoing initial harmonisation, and previously harmonised documents subject to revision and update. For more information visit the VICH website (http://www.vichsec.org/).

Legislative Framework

Regulations and Directives

The EU has two primary types of legislative acts: regulations and directives.

Following publication, a regulation becomes immediately enforceable in all Member States simultaneously as it does not have to be transposed into national law. Directives must be incorporated into the national law of each individual Member State; consequently, dates of implementation can differ from country to country, and the final text can differ providing the aims of the legislation are met (for example it can be supplemented with national rules).

Chapter 33

Legislative History

Since the veterinary directives[14, 15] were introduced in 1981, there has been a legal framework to harmonise procedures and requirements across the EU Member States. The directives have been amended and extended on a number of occasions. During the late 1990s, the 1981 directives and all the subsequent amendments were consolidated through a process called "codification"[16] into Directive 2001/82/EC, in order to improve the transparency of the veterinary medicines legislation. This also paved the way for a major review of the legislation in 2001–03, which resulted in Directive 2001/82/EC being amended further by Directives 2004/28/EC and 2009/9/EC.

In a move partly inspired by the need to establish a single EU biotechnology product assessment system, a regulation describing a centralised registration system was published in 1993.[17] The basic legal framework was completed in 1995, when procedures for examining variations to national and centralised marketing authorisations (MAs) were established.

The legislative framework is slowly harmonising the Member States' different registration systems and requirements. Member States have been actively encouraged to trust and accept the opinions of the Competent Authorities in other states. The 1981 directives introduced a "mutual recognition" procedure whereby a company could request Member States to recognise the MA granted by another Member State. The 2004 directive took this procedure a step further with the introduction of a "decentralised" procedure, whereby all the Member States involved in an MAA can contribute to the initial scientific assessment process. These procedures are described in more detail later.

The system has also evolved to include immunological and homeopathic products, and to lay down the principles of Good Manufacturing Practice (GMP).[18]

The current legal texts and ancillary legislation are listed in **Table 33-1**. The full texts of these documents are published in *Volume 5* of *The Rules Governing Medicinal Products in the European Union*. Provisions that extend the EEA to include Iceland, Liechtenstein and Norway with the EU Member States are outlined in the relevant sections of *Volume 5* and *Volume 6A*.

Revision and Update of the Legislation

The legislation harmonising EU registration procedures and requirements includes clauses that require the European Commission to review and publish a report on the functioning of the legislation within at least 10 years of its adoption. Since the mid-2000s, any proposal for significant legislation must be preceded by an impact assessment. This process can take two years. If necessary, the European Commission will publish proposals for new legislation. These proposals will then enter the European Parliament and European Council co-decision procedure, which can take a further one or two years.

The 2001–03 review resulted in the following key changes:
- increased EMA responsibilities and adapted EMA structures to an expanded EU
- improved Scientific Advice procedure
- strengthened the pharmacovigilance system
- improved Mutual Recognition Procedure for granting MAs
- introduction of the Decentralised Procedure for granting MAs
- shortened the European Commission decision-making procedure (Centralised Procedure)
- more focus on benefit:risk assessment in the scientific assessment process
- loss of data protection for extending products to additional species

A new review of the legislation governing veterinary medicinal products was initiated in 2010 (four years before the 10-year deadline). The main drivers behind this review are the need for simplification of the MA procedures, a reduction in administrative burdens for both regulatory authorities and companies, and to improve data protection to stimulate innovation.[19, 20] The main goal of these objectives is to increase the availability of authorised veterinary medicinal products in all EU Member States. Due to the length of the process, new legislation will not be adopted before late 2014 or 2015.

Registration Procedures

An MA granted by a Competent Authority is required before a veterinary medicinal product may be marketed in any EU Member State.

MAs are only granted to applicants established within the European Community, i.e., within one of the 27 Member States of the EU plus Norway, Iceland and Liechtenstein (European Economic Area (EEA)).

Choice of Procedure

There are four procedures by which veterinary MAs may be obtained within Europe:
- National Procedure—This procedure is used to obtain a single national authorisation in one Member State. This procedure is normally used when an applicant wishes to market in one Member State only.
- Mutual Recognition Procedure—This system may be used when an MA already exists in one Member State. The procedure allows an applicant to obtain further national authorisations by concurrently requesting "mutual recognition" of the first MA in a number of other Member States.

- Decentralised Procedure—This system may be used for products without an existing authorisation. The procedure allows an applicant to simultaneously request national authorisations in several or all Member States.
- Centralised Procedure—This system involves a single application to the EMA that results in a single, pan-European MA with a single trade name. Access to this procedure is restricted to biotech (for which it is mandatory) and innovative products (for which it is optional).

Certain types of products must be authorised using the Centralised Procedure, but for all others, the choice of procedure is dependent on the target market and marketing objectives (including the flexibility to choose one or more trade names).

Short Descriptions of the Procedures

A full description of each procedure can be found in *The Rules Governing Medicinal Products in the European Union, Volume 6A*. A short summary of each procedure is provided below.

Applications to a Single Member State (National Procedure)

Applicants wishing to obtain a veterinary MA in just one Member State may submit an application to that Member State's Competent Authority in the national language. This procedure is useful for small companies with local distribution networks or for products for diseases prevalent in only one country. The dossier is assessed by the national Competent Authority, following the procedures described in *The Rules Governing Medicinal Products in the European Union, Volume 6A* and any appropriate national legislation. This procedure may be used for all products except those listed in the Annex of Regulation (EC) No 726/2004.[21]

The product dossier is submitted to the national Competent Authority. Following a validation period to confirm that all legislative requirements have been fulfilled, the Competent Authority evaluates the data and produces an assessment report, usually accompanied by a list of questions. Once the applicant has answered the questions, a national MA is either issued or refused. The timeline set for the national Competent Authority to complete this process is 210 days; the period during which the applicant assembles the responses to questions is in addition to this period.

Applications to Two or More Member States

Applicants wishing to obtain veterinary MAs in more than one Member State are obliged to use either the Mutual Recognition Procedure or the Decentralised Procedure. These procedures may be used for all products except those listed in the Annex of Regulation (EC) No 726/2004.[21]

Mutual Recognition Procedure

The Mutual Recognition Procedure (MRP) is normally used when a medicine has already been authorised in one (or more) EU Member State(s). Further MAs can then be sought from other EU Member States in a procedure whereby the countries concerned agree to recognise the validity of the original MA. Agreement must be given unless the Member State can justify that the authorisation of the veterinary medicinal product may present a potential serious risk to human or animal health or the environment.

As this requires two separate steps (i.e., the original authorisation procedure followed by the Mutual Recognition Procedure), the overall timeline is longer. If there is no existing MA, the applicant is expected to use the Decentralised Procedure, with the added benefit of a shorter timeline. The two phases run to a strict timetable.

- Phase 1—The National Procedure already will have been completed (210 days). The Member State where the existing MA is held is requested by the applicant to produce an updated European assessment report (90 days). This Member State becomes known as the Reference Member State (RMS). The applicant also has to update the dossier in light of the questions from the national phase.
- Phase 2—The applicant selects other Member States where MAs are required; these are known as the Concerned Member States (CMS). The applicant sends identical copies of the updated dossier to the RMS and all CMS, requesting that the MA be mutually recognised by the CMS Competent Authorities. The RMS sends copies of the updated assessment report to the CMS, together with the approved Summary of Product Characteristics (SmPC), labelling and package leaflet. After a validation phase of 14 days, during which the availability of all necessary documentation and translations and payment of fees are verified, the CMS then have 90 days to agree to mutually recognise the opinion and recommendations of the RMS. The CMS frequently will produce their own lists of questions, which should be limited to issues of serious risk, and the time available for the applicant to supply answers is short (10 days).

If the CMS all agree to authorise the product, the procedure closes on Day 90. If full agreement is not reached, the procedure is extended to allow further discussion (see Resolving Disagreements below).

The Mutual Recognition Procedure is an intense, time-limited process, during which difficulties can arise due to differences in the interpretation of the requirements by the CMS. To facilitate the process, the Veterinary Mutual Recognition Facilitation Group (VMRFG) was created in 1997 as an informal discussion forum for both technical and procedural issues. The 2004 revision to the directive established the CMDv, which officially replaced the informal VMRFG. The VMRFG/CMDv have produced a number of guidance documents covering timelines and best practice;[22, 23] the group also supplies answers to procedural questions from the pharmaceutical industry (these documents are accessible via the HMA/CMDv website).[24]

The applicant must submit final translations of the product literature within five days of the close of the procedure. The Member States are then expected to issue a national MA within 30 days of receipt of the final translations of the product literature from the applicant.

Decentralised Procedure
The Decentralised Procedure may be used to obtain an MA for a veterinary medicinal product that has not yet received an authorisation in any Member State. The application is sent simultaneously to all EU Member States that are to be included in the procedure. One Member State is nominated as the RMS; this state supplies an assessment report and guides the application through the procedure. There are 14 days set for validation of the application and then "assessment step 1" starts. A period of 70 days is available for the RMS to conduct the scientific assessment and provide a preliminary assessment report, which is circulated to all the CMS. Comments from the CMS must be supplied by Day 100, and a single list of questions is sent to the applicant by Day 105. At this point, the time clock is stopped pending receipt of the responses. The applicant normally is expected to submit responses with three months, and then the clock restarts. The RMS must then submit the updated assessment report to all CMS by Day 120, together with the approved SmPC, labelling and package leaflet.

"Assessment step 2" starts on Day 120 and runs to a 90-day time clock, ending on Day 210. During this time, issues relating to the SmPC, packaging and labelling texts must be settled. The CMS have until Day 145 to raise issues about matters that remain unresolved. The applicant has 20 days to supply suitable responses. The application then goes forward to discussion, if necessary, at the CMDv meeting on Days 197–198, but normally the discussion takes place using electronic virtual meetings on the Monday and/or Tuesday after the CMDv meeting (Days 201–202) to enable the appropriate national experts to participate. By Day 205, all CMS should give their final opinion, and the final drafts of the SmPC, labelling and package insert should be agreed if not done previously.

If the CMS all agree to authorise the product, the procedure closes on Day 210. If full agreement is not reached, the procedure is extended to allow further discussion (see Resolving Disagreements below), and the RMS circulates a list of Member States in favour of and opposed to granting an authorisation.

The Member States are then expected to issue national MAs within 30 days of receipt of the final translations of the product literature from the applicant.

Resolving Disagreements in the MRP or DCP
Resolving Issues by Discussion (CMDv Referral)
Although Member States are expected to mutually recognise the RMS assessment and only raise objections if there are serious public health concerns, in practice, CMS frequently raise commonplace, non-serious matters, particularly if they are following a national precedent. CMS questions and objections should be sent to the RMS by Day 54 of the 90-day "assessment step 2" period. The applicant must supply answers by Day 65. The RMS will actively coordinate dialogue between the applicant and any CMS that still have concerns.

If no agreement can be reached by Day 90 or 210, a further discussion period of 60 days is triggered involving the entire CMDv. The CMS must use their best endeavours to reach agreement. No clock stop is possible, and the applicant may request an oral hearing. If agreement is reached after this 60-day period, the procedure is closed (now Day 270); if not, the issue is referred to CVMP for arbitration.

Resolving Issues by Arbitration (CVMP Referral)
If an agreement cannot be reached during the 60-day CMDv referral period, the disputed point is referred to EMA for arbitration by the CVMP referral procedure. This process cannot be stopped even if the applicant withdraws the application from any CMS. From receipt of the detailed description of the issue, CVMP has 60 days to deliver an opinion. If CVMP decides the objection is valid, the application is rejected and the applicant loses the authorisation in the RMS (MRP) or the procedure is closed (DCP). If the objection is not considered valid, the CMS must approve and authorise the product. The costs for the arbitration procedure are paid by the applicant.

Centralised Procedure
Summary of the Centralised Procedure
EMA is responsible for organising and conducting the Centralised Procedure. This procedure leads to a single MA that is valid in all Member States across the EU. The Centralised Procedure is compulsory for medicinal products derived from biotechnology and for the product groups listed in the Annex to Regulation (EC) No 724/2004. Companies can also access this procedure for new products that fall within the definition of "innovative" provided in Article 3 of the regulation.

Applications through the Centralised Procedure are submitted directly to EMA. Evaluation by CVMP follows a similar procedure to those above with a 210-day timeline, normally interrupted with a list of questions to the applicant. At the end of 210 days, the committee adopts an opinion on whether the medicine should be marketed. This opinion is then transmitted to the European Commission, which issues a formal Commission Decision on the authorisation of the product. This decision must be approved by the Commission's Standing Committee on veterinary medicines (this is normally a written procedure, taking approximately two months).

The applicant is then expected to submit the final translations of the product literature for all 27 Member States.

More detail on each of the key steps is given below.

EMA Presubmission Guidance
EMA strongly advises all applicants to view the presubmission guidance published on its website.[25] The guidance addresses a number of questions commonly asked by Centralised Procedure users. It provides an overview of EMA's position on issues typically encountered during the course of presubmission meetings. EMA also emphasises the importance of presubmission meetings with potential applicants. These meetings, which should take place four to six months prior to the anticipated submission date, are an opportunity to obtain procedural, regulatory and legal advice from EMA. Scientific Advice is also available from EMA/CVMP; it is organised through a separate, formal procedure.

After applicants have notified EMA of their intention to submit an application, members of CVMP are assigned as rapporteur and co-rapporteur to the application.

Scientific Assessment Process
Upon submission to EMA, the application is validated and the procedure initiated. A rapporteur and co-rapporteur are appointed from different Member States. The primary responsibilities of the rapporteur and co-rapporteur are the coordination of the scientific assessment and evaluation of the application and the production of draft and final assessment reports. The rapporteur co-opts a team for quality, safety and efficacy assessment, which also may include input from a scientific advisory group (SAG). EMA will appoint a project manager, whose primary role is to provide technical, scientific, legal and regulatory assistance to the rapporteur and the co-rapporteur, CVMP and the applicant during the procedure.

The rapporteur produces a draft assessment report by Day 70 and sends this to the co-rapporteur, who produces a critique of the assessment report by Day 85. Comments from other CVMP members can be submitted up to Day 100. The updated assessment report and a list of questions must be sent to the applicant by Day 120, and the clock is stopped. The applicant is expected to respond within six months, and the clock is restarted when the responses are received. In addition, an oral hearing may be required to elucidate some open questions.

The rapporteur then produces a final assessment report for evaluation by CVMP. CVMP must deliver an opinion, by majority vote if necessary, on whether to grant or refuse the MA within 210 days from the start of the procedure.

After Day 210, the applicant is required to submit product literature (SmPC, package leaflet, package labels) in all official EU languages.

Following adoption of a positive opinion, EMA has 30 days to forward CVMP's opinion to the European Commission, as it is this body that makes the final decision. The following documents are appended to the opinion:
- SmPC
- MA, conditions of supply and use, specific obligations
- labelling and package leaflet

The Decision-making Procedure
The European Commission confirms that the MA complies with Community law and converts the EMA/CVMP recommendations into a binding decision. A registration number, which must be placed on the package materials, is issued. This decision-making procedure[26] takes approximately two months, and comprises the following steps:
- A draft decision is prepared by the European Commission, DG Health and Consumers (30 days).
- Various European Commission directorates-general are consulted (10 days).
- A draft decision is given to the Standing Committee on Veterinary Medicinal Products (15 days for linguistic comments, 30 days for scientific and technical comments).
- A plenary meeting of the standing committee may be held to discuss any comments received.
- The agreed draft decision is forwarded to the Commission's secretariat-general for adoption.
- After final approval by the commissioner for DG Health and Consumers, the secretariat-general notifies Member States and the MAH in the official European languages.

A Community MA is issued to a single MAH, which is responsible for placing the medicinal product on the market, either directly or via a designated agent. The product will be required to have a single trade name unless the applicant can convince the European Commission that exceptional circumstances create a need for two or more trade names. An eight-year data protection period applies following issue of the MA, followed by a two-year market protection period.

Appeals Procedure
Applicants may appeal any CVMP opinion provided they notify EMA in writing of their intention to appeal within 15 days of receipt of the opinion. The applicant must submit detailed grounds for the appeal to EMA within 60 days.

CVMP will issue a final opinion within a further 60 days, after considering the grounds for appeal and may permit the applicant an oral hearing.

Product Literature and Translations
The SmPC, package leaflet, container label and the texts on any secondary packaging (e.g., carton) are known as the product literature. EMA supplies the outlines for the SmPC, label, carton and package leaflet in each official language. The documents, known as the "QRD templates," are located on the EMA website.[27]

The product literature is an integral part of the application, and there is a specific procedure for review and approval in all the official languages by EMA and the Competent Authorities—the linguistic review process. The linguistic review process ensures high-quality translations and consistent product information for centrally authorised products.

There are 24 official languages in the EU. Translations are, therefore, a major cost in both time and money. This is a significant burden for products with small veterinary markets and for companies that have medicinal products with several dosage forms and sizes, leading to multiple packages and leaflets. This high burden has been identified as an issue to be addressed in the next review of the legislation (2010–14). Over-stickers are prohibited under GMP legislation.[28] Combining languages to create multilingual packs can help overcome the problem of small print runs and reduce costs.

Blue Box
The "blue box" is used on the labelling for centrally authorised products. Certain information specific to a particular Member State (e.g., the legal status for supply and safety symbols required by national legislation) must be clearly identified by placing it in a blue box on the pack. Full details on the blue box requirements are found in *The Rules Governing Medicinal Products in the European Union, Volume 6A*, Chapter 6. Member States revise their requirements from time to time, so the information should be checked for each application. For example, it may no longer be necessary to use the colour blue.

European Competent Authorities Responsible for Authorisation of Veterinary Medicines

European Medicines Agency (EMA)
EMA and the centralised authorisation procedure were established in 1995 by Council Regulation (EC) No 2390/93.[29] EMA's structure, responsibilities and name were updated in May 2004 by Regulation (EC) No 726/2004.[30] In 2010, in recognition of its increased responsibilities, the name of the agency was changed from European Medicines Evaluation Agency (EMEA) to European Medicines Agency (EMA).

EMA is located in London and is responsible for coordinating the existing scientific resources put at its disposal by Member States' Competent Authorities to evaluate and supervise medicinal products via the Centralised Procedure. EMA also is responsible for providing scientific advice on quality, safety and efficacy; delivering scientific opinions on centralised MAs for both human and veterinary products; and establishing maximum residue levels (MRLs) for all substances with pharmacological activity. These responsibilities are carried out by CVMP, which is comprised of one scientific expert from each Member State and has the option of co-opting up to five additional experts selected for their specific scientific competence.

EMA also provides presubmission scientific guidance and independent arbitration in the event of disputes occurring in the Mutual Recognition or Decentralised Procedures. The CVMP working groups are responsible for elaborating specific guidelines on fulfilling the detailed requirements for quality, safety and efficacy data.

National Competent Authorities
Each EU Member State has an established national Competent Authority, either as an independent agency or as part of the Ministry of Health. While the majority supervise both human and veterinary medicinal products, albeit in separate departments, several countries (France, Germany, the Netherlands and the UK) have completely separate agencies responsible for the control of veterinary medicines. In some cases, the agency may be under the control of a different ministry. For example, in the UK, veterinary products are under the control of the Department of the Environment, Food and Rural Affairs. In a small number of Member States (Finland, Germany and Ireland), veterinary pharmaceuticals are under the supervision of the Ministry of Health, while veterinary immunological products are regulated by a different agency such as the Ministry or Department of Agriculture. The Competent Authority for each Member State (with the standard country abbreviation) within the EU and the wider EEA is listed in **Table 33-2**. These details are also published in *The Rules Governing Medicinal Products in the European Union, Volume 6A*, Chapter 7 and on the HMA website.[31]

Legal Bases of Applications
The legal requirements and procedures for applying for an MA are set out in Directive 2001/82/EC, as amended by Directive 2004/28/EC. Normally, a full dossier is required (Article 12(3) of the directive). However, there are certain exemptions described in Article 13 of the directive. For clarity, applicants are asked to specify the "legal basis" of their application (i.e., Article 12 or Article 13) in the application form. The following legal bases are available (and are described in more detail in the next section):

- according to Article 12(3), a complete and independent application requiring a full dossier

- according to Article 13, application for a generic/hybrid/similar biological application requiring an abridged dossier

    Applications under Article 13 are classified further, as follows:
    o according to Article 13(1), relating to a generic veterinary medicinal product
    o according to Article 13(3), relating to a "hybrid" application
    o according to Article 13(4), relating to a similar biological application
    o according to Article 13a, an application relying on well-established use as a veterinary medicine, supported by bibliography
    o according to Article 13b, fixed combination products
    o according to Article 13c, application with informed consent of the MAH
    o according to Article 13d, application for an immunological product where certain trial results are omitted

Generic Veterinary Medicinal Products

A "generic veterinary medicinal product" is defined in Article 13(2)(b) of Council Directive 2001/82/EC, as amended, as follows:

"A 'generic medicinal product' shall mean a medicinal product which has the same qualitative and quantitative composition in active substance and the same pharmaceutical form as the reference medicinal product, and whose bioequivalence with the reference medicinal product has been demonstrated by appropriate bioavailability studies. The different salts, esters, ethers, isomer, mixtures of isomers, complexes or derivatives of an active substance shall be considered to be the same actives substance, unless they differ significantly in properties with regard to safety and/or efficacy. In such cases additional information intended to provide proof of the safety and/or efficacy of the various salts, esters or derivatives of an authorised active substance must be supplied by the applicant. The various immediate-release oral pharmaceutical forms shall be considered to be one and the same pharmaceutical form. Bioavailability studies need not be required of the applicant if he can demonstrate that the generic medicinal product meets the relevant criteria as defined in the appropriate detailed guidelines."

Applications under Article 13 for generic products may be made when the reference medicinal product (RMP) has been authorised for a minimum of eight years in a Member State or the Community. However, a further period of two years must elapse before the generic medicine can be placed on the market. The applicant is not required to provide safety and residue test results or preclinical and clinical trial results for generic applications. However, the applicant must demonstrate bioequivalence and that the active substance has the same impurity profile as the RMP. A full user safety assessment and environmental risk assessment also are required for the generic product.

A change introduced by Directive 2004/28/EC now allows generic applications to be made in Member States where the RMP is not already authorised. This is known as the European Reference Product concept. However, a Competent Authority may object to this, particularly if it previously has rejected an MAA for the reference product. This has led to a significant number of referrals, and such a course of action should be discussed with the Member States concerned before proceeding.

The applicant may refer to the RMP under Article 13a ("well-established use") or Article 13c (with the MAH's permission, "informed consent"). In both cases, a complete set of quality data (Part 2) is required. The requirement for safety and efficacy data is minimal, as cross-reference to the RMP data set is permitted.

The RMP must always be supported by a full dossier; it is not possible to make reference to another generic or abridged dossier.

For fixed combination products containing known active substances (Article 13b), efficacy data on the individual substances are not required; preclinical and clinical data on the combination only are required.

Fees

Mutual Recognition, Decentralised and National Procedures

Fees must be paid for all procedures, and each Member State has its own system for calculating the fees required for a particular application. Information on the fee required and the method of payment is supplied on the Competent Authority websites (links to these are available from the HMA/CMDv website), but some sites are not easy to navigate and not all are written in English. The majority of Member States require payment before submission with the proof of payment included in the documentation.

Prospective applicants should contact each Member State concerned to confirm the fee required. Information on the payment procedures and bank details for each Member State are given in *The Rules Governing Medicinal Products in the European Union, Volume 6A*, Chapter 7. These should be checked regularly, as changes to addresses and account numbers do occur.

Centralised Procedure

The European Commission sets the EMA fees for applications through the Centralised Procedure. In exceptional circumstances or for imperative public and animal health

Table 33-2. Competent Authorities for the Regulation of Veterinary Medicinal Products in the EEA

Member State		Agency name
Austria	AT	Agentur fur Gesundheit und Ernahrungssicherheit GmbH
Belgium	BE	Federal Agency for Medicines & Healthcare Products
Bulgaria	BG	Institute for Control of Veterinary Medicinal Products
Cyprus	CY	Ministry of Agriculture, Natural Resources and Environment
Czech Republic	CZ	Ústav pro státní kontrolu veterinárních biopreparátu a léciv (Institute for the State Control of Veterinary Biologicals and Medicaments)
Denmark	DK	Lægemiddelstyrelsen (Danish Medicines Agency)
Estonia	EE	Ravimiamet (State Agency of Medicines)
Finland	FI	The Finnish Medicines Agency (Fimea)
France	FR	AFSSA-ANMV Agence Nationale du Médicament Vétérinaire
Germany	DE	Bundasamt für Verbraucherschutz und Lebensmittelsicherheit (BVL) (Pharmaceuticals) Paul-Ehrlich-Institut (Immunologicals)
Greece	EL	National Organization for Medicines
Hungary	HU	Mezögazdasági Szakigazgatási Hivatal Állatgyógyászati Termékek Igazgatósága (Central Agricultural Office Directorate of Veterinary Medicinal Products)
Ireland	IE	Bord Leigheasra nah Eireann (Irish Medicines Board)
Iceland	IS	Lyfjastofnun (The Icelandic Medicines Control Agency)
Italy	IT	Ministero della Salute - Dipartimento della Sanità Pubblica Veterinaria, della sicurezza alimentare e degli organi collegiali per la tutela della salute - Direzione generale della sanità animale e dei farmaci veterinari
Latvia	LV	Latvian State Agency of Medicines
Liechtenstein		Liechtenstein National Administration, Office of Health
Lithuania	LT	National Food and Veterinary Risk Assessment Institute
Luxemburg	LU	Division de la Pharmacie et des Médicaments, Ministry of Health
Malta	MT	Medicines Regulatory Unit, Ministry for Food, Agriculture and Fisheries
Netherlands	NL	College ter Beoordeling van Geneesmiddelen (Medicines Evaluation Board, Veterinary Medicinal Products Unit)
Norway	NO	Statens legemiddelverk (Norwegian Medicines Agency)
Poland	PL	Urzad Rejestracji Produktów Leczniczych, Wyrobów Medycznych, I Produktów Biobójczych (Office of Medicinal Products, Medical Devices and Biocides)
Portugal	PT	Direção Geral de Alimentação e Veterinaria - DGAV
Romania	RO	Institutul pentru Controlul Produselor Biologice si Medicamentelor de Uz Veterinar (Institute for Control of Biological Products and Veterinary Medicines)
Slovak Republic	SK	Ústav štátnej kontroly veterinárnych bioparátov a lieciv Institute for State Control of Veterinary Biologicals and Medicaments
Slovenia	SL	Javna Agencija Republike Slovenija Za Zdravila in Medicinske Pripomocke (Agency for Medicinal Products and Medical Devices)
Spain	ES	Ministerio de Sanidad y Consumo—Agencia Española de Medicamentos y Productos Sanitarios (Spanish Agency of Medicines and Health Products)
Sweden	SE	Läkemedelsverket (Medical Products Agency)
UK	UK	Veterinary Medicines Directorate (VMD)
EU		European Medicines Agency (EMA)

reasons, EMA may grant fee waivers or reductions. Any fee waiver or reduction requests should be sent to EMA with the appropriate justification at least two months prior to submission using the following criteria:

a) New Product for Major Species
- The product is indicated for a rare disease or circumstance.
- No other product is licensed in the Community for this claim.
- Control of the disease(s) indicated is imperative for animal health, and possibly for human health.

b) New Product for Minor Species
- The product is for a specific claim (not necessarily a rare disease or circumstance).

- The product is not already authorised for a similar claim in another species.
- No other product is licensed in the Community for this claim in this species.
- Control of the disease is imperative for the health of the minor species concerned.

Small or medium-sized enterprises (SMEs) can register for SME status,[32] thereby allowing a reduction in fees or deferred payment. Information can be found on the EMA website.[33] The fees are periodically updated and published in a European Commission Regulation (the most recent is Commission Regulation (EC) No 249/2009).

Data Requirements

Each of the four procedures requires the same data, which must be submitted in four separate parts for pharmaceutical products and six for immunologicals.
- Part 1—application form and administrative data; SmPC, packaging and labelling texts; critical summaries
- Part 2—quality documentation, comprising the pharmaceutical (physicochemical, biological or microbiological) information
- Part 3—safety documentation, comprising pharmacological and toxicological studies, user safety assessment and environmental risk assessment (Part 3A) and residue depletion studies (Part 3B); Part 3B is not a requirement for immunological products
- Part 4—efficacy documentation, comprising preclinical studies and clinical field trials
- Part 5 (immunologicals only)—particulars and documents associated with laboratory and field studies
- Part 6 (immunologicals only)—bibliographic references

Data requirements are specified in the Annex to Directive 2001/82/EC, as amended by Directive 2009/9/EC. The introduction to the annex states, "All information which is relevant to the evaluation of the medicinal product concerned shall be included in the application, whether favourable or unfavourable to the product. In particular, all relevant details shall be given of any incomplete or abandoned pharmaco-toxicological or clinical studies relating to the product."

Differences Between Human and Veterinary Dossiers

The quality, safety and efficacy procedures and standards applicable to veterinary medicinal products within the EU parallel those for human medicinal products wherever possible. However, there are some fundamental differences in both the safety and efficacy parts of the dossier.

The documentation required for Part 2 (Quality) is virtually identical for both human and veterinary products. There are specific veterinary guidelines defining product quality but a great many are identical to those used for human medicines. In the absence of a veterinary equivalent, pharmaceutical assessors will normally refer to the human guidelines. For transmissible spongiform encephalopathy compliance, there are strict rules concerning the use of ingredients of ruminant origin in medicinal products, in particular, when substances of bovine origin are used for bovine medicinal products.

Substantial differences in documentation occur in Part 3 (Safety) of the dossier. The safety data required for veterinary medicinal products are divided into two files:
- Part 3A: active substance toxicology data, target animal tolerance, user safety and environmental risk information
- Part 3B: drug residues documentation

In Part 3A, the information necessary to demonstrate the active substance's basic toxicological properties is the same for both human and veterinary products. However, veterinary products require specific studies on metabolism and excretion in each target species. Operator/user safety is a significant issue for all products and assumes greater importance in certain product classes, for example, ectoparasiticides. A detailed user safety risk assessment, written in accordance with the CVMP guideline[34] and considering all indicated species, routes of administration and patterns of use, is required for each application.

A veterinary product is also subject to a more rigorous environmental risk assessment (ERA) than a human medicine. The environment can be directly contaminated by an active substance and/or its metabolites by excretion directly to pasture by livestock or by application of manure to land. In addition, a number of active substances used for veterinary medicines are authorised as pesticides, so it is necessary for the Competent Authorities to examine the potential for cumulative effects. The guidelines that govern the format and content of the ERA for conventional veterinary medicinal products are internationally harmonised by VICH.[35–37] A specific guideline exists for ERAs of veterinary medicinal products consisting of, or containing, genetically modified organisms.

Part 3B has no comparable document in applications for human medicinal products.

The residue file, necessary for all products intended for administration to food producing species, contains:
- studies on residue depletion in the appropriate tissues (milk, eggs and honey are also considered as "tissues" in this context)
- confirmation of the marker residue, as this is not always the active substance
- MRL information

- methodology for residue(s) analysis in the appropriate tissue(s)
- proposed post-therapy withdrawal period to be implemented before any animal product may be collected for human consumption

Part 4 (Efficacy) requirements are similar for the veterinary and human sectors. The efficacy file contains two sections: Part 4A, comprising preclinical/pharmacological information and Part 4B, clinical trials. The third section for human products, "other information," is not applicable to veterinary medicines. The preclinical section for a veterinary medicine must include data on target species safety (tolerance to the drug). For veterinary antimicrobial or anthelmintic products, the geographic distribution and existing level of resistance in the disease organism population must be defined. Identification of the factors influencing selection pressure and the potential for further development of resistant strains also must be considered.

Applications for veterinary immunological medicinal products have two further parts: Part 5 contains particulars and documents relating to laboratory testing and field studies; Part 6 is for any bibliographic references quoted in the critical summaries.

Specific Quality (Part 2) Issues

European Pharmacopoeia

A second complementary dimension to European harmonisation is the publication of a comprehensive set of substance monographs by the *European Pharmacopoeia* (*PhEur*). Established in 1964, the purpose of the *PhEur* is to promote public health and a single market by providing common quality standards for active substances, excipients, pharmaceutical preparations, methods of analysis and packaging materials for human and veterinary medical use. Unlike guidelines, the monographs are legally binding. Any substance in a medicinal product's composition must comply with the relevant monograph. To facilitate this, an active substance manufacturer can submit a dossier to the European Department for the Quality of Medicines (EDQM), which will confirm validation and issue a certificate of compliance with the *PhEur*. The certificate, known as Certification of Suitability to the Monographs of the European Pharmacopoeia, can be included in any MAA and obviate the need to supply detailed descriptions of synthesis, manufacturing processes and analytical methods.

Active Substance Master File

In Part 2 of the dossier, the applicant is required to submit details of the active substance manufacturing method or route of synthesis and quality control procedures. However, this information may be confidential if the manufacturer is a different legal entity than the applicant. To overcome this difficulty, the applicant and manufacturer must work together to ensure that all relevant information required for Part 2 is provided in the form of an Active Substance Master File (ASMF).

The ASMF frequently is produced as two documents:
- a "closed" part containing the full package of information on the active substance
- an "open" part, which comprises the non-confidential information

The complete closed part of the ASMF is submitted directly to the Competent Authorities by the manufacturer, thereby maintaining confidentiality. The manufacturer must ensure that the closed part is accompanied by a separate critical summary. The applicant receives a copy of the open part to submit as part of its MAA dossier. A manufacturer's letter of consent (letter of access) authorising the use of the ASMF for a specific application also is required by the applicant for inclusion in the dossier.

Common Technical Document

Use of the Common Technical Document (CTD) enables a single dossier for a human medicinal product to be submitted to the Competent Authorities throughout the EU, US and Japan. However, the CTD system is not used for authorisation of veterinary medicinal products within the EU. In 2001, the VICH Steering Committee discussed a concept paper for a veterinary CTD but concluded that harmonisation of guidelines should be given priority. A veterinary CTD will not be established in the foreseeable future. However, it is possible to submit an ASMF in CTD format, particularly where the active substance is also used in human medicine(s). A document providing detailed cross-reference between the CTD and the appropriate sections in the *Notice to Applicants* is an essential component of such an application.

Transmissible Spongiform Encephalopathies

The applicant must demonstrate that the starting materials are manufactured in such a way as to minimise the risk of transmission of animal spongiform encephalopathies. The means of doing so include a number of control measures related to the sources and quality control of the starting materials and manufacturing process design and control. The relevant guideline is EMA/410/01-Rev. 3.[38]

Residual Solvents

The applicant must demonstrate that residual solvent levels in both new and existing products comply with precise limits, which are specified in EMEA/CVMP/423/01-Final.[39] Three classes of solvent are defined:
- Class I—known to be hazardous to human health and the environment
  - use of Class I solvents is to be avoided

- Class II—suspected of significant but reversible toxicity
  - o Class II solvents are permitted in limited amounts
- Class III—considered to have low toxic potential

Genetically Modified Organisms

An MAA for a veterinary medicinal product containing a genetically modified organism (GMO), as defined by Article 2 (2) of Directive 2001/18/EC, must be made through the Centralised Procedure. In addition to the letter of intent to submit, the applicant must provide a confirmation of compliance with all the obligations of the above directive. The application must be accompanied by:
- a copy of any written Competent Authority consent to the deliberate environmental release of the GMO for research and development purposes, provided by Part B of Directive 2001/18/EEC
- a complete technical dossier supplying the information requested in Annexes II and III of Directive 2001/18/EEC and the ERA resulting from this information
- results of any investigations performed for research or development

Postauthorisation Phase

MA Renewal

MAs issued within the European Community are initially valid for five years. After that time, the authorisation may be renewed based on a reevaluation of the risk:benefit balance. Renewal requirements vary among the Competent Authorities, but will be based on a review of the risk:benefit assessment derived from the complete set of quality, safety and efficacy documentation, including all variations and submissions made under pharmacovigilance requirements since the MA was granted. Once renewed, the authorisation will be valid for an unlimited period. However, a Competent Authority may suspend, revoke or vary an MA at any time when justified by a safety issue, e.g., following the evaluation of pharmacovigilance data.

Sunset Clause

Revocation of the MA will occur if any product is not marketed for a period of three years (unless there are exceptional circumstances); this is known as the "sunset clause."

Variations to Marketing Authorisations

Any required modifications to an MA must be made by formal submission of an application for MA variation. The original variation regulations, Commission Regulation (EC) No 541/95 of 10 March 1995 and Commission Regulation (EC) No 542/95 of 10 March 1995, were replaced in 2003 by Commission Regulation (EC) No 1084/2003[40] for the Mutual Recognition Procedure and Commission Regulation (EC) No 1085/2003[41] for the Centralised Procedure. Both of these have recently been superseded by a single regulation, Commission Regulation (EC) No 1234/2008.[42] Variations are classified into five categories by this regulation:
- minor variations of Type IA
- minor variations of Type IB
- major variations of Type II
- extensions
- urgent safety restrictions

A single submission can cover more than one variation. Secondary changes arising directly from the primary variation (consequential changes) can be made simultaneously, and there is now a system of "grouping" variations and "work sharing." The applicant is advised to seek advice from the relevant Competent Authority on the best way to compile a series of variations as there can be major cost implications.

Maximum Residue Limits

Introduction

The primary objective of pharmaceutical legislation is to protect public health, including the health of consumers of foodstuffs of animal origin. Therefore, safety standards must be set for foodstuffs obtained from animals treated with veterinary medicines to ensure that residues of the medicine or their metabolites that might also constitute a potential health hazard are not present.

Before any MA can be issued for a veterinary medicinal product intended for a food producing species, all pharmacologically active substances contained in the product must undergo a safety and residue evaluation under Regulation (EC) No 470/2009 of 6 May 2009,[43] which replaced Regulation (EC) No 2377/90.

Following the adoption of the new regulation, all the substances listed in a series of five annexes to the previous regulation were re-assembled in a single annex that listed them in alphabetical order; this single annex was published as Commission Regulation (EU) 37/2010 of 22 December 2009.[44] The annex contains two tables: Table 1 of the annex lists substances with maximum residue limits (MRLs), substances with provisional MRLs and substances for which no MRL is necessary; Table 2 lists substances prohibited for use in food-producing animals because a safe MRL cannot be established.

"Food-producing animals" are defined as those bred, raised, kept, slaughtered or harvested for the purposes of producing food. **Table 33-3** lists species that are considered "food producing" in the EU.

All active substances are considered to be pharmacologically active and, depending on the product, some excipients may also require assessment for potential residues.

The new regulation introduced the legal basis for the European Commission to take over without a further risk assessment those Codex Alimentarius MRLs it has supported in the relevant Codex Alimentarius Commission meetings. The new regulation also introduced the legal basis for an MRL to be extrapolated to another species or tissue in the interest of helping to increase the availability of products for minor food-producing species (see section on Minor Uses and Minor Species).

How an MRL is established is described in the next section. At the conclusion of the MRL procedure, the name of the substance is published and added to the annex (in a Commission regulation amending the Annex to Regulation (EU) No 37/2010), together with the marker residue (if different from the parent substance), and the limits set.

There is also a list of substances considered as falling outside the scope of Regulation (EC) No 470/2009 with regard to residues of veterinary medicinal products in foodstuffs of animal origin.[45] This "out-of-scope list" contains substances that may be considered normal foodstuffs, substances of natural origin and excipients, and is available from the European Commission DG Health and Consumers website (public health/veterinary medicines/MRLs).

Establishment of MRLs

Regulation (EC) No 470/2009 defines "residues of pharmacologically active substances" as all pharmacologically active substances, expressed in mg/kg or µg/kg on a fresh weight basis, whether active substances, excipients or degradation products and their metabolites that remain in food obtained from animals.

MRLs are derived from a safety file containing toxicology data and a residue file, comprising data on the nature, magnitude, metabolism and depletion of the particular residue(s) concerned. Additional residue depletion studies or bioequivalence studies generally are required to establish a withdrawal period.

Toxicological studies investigate acute, subchronic and chronic toxicity; reproductive toxicity; mutagenicity; carcinogenicity; and other effects such as immuntoxicity, effects on human gut flora and effects on food processing microorganisms. The residue file contains studies investigating product absorption, metabolism, distribution and excretion in the target species, together with target animal tissue residue distribution and depletion studies. An analytical method suitable for detecting the parent compound and marker residues in the appropriate target tissue must be developed and validated for each substance. This method may form the basis of the method used in the national residue surveillance programme.

Calculating an Acceptable Daily Intake

The toxicological information is used to determine a "no observable adverse effect level" (NOAEL), which is the highest drug dose at which there are no observable adverse effects in the most sensitive animal species. The NOAEL is used to calculate the compound's acceptable daily intake (ADI). The ADI is an estimate of the amount a person can ingest daily over a lifetime that, on the basis of all known facts and with some certainty, will cause no risk to health. Typically, the ADI will include a large safety factor of 100 or more, depending on the particular substance. Antimicrobial residue risks are assessed by establishing a microbiological ADI that excludes adverse effects on human gut flora.

Table 33-3. Food-producing Species

Major species	Minor species
Cattle—meat and milk	Sheep—milk
Sheep—meat	Goats—meat and milk
Pigs	Deer
Chickens—meat and eggs	Other mammalian species (horse, rabbit)
Salmonidae	Other avian species
	Other fish species
	Bees—honey

Determination of the Maximum Residue Limits

Transforming the ADI into an MRL requires the following steps:

1. The total residue distribution and depletion from the edible tissues of the treated animal species are investigated; total residues represent the sum of the remaining unmetabolised parent compound and all its metabolites.
2. The composition of the residues is studied to identify a marker residue.
3. The ADI is distributed appropriately among the different animal produce that makes up the "daily food basket"—muscle, liver, kidney, fat, milk, eggs and honey—to determine an MRL for each edible tissue. The MRLs are allocated so that the total amount of residues does not exceed the ADI.

The daily food basket uses arbitrarily high, fixed values to ensure protection of the majority of consumers. To exceed an ADI in relation to a particular substance, a person would need to consume more than 500g of meat (including offal and fat), 1.5 litres of milk, two eggs and 20g of honey, each containing residues at the MRL, every day, for life.

Determination of the Withdrawal Period

The rate of residue depletion for the appropriate tissue is investigated under controlled field conditions. For this, it is necessary to have developed and validated an analytical method that can quantify the selected marker residue. The marker residue is frequently the parent compound but may be one of the major metabolites. The results from the residue depletion study are used to set the withdrawal period: the time required after the last treatment for the level of residues to fall below the MRL fixed for the various tissues. It is only after this period has elapsed that animal produce can be collected for human consumption.

The withdrawal periods for meat and milk should be calculated by a suitable statistical method. The aim is to set a withdrawal time that ensures no sample obtained by random field monitoring will violate the MRL. Therefore, the statistics are applied to derive a 95% tolerance and a 95% level of confidence.

The following worst-case scenarios and safety margins are applied with the aim of minimising any potential risk to consumers:
- use of the NOAEL from the most sensitive species and the most appropriate study (pharmacology or toxicology)
- selection of the last test concentration to show no effect at the NOAEL (the true NOAEL will fall between this concentration and the previous concentration)
- use of large safety factors (typically x100 or more depending on the particular substance)
- assumption that the maximum permitted residue level is eaten every day of one's life
- assumption that everybody consumes the entire food basket every day
- statistical calculation of the withdrawal period using high confidence levels

The Procedure
An application for establishment of an MRL must be submitted to EMA at least six months before the intended MAA submission date. Approximately three months before submission, the applicant should notify EMA in writing of its intention to submit an MRL application. EMA will then appoint a rapporteur and co-rapporteur.

The format required and the data to be included for an MRL application are described in *The Rules Governing Medicinal Products in the European Union, Volume 8*. The data requirements are equivalent to Part 3 of an MAA for a product for a food-producing animal. The dossier should be presented in two separate parts: a safety file and a residues file, each containing an expert report. Following submission, a period of 10 days is allowed for validation of the application. The rapporteur and CVMP must then complete their assessment and prepare a summary report within 120 days. If the applicant is required to supply further information, the assessment clock will be stopped at this point.

At the end of the procedure, CVMP produces an opinion. It is possible to appeal this opinion and request a hearing within 15 days of receiving the notification. After this period, the opinion becomes final and is transmitted within 30 days by EMA to the European Commission. The Commission prepares a draft regulation to incorporate the substance into the appropriate annex of Council Regulation (EEC) No 470/2009 and sends it to the Standing Committee on Veterinary Medicinal Products for adoption (N.B. It is important to note that this is a committee of the Commission, composed of government experts from the Member States; it is not the same as EMA's CVMP).

Minor Uses and Minor Species
European legislation defines the "major animal species" as cattle, pigs, sheep, chickens and *Salmonidae*. Any other animal species is considered to be "minor." With the high cost of developing, licensing and maintaining veterinary medicines, product development for a minor species or a minor use in a major species is often not financially feasible. Consequently, new products often are developed only for major species. As a result, there is a significant shortfall in the number of authorised veterinary medicines available for minor species. Since 1999, there has been a wide-ranging debate on how the regulations and procedures impact the availability of veterinary medicinal products in the EU.

Responding to this issue, the first CVMP initiative was to investigate the possibility of extrapolating MRL data from major to minor species based on a pragmatic risk assessment.[46] This has since obtained a legal basis in the recent new MRL regulation. The second CVMP initiative developed a position paper on the availability of products for minor use, minor species (MUMS).[47] The principal recommendation was for the CVMP working groups for quality, safety, efficacy and biological products to examine the ways in which data requirements for MUMS products could be reduced without negatively affecting consumer safety. This resulted in several guidelines (see **Table 33-4**).

In addition, several existing legislative provisions and independent initiatives address specific areas of the problem. These are summarised in the following paragraphs.

Existing Legislative Provisions for Minor Species in Directive 2001/82/EC, as Amended
Article 4.2 of Directive 2001/82/EC, as amended, allows Member States to permit exemption from the need for an MA for certain veterinary medicinal products intended solely for aquarium fish, caged birds, homing pigeons, terrarium animals, small rodents, ferrets and rabbits kept exclusively as pets. Products containing antimicrobial or psychotropic substances are not included in this exemption, and an MA is required for these products for all species.

Where the Health Situation so Requires
Article 7 of Directive 2001/82/EC, as amended, provides Member States with an interesting provision that allows a Member State to authorise the marketing or administration of a veterinary medicinal product authorised in another EU Member State "if the health situation so requires."

The Cascade Provision

To avoid causing unacceptable suffering to animals, Article 10 (for companion animals and *equidae* declared not for human consumption) and Article 11 (for food-producing animals) of Directive 2001/82/EC provide that, where no authorised medicinal product exists for a condition, Member States may exceptionally permit a veterinary surgeon or someone under his or her direct personal responsibility to administer the following to an animal or small number of animals on a particular holding:

a) a veterinary medicinal product authorised within that Member State for use in another animal species or for another condition in the same animal species

b) if there is no product such as referred to in point a), a human medicinal product authorised for use in the Member State or a veterinary medicinal product authorised in another Member State for use in the same species for the condition in question or for another condition

c) if there is no product such as referred to in point b), a veterinary medicinal product prepared extemporaneously by a person authorised to do so under national legislation in accordance with the terms of a veterinary prescription

These provisions shall apply provided the medicinal product, where administered to food-producing animals, contains only substances that have an established MRL. This decision tree is known as the "cascade"[48] and allows minor species or minor indications in any species to be treated; however, it should be used only in exceptional circumstances.

A veterinary surgeon prescribing for, or administering a medicine to, food-producing animals under the cascade is required to specify an appropriate period before the food stuff may be consumed (withdrawal period). When setting the withdrawal period, a veterinary surgeon must take into account known information about the use of the product on the authorised species when prescribing under the cascade. Unless the medicinal product's label indicates a withdrawal period for the species concerned, this should not be less than:

- 7 days for eggs and milk
- 28 days for meat from poultry and mammals
- 500 degree days for meat from fish (degree day: the withdrawal period for fish depends on the water temperature; at a water temperature of 10°C, the withdrawal period is 50 days; at a water temperature of 5°C, the withdrawal period is 100 days, etc.)
- in addition the Commission shall establish a list of substances essential for the treatment of *equidae* and for which the withdrawal period shall be not less than six months

Clinical Requirements and Exceptional Circumstances

Exceptional circumstances are mentioned twice in the body of Directive 2001/82/EC, as amended, to allow clinical trials to be omitted for objective and verifiable reasons.

First, Article 13d provides derogation from Article 12(3)(j) of Directive 2001/82/EC for immunological veterinary medicinal products under exceptional circumstances, whereby the applicant shall not be required to provide results of certain field trials on the target species if these trials cannot be carried out for duly substantiated reasons, in particular on account of other Community provisions.

Second, Article 26.3 introduces the notion of exceptional circumstances under which an authorisation may be granted for objective and verifiable reasons. More information on this is found in the Annex to Directive 2001/82/EC, as amended, which describes basic MAA data requirements. This annex was updated in 2009 by Commission Directive 2009/9/EC. Title III outlines the requirements for a few specific MAAs. One of these is applications in exceptional circumstances, whereby, if the applicant demonstrates an inability to provide comprehensive efficacy and safety data under normal conditions of use (e.g., if the indication is rare or current scientific knowledge is insufficient), the Competent Authority can grant an MA subject to specific obligations on the applicant. These obligations will, in particular, concern ensuring the safety of the product, such as an enhanced pharmacovigilance plan; the product can be supplied only on a veterinary prescription and the package leaflet must inform the veterinarian that the data are incomplete.

Establishment of Maximum Residue Limits for Minor Species

CVMP has adopted guidelines on establishing MRLs for *Salmonidae* and other fin fish[49] and for minor species.[50] The guidelines permit the use of *in vitro* models for qualitatively extrapolating the marker residue and plasma kinetics studies as an alternative to residue studies, and the use of residue studies with a limited number of animals and no statistical evaluation. The validation requirements of an analytical method for residue in minor species' tissues were marginally reduced.

The guideline also permits extrapolation of an MRL established for a major species to the corresponding minor species, i.e., an MRL for cattle or sheep meat may be extrapolated to other ruminant meat. There is, however, a provision that an appropriate residue depletion study be conducted in the minor species. This study must show that the marker residue can be detected and used in practice in residue monitoring programmes.

Since publishing the above guidelines, CVMP has developed a scientific basis for extrapolating MRLs from major to minor species, providing certain conditions are met.[51] In this case, if data from three major species are available, the MRLs may be extended to cover all food-producing species.

Table 33-4. MUMS Guidelines

Topic	Reference Number
Note regarding CVMP Guidelines on data requirements for veterinary medicinal products intended for minor uses or minor species	EMEA/CVMP/133672/2005 Rev.1
Guideline on quality data requirements for veterinary medicinal products intended for minor uses or minor species	EMEA/CVMP/QWP/128710/2004
Guideline on safety and residue data requirements for veterinary medicinal products intended for minor uses or minor species	EMEA/CVMP/SWP/66781/2005
Note for Guidance on the establishment of MRLs for Salmonidae and other fin fish	EMEA/CVMP/153b/97
Guideline on efficacy and target animal safety data requirements for veterinary medicinal products intended for minor uses or minor species	EMEA/CVMP/EWP/117899/2004
Points to Consider regarding efficacy requirements for minor species and minor indications	EMEA/CVMP/610/01
Guideline on data requirements for immunological veterinary medicinal products intended for minor use or minor species	EMEA/CVMP/IWP/123243/2006 Rev. 2

Several MRLs have been successfully extrapolated since this guideline came into effect.[52,53]

Pharmacovigilance

Introduction

"Pharmacovigilance" is defined by the World Health Organization as the science and activities relating to the detection, assessment, understanding and prevention of adverse effects or any other drug-related problems.

Pharmacovigilance for all medicinal products within the EU became a legal requirement under Council Regulation (EEC) No 2309/93, as amended, and Directive 2001/82/EC, as amended. Council Regulation (EEC) No 2309/93 has since been replaced by Regulation (EC) No 726/2004, which *inter alia* tightened the pharmacovigilance requirements.

Pharmacovigilance includes information on suspected adverse drug reactions (SADR) in treated animals, suspected lack of expected efficacy (SLEE), human reactions, violations of approved residues and environmental incidents.

It is the MAH's responsibility to provide evidence of quality, safety and efficacy prior to introducing a medicinal product onto the market. This responsibility continues throughout the product lifecycle through pharmacovigilance requirements, which fall into three categories:
- recording and reporting SADRs
- compiling and submitting periodic safety update reports (PSURs)
- performing/carrying out postauthorisation safety studies

These obligations apply to all veterinary medicinal products in the EU, regardless of the date of authorisation or the authorisation procedure used.

The Competent Authorities and EMA have a responsibility to collect and evaluate pharmacovigilance reports submitted by the MAH, veterinarians and the general public. The framework provided by the Competent Authorities for collecting, evaluating and collating information includes guidance documents for both MAHs and Competent Authorities on the scope and format of pharmacovigilance reports, electronic submissions and conduct of postmarketing surveillance studies. The guidelines are presented in *The Rules Governing Medicinal Products in the European Union, Volume 9*. Volume 9b relates specifically to veterinary medicinal products guidelines (updated in October 2011) that have been harmonised within the VICH regions.

Communication Network

EudraVigilance Veterinary is the European data processing network and database management system for the exchange, processing and evaluation of SADRs related to veterinary medicinal products authorised in the EEA. The system has its own website[54] and a series of dedicated guidance documents.

Suspected Adverse Drug Reactions

An SADR is defined as "a reaction which is harmful and unintended and which occurs at doses normally used in animals for prophylaxis, diagnosis or treatment of disease or the modification of physiological function."

The MAH is required to maintain a system for collecting and collating reports of such reactions with the aim of preparing and submitting SADR reports and follow-up information to the Member State Competent Authority and/or EMA, where applicable.

Reports must include:
- identifiable source

Chapter 33

- animal details and human details for human reactions to veterinary medicinal products
- product name and MA number
- information on the reaction

CVMP has devised a list of clinical terms to be used in pharmacovigilance reports. This is known as the Veterinary Dictionary for Drug Regulatory Activities (VeDDRA).[55]

PSURs

PSURs provide the Competent Authorities and/or EMA with a review of global information on a product's quality, safety and efficacy. These reports are required every six months during the first two years after an MA is issued, annually in years three and four, then every three years for the lifetime of the product. Electronic reporting is encouraged, and database systems specifically designed for this purpose are available.

Each PSUR must cover the period since the last report and be submitted within 60 days after the cut-off point (known as the data-lock point). The data-lock point is determined by the EU birth date, which is the date of the product's first MA in the EU. The date may be adjusted by up to six months to allow for harmonisation of the date across several national authorisations of the same product.

PSURs should be written in English, unless it is a national authorisation, in which case the national language is acceptable. All PSURs should follow the EMA-specified format and must include the following:
- MAH and product details
- SmPC
- regulatory/MAH update (global update of safety action taken)
- sales volume and SADR incidence (the incidence is the number of animals reacting during a period expressed as a percentage of the number of doses sold during the period)
- individual case histories and reports and summary table (standard forms are available)
- SADRs and overview
- safety evaluation
- additional information received after the data-lock point (if necessary)

Postmarket Surveillance Studies

Responsibilities for postmarket surveillance studies are shared by the Competent Authorities and the MAH. The guideline describing the conduct of these studies is EMEA/CVMP/044/99.[56] Postmarket surveillance requirements may be defined at the time of granting the MA or may be required following the evaluation of postmarket periodic safety update data.

Future Trends in Pharmacovigilance

To compensate for less emphasis on five-yearly renewals, and in response to crises within the human medicines sector, the importance of pharmacovigilance has increased. The 2004 revised regulation increased EMA's responsibilities in allowing central coordination, including a central pharmacovigilance database, and by increasing the frequency of reporting to every three years. VICH has developed internationally harmonised guidelines in the following areas:

- *Management of Adverse Event Reporting* (VICH GL24)
- *Management of Periodic Summary Update Reports* (VICH G29)
- *Controlled List of Terms* (VICH GL30)
- *Electronic Standards for Transfer of Data* (VICH GL35) – not yet finalised
- *Data Elements for Submission of Adverse Event Reports* (VICH GL42)
- Recommendations on causality assessment

The focus on strengthening pharmacovigilance procedures has turned this regulatory area into one of high administrative burden for the veterinary sector. During the forthcoming review of the legislation, changes are expected to the chapter on pharmacovigilance.[57] It will be particularly important to avoid a disproportionately high administrative burden in future legislation by ensuring the limited resources of the veterinary sector are focused on areas of identifiable risk (such as new products with unknown actives). It also will be necessary to ensure the new legislation on pharmacovigilance is carefully tailored to the size and nature of the risks in the veterinary sector, which are very different to those in the human medicines sector.

Manufacturing and Product Control Requirements

GMP

GMP is applicable to both human and veterinary medicinal products.

In 1991, the European Commission adopted two directives, Directive 91/356/EEC (human products) and Directive 91/412/EEC[58] (veterinary products), that defined manufacturing standards within the EEC for medicinal products. GMP guidelines were established based on these directives. The complete set of requirements is presented in *The Rules Governing Medicinal Products in the European Union, Volume 4,* available from the European Commission—DG Health and Consumers.[59] Within this volume, two annexes define the specific veterinary product requirements and exceptions: Annex 4 "Manufacture of veterinary medicinal products other than immunologicals" and Annex 5 "Manufacture of immunological veterinary medicinal products." Annex 4 includes GMP adaptations for medicated feedstuffs, premixes, ectoparasiticides and veterinary medicinal products containing penicillin.

In 2005, starting materials used as active substances also became subject to GMP requirements. There is one exception: in the case of ectoparasiticides for veterinary use, *Volume 4* states, "other standards than these guidelines, that ensure that the material is of appropriate quality, may be used."

Sterile Veterinary Medicinal Products

Sterile products are classified via grades according to airborne particulate contamination, microbiological limits and standard operating procedures. Consideration should be given to Annex 1 of *Volume 4*, "Manufacture of Sterile Medicinal Products," to ensure compliance with the guidelines.

Where accepted by the relevant Competent Authorities, terminally sterilised veterinary medicinal products may be manufactured in a clean area of lower grade than that specified in Annex 1, but at least a grade D environment is mandatory.

Immunological Veterinary Medicinal Products

The requirements for manufacturing immunological veterinary medicinal products are specified in Annex 5 of *Volume 4*. The manufacture of these products requires special regulation due to the low volumes produced, the high risk of contamination and cross-contamination and the risk of environmental contamination. Areas specifically addressed in Annex 5 include starting materials, production, quality control, personnel, premises, equipment, animals/animal housing and disinfection/waste disposal.

Medicated Feedstuffs and Premixes

A "medicated feedstuff" is defined as any mixture of a veterinary medicinal product or products and feed or feeds that is ready prepared for marketing and intended to be fed to animals without further processing because of its curative or preventative properties or other properties as a medicinal product covered by Article 1 (2) of Directive 2001/82/EC, as amended.

A premix for medicated feedstuffs is any veterinary medicinal product prepared in advance with a view to the subsequent preparation of medicated feedstuffs.

Adequate pest control programs, cross-contamination prevention, dedicated/buffered production areas, specialised cleaning and standardisation of operations that may affect active ingredient stability are additional requirements to be considered in relation to medicated feedstuffs. Recently, the European Commission has also adopted legislation governing the acceptable levels of carry-over of the active ingredient from a medicated feed to a subsequent non-medicated feed manufactured in the same plant.

Ectoparasiticides

Ectoparasiticides for external application to animals that are veterinary medicinal products may be produced and filled on a campaign basis in areas dedicated to the production of pesticides. However, other categories of veterinary medicinal product should not be produced in such areas. Adequate validated cleaning methods should be employed to prevent cross-contamination, and steps should be taken to ensure secure storage of the veterinary medicinal product in accordance with the guide.

Veterinary Medicinal Products Containing Penicillin

Although desirable, veterinary medicinal products containing penicillin are no longer required to be manufactured in dedicated, self-contained facilities in the case of facilities dedicated to the manufacture of veterinary medicinal products only. However, all necessary measures should be taken to avoid cross-contamination and risk to operator safety in accordance with the guide. In such circumstances, penicillin-containing products should be manufactured on a campaign basis and should be followed by appropriate decontamination and cleaning processes.

Sample Retention

Retention of samples under appropriate storage conditions is required under GMP. However, if the size or volume of the product is such that it reduces the feasibility of such retention in the final packaging, auxiliary packaging may be used. Manufacturers should retain a representative sample of each batch and ensure that the auxiliary storage container is composed from the same material as the marketing container.

Summary

This chapter describes the background history for the procedures currently required for the authorisation of veterinary medicinal products within the EU. The four MAA types currently available—Centralised, Mutual Recognition, Decentralised and National—are explained and information supplied on the sources of information that will specify the data requirements and application format. The differences between the application content for human and veterinary medicines are also discussed. The names of the Competent Authorities for all EU Member States are provided together with an extensive list of references comprising European veterinary medicines legislation, guidance documents and website addresses that should be consulted prior to making any application.

Information is also included on the issues associated with obtaining and maintaining MAs within the EU: minor uses and minor species; variations and renewal of authorisations; food-producing species, MRLs and withdrawal periods; the data requirements and differences between human medicinal products; pharmacovigilance; the cascade; and GMP.

Note has also been made that the European legislation governing the MA of veterinary medicinal products is currently undergoing a major review. It is anticipated that new legislation will be published sometime after 2014.

References

1. Clayton R. "Veterinary medicines legislative review—The big debate—IFAH-Europe Annual Conference, Brussels, 16 June 2011." *Regulatory Rapporteur*, September 2011, Vol 8, No 9, pp. 29–31. www.topra.org.
2. Clayton R. "The review of the veterinary medicines legislation: An update." *Regulatory Rapporteur*, February 2012, Vol 9, No 2, pp. 4-7. TOPRA website. www.topra.org/sites/default/files/regrapart/1/4065/the_review_of_the_veterinary_medicines_legislation__an_update__rick_clayton.pdf. Accessed 4 June 2012.
3. Directive 2001/82/EC of the European Parliament and the Council of 6 November 2001 on the Community code relating to veterinary medicinal products. EUR-Lex website. http://eur-lex.europa.eu/LexUriServ/LexUriServ.do?uri=CONSLEG:2001L0082:20090807:EN:PDF. Accessed 4 June 2012.
4. Directive 2004/28/EC of the European Parliament and the Council of 31 March 2004 on the Community code relating to veterinary medicinal products. EUR-Lex website. http://eur-lex.europa.eu/LexUriServ/LexUriServ.do?uri=CELEX:32004L0028:EN:HTML. Accessed 4 June 2012.
5. Council Directive 2009/9/EC of 10 February 2009 amending Directive 2001/82/EC of the European Parliament and of the Council on the Community Code relating to medicinal products for veterinary use. EUR-Lex website. http://eur-lex.europa.eu/LexUriServ/LexUriServ.do?uri=OJ:L:2009:044:0062:0078:EN:PDF. Accessed 4 June 2012.
6. CMDv. EMEA/CMDv/20106/2008, Questions and Answers from Member States—Authorisaton of ectoparasiticidal collars companion animals. HMA website. www.hma.eu/uploads/media/47a_Authorisation_of_ectoparasiticidal_collars_for_companion_animals_-_EMEA-CMDv-20106-2008_01.pdf. Accessed 4 June 2012.
7. Veterinary Mutual Recognition Facilitation Group, VMRF/060/03, *Classification of teat dips in Member States.* (April 2003). HMA website. www.hma.eu/uploads/media/VMRF_060_03.pdf. Accessed 4 June 2012.
8. Veterinary Mutual Recognition Facilitation Group, VMRF/086/98, *Colostrum and Colostrum Substitutes,* (September 1998). HMA website. www.hma.eu/uploads/media/VMRF_086_01.pdf. Accessed 4 June 2012.
9. Directive 98/8/EC of the European Parliament and of the Council of 16 February 1998 concerning the placing of biocidal products on the market. EUR-Lex website. http://eur-lex.europa.eu/LexUriServ/LexUriServ.do?uri=OJ:L:1998:123:0001:0063:EN:PDF. Accessed 4 June 2012.
10. European Commission, DG Health and Consumers, EC webpage: http://ec.europa.eu/health/documents/eudralex/index_en.htm. Accessed 4 June 2012.
11. European Medicines Agency (EMA) website: www.ema.europa.eu/ema/. Accessed 4 June 2012.
12. Heads of Medicines Agencies (HMA) website: www.hma.eu/. Accessed 4 June 2012.
13. Clayton R., Zänker S. "International Harmonisation of standards for veterinary medicinal products." *Regulatory Affairs Journal.* 2000;11(3):174-177.
14. Council Directive 81/851 EEC of 28 September 1981 on the approximation of the laws of the Member States relating to veterinary medicinal products. EUR-Lex website. http://eur-lex.europa.eu/LexUriServ/LexUriServ.do?uri=CONSLEG:2001L0082:20040430:EN:PDF. Accessed 4 June 2012.
15. Council Directive 81/852 EEC of 28 September 1981 on the approximation of the laws of the Member States relating to analytical, pharmacotoxicological and clinical standards and protocols in respect of the testing of veterinary medicinal products. EUR-Lex website. http://eur-lex.europa.eu/LexUriServ/LexUriServ.do?uri=CELEX:31981L0852:en:NOT. Accessed 4 June 2012.
16. Clayton R. "Veterinary Medicines Legislation: Codification." *Regulatory Affairs Journal.* 2001;12(2):127-130.
17. Council Regulation (EEC) No 2309/93 of 22 July 1993 laying down Community procedures for the authorisation and supervision of medicinal products for human and veterinary use and establishing a European Agency of the evaluation of medicinal products. EUR-Lex website. http://eur-lex.europa.eu/LexUriServ/LexUriServ.do?uri=CELEX:31993R2309:en:HTML. Accessed 4 June 2012.
18. Commission Directive 91/412/EEC of 23 July 1991 laying down the principles and guidelines of good manufacturing practice for veterinary medicinal products. EC website. http://ec.europa.eu/health/files/eudralex/vol-5/dir_1991_412/dir_1991_412_en.pdf. Accessed 4 June 2012.
19. Op cit 1.
20. Op cit 2.
21. Regulation (EC) No 726/2004 of the European Parliament and of the Council of 31 March 2004 laying down Community procedures for the authorisation and supervision of medicinal products for human and veterinary use and establishing a European Medicines Agency. EUR-Lex website. http://eur-lex.europa.eu/LexUriServ/LexUriServ.do?uri=OJ:L:2004:136:0001:0033:en:PDF. Accessed 4 June 2012.
22. Co-ordination Group for Mutual Recognition and Decentralised Procedures, Veterinary, EMEA/CMDv/83618/2006, *Best Practice Guide for Mutual Recognition Procedure*, Edition 03 (16 July 2010). HMA website. www.hma.eu/uploads/media/BPG-001-03_FINAL_-_MRP_EMEA-CMDv-83618-2006.pdf. Accessed 4 June 2012.
23. Co-ordination Group for Mutual Recognition and Decentralised Procedures, Veterinary, EMEA/CMDv/63793/2006, *Best Practice Guide for Veterinary Decentralised Procedure*, Edition 04 (15 July 2010). HMA website. www.hma.eu/uploads/media/CMDv_BPG-002-04_DC_EMA-CMDv-63793-2006_Final.pdf. Accessed 4 June 2012.
24. Co-ordination Group for Mutual Recognition and Decentralised Procedures, Veterinary (CMDv) website: www.hma.eu/cmdv.html. Accessed 4 June 2012.
25. Op cit 11.
26. Clayton R, Brinkman D, Zänker S. "The Review Proposals for the Decision Making Process and What It Really Means." *Regulatory Affairs Journal.* 2001;12(12):975-981.
27. Quality Review of Documents templates. EMA website. www.ema.europa.eu/ema/index.jsp?curl=pages/regulation/document_listing/document_listing_000185.jsp&mid=WC0b01ac058002d9b0. Accessed 4 June 2012.
28. Op cit 18.
29. Op cit 17.
30. Op cit 21.
31. Op cit 12.
32. Commission Regulation (EC) No 2049/2005 laying down, pursuant to Regulation (EC) No. 726/2004 of the European Parliament and of the Council, rules regarding the payment of fees to, and the receipt of administrative assistance from, the European Medicines Agency by micro, small and medium-sized enterprises. EC website. http://ec.europa.eu/health/files/eudralex/vol-1/reg_2005_2049/reg_2005_2049_en.pdf. Accessed 4 June 2012.
33. User Guide for Micro, Small and Medium-sized Enterprises (SMEs) on the administrative and procedural aspects of the provisions laid down in Regulation (EC) 726/2004, that are of particular relevance

to SMEs (2009). EMA website. www.ema.europa.eu/docs/en_GB/document_library/Regulatory_and_procedural_guideline/2009/10/WC500004134.pdf. Accessed 4 June 2012.
34. EMA/CVMP/543/03-Rev.1, *Guideline on user safety for pharmaceutical veterinary medicinal products.* EMA website. www.ema.europa.eu/docs/en_GB/document_library/Scientific_guideline/2010/03/WC500077971.pdf. Accessed 4 June 2012.
35. VICH GL6, *Environmental Impact Assessment (EIA) for Veterinary Medicinal Products (VMPs) - Phase I.* VICH website. www.vichsec.org/pdf/2000/Gl06_st7.pdf. Accessed 4 June 2012.
36. VICH GL38, *Environmental Impact Assessment for Veterinary Medicinal Products Phase II Guidance.* VICH website. www.vichsec.org/pdf/10_2004/GL38_st7.pdf. Accessed 4 June 2012.
37. EMEA/CVMP/ERA/418282/2005-Rev.1, *Revised Guideline on Environmental Impact Assessment for veterinary medicinal products. In support of the VICH guidelines GL 6 and GL 38.* EMA website. www.ema.europa.eu/docs/en_GB/document_library/Scientific_guideline/2009/10/WC500004389.pdf. Accessed 4 June 2012.
38. EMA/410/01-Rev.3, *Note for guidance on minimising the risk of transmitting animal spongiform encephalopathy agents via human and veterinary medicinal products* (2011). EUR-Lex website. http://eur-lex.europa.eu/LexUriServ/LexUriServ.do?uri=OJ:C:2011:073:0001:0018:EN:PDF. Accessed 4 June 2012.
39. EMEA/CVMP/423/01-Final, *Application of the VICH guideline on residual solvents to veterinary medicinal products containing existing active substances* (May 2001). EMA website. www.ema.europa.eu/docs/en_GB/document_library/Scientific_guideline/2009/10/WC500004300.pdf. Accessed 4 June 2012.
40. Commission Regulation (EC) No 1084/2003 of 3 June 2003 concerning the examination of variations to the terms of a marketing authorisation for medicinal products for human use and veterinary medicinal products granted by a competent authority of a Member State. EUR-Lex website. http://eur-lex.europa.eu/LexUriServ/LexUriServ.do?uri=OJ:L:2008:334:0007:0024:en:PDF. Accessed 4 June 2012.
41. Commission Regulation (EC) No 1085/2003 of 3 June 2003 concerning the examination of variations to the terms of a marketing authorisation for medicinal products for human use and veterinary medicinal products falling within the scope of Council Regulation (EEC) No. 2309/93. EUR-Lex website. http://eur-lex.europa.eu/LexUriServ/LexUriServ.do?uri=OJ:L:2008:334:0007:0024:en:PDF. Accessed 4 June 2012.
42. Commission Regulation (EC) No 1234/2008 of 24 November 2008 concerning the examination of variations to the terms of marketing authorisations for medicinal products for human use and veterinary medicinal products. EUR-Lex website. http://eur-lex.europa.eu/LexUriServ/LexUriServ.do?uri=OJ:L:2008:334:0007:0024:en:PDF. Accessed 4 June 2012.
43. Regulation (EC) No 470/2009 of 6 May 2009 laying down Community procedures for the establishment of residue limits of pharmacologically active substances in foodstuffs of animal origin, repealing Council Regulation (EEC) No 2377/90 and amending Directive 2001/82/EC of the European Parliament and of the Council and Regulation (EC) No. 726/2004 of the European Parliament and of the Council. EUR-Lex website. http://eur-lex.europa.eu/LexUriServ/LexUriServ.do?uri=OJ:L:2009:152:0011:0022:en:PDF. Accessed 4 June 2012.
44. Commission Regulation (EU) No 37/2010 of 22 December 2009 on pharmacologically active substances and their classification regarding maximum residue limits in foodstuffs of animal origin. EUR-Lex website. http://ec.europa.eu/health/files/eudralex/vol-5/reg_2010_37/reg_2010_37_en.pdf. Accessed 4 June 2012.
45. EMEA/CVMP/519714/2009-Rev 10, List of substances considered as not falling within the scope of Regulation (EC) No. 470/2009, with regard to residues of veterinary medicinal products in foodstuffs of animal origin. EMA website. www.ema.europa.eu/docs/en_GB/document_library/Regulatory_and_procedural_guideline/2009/10/WC500004958.pdf. Accessed 4 June 2012.
46. COM (2000) 806, *Communication from the Commission to the Council and the European Parliament—Availability of Veterinary Medicinal Products* (Brussels, 5 December 2000). EUR-Lex website. http://eur-lex.europa.eu/LexUriServ/LexUriServ.do?uri=COM:2000:0806:FIN:EN:PDF. Accessed 4 June 2012.
47. EMEA/CVMP/477/03, *Position paper regarding the availability of products for minor uses and minor species (MUMS)* (14 July 2004). Federation of Veterinarians in Europe website. www.fve.org/veterinary/pdf/medicines/emea_position_paper_mums_2004.pdf. Accessed 4 June 2012.
48. *Guidance on the use of the Cascade.* Veterinary Medicines Guidance Note No. 13. Veterinary Medicines Directorate, 2011. UK Department for Environment, Food and Rural Affairs website. www.vmd.defra.gov.uk/pdf/vmgn/VMGNote13.pdf. Accessed 4 June 2012.
49. CVMP/153b/97, *Note for guidance on the establishment of maximum residue limits for* salmonidae *and other fin fish,* (CVMP adopted 15 January 1998). EMA website. www.ema.europa.eu/docs/en_GB/document_library/Scientific_guideline/2009/10/WC500004584.pdf. Accessed 4 June 2012.
50. EMEA/CVMP/SWP/66781/2005, *Guideline on Safety and residue data requirements for veterinary medicinal products intended for minor uses or minor species,* (CVMP adopted 20 July 2006). EMA website. www.ema.europa.eu/docs/en_GB/document_library/Scientific_guideline/2009/10/WC500004581.pdf. Accessed 4 June 2012.
51. EMEA/CVMP/187/00, *Note for guidance on the risk analysis approach for residues of veterinary medicinal products in food of animal origin* (10 January 2001). EMA website. www.ema.europa.eu/docs/en_GB/document_library/Scientific_guideline/2009/10/WC500004534.pdf. Accessed 4 June 2012.
52. EMEA/CVMP/069/02, *Implementation of the note for guidance on the risk analysis approach for residues of veterinary medicinal products in food of animal origin* (10 January 2002). EMA website. www.ema.europa.eu/docs/en_GB/document_library/Scientific_guideline/2009/10/WC500004535.pdf. Accessed 4 June 2012.
53. EMEA/CVMP/457/03, *Position Paper regarding the availability of veterinary medicinal products—extrapolation of MRLs* (10 December 2003). EMA website. www.ema.europa.eu/docs/en_GB/document_library/Position_statement/2009/10/WC500005164.pdf. Accessed 4 June 2012.
54. EudraVigilance Veterinary website. http://eudravigilance.ema.europa.eu/veterinary/index.html. Accessed 4 June 2012.
55. EMEA/CVMP/10418/2009-Rev 3. Combined VeDDRA List of Clinical Terms for Reporting Suspected Adverse Reactions in animals and humans. EMA website. www.ema.europa.eu/docs/en_GB/document_library/Scientific_guideline/2010/07/WC500094802.pdf. Accessed 4 June 2012.
56. EMEA/CVMP/044/99, *Guideline for the Conduct of Post Marketing Surveillance Studies of Veterinary Medicinal Products,* (CVMP adopted 19 April 2000). EMA website. www.ema.europa.eu/docs/en_GB/document_library/Scientific_guideline/2009/10/WC500005043.pdf. Accessed 4 June 2012.
57. Meillerais S. "A proposal to amend the veterinary pharmacovigilance legislation by means of the principles of 'Better Regulation'." *Regulatory Rapporteur,* November 2011, Vol 8, No 11, pp. 21–25. www.topra.org
58. Op cit 18.
59. Op cit 10.

Regulatory Affairs Comparative Matrix of the Regulations Across Product Lines

Authorities		
	Source*	*Authorities and Standards Organisations*
Devices	www.cen.eu http://meddev.net/ http://eur-lex.europa.eu www.ghtf.org/ www.imdrf.org/ www.iso.org www.iec.ch www.newapproach.org	European Committee for Standardisation European Commission—Enterprise—Medical Devices EUR-Lex—European law and other documentation Global Harmonization Task Force/International Medical Device Regulators Forum International Organization for Standardization International Electrotechnical Commission New Approach Directives and related harmonised standards
Drugs	www.edqm.eu www.ema.europa.eu www.europarl.eu.int http://ec.europa.eu http://ue.eu.int http://eur-lex.europa.eu www.ich.org/ www.hma.eu www.who.int/	European Directorate for the Quality of Medicines and HealthCare European Medicines Agency (EMA) European Parliament European Commission Council of the European Union EUR-Lex—European law and other documentation International Conference on Harmonisation Heads of Medicines Agencies World Health Organization
Biologics		**Same as drugs**

*These websites are accurate at the time of publication (15 June 2012).

Regulatory Affairs Comparative Matrix of the Regulations Across Product Lines

Major Regulations and Directives		
	Source	Directives and Regulations
Devices		• Directive 2007/47/EC amending Directive 90/385/EEC, Directive 93/42/EEC and Directive 98/8/EC • Medical Devices Directive (MDD) Directive 93/42/EEC • Active Implantable Medical Device Directive (AIMDD) Directive 90/385/EEC • In Vitro Diagnostic Device Directive (IVDD) Directive 98/79/EC • Blood Directive 2002/98/EC

Drugs		*The Rules Governing Medicinal Products in the European Union*: Medicinal Products for Human and Veterinary Use list both pharmaceutical legislation (Volumes 1 & 5) and various guidance documents (Volumes 2-4 and 6-10) (Volume # below)
		• Legislation:
		  ○ *Volume 1 EU pharmaceutical legislation for medicinal products for human use*
		  ○ *Volume 5 EU pharmaceutical legislation for medicinal products for veterinary use*
		• Guidelines:
		  ○ *Volume 2 Notice to applicants and regulatory guidelines for medicinal products for human use*
		  ○ *Volume 3 Scientific guidelines for medicinal products for human use*
		  ○ *Volume 4 Guidelines for good manufacturing practices for medicinal products for human and veterinary use*
		  ○ *Volume 6 Notice to applicants and regulatory guidelines for medicinal products for veterinary use*
		  ○ *Volume 7 Scientific guidelines for medicinal products for veterinary use*
		  ○ *Volume 8 Maximum residue limits*
		  ○ *Volume 9 Guidelines for pharmacovigilance for medicinal products for human and veterinary use*
		  ○ *Volume 10 Guidelines for clinical trials*
		Medicinal products for paediatric use, orphan, herbal medicinal products and advanced therapies are governed by specific rules.
		
		Directives and Regulations
		• Council Directive 2001/83/EC on the Community code relating to medicinal products of human use, as amended by:
		  ○ Directive 2002/98/EC
		  ○ Directive 2003/63/EC
		  ○ Directive 2004/24/EC
		  ○ Directive 2004/27/EC
		  ○ Regulation (EC) No 1901/2006
		  ○ Regulation (EC) No 1394/2007
		  ○ Directive 2008/29/EC
		  ○ Directive 2009/53/EC
		  ○ Directive 2009/120/EC
		  ○ Directive 2010/84/EU
		• Directive 2001/82/EC on the Community code relating to veterinary medicinal products, as amended by:
		  ○ Directive 2004/28/EC
		  ○ Directive 2009/9/EC
		  ○ Regulation (EC) No 470/2009
		  ○ Directive 2009/53/EC
		  ○ Regulation (EC) No 596/2009
		• Commission Regulation (EC) No 540/95—Reporting Serious Adverse Reactions
		• Commission Regulation (EU) No 1235/2010 amending Regulation (EC) No 726/2004
		
		• All ICH Guidelines

Biologics		**Same as drugs**

Regulatory Affairs Comparative Matrix of the Regulations Across Product Lines

Product Classification		
	Source	*Product Classification*

Devices	Directive 93/42/EEC and Directive 90/385/EEC Amended by Directive 2007/47FEC and Directive 98/79/EC	**Active Implantable Medical Devices**—all one classification
		
		Medical Device Classification
		• Class I—nonsterile, non-measuring
		• Class I sterile and/or Class I with a measuring function
		• Class IIa
		• Class IIb
		• Class III
		
		IVD Classification
		• Annex II List A and List B devices
		• Self-testing devices
		• Non-Annex II and Non-self-testing devices ("Other" IVDs)
		
		CE Marking
		• Symbolises the conformity of a product with the applicable European Community requirements imposed on the manufacturer
		• A declaration by the person responsible that the product conforms to all applicable Community provisions and the appropriate Conformity Assessment Procedures have been completed
		• CE Mark must be on the label when conforming products are placed on the market
		• CE Mark must be on the device itself or the sterile pack (where practicable and appropriate)
		• CE Mark must also be included on the instructions for use
		• CE Mark must:
		   ○ be legible
		   ○ be visible
		   ○ be indelible
		   ○ include Notified Body Number (except Class I and non-Annex II/non-self-testing IVDs)
		   ○ be in the exact proportions given in the directive
		• Custom-made and devices used in clinical trials need not bear the CE Mark
		
		Classification of Medical Devices is Based Upon:
		• Device's intended purpose
		• Duration of contact with patient
		   ○ transient—normally intended for continuous use for less than 60 minutes
		   ○ short-term—normally intended for continuous use for not more than 30 days
		   ○ long-term—normally intended for continuous use for more than 30 days
		• Invasiveness of device
		   ○ body orifice
		   ○ surgically invasive device—which penetrates inside the body through the surface of the body
		• Implantability of device
		• Active device (power source)
		• Devices incorporating a measuring function
		• In vitro diagnostic device
		
		Classification Rules—Applicable only to medical devices under Directive 93/42/EEC; to determine the class, apply the highest class for the characteristics or a combination of characteristics of the medical device:
		• noninvasive device—Rules 1, 2, 3, 4
		• invasive device—Rules 5, 6, 7, 8
		• active devices—Add Rules 9, 10, 11, 12
		• special rules—Rules 13, 14, 15, 16, 17, 18

Regulatory Affairs Professionals Society

Regulatory Affairs Comparative Matrix of the Regulations Across Product Lines

Product Classification

	Source	Product Classification
		The Rules (see full rules for exceptions) • Rule 1—Either does not touch patient or contacts only intact skin—Class I • Rule 2—All noninvasive devices intended for channelling or storing blood, body liquids or tissues, liquids or gases for the purpose of eventual infusion, administration or introduction into the body are Class IIa • Rule 3—All noninvasive devices intended for modifying the biological or chemical composition of blood, other body liquids or other liquids intended for infusion into the body are Class IIb • Rule 4—All noninvasive devices that come into contact with injured skin are in Class I if they are intended to be used as mechanical barriers, for compression or for absorption of exudates, or are in Class IIb if they are intended to be used principally with wounds that have breached the dermis and can only be healed by secondary intent • Rule 5—All invasive devices with respect to body orifices, other than surgically invasive devices, and that are not intended for connection to any active medical device are in Class I if they are intended for transient use, in Class IIa if they are intended for short-term use and in Class IIb if they are intended for long-term use • Rule 6—All surgically invasive devices intended for transient use are in Class IIa • Rule 7—All surgically invasive devices intended for short-term use are in Class IIa • Rule 8—All implantable devices and long-term surgically invasive devices are in Class IIb • Rule 9—All active therapeutic devices intended to administer or exchange energy are in Class IIa • Rule 10—All active devices intended for diagnosis are in Class IIa • Rule 11—All active devices intended to administer and/or remove medicines, body liquids or other substances to or from the body are in Class IIa • Rule 12—All other active devices are in Class I • Rule 13—All devices incorporating, as an integral part, a substance which, if used separately, can be considered to be a medicinal product as defined in Article 1 of Directive 65/65/EEC, and which is liable to act on the human body with action ancillary to that of the device, are in Class III • Rule 14—All devices used for contraception or the prevention of the transmission of sexually transmitted diseases are in Class IIb • Rule 15—All devices intended specifically to be used for disinfecting, cleaning, rinsing or, when appropriate, hydrating contact lenses are in Class IIb; those intended specifically for disinfecting medical devices are in Class IIa • Rule 16—Non-active devices specifically intended for recording of X-ray diagnostic images are in Class IIa • Rule 17—All devices manufactured utilising animal tissues or derivatives rendered non-viable are Class III except where such devices are intended to come in contact with intact skin only • Rule 18—Blood bags are in Class IIb
Drugs	Directive 2001/83/EC, as amended Directive 2001/82/EC, as amended	**Prescription Only** • are likely to present a danger either directly or indirectly, even when used correctly, if utilised without medical supervision or • are frequently and to a very wide extent used incorrectly, and as a result are likely to present a direct or indirect danger to human health or • contain substances or preparations thereof, the activity and/or side effects of which require further investigation or • are normally prescribed by a doctor to be administered parenterally **Nonprescription** • all drugs not subject to prescription (such as OTC) **Other Medicinal Products Include:** • orphan • herbal • medicinal products for paediatric use • advanced therapy medicinal products • veterinary medicinal products • radiopharmaceuticals
Biologics		**Same as drugs**

Format and Content of Applications

	Source	Format and Content of Applications

Devices	Directive 93/42/EEC and Directive 90/385/EEC Amended by Directive 2007/47/EC and Directive 98/79/EC
	
	ISO 14155
		Quality System Application to Notified Body Requirements
		• manufacturer name and address
		• class or category of products to be manufactured
		• statement that no application has been lodged with another Notified Body for the same product-related quality system
		• quality system documentation
		• how the manufacturer will fulfil the approved quality system obligations
		• how the manufacturer will maintain the approved quality system to ensure adequacy and efficacy
		• how the manufacturer will institute and maintain the postmarketing surveillance system
		• the manufacturer must ensure that products conform to the directive provisions and apply them at every stage from design to final controls through quality objectives, organisation of the business, procedures for monitoring and verifying the design of the products, inspection and quality assurance techniques, and appropriate tests and trials before, during and after manufacture
		
		Clinical Trial Documentation
		• A statement must be made to the Competent Authority of the Member State(s) where the trials are to take place prior to commencement of clinical trials, containing the following elements (in addition to elements required in application below):
		    ○ data allowing the devices to be identified
		    ○ an investigational plan identifying the purpose, scope and number of devices concerned
		    ○ name and doctor of institution responsible for the investigation
		    ○ the place, date of commencement and duration scheduled for the investigations
		    ○ a statement affirming the device in question complies with the Essential Requirements and stating what precautions have been used to protect the health and safety of the patient
		
		Design Dossier Application to Notified Body (Class 3, Annex II, List A and Self-testing IVDs)
		• manufacturer name and address
		• Authorised Representative name and address (if applicable)
		• a written declaration that the application has not been made to another Notified Body
		• general description of the device
		• design drawings
		• methods of manufacture envisioned (sterilisation, diagrams of parts, subassemblies, circuits, etc.)
		• description and explanations necessary for understanding the drawings and diagrams and the operation of the product
		• results of design calculations, investigations and technical tests carried out
		• design specifications, including standards applied
		• if standards are not being used, describe the test methods used
		• clinical trial data
		• draft instruction leaflet
		• additional data requested by Notified Body
		
		Modification to Device Design
		• The Notified Body issuing the EC Design Examination Certification or EC Type-Examination Certificate shall be notified of any modifications made to the approved design.
		• Supplementary approval must be obtained for any design modifications.
		
		Possible Decision Outcome From Notified Body
		• If the dossier complies with all relevant provisions of the directive, the device will be allowed to be placed on the market and an EC Design Examination Certification shall be issued. The certification shall contain:
		    ○ conclusions of the examination
		    ○ conditions of its validity
		    ○ data needed for identification of the approved design
		    ○ description of the product's intended use
		• Allowed to be placed on the market with restrictions
		• Refusal to allow the device to be placed on the market

Regulatory Affairs Comparative Matrix of the Regulations Across Product Lines

Format and Content of Applications		
	Source	Format and Content of Applications
		Renewal of the EC Design Examination Certification is applied for every five years. For restrictions and refusals, remedies are allowed. **CE Marking** • Once necessary Notified Body certificates are in place for quality systems and product evaluation and the necessary Technical Documentation is in place, the manufacturer will be able to sign a Declaration of Conformity and CE mark the product. • Class I medical devices or non-Annex II, non-self-testing IVDs may be self-declared to conform to the requirements of the necessary directive and placed on the market directly without intervention from a Notified Body.

Drugs	Directive 2001/83/EC, as amended
	
	Volume 2B, Notice to Applicants, Presentation and content of the dossier
		European Dossier
		
		Common Technical Document (CTD)
		The CTD is organised into five Modules. Module 1 is region specific. Modules 2, 3, 4 and 5 are intended to be common for all regions.
		• **Module I: Administrative and Prescribing Information**
		   ○ Comprehensive Table of Contents
		   ○ Country Specific Information
		   ○ Application Form
		   ○ Summary of Product Characteristics (SmPC), Labelling and Package Leaflet
		   ○ Information about the Experts
		   ○ Pharmacovigilance system description
		   ○ Risk management plan
		   ○ Environmental Assessment Risk
		
		• **Module 2: Common Technical Document Summaries**
		   ○ Table of Contents (Modules 2–5)
		   ○ Introduction
		   ○ Quality Overall Summary
		   ○ Nonclinical Overview
		   ○ Clinical Overview
		   ○ Nonclinical Written and Tabulated Summary
		      - Pharmacology
		      - Pharmacokinetics
		      - Toxicology
		   ○ Clinical Summary
		      - Biopharmaceutics and Associated Analytical Methods
		      - Clinical Pharmacology Studies
		      - Clinical Efficacy
		      - Clinical Safety
		      - Synopses of Individual Studies
		
		• **Module 3: Quality**
		   ○ Table of Contents (Module 3)
		   ○ Body of Data
		   ○ Literature References
		
		• **Module 4: Nonclinical Study Reports**
		   ○ Table of Contents (Module 4)
		   ○ Study Reports
		   ○ Literature References
		
		• **Module 5: Clinical Study Reports**
		   ○ Table of Contents (Module 5)
		   ○ Tabular Listing of All Clinical Studies
		   ○ Clinical Study Reports
		   ○ Literature References

Format and Content of Applications

	Source	Format and Content of Applications

	ICH: M4 (M4Q, M4E, M4S)— Common Technical Document	**Application Renewals**
		• A renewal application should be submitted no later than six months before the end of the five-year period. The following documentation should be submitted:
		    ○ an updated CTD: Module I, including current manufacturing authorisation and SmPC and other information such as dates of authorisation in all Member States, chronological list of all the variations of any type approved since the grant of the marketing authorisation or last renewal, including the CHMP opinion number
		    ○ an updated Module 2 (2.3 Quality overview and 2.5 Clinical overview)
		    ○ Module 5: Required PSURs, including all relevant pharmacovigilance data and proposals for any subsequent changes in the SmPC
		    ○ update of studies requested in the CHMP opinion

Biologics	Volume 2B, Notice to Applicants	**Same as drugs (with some specific extra information)** Extra information required for biotech products covers such topics as schematic amino acid sequence, cell bank and cell culture, harvest(s), purification and modification reactions, filling, storage and shipping conditions, among others.

Regulatory Affairs Comparative Matrix of the Regulations Across Product Lines

Marketing Authorisation Procedures			
		Source	Marketing Authorisation Procedures
	Devices	Directive 93/42/EEC and Directive 90/385/EEC Amended by Directive 2007/47/EC and Directive 98/79/EC	CE marking is the only prerequisite to placing products on the EU market. While it is necessary to communicate with the national Competent Authorities when placing medical devices on the market—including all Class I and custom-made devices and, in some countries, Class IIa, Class IIb and Class III devices—this communication does not constitute or convey approval by these authorities.

Regulatory Affairs Comparative Matrix of the Regulations Across Product Lines

Marketing Authorisation Procedures

	Source	Marketing Authorisation Procedures
Drugs	Directive 2001/83/EC, as amended Regulation (EC) No 726/2004	**Marketing Authorisation Exempted for:** • medicinal products prepared on the basis of magisterial or official formula • medicinal products intended for research or clinical trials • intermediate products intended for further processing by an authorised manufacturer **Four Routes for Marketing Authorisation: National, Mutual Recognition, Decentralised and Centralised** **National Procedure** for Member States of European Union • Submit a marketing authorisation application (MAA) to only one Member State (usually targeted for the initial marketing authorisation or as a basis for the application to be mutually recognised by other Member States). • If recognition of the national authorisation is requested in another Member State, the Mutual Recognition procedure must be used. The Reference Member State (RMS) is the first Member State to which an application is submitted. Once marketing authorisation (MA) has been granted by the RMS, identical applications can be submitted to the Concerned Member States (CMS) requesting them to mutually recognise the MA already granted. An identical dossier translated into the language of the CMS should be submitted. **Mutual Recognition Procedure** • Submit an MAA in one Member State and, once the MA has been granted (serial), make applications in other Member States concerned requesting them to mutually recognise the MA already granted. Timeframe • RMS has 210 days from receipt of the application to issue a decision. • If the parallel procedure is used, CMS can suspend their decision until the RMS decision is issued. • CMS have 90 days to mutually recognise the RMS authorisation once the marketing authorisation holder (MAH) applies; CMS can also mutually recognise an application within 90 days without the MAH's request. MAH Must Ensure: • dossier is identical (including any approved variations) to that accepted by the RMS, or identify any additions • summary of product characteristics (SmPC) is identical • dossier and SmPC as submitted are identical in all CMS The Centralised Procedure may be used if concerns are raised that cannot be resolved within the 90-day period for mutual recognition.
	Regulation (EC) No 726/2004	**Decentralised Procedure** The Decentralised Procedure is used for medicinal products for which there is no existing MA in any EU Member State at the time of application. It covers all medicinal products not authorised in the EU (for which the Centralised Procedure is not mandatory). Like the Mutual Recognition Procedure, the applicant can select the RMS and list the CMS. The Decentralised Procedure was introduced by Directive 2004/27/EC. **Centralised Procedure** Council Regulation (EEC) No 2309/93 (now replaced by Regulation (EC) No 726/2004) created a centralised community procedure for the authorisation of medicinal products and established the European Medicines Agency (EMA). An MA granted under the Centralised Procedure is valid for the entire Community market.

	Regulation (EC) No 1234/2008	• *Obligatory* for:
		   ◦ Medicinal products developed by means of biotechnological processes such as:
		      - recombinant DNA technology
		      - hybridoma and monoclonal antibody methods
		   ◦ veterinary medicinal products, including those not derived from biotechnology, intended primarily for use as performance enhancers
		   ◦ orphan medicinal products

Regulatory Affairs Professionals Society

Regulatory Affairs Comparative Matrix of the Regulations Across Product Lines

	Marketing Authorisation Procedures	
	Source	Marketing Authorisation Procedures
		<ul><li>medicinal products containing a new active substance intended for the treatment of - acquired immune deficiency syndrome (AIDS) - cancer - neurodegenerative disorders - diabetes</li></ul>• *Optional* for the following, where it can be demonstrated that central registration is an added value for the community:<ul><li>innovative products</li><li>has a significant benefit for the society; this also applies to OTC products intended for human use</li></ul>**Submission and Dossier Evaluation** • Submit an application to EMA in all official EU languages. • Scientific evaluation is carried out by Committee for Medicinal Products for Human Use (CHMP), which prepares and issues a scientific opinion within 210 days after receiving the dossier. • The opinion is sent to the European Commission, which drafts a decision and consults with a Standing Committee. **Potential Decisions** • product is approvable • product would be approvable • major deficiencies identified and approval unlikely (this can be appealed within 15 days) Usually, the European Commission will adopt the decision. If favourable, an MA will be granted. The Community Marketing Authorisation is valid in all Member States and confers the same rights and obligations in each of the Member States as if granted by that Member State. **Variations to an Approved Marketing Authorisation** **Type IA and Type IB** Type IA notifications are listed in Annex II of Regulation (EC) No 1234/2008. A variation that is not an extension and whose classification is undetermined after application of the rules provided for in Regulation (EC) No 1234/2008 shall by default be considered a minor variation of Type IB. These types of variations concern an amendment to the contents of a document as they were at the moment of the decision on the marketing authorisation. **Type II** Any change to the documentation proposed by the MAH, which is not a Type IA or Type IB notification and is not regarded as an extension to the MA, is considered a Type II variation. Changes that require a new application procedure are defined in Annex II of the regulations. Type II variations are listed in Annex II of Regulation (EC) No 1234/2008. **Urgent Safety Restriction** An Urgent Safety Restriction can only be used by the applicant or holder of a certificate of registration to amend the package insert of a medicinal product based on new information that has a bearing on the safe use of the product. It involves an interim change to product information by the MAH restricting the indication(s), and/or dosage, and/or target species of the medicinal product; or adding a contraindication and/or warning due to new information having a bearing on the safe use of the product. Such an urgent safety restriction may be imposed by either the MAH or by the Competent Authorities. **Extension Applications** An application for an extension to the MA can be made, provided the conditions reflected in Annex I of Regulation (EC) No 1234/2008 are met. These applications fall outside the scope of the definition of a variation to an MA and, consequently, such applications are examined by the Competent Authority/Community in accordance with the procedure for granting of a new MA. An extension or a modification of the existing MA will, therefore, have to be granted by the Competent Authority/Community. Further guidance on whether a change leads to a new application or variation can be found in the EC guidance, *Categorisation of New Application Versus Variations Applications*. **Action by Application** The detailed actions for each type of variation and procedure are listed in Regulation (EC) No 1234/2008.

Marketing Authorisation Procedures

	Source	Marketing Authorisation Procedures

Biologics	Directive 2001/83/EC, as amended Annex of Regulation (EC) No 726/2004	New biologics can be submitted through the Mutual Recognition or Centralised Procedure like drugs (see above) with some restrictions (below).
		
		Centralised Procedure is *Optional* for:
		• innovative products with a clear added value
		• product that has a significant benefit for the society; this also applies to OTC products intended for human use
		
		Centralised Procedure is *Obligatory* for:
		• Medicinal products developed by means of biotechnological processes such as:
		   o recombinant DNA technology
		   o hybridoma and monoclonal antibody methods
		• Veterinary medicinal products, including those not derived from biotechnology, intended primarily for use as performance enhancers
		• Orphan medicinal products
		• Medicinal products containing a new active substance intended for the treatment of
		   o acquired immune deficiency syndrome (AIDS)
		   o cancer
		   o neurodegenerative disorders, and
		   o diabetes
		
		Variations/Changes (same as drugs)

Regulatory Affairs Comparative Matrix of the Regulations Across Product Lines

Requirements for Clinical Investigations/Investigators (GCP)		
	Source	Requirements for Clinical Investigations
Devices	ISO 14155 Directive 93/42/EEC and Directive 90/385/EEC Amended by Directive 2007/47/EC and Directive 98/79/EC	**Notification/Approval Prior to Trial Initiation** • The manufacturer or Authorised Representative must submit a statement to the Competent Authority of its intention to conduct a clinical trial with a medical device 60 days prior to commencement. • A clinical trial can begin 60 days after notification unless the Competent Authorities have notified the manufacturer that clinical trials cannot begin. • No clinical trial can begin until Ethics Committee approval is also obtained. **Purpose of a Clinical Investigation** • Verify that, under normal conditions of use, the device's performance complies with the conditions indicated in the statement required for clinical investigations. • Determine any undesirable side effects, under normal conditions of use, and assess whether they are acceptable risks with regard to the device's intended performance. **Ethics** • All clinical trials must be conducted according to the Declaration of Helsinki. **Methods** • Investigational plan must be designed to confirm or refute the claim for the device. • An adequate number of observations should be included to guarantee the scientific validity of the conclusions. • Procedures used to perform the investigation must be appropriate to the device being investigated. • The clinical investigation must have equivalent circumstances to the device's normal conditions of use. • All features, including the device's safety and performance and its effects on patients, must be examined. • All adverse events should be recorded. • The clinical investigation should be performed by a qualified medical specialist in an appropriate environment. • The qualified medical specialist shall have access to the technical data regarding the device. **Literature Review as Basis for Approval (for nonimplantable or devices equivalent to existing CE-marked devices)** • identify hazards in the clinical part of the risk analysis • published literature should be taken from recognised scientific publications including unfavourable and favourable data • other scientific data including in vitro and bench testing • documented expert opinions • description of the device and any variants • product specifications • data that may have been submitted to regulatory bodies for approval **Adverse Event Reporting** All serious adverse events must be fully recorded and immediately notified to all Competent Authorities of the Member States in which the clinical investigation is being performed.

Regulatory Affairs Comparative Matrix of the Regulations Across Product Lines

Requirements for Clinical Investigations/Investigators (GCP)

	Source	Requirements for Clinical Investigations

Drugs	*Clinical Trials Directive 2001/20/EC*
	
	Directive 2001/83/EC, as amended
	ICH E1, E2A, E2B, E2F, E3, E4, E5, E6, E7, E8, E9, E10, E11
		Protection of Subjects
		• Right to privacy, integrity and withdrawal at any time is required.
		• For children and incapacitated adults, legal representative consent is required and can be revoked at any time (no incentives are allowed in this population).
		• Provision should be taken to minimise pain, fear, risk and distress.
		• All clinical trials must be conducted according to the Declaration of Helsinki.
		
		Ethics Committee Responsibilities
		• Review of trial design
		• Review trial risk:benefit evaluation
		• Review of informed consent
		• Review Investigator's Brochure and protocol
		• Review patient recruitment
		• Review quality of investigator, staff and facilities
		• Provision for compensation in case of injury
		• Review all information provided to patient before consent
		• Review of patient or investigator incentives
		• An opinion will be issued in 60 days after a valid application is received
		   ○ The clock stops if additional information is requested from the sponsor.
		• Metacentre trials in one Member State can obtain one Ethics Committee approval
		• Multi-state trials require a single Ethics Committee opinion per Member State
		
		Regulatory Notification/Approval Prior to Trial Initiation
		• Parallel notification/submission of regulatory authority and Ethics Committee is allowed.
		• No clinical trial can begin until Ethics Committee approval is obtained.
		• The regulatory authority has 60 days from the submission of a valid dossier to notify the sponsor of no objections or nonacceptance of dossier.
		   ○ If no objections are raised after 60 days, the trial shall be authorised.
		   ○ If grounds for nonacceptance are issued, a sponsor can file a one-time amendment.
		   ○ If no amendment is filed, the request is rejected.
		• The notification time cannot be extended except for certain biologic products (see below).
		
		Conduct of Trials
		• Substantial protocol amendments need both regulatory and Ethics Committee approval before being implemented. Substantial amendments include:
		   ○ safety
		   ○ interpretation of scientific documents
		   ○ duration of the trial
		   ○ number of doses
		   ○ clinical/biological examinations
		• Ethics Committee opinion on amendments should be issued in 35 days.
		• End of clinical trial—Competent Authorities and Ethics Committee need to be notified of the end of a clinical trial within 90 days.
		• Early termination of a clinical trial—Competent Authorities and Ethics Committee need to be notified of the early termination of a clinical trial within 15 days.
		• Trial must comply with Good Clinical Practice (GCP).

Regulatory Affairs Comparative Matrix of the Regulations Across Product Lines

Requirements for Clinical Investigations/Investigators (GCP)		
	Source	Requirements for Clinical Investigations
		Suspension of a Trial • A trial may be prohibited or suspended if the Member State has doubts about the trial's safety or scientific validity or if the conditions for the request for authorisation are not being met. • Unless there is imminent risk, the sponsor or investigator will be given a week to respond to the matter. • If the Competent Authority has objective grounds for considering that the sponsor or investigator or any other person involved in the conduct of the clinical trial is no longer meeting his obligations, it shall inform the sponsor or investigator of the actions needed to remedy the situation. The Competent Authority also will notify the Ethics Committee and the other Competent Authorities of its actions. **Manufacture of Clinical Supplies (See GMP Section)** • Clinical supply manufacturer must comply with GMP requirements. • A manufacturing authorisation should have been granted. • Import/free movement is authorised upon certification by a Qualified Person. **Adverse Event Reporting** • The investigator shall report all serious adverse events to the sponsor immediately, except those that the protocol or Investigator's Brochure identifies as not requiring immediate reporting. • The immediate report shall be followed by detailed, written reports. • The immediate and follow-up written reports shall identify subjects by unique code numbers. • Adverse events or laboratory abnormalities identified in the protocol as critical to safety evaluations shall be reported to the sponsor according to the reporting requirements and within the time periods specified within the protocol. • Detailed records shall be kept for all adverse events; these records shall be submitted to the Member States (if requested) in whose territory the clinical trial is being conducted. **Serious Adverse Reaction Notification** • The sponsor shall ensure that all relevant information about serious unexpected adverse reactions that are fatal or life-threatening is recorded and reported as soon as possible to the Competent Authorities in all Member States concerned and to the Ethics Committee, no later than seven days after learning about the event, and a follow-up report with all relevant information is submitted within an additional eight days. • All other serious adverse reactions shall be reported to the Competent Authorities in all Member States concerned and to the Ethics Committee, as soon as possible but with a maximum of 15 days after the sponsor first learns of the event. • Each Member State shall ensure that all suspected unexpected serious adverse reactions are recorded. • The sponsor shall inform all investigators of unexpected serious adverse reactions. • Once a year, during the conduct of the clinical trial, the sponsor shall provide the Member States and Ethics Committee in whose territory the clinical trial is being conducted with a list of all suspected serious adverse reactions that have occurred during the period and a report of the subjects' safety (Development Safety Update Report (DSUR)).

Requirements for Clinical Investigations/Investigators (GCP)

	Source	Requirements for Clinical Investigations
Biologics	*Clinical Trials Directive 2001/20/EC* *Directive 2001/83/EC, as amended*	**Same as drugs (except where noted below)** **Ethics Committee Responsibilities** • An opinion will be issued 60 days after a valid application is received, except for gene or cell therapy where an extension of 30 days is granted. • There is no set time limit for clinical trial notification for clinical trials involving gene therapy, cell therapy, xenogeneic cell therapy, biotechnology-derived or any biological product. • A trial cannot begin until a favourable opinion is issued by an Ethics Committee. **Notification/Approval Prior to Trial Initiation** • A dossier can be submitted to the Competent Authorities at the same time it is submitted to the Ethics Committee. • For classic medicinal products, a clinical trial can be initiated 60 days after submission of the dossier. • Regulatory authorisation is needed to begin a clinical trial and is granted within 90 days for gene therapy, cell therapy products, genetically modified organisms and xenogeneic cell therapy medicinal products, unless the clock is stopped for additional information requests. An additional 90 days may be added to this timeline if experts are consulted.

Reporting/Recordkeeping Requirements for Clinical Investigators and Sponsors

	Source	Reporting/Recordkeeping Requirements for Clinical Investigators
Devices	ISO 14155	• ISO 14155-1 states that it should be the sponsor's responsibility to "collect, store, guard and ensure completion by relevant parties of all the documentation from clinical investigations. This shall include: 　o clinical Investigator's Brochure 　o clinical investigation plan 　o CVs for all investigators 　o name of the institution(s) where investigation will be held 　o Ethics Committee opinion 　o correspondence with authorities 　o agreements between sponsor and investigator 　o informed consent forms 　o case report forms 　o forms for reporting adverse incidents 　o names/contact details of monitor(s) 　o copies of signed and dated case report forms 　o records of any adverse incidents reported during the investigation 　o statistical analyses and underlying supporting data 　o final report • Arrangements for the storage of such records should be part of the sponsor/investigator agreement. • Since this type of data supports the information put into the Technical File for devices, it should be retained for at least the same length of time as the rest of the Technical File (i.e., the lifetime of the device plus five years minimum). The sponsor should therefore specify the retention period required.
Drugs	Directive 2001/83/EC, as amended	General • The sponsor shall arrange with the investigator for the retention of patient identification codes for at least 15 years after the completion or discontinuation of the trial. • Patient files and source data shall be kept for the maximum period of time permitted by the hospital, institution or private practice. • The sponsor or other owner of the data shall retain all other documentation pertaining to the trial for as long as the product is authorised and shall include: 　o clinical protocol 　o details of the investigational product, including the reference medicinal product and/or the placebo used 　o Standard Operating Procedures 　o all written opinions on the protocol and procedures 　o Investigator's Brochure 　o case report forms on each trial subject 　o final study report 　o audit certificate(s), if available • The final report shall be retained by the sponsor or subsequent owner for five years after the product is no longer authorised (discontinued marketing).
Biologics		Same as drugs

Packaging and Labelling

	Source	Labelling

Devices	Directive 93/42/EEC and Directive 90/385/EEC Amended by Directive 2007/47/EC and Directive 98/79/EC
	
	ISO/TC 210 *Medical Device Symbols*
	
	CEN/TC 257 *Symbols for Medical Devices*
	
	ISO/TC 145 ISO 7000 *Graphical Symbols*
	
	ISO 15223-1:2007
	ISO 15223-2:2010
	
	EN 980:2008
	
	Guidance on Labelling for Medical Devices (GHTF)
	
	AIMDD Annex 1 Essential requirements 12–15
	
	MDD Annex 1 Essential requirement 13
	
	IVDD Annex 1 Essential requirement 8
		Information Supplied By the Manufacturer Must Include:
		
		Labelling on device, outer packaging and instructions for use must include:
		• manufacturer name or trade name and address
		• if imported into the Community
		• Authorised Representative (if appropriate)
		• device and packaging contents identification
		• "Sterile" when appropriate
		• batch code or serial number preceded by the word, "LOT"
		• use-by date specified by year and month
		• indication that the device is for single use (if appropriate)
		• "Custom-made device" if the device is custom made
		• "Exclusively for clinical investigations" if device is intended for clinical investigations
		• any special storage and/or handling conditions
		• any special operating instructions
		• any warnings and/or precautions to take
		• year of manufacture for active devices (this may be included in the serial or batch number)
		• sterilisation method (where applicable)
		• intended purpose of the device (unless obvious)
		• identification of device components (when reasonable and practical)
		
		Instructions for Use
		• may be omitted for Class I and Class IIa devices if the manufacturer can ensure that they can be used safely without instructions
		
		In addition to requirements (above), labelling must contain, when practical:
		• device performance standards
		• undesirable side effects
		• whether the device must be installed or used with other components in order to operate as required for its intended purpose
		• how to verify the device is properly installed and can operate safely and correctly
		• nature and frequency of needed maintenance, including calibration needed to ensure that the device operates properly and safely at all times
		• information on how to avoid certain risks in connection with implantation of devices (where appropriate)
		• if the device is reusable, how to process the device to allow for re-use
		
		Use-By Date
		• All medical devices must contain a statement about any time limitations on their safe use.
		• The "use-by" time limit relates to the period before the first use of the device and does not relate to the number or period of subsequent uses.
		• The manufacturer must demonstrate via relevant performance that device characteristics are maintained over the claimed shelf-life reflected by the "use-by" date, by:
		   ○ prospective studies on accelerated aging, validated with real time degradation correlation
		   ○ retrospective studies using real time experience, involving testing of stored samples, review of complaints history or published literature
		• The lack of a "use-by" date implicitly implies that the product has an infinite shelf life.

Regulatory Affairs Comparative Matrix of the Regulations Across Product Lines

Packaging and Labelling		
	Source	Labelling

Drugs	Directive 2001/83/EC, as amended
	
	ICH Q7 *Good Manufacturing Practices for Active Pharmaceutical Ingredients*
		Controlled at the National Level
		
		All labelling should be easily legible, clearly comprehensible and indelible and shall appear in the official language(s) of the Member State where the medicinal product is placed on the market.
		
		Investigational Products
		• Particulars must be in at least the language of the Member State on outer packaging and on the immediate packaging if there is no outer packaging.
		
		Outer Pack Required Information
		• product name (trade name, international nonproprietary name)
		• strength
		• pharmaceutical form
		• qualitative and quantitative composition of active ingredients
		• qualitative list of excipients
		• method and route of administration
		• expiry date in clear terms (month/year)
		• storage conditions
		• precautions for disposal of unused product or waste materials
		• MAH name and address
		• special warnings (e.g., "keep out of reach of children")
		• manufacturer's batch number
		• marketing authorisation number
		• instructions for self-medication (where applicable)
		• may include symbols or pictograms designed to clarify certain information
		• trade name and strength in Braille
		
		Minimum Requirement on Immediate Packaging
		• product trade name
		• strength and route of administration
		• method of administration
		• expiry date of the batch
		• batch number
		• contents (weight, volume and dosage)
		
		Package or User Leaflet Must Contain:
		• Product identification (name and common name)
		• Strength
		• Quantitative composition of the active ingredient
		• Quantitative list of excipients
		• Contents per dose
		• Product's group
		• MAH name and address
		• Therapeutic indications
		• Contraindications
		• Precautions
		• Interactions
		• Warnings
		• Instructions for Use
		   o dosage
		   o method
		   o frequency
		   o overdose
		   o side effects
		   o warning regarding expiry and storage
		   o date of last revision

Packaging and Labelling

	Source	Labelling

		Centralised Procedure Marketing Authorisation
		• Package leaflet and all packaging materials must be identical except for language.
		• Identical colour schemes, layout and design must be used across the EU.
		• Information specific to Member State is allowed on outer pack inside a blue box.
		
		Mutual Recognition Marketing Authorisation
		• Minor differences are accepted among the package leaflet, packaging and labelling materials.
		• The SmPC (between applications) needs to be identical except the:
		    ○ MAH
		    ○ authorisation number
		    ○ pack-size presentation used in the specific country
		• **Differences are accepted for:**
		    ○ label
		    ○ package/patient leaflet
		    ○ outer pack

Biologics		**Same as drugs**

Regulatory Affairs Comparative Matrix of the Regulations Across Product Lines

Promotion and Advertising		
	Source	Promotion and Advertising
Devices	No specific documented requirements	Marketing claims must match those in the clinical trial and technical documentation. Advertising is regulated in some countries through the national transpositions of the directives.

Drugs	Directive 2001/83/EC, as amended	Controlled at the National Level
		
		Advertising Directive Covers
		• Advertising to healthcare professionals and suppliers
		  ○ compliance with the product's SmPC
		  ○ compliance with supply classification
		• Behaviour of sales representatives
		  ○ representatives need to be trained correctly
		  ○ they shall supply the SmPC to the physician
		  ○ they shall supply information on price and reimbursement to the physician
		• Supply of samples to physicians
		  ○ is limited
		  ○ written request from the physician is needed
		  ○ only the smallest pack size available labelled, "Free Sample—Not for Sale" will be provided
		  ○ all samples need to be traceable
		• Advantages granted to physicians encouraging prescriptions
		• Sponsorship of meetings and participation by healthcare professionals including travel expenses
		
		A company must provide to the authority models of advertisement issued by the company, stating to whom it was sent and how the advertisement was distributed.
		
		Advertising prescription products to the public is prohibited.

Biologics		**Same as drugs**

Postmarketing Surveillance and Pharmacovigilance

	Source	Form	Postmarketing Surveillance and Pharmacovigilance

Devices	*Guideline on the Medical Device Vigilance System (MEDDEV 2.12/1)*
	
	Clinical Evaluation— Postmarket Clinical Follow-up (MEDDEV 2.12/2)
	
	Guidance on how to handle information concerning vigilance reports related to medical devices
	
	Volume 9, Pharmacovigilance
			Postmarketing surveillance covers the requirement to have a proactive systematic procedure in place to gather information about the product in its postmarketing phase. This should include a process on how to handle vigilance incidents that need to be reported to the Competent Authorities.
			
			Postmarketing surveillance data can come from complaint monitoring, feedback from sales representatives, reports from regulatory authorities, literature reviews and service/repair information.
			
			For vigilance incidents, the manufacturer makes an initial report to the Competent Authority for recording and evaluation. Each initial report should lead to a final report, but not every initial report will lead to a corrective action.
			
			Corrective action includes:
			• device recall
			• issue of Advisory Notice
			• additional surveillance/modification of devices in use
			• modification to future device design
			• components or manufacturing process
			• modification to labelling or instructions for use
			
			Submit a vigilance report to the Competent Authority when:
			• An incident (or potential incident) has occurred that led to:
			   ○ a death
			   ○ a serious deterioration in health (the determination of serious should be made in consultation with a medical practitioner)
			      - life-threatening illness or injury
			      - permanent impairment of a body function or permanent damage to a body structure
			      - condition necessitating medical or surgical intervention to prevent permanent impairment of a body function or permanent damage to a body structure
			• The manufacturer's device is associated with the incident:
			   ○ incident led, or might have led, to one of the following outcomes:
			      - death of a patient, user or other person
			      - serious injury of a patient, user or other person
			
			A vigilance report does not need to be submitted when:
			• adverse incident is caused by patient conditions (e.g., pre-existing conditions)
			• service life of medical device exceeded
			• protection against a fault functioned correctly
			• remote likelihood of occurrence of death or serious injury
			• expected and foreseeable side effects
			• adverse incident described in advisory notice
			• reporting exemption granted by Competent Authority
			
			An Initial Report must contain:
			• Manufacturer's name, address, contact point, telephone and fax number
			• Date the incident came to the attention of the manufacturer
			• Medical device
			   ○ commercial name
			   ○ catalogue number/model
			   ○ serial/batch/lot number
			   ○ software version
			   ○ identification number of the Notified Body involved in the Conformity Assessment Procedure (if any) and the dates of attestation(s)

Postmarketing Surveillance and Pharmacovigilance

Source	Form	Postmarketing Surveillance and Pharmacovigilance
		<ul><li>Associated devices and/or accessories involved in the incident</li><li>Details of the incident (to the extent known) including date, patient and user outcome</li><li>Current location of the device involved in the incident (if known)</li><li>Contact point of user where incident occurred</li><li>Manufacturer's preliminary investigation and comments</li><li>Manufacturer's proposed next action and timeframe</li><li>Statement of whether the manufacturer is aware of similar incidents having an impact on the current report, and when and to whom these were reported</li><li>Any other EEA state in which the device is known to be on sale</li></ul> **Reporting Time Frames (based on the guidelines)** Incidents: 10 Calendar Days Near Incidents: 30 Calendar Days **Typical events are:**<ul><li>malfunction or deterioration in the characteristics of performance</li><li>inadequate design or manufacture</li><li>inaccuracy of labelling, Instructions for Use and/or promotional materials</li><li>significant health concern</li><li>other information becoming available</li></ul> If the initial report is made by telephone or fax, it must be followed up by a written confirmation (hard copy posted to Competent Authority). The Competent Authority will acknowledge receipt of the report. Reports can be made to the manufacturer or the Competent Authority or both. Member States may supplement reports received from manufacturers with reports from other sources.

Regulatory Affairs Comparative Matrix of the Regulations Across Product Lines

Postmarketing Surveillance and Pharmacovigilance

	Source	Form	Postmarketing Surveillance and Pharmacovigilance
Drugs	Directive 2001/83/EC, as amended, including Directive 2010/84/EU as regards Pharmacovigilance Regulation (EU) No 1235/2010 amending, as regards pharmacovigilance of medicinal products for human use, Regulation (EC) No 726/2004 ICH E2A: *Clinical Safety Data Management*	Individual Case Safety Reports (ICSRs)	**System Requirements and Non-compliance** All MAHs must have an appropriate pharmacovigilance system in place (with the 2010 regulation, must have a Pharmacovigilance System Master File (PSMF) permanently available for submission or inspection by the national Competent Authority). The system should be capable of: • expedited reporting • periodic safety update reporting • responding to requests for information from Competent Authorities • handling urgent safety restrictions for safety variations • continuously monitoring the authorised medicinal product's safety profile and notifying Competent Authorities and healthcare professionals of changes to the product's benefits/risks • meeting CHMP commitments (where MAHs hold a centralised marketing authorisation) • internal audit of the pharmacovigilance system **Qualified Person Responsible for Pharmacovigilance** Person responsible for placing a medicinal product on the market shall have a qualified person for pharmacovigilance. This person shall be responsible for: • establishing and maintaining a system to ensure that all suspected adverse reactions are reported • preparing a report within 15 days to the Competent Authorities • addressing any requests made for additional information by the Competent Authorities **Serious Adverse Reaction** An adverse reaction that: • results in death • is life-threatening • requires in-patient hospitalisation or prolongation of existing hospitalisation • results in persistent or significant disability or incapacity • is a congenital anomaly/birth defect **Unexpected Adverse Reaction** An adverse reaction, the nature, severity or outcome of which is not consistent with the SmPC. **Expedited Adverse Drug Reactions** • MAHs are required to report all suspected serious adverse drug reactions (causal relationship) occurring within and outside of the EU and Member States within 15 days through the EudraVigilance system, EU's electronic database for suspected adverse reactions. **PSURs** A periodic safety update report (PSUR) is intended to provide an update of a medicinal product's worldwide safety experience to Competent Authorities at defined times, postauthorisation. A worldwide safety update summary should be prepared and submitted to the Competent Authorities and EMA for all medicinal products authorised at the following intervals unless the MA makes different provisions: • at least every six months during the first two years following authorisation • every six months during the first two years after being placed on the market • once a year for the following two years • afterward, every three years or as requested by the Competent Authority Each safety report should cover the period of time since the last update report and should be submitted within 60 days of the data-lock point.
Biologics			Same as drugs

Regulatory Affairs Professionals Society

Quality Management Systems/Good Manufacturing Practices (GMPs)

	Source	GMP

Devices	ISO 9001:2000
	
	ISO 13488:1996
	
	ISO 13485:2003
	
	Regulatory Auditing of Quality Management Systems of Medical Device Manufacturers (www.ghtf.org: SG4/84:2010, SG4/83:2010, SG4/N30:2010, SG4/N28R4:2008, SG4/N33R16:2007, SG4 (00) 3)
	
	ISO 19011:2011 *Guidelines for auditing management systems*
	
	ISO 9000:2000 *Quality Management Systems—Fundamentals and Vocabulary*
	
	ISO 14971 *Application of Risk Management to Medical Devices*
	
	Council Directive 90/385/EEC
	
	Directive 93/42/EEC and Directive 90/385/EEC Amended by Directive 2007/47/EC and Directive 98/79/EC
	
	EN 980 *Symbols to be used in labelling of medical devices*
		A manufacturer must be audited by a Notified Body (for all AIMDs, Class I sterile and Class I with measuring function, Class IIa, Class IIb and Class III medical devices, and Annex II listed and self-test IVDs) to ensure compliance with the quality system.
		
		Quality System
		Mandatory documented procedures and mandatory records in accordance with ISO 13485/13488:1996.
		
		Design
		• devices must be designed to minimise risk
		• all devices must be designed to comply with the Essential Requirements of the applicable directive(s)
		• manufacturing, storage and quality control criteria
		• quality control
		
		Symbols
		• "Sterile" (on a sterile pack)
		• sterilisation method
		• "Do not re-use"
		• lot or serial number
		• use by date
		• manufacturer
		
		Device Technical Documentation
		• product documentation and related data
		• description of the device and any variants
		• product specifications
		• data that may have been submitted to regulatory bodies for approval
		
		Risk Analysis
		• identification and documentation of any potential hazards that may exist with the device design and how that risk has been minimised or eliminated
		• record of how long the device has been in use, number of units sold, and number and classification of complaints received
		• critical appraisal of the scientific literature
		
		Documentation must uniformly interpret quality policies and procedures, such as quality programs, quality plans, quality manuals and quality records. Documentation must include:
		• manufacturer's quality objectives
		• organisational structure of business
		• procedures for monitoring and verifying product design
		• appropriate tests used before, during and after production
		
		The manufacturer shall inform the Notified Body of any plans to alter the system.
		
		Design changes should be reported to the Notified Body when "substantial" or "significant."
		• All changes made to a device should be documented and classified as substantial or not substantial.
		• Changes considered "substantial" are:
		   o product changes that would affect conformity with the Essential Requirements or the conditions prescribed for the intended use
		   o changes to the quality system that would affect compliance of the device or would mean an addition to the product range covered by the quality system
		• The manufacturer shall inform the Notified Body of all planned substantial changes.
		
		All documents must be kept for five years after the last date of manufacture of the product. All records should be kept for the foreseen device lifetime but not less than two years from the date of delivery.

Regulatory Affairs Comparative Matrix of the Regulations Across Product Lines

Quality Management Systems/Good Manufacturing Practices (GMPs)		
	Source	GMP
Drugs	*Volume 4, Good manufacturing practice (GMP) Guidelines* Directive 2001/83/EC and 2001/82/EC, as amended. Directive 2003/94/EC Directive 91/412/EEC ICH Q1A, Q1B, Q1C, Q1D, Q1E, Q1F, Q2(R1), Q3A, Q3C, Q6A, Q6B, Q7, Q8, Q9, Q10 Directive 2001/83/EC, as amended	Manufacturing authorisation is granted/maintained by the authority of the Member State. A Manufacturing Authorisation Application is granted for specific products and the facilities specified for their production. **GMP Requirements** • quality management (quality assurance, quality control) • personnel (key personnel, training, personnel hygiene) • documentation (required documents, specifications for starting and packing materials, specifications for intermediate and bulk products, specifications for finished products, manufacturing and validation processes, manufacturing formulae and processing instructions, packaging instructions, batch processing records, batch packaging records, procedures and records for: receipt, sampling and testing) • production (prevention of cross-contamination in production, validation, starting materials, processing operations: intermediate and bulk products, packaging materials, packaging operations, finished products, and rejected, recovered and returned materials) • quality control (good quality control laboratory practice, documentation, sampling, testing) • contract manufacture and analysis (the contract giver, the contract acceptor, the contract) • complaints and recalls • self inspection **GMP Requirements for Investigational Medicinal Products** • quality management (quality assurance, quality control) • personnel (key personnel, training, personnel hygiene) • premises and equipment • documentation (order, product specification file, manufacturing formulae and processing instructions, packaging instructions, labelling instructions, and manufacturing and packaging batch records) • production (starting materials, manufacturing operations, principles applicable to comparator product, randomisation code) • quality control • release of batches • free movement • contract manufacturer and contract analysis • complaints • recalls and returns • shipping, returns, destruction **Manufacturing authorisation** is based on compliance with the following: • identification of the medicinal product and pharmaceutical forms to be manufactured • name and address of manufacturing and control plants • suitability and adequacy of the facilities • equipment and premises must comply with legal requirements (production, control and storage) • have at the manufacturer's disposal the services of a Qualified Person, a staff complying with the manufacturing and control requirements of the Member State where the facilities are located • informing the authorities of any proposed changes to the product qualified person, facilities, equipment, processes, etc. • giving the Qualified Person the tools needed to fulfil his responsibilities • complying with the principles of GMP applicable in the EU The decision to grant manufacturing authorisation shall take place within 90 days of the initial application. All decisions regarding applications for changes to the current authorisation shall be made within 30 days. The clock will stop if the authority asks for additional information from the applicant.

Regulatory Affairs Comparative Matrix of the Regulations Across Product Lines

Quality Management Systems/Good Manufacturing Practices (GMPs)		
	Source	GMP

		Distribution
		• A distribution authorisation is needed to hold, supply or export medicinal products.
		• Member States grant distribution authorisations.
		• A distributor must comply with the following specific conditions:
		   o appropriate facilities and equipment to ensure adequate storage and distribution of the product
		   o a Qualified Person
		• A distributor can distribute products to all Member States.
		
		Qualified Person
		• A manufacturer must have at its disposal the permanent services of a Qualified Person who:
		   o ensures and certifies that each lot manufactured is produced in accordance with the manufacturing authorisation and that these certifications are recorded in a register that is to be made available during an inspection
		   o controls the quality of imported product

Biologics	*Volume 4, Good Manufacturing Practice (GMP) Guidelines* ICH same as drugs plus Q5A – Q5E	**Same as drugs, including:** **Biological Medicinal Products for Human Use** (microbial cultures, recombinant DNA or hybridoma techniques, extraction from biological tissues and propagation of live agents in embryos or animals) • personnel • premises and equipment • animal quarters and care • documentation (specifications for starting materials, specifications required for intermediate and bulk biological medicinal products) • production (starting materials, seed lot and cell bank system, operating principles) • quality control **Manufacturer of Radiopharmaceuticals** • personnel • premises and equipment • production • quality control • distribution and recalls **Manufacturer of Products Derived from Human Blood or Human Plasma** • quality management (quality assurance, blood collection control and procedures) • premises and equipment • blood collection • production and quality control (storage of blood products, testing, cleaning procedures, labelling, method validation) • fractionation/purification procedures (precipitation methods, solid phase and filtration methods) • retention of samples (kept for one year after expiry date with longest shelf-life) • cellular products and whole blood (quality monitoring, visual inspection)

Complaints

	Source	Complaints
Devices	*Guidance on the Quality Systems for the Design and Manufacture of Medical Devices* (GHTF) ISO 13485:2003, Clause 8.5.1	Any complaint received from the supplier about a product that either fails to conform to its specification or conforms to its specification but nevertheless causes a problem in use shall be recorded and investigated. **Complaint documentation system should include:**<ul><li>establish responsibility for complaint handling system</li><li>complaint evaluation</li><li>records and statistical summaries, to determine the major causes of complaints</li><li>documentation of any corrective action taken</li><li>desegregation and disposition, or reprocessing, of customer returns and faulty stock (with special attention given to decontamination)</li><li>filing of customer correspondence and other relevant records; define retention time for these items</li><li>determine if a death or serious injury occurred</li></ul>**Complaint and investigation documentation should include:**<ul><li>Product name</li><li>Date the complaint was received</li><li>Any control number used</li><li>Complainant name and address</li><li>Nature of the complaint</li><li>Results of the investigation including:<ul><li>corrective action taken</li><li>justification if no action was taken</li><li>dates of investigation</li><li>name of investigator</li><li>the reply (if any) to the complainant</li></ul></li></ul>

Regulatory Affairs Comparative Matrix of the Regulations Across Product Lines

Complaints

	Source	Complaints
Drugs	Directive 2001/83/EC, as amended Directive 2003/94/EC ICH Q7 *Good Manufacturing Practices for Active Pharmaceutical Ingredients*	All complaints and other information concerning potentially defective products must be reviewed carefully according to written procedures. **Complaint documentation system should include:** • designated person responsible for handling complaints and deciding measures to be taken, with sufficient supporting staff • written procedure describing the action to be taken, including the need to consider a recall (for a complaint concerning a possible product defect) • procedure for recording a complaint concerning a product defect with all the original details and a thorough investigation • if a product defect is discovered or suspected in a batch, consideration should be given to checking other batches in order to determine whether they are also affected • all decisions and measures taken as the result of a complaint should be recorded and referenced to the corresponding batch records • complaint records should be reviewed regularly for any indication of specific or recurring problems requiring attention and possibly the recall of marketed products • Competent Authorities should be informed if a manufacturer is considering action following possibly faulty manufacture, product deterioration or any other serious quality problems with a product **Complaint records should include:** • complainant name (title, where appropriate) and address • phone number of person submitting the complaint • date complaint is received • product name • complaint nature (including name and batch number) • action initially taken (including dates and identity of person taking the action) • any follow-up action taken • response provided to the originator of complaint (including date response sent) • final decision on intermediate, or batch or lot • results of the investigation including corrective action taken Records of complaints should be retained to evaluate trends, product-related frequencies and severity with a view to taking additional and, if appropriate, immediate corrective action. In the event of a serious or potentially life-threatening situation, local, national and/or international authorities should be informed and their advice sought. **Investigational Products** The conclusions of any investigation carried out in relation to a complaint should be discussed between the manufacturer and sponsor to assess any potential impact on the trial and on the product development.
Biologics		Same as drugs

Quality System Assessment/Inspection

	Source	Quality System Assessment/Inspection
Devices	*Regulatory Auditing of Quality Management Systems of Medical Device Manufacturers* (www.ghtf.org: SG4/84:2010, SG4/83:2010, SG4/N30:2010, SG4/N28R4:2008, SG4/N33R16:2007, SG4 (00) 3)	The manufacturer shall authorise the Notified Body to carry out all necessary inspections and shall supply it with all appropriate information, including: • quality system documentation • data stipulated in quality system relating to design, e.g., result of analyses, calculations, tests, etc. • data stipulated in quality system relating to manufacture, e.g., reports concerning inspections, tests, standardisations/calibrations and staff qualifications The Notified Body shall periodically carry out appropriate inspections and evaluations to ascertain whether the manufacturer is applying the approved quality systems. The manufacturer will receive a written evaluation report of the inspection from the Notified Body. The Notified Body may conduct an inspection of the manufacturer without notice. **Audits** A manufacturer will be audited to ensure compliance to the quality system. There are four types of audits: • initial audit • surveillance audit • special audit • unannounced audit
Drugs	Directive 2001/83/EC, as amended Regulation (EC) No 726/2004	**Good Clinical Practice/Manufacturing Audits** • The Competent Authority of a Member State can inspect: 　o clinical trial/investigator's site 　o investigational product manufacturing site 　o laboratory used for analysis during the clinical trial 　o sponsor's premises • A report will be prepared after the inspection and made available to the sponsor. • Inspection findings will be shared and recognised by all Member States. **GMP Inspections** for manufacturing sites and control laboratories are regularly carried out by national authority representatives: • Manufacturing plant and equipment are inspected. • Inspectors may take samples. • Inspectors may review relevant documents and control processes to validate that medicinal product is being manufactured in accordance with marketing authorisation. **Inspections required for:** • intermediate products • finished products • NOT for starting materials and excipients **Outcome of an inspection:** • written report is prepared and sent to manufacturer • a decision on granting or maintaining the manufacturing authorisation is made
Biologics		Same as drugs

Regulatory Affairs Comparative Matrix of the Regulations Across Product Lines

Traceability Requirements

	Source	Traceability Requirements
Devices	EN ISO 13485; 7.5.3 Directive 93/42/EEC and Directive 90/385/EEC Amended by Directive 2007/47/EC and Directive 98/79/EC	Product traceability involves the ability to trace the history, application or location of an item or activity by means of recorded identification. Each individual product must have an identifier (e.g., serial number, date code, batch code, lot number, etc.) unique to the source of operation. Separate identifiers are required for changes in operative personnel, raw materials, tooling; new or different machine set-ups; changes in process methods, etc. The product should be traceable up to the point of device use or implantation. Traceability records should be maintained throughout the product's lifetime.

Drugs	ICH Q7 *Good Manufacturing Practices for Active Pharmaceutical Ingredients*
	
	Volume 4, Good Manufacturing Practice for Active Pharmaceutical Ingredients
		Product Samples
		All samples distributed to physicians need to be traceable.
		
		Record Maintenance
		• Blending process batch records should allow traceability back to the individual batches that make up the blend.
		• Manufacturer name; identity and quantity of each batch shipment of raw materials, intermediates, or labelling and packaging materials for APIs; supplier name; supplier's control number(s), if known, or other identification number; the number allocated on receipt; and the date of receipt must be recorded, along with:
		   ○ results of any test or examination performed and the conclusions derived from this
		   ○ records tracing the use of materials
		   ○ documentation of API labelling and packaging materials examination and review for conformity with established specifications
		   ○ final decision regarding rejected raw materials, intermediates or API labelling and packaging materials

Biologics		**Same as drugs (except where noted below)** Donations from blood/plasma collection establishments to the manufacturer need to be traceable.

Import/Export Requirements

	Source	Import/Export Requirements
Devices		No additional requirements. Products must be CE marked to come into the EU. In some countries, importers must hold a licence or authorisation issued by the national authorities to retrieve devices from customs when the devices originate outside the EU.

Drugs	Directive 2001/83/EC, as amended	**Import**
		A manufacturing authorisation, called an import authorisation, is required for importing medicinal products or intermediates from a country outside the EU. An import authorisation is granted by the competencies of the Member States. Importing authorisation is also required for products being brought into the EU for exportation outside the EU.
		
		Any batch of medicinal products imported into the EU must be batch tested by an independent laboratory and found to be within relative specifications before it can be used in the EU.
		
		Investigational Drug
		GMP must be applied to the manufacturer of products used in clinical trials. Product batches imported from a country outside the EU need to be certified by a Qualified Person. Some Member States will accept certification, without further retesting, if a Qualified Person formally releases the batch.
		
		Parallel Import
		Parallel import is the import of medicinal product from one Member State into another Member State. To use parallel import, the products must be therapeutically equivalent, and a valid MA must be in place in both the importing and exporting Member States.
		
		Export
		• To export a product from the EU, a manufacturer's authorisation must be held, but a marketing authorisation is not a requirement.
		• Manufacturer must request/apply for certification from a Member State that the product being exported complies with the MA by supplying the Member State with:
		  ○ SmPC (if product is authorised)
		  or
		  ○ declaration explaining why no marketing authorisation is available

Biologics		**Same as drugs**

Regulatory Affairs Comparative Matrix of the Regulations Across Product Lines

Product Recalls

	Source	Product Recalls

Devices	ISO 13485:2003
	
	Guidance on the Quality Systems for the Design and Manufacture of Medical Devices (GHTF)
		Where there is risk of death or serious deterioration of the state of health, a recall is implemented by:
		• returning a medical device to the supplier
		• supplier modification of the device at the site of installation
		• exchanging the device
		• destroying the device
		
		A manufacturer must notify the Competent Authority via the vigilance system of any technical or medical reason for a systemic recall.
		
		Removal from the market for purely commercial reasons is not considered a recall.
		
		When implementing recalls, the manufacturer shall:
		• Issue an advisory notice or recall which will provide:
		   ○ medical device description and model designation
		   ○ serial numbers or other identification (batch or lot numbers) of the medical device concerned
		   ○ reason for the issue of a notice/recall
		   ○ advice on possible hazards and consequent action(s) to be taken
		• Monitor the progress of the recall and reconcile the number of products received
		• Send a copy of the advisory notice to Competent Authorities in the applicable countries
		   ○ for Class II and III devices, the Notified Body which attested to the CE Mark shall be notified
		   ○ for Class I devices, only the Competent Authority where the manufacturer is located shall be notified
		   ○ when a serious deterioration in health occurs (the determination of serious should be made in consultation with a medical practitioner)

Product Recalls

	Source	Product Recalls
Drugs	Directive 2001/83/EC, as amended ICH Q7 *Good Manufacturing Practices for Active Pharmaceutical Ingredients*	**General** • To provide for all contingencies, a system should be designed to recall from the market, if necessary—promptly and effectively—products known or suspected to be defective. • There should be established written procedures, regularly checked and updated when necessary, to organise any recall activity. • The recall procedure should designate who should be involved in evaluating the information, how a recall should be initiated, who should be informed about the recall, and how the recalled material should be treated. • A person should be designated as responsible for executing and coordinating recalls and should be supported by sufficient staff to handle all aspects of recalls with the appropriate degree of urgency. • Recall operations should be capable of being initiated promptly and at any time. • Distribution records should be readily available to the person(s) responsible for recalls and should contain sufficient information on wholesalers and directly supplied customers (with addresses, phone and/or fax numbers inside and outside working hours, batches and amounts delivered), including those for exported products and medical samples. • Recalled products should be identified and stored separately in a secure area while awaiting a decision on their fate. • Recall process progress should be recorded and a final report issued, including a reconciliation between the delivered and recovered quantities of products. • Recall arrangements' effectiveness should be evaluated periodically. • All Competent Authorities of all countries to which products may have been distributed should be informed promptly if products are intended to be recalled because they are, or are suspected of being defective. **Investigational Products** Procedures for retrieving investigational medicinal products and documenting this retrieval (e.g., for defective products recall, returns after trial completion or expired products return) should be in place. This should be understood by the sponsor, investigator and monitor in addition to the person(s) responsible for recalls. **Recall Classification** **Class 1:** Defects that are potentially life-threatening or could cause serious risk to health: • wrong product (label and contents are different product) • correct product but wrong strength, with serious medical consequences • microbial contamination of sterile injectable or ophthalmic product • chemical contamination with serious medical consequences **Class 2:** Defects that could cause illness or mistreatment but are not Class 1: • mislabelling (wrong or missing text or figures, wrong or missing batch numbers or expiry date) • missing or incorrect information (leaflets or inserts) • microbial contamination of noninjectable, nonophthalmic sterile product with medical consequences • chemical/physical contamination **Class 3:** Defects that may not pose a significant hazard to health but where a recall has been initiated for other reasons, not necessarily required by the Competent Authority, but are not Class 1 or 2: • faulty packaging • faulty closure • contamination (microbial spoilage)
Biologics		**Same as drugs**

Regulatory Affairs Comparative Matrix of the Regulations Across Product Lines

Product Withdrawal		
	Source	Product Withdrawal
Devices	AIMDD Article 14, as amended MDD Article 19, as amended IVDD Article 18	**Withdrawal by a Member State or Community** Member State may withdraw medical devices from the market at any time • If time allows (due to safety concerns) the Member State will notify the manufacturer (or Authorised Representative) of the reasons for the product withdrawal and the available remedies and time limits to which the remedies are subject. • If time does not allow, the Member State can withdraw the product first and then notify the manufacturer (or Authorised Representative) of the reasons for the product withdrawal.
Drugs	Directive 2001/83/EC, as amended	**Withdrawal by a Member State or Community** Member States shall take all appropriate measures to ensure that the supply of the medicinal product shall be prohibited and the medicinal product withdrawn from the market if: • the medicinal product proves to be harmful under normal conditions of use or • it is lacking in therapeutic efficacy or • its qualitative and quantitative composition is not as declared or • the controls on the medicinal product and/or on the ingredients and the controls at an intermediate stage of the manufacturing process have not been carried out or if some other requirement or obligation relating to the grant of the manufacturing authorisation has not been fulfilled Member States can decide to refuse or revoke a marketing authorisation or withdraw a product from the market. This decision and the reasons for it are sent to EMA. Any Member State, due to public health concerns (such as adverse drug reactions which present an unacceptable level of risk under normal conditions of use) can suspend or withdraw the medicinal product and refer the matter to CHMP for a decision. The MAH shall notify the Member States concerned of any action taken to suspend the marketing of a product or to withdraw the product from the market, together with the reasons for such action if the latter concerns the efficacy of the product or the protection of public health. CHMP shall annually publish a list of medicinal products that are prohibited in the Community.
Biologics	Directive 2001/83/EC, as amended	**Same as drugs (except where noted below)** The Competent Authority may limit the prohibition to supply the product, or its withdrawal from the market, to those batches that are the subject of dispute.

Retention of Product Samples		
	Source	Retention of Product Samples
Devices		No documented requirements. The need for retained samples is the manufacturer's decision.
Drugs	ICH Q7 *Good Manufacturing Practices for Active Pharmaceutical Ingredients*	Samples from each batch are to be retained for one year after the expiry date of the batch assigned by the manufacturer, or for three years after distribution of the batch, whichever is longer. For active pharmaceutical ingredients (APIs) with retest dates, similar reserve samples should be retained for three years after the batch is completely distributed by the manufacturer. The reserved samples should be stored in the same packaging system in which the API is stored or in one that is equivalent to or more protective than the marketed packaging system. Sufficient quantities should be retained to conduct at least two full compendial analyses or, when there is no pharmacopoeial monograph, two full specification analyses.
Biologics	Directive 2001/83/EC, as amended	**Same as drugs (except where noted below)** Samples of each pool of plasma should be stored under suitable conditions for at least one year after the expiry date of the finished product with the longest shelf life. Member States may require samples of each bulk and finished product batch of certain immunological products (vaccines, toxins, serums, allergens) and products derived from human blood and plasma to be submitted to and controlled by an official laboratory of a Member State prior to being placed on the market. The batch should be released by the Official Medicines Control Laboratory (OMCL) of a Member State within 60 days; other Member States are not allowed to control the same batch and should recognise the certificate issued by the first OMCL stating that the batch complies with the approved specifications.

… Regulatory Affairs Comparative Matrix of the Regulations Across Product Lines

Glossary

A

Abridged Application
An application for marketing authorisation that, based upon demonstrating essential similarity or by detailed references to published scientific literature, does not contain the results of pharmacological and toxicological tests or the results of clinical trials.

Acquis Communautaire
Usually just referred to as the *Acquis*, it is the collection of European laws to which all EU Member States must adhere.

Active Implantable Medical Devices Directive
(*AIMDD*) First EU medical device legislation; sets general requirements relating to the design, construction and CE-marking of these devices and their accessories.

ADR
Adverse Drug Reaction

Advanced Therapy Medicinal Product
(ATMP) A medicinal product that is either a gene therapy medicinal product as defined in Part IV of Annex 1 to Directive 2001/83/EC, a somatic cell therapy medicinal product as defined in Part IV of Annex 1 to Directive 2001/83/EC or a tissue engineered product as defined in Article 2 1 (b) of the *ATMP Regulation*.

Adverse Event
Any untoward medical occurrence, unintended disease or injury or untoward clinical signs (including abnormal laboratory findings) in subjects, users or other persons, whether or not related to the investigational medical device. (EN 14155)

AESGP
Association Européenne des Spécialités Pharmaceutiques Grand Public, Association of the European Self-medication Industry

AIMDD
See *Active Implantable Medical Devices Directive*

Applicant
See Marketing Authorisation applicant

Arbitration Rapporteur
Under the Mutual Recognition Procedure, the CHMP member appointed to prepare a report after notification by the Reference and Concerned Member States that there are serious public health issues remaining related to the product at the end of the MRP's 90-day clarification and dialogue phase.

Assessment Report
The assessment of the medicinal product by the Reference Member State, including the reasons for its conclusions during the Mutual Recognition Procedure. During the Centralised Procedure, the CHMP prepares an assessment report released as the EPAR.

ATC
Anatomical Therapeutic Chemical (classification of drugs)

ATMP
See Advanced Therapy Medicinal Product.

Glossary

B

Bibliographic Application
Also known as "well-established use applications." The applicant prepares a product dossier based upon literature available in the public domain. The drug product concerned needs to have been on the market for at least 10 years. This type of application is especially important to the newer Member States as it allows them to keep their current generic products on the market where no reference product exists.

Blue Box
The area into which country-specific text is usually placed on packaging materials and leaflets for medicinal products approved via the Centralised Procedure.

C

CADREAC
See Collaboration Agreement of Drug Regulatory Authorities in European Union Associated Countries

CAPs
Conformity Assessment Procedures; see Conformity Assessment

CAT
See Committee for Advanced Therapies

CE Mark
European conformity, *Conformité Européenne*, mark. Mandatory European mark for products falling under one of the New Approach directives (including medical devices) to indicate conformity with the essential health and safety requirements.

CEN
See European Committee for Standardization.

CENELEC
See European Committee for Electrotechnical Standardization

Centralised Procedure
Submission of a dossier to EMA to obtain marketing authorisation from the European Commission that is valid in all EU Member States. The Centralised Procedure is compulsory for orphan medicinal products; any medicinal product for human use containing an entirely new active substance; those manufactured using biotechnological processes; and medicinal products for the treatment of AIDS, cancer, neurodegenerative disorders, autoimmune diseases and other immune dysfunctions and viral diseases or diabetes. It also may be used on a voluntary basis for other innovative products. Products are assessed by the CHMP (human) and CVMP (veterinary). Individual Member States may prohibit the marketing of an approved veterinary product based upon epidemiological considerations.

CEP
Certificate of European Pharmacopoeia. See Certificate of Suitability.

Certificate of Suitability
(CEP) Certificate granted by the Certification Secretariat of the EDQM certifying that a substance's quality is suitably controlled by the relevant monographs of the European Pharmacopoeia with, if necessary, an annex appended. A CEP can be granted for active substances or excipients and for substances or preparations with risk of transmitting agents of animal spongiform encephalopathies.

CHMP
See Committee for Medicinal Products for Human Use

CIOMS
Council for International Organisations of Medical Sciences

Clinical Investigation Plan
Document that states the rationale, objectives, design and proposed analysis, methodology, monitoring, conduct and recordkeeping of the clinical investigation. (EN 14155)

Clinical Trials Directive
Directive setting analytical, pharmatoxicological and clinical standards and protocol requirements for clinical trials.

CMDh
See Coordination Group for Mutual Recognition and Decentralised Procedures (human).

CMDv
See Coordination Group for Mutual Recognition and Decentralised Procedures (veterinary).

CMS
See Concerned Member State

Co-decision Procedure
Procedure by which the Council of the European Union and the European Parliament—the two institutions responsible for EU legislation—adopt legislative acts. It applies to virtually all legislation regarding pharmaceutical law.

COE
See Council of the European Union

Collaboration Agreement of Drug Regulatory Authorities in European Union Associated Countries
(CADREAC) CADREAC's mission was to facilitate smooth transition of regulatory conditions in EU-associated countries to achieve regulatory standards required by *Acquis Communautaire*. Signatories of CADREAC (first phase) were state regulatory authorities for human medicinal products of countries in Central, Eastern and Southern Europe, i.e., Cyprus, Czech Republic, Estonia, Hungary, Latvia, Lithuania, Poland, Slovak Republic, Slovenia and Turkey. (See also new CADREAC)

Committee for Advanced Therapies
(CAT) A multidisciplinary committee advising EMA, comprising the best available experts in Europe to assess the quality, safety and efficacy of ATMPs, and to follow scientific developments in the field.

Committee for Medicinal Products for Human Use
(CHMP) A committee that provides scientific advice to EMA on questions relating to the evaluation of medicinal products for Human Use. Formerly, the CPMP—Committee for Proprietary Medicinal Products.

Committee for Orphan Medicinal Products
(COMP) A committee that provides scientific advice to EMA on questions relating to the designation of "orphan drugs" for rare diseases.

Committee for Veterinary Medicinal Products
(CVMP) A committee that provides scientific advice to EMA on questions relating to the evaluation of veterinary medicinal products.

Committee on Herbal Medicinal Products
(HMPC) A committee that provides scientific advice to EMA on questions relating to herbal medicinal products.

COMP
See Committee for Orphan Medicinal Products

Competent Authority
For medicinal products, a Member State's governmental body responsible for authorising and supervising such products. For medical devices, the organisation authorised by a Member State's government to act on its behalf to ensure that all medical devices meet the essential requirements laid down in the medical device directives.

Concerned Member State
(CMS) A Member State included in a Mutual Recognition Procedure application.

Conformity Assessment
The systematic examination of evidence generated and procedures undertaken by the manufacturer, under requirements established by the regulatory authority, to determine that a medical device is safe and performs as intended by the manufacturer and, therefore, conforms to the Essential Principles of Safety and Performance for Medical Devices.

Coordination Group for Mutual Recognition and Decentralised Procedures (human)
(CMDh) Coordinates and facilitates the operation of the Decentralised and Mutual Recognition Procedures for medicinal products for human use.

Coordination Group for Mutual Recognition and Decentralised Procedures (veterinary)
(CMDv) Coordinates and facilitates the operation of the Decentralised and Mutual Recognition Procedures for medicinal products for veterinary use.

COREPER
Comité des Représentants Permanents, Committee of Permanent Representatives from Member States that advises the Council of the European Union.

Council of the European Union
Sometimes referred to as the Council of Ministers, it is the EU's main decision-making institution and final legislative authority. It comprises one representative per Member State. The representative is usually a government minister and varies depending upon the matters being discussed, e.g., the Minister for Health for pharmaceutical issues.

CTD
Common Technical Document

CVMP
See Committee for Veterinary Medicinal Products

D

Decentralised Procedure
Procedure that may be used for medicinal products for which there is no existing Marketing Authorisation in any EU Member State. The applicant can select the Reference Member State and list the Concerned Member States.

Directive
A European Commission decision that is binding upon Commission institutions and Member States, and must be transposed into national legislation. However, the way in which it is implemented is left to the discretion of individual Member States.

DMF
Drug Master File

Glossary

E

ECJ
European Court of Justice

eCTD
Electronic Common Technical Document

EDQM
See European Directorate of Quality of Medicines and Healthcare

EEA
See European Economic Area

EEC
See European Economic Community

EFPIA
European Federation of Pharmaceutical Industries and Associations

EFTA
European Free Trade Association, composed of Iceland, Liechtenstein, Norway and Switzerland.

EGA
European Generic Medicines Association

EMA
See European Medicines Agency

EN
See European Standard

Enterprise Directorate-General
Enterprise DGs are the principal administrative agencies of the European Commission. Their objective is to supply policy ideas that promote a supportive business environment for all European enterprises—including pharmaceutical companies.

EPAR
See European Public Assessment Report

Essential Requirements
Technical requirements defined in each New Approach directive (usually Annex 1) with which a product must comply to qualify for CE marking.

Essential Similarity
According to the European Court of Justice, a medicinal product is essentially similar to another product if it has: the same quantitative and qualitative composition of active substance(s); the same dosage form; and the same bioequivalence, documented by a corresponding bioavailability.

Ethics Committee
Independent body whose responsibility it is to review clinical investigations in order to protect the rights, safety and wellbeing of human subjects participating in a clinical investigation.

EU
See European Union

Eudralex
Compilation of EU pharmaceutical legislation and guidelines accessible from the European Commission Pharmaceuticals Unit website.

EudraVigilance
A data processing network and management system for reporting and evaluating suspected adverse reactions during the development and following the marketing authorisation of medicinal products in the European Economic Area (EEA).

European Medicines Agency
(EMA) The agency responsible for coordinating the scientific evaluation of the safety, efficacy and quality of human and veterinary medicinal products that undergo the Centralised Procedure as well as for arbitration during the Mutual Recognition Procedure. It comprises the CHMP, CVMP, COMP, CAT, HMPC, PDCO, a Secretariat, the Executive Director and a Management Board.

European Commission
The executive branch of the European Union, composed of 27 commissioners led by a Commission President. The body is responsible for proposing legislation, implementing decisions, upholding the Union's treaties and the general day-to-day operation of the EU.

European Committee for Electrotechnical Standardization
(CENELEC) EU standards body that establishes voluntary electrotechnical standards.

European Committee for Standardization
(CEN) *Comité Européen de Normalisation*, promotes voluntary harmonisation of European technical standards across a wide range of products, processes and appliances.

European Community
The collective body formerly designated as the European Economic Community (EEC). The plural term European Communities is also widely used.

European Council
Comprised of the heads of state of governments of the EU Member States, the Council meets regularly. It is the most senior manifestation of the Council of the European Union.

European Directorate of Quality of Medicines and Healthcare
(EDQM) Part of the administrative structure of the Council of Europe, its responsibilities include the Technical Secretariat of the European Pharmacopoeia Commission, the unit for certifying the suitability of Ph.Eur. monographs, developing the European network of the Official Medicines Control Laboratories (OMCL) and providing the secretariat for this network.

European Economic Area
(EEA) A free-trade area, in all but agriculture, comprising the Member States of the EU plus Iceland, Liechtenstein and Norway. Previously called the European Economic Space.

European Economic Community
(EEC) One of three communities created by the Treaties of Rome in 1957 to establish a common market. The 1967 merger of the EEC, Customs Union and European Atomic Energy Community created the European Communities. Precursor to the European Union.

European Federation of Pharmaceutical Industries and Associations
(EFPIA) Represents more than 2,000 pharmaceutical companies involved in research, development and manufacturing medicinal products for human use in Europe.

European Parliament
The directly elected parliamentary body of the European Union. Together with the Council of the European Union (the Council), it forms the bicameral legislative branch of the Union's institutions. The highest EU legislative body.

European Pharmacopoeia
(PhEur) *Pharmacopée Européenne* is a pharmacopoeia whose monographs are common to all concerned European nations.

European Police Office
(Europol) European Union law enforcement organisation that handles criminal intelligence. It assists Member States' law enforcement authorities in fighting organised crime. It was established in 1992 as the European Drugs Unit to aid in controlling illegal drug-related activities.

European Public Assessment Report
(EPAR) Report on CHMP's scientific conclusion at the end of the centralised evaluation process, summarising the grounds for the CHMP opinion on granting a marketing authorisation for a specific medicinal product. EMA makes this information available to the public after deleting commercially confidential information.

European Standard
(EN) Standards that are harmonised across the EU whose use, in theory, is voluntary. They address product health or safety aspects, as well as such other characteristics as durability, appearance, quality levels or even cultural preferences. These standards may be test methods or measurement guides.

European Union
(EU) Political body comprising 27 Members States established by the 1993 *Treaty of Maastricht*. It is the de facto successor to the European Economic Community founded in 1957 by the *Treaty of Rome*.

Expert Report
Report drawn up for a Marketing Authorisation applicant by an expert, on the applicant's behalf, on the quality (chemical, pharmaceutical and biological documentation), safety (pharmacotoxicological) or efficacy (clinical) of a medicinal product, including a tabulation, written summary (optional) and critical discussion of the product's properties. The clinical and nonclinical Expert Report has been replaced in the Common Technical Document by the respective overviews (modules 2.4 and 2.5).

G

GCP
Good Clinical Practice

Genetically Modified Organism
(GMO) An organism in which the genetic material has been altered in a way that does not occur naturally by mating and/or natural recombination.

GLP
Good Laboratory Practice

GMO
See Genetically Modified Organism

GMP
Good Manufacturing Practice

H

HMPC
See Committee on Herbal Medicinal Products

I

ICH
International Conference on Harmonisation of Technical Requirements for Registration of Pharmaceuticals for Human Use

Glossary

IFPMA
International Federation of Pharmaceutical Manufacturers' Associations

IFU
Instructions for use—applies to medical devices

In Vitro Diagnostic Devices Directive (IVDD)
Covers devices used in vitro for to examine specimens derived from the human body, including reagents, instruments and specimen receptacles.

INN
International Nonproprietary Name

ISO
International Organization for Standardization

IVDD
See In Vitro Diagnostic Devices Directive

L

LOA
Letter of Access

M

MAA
See Marketing Authorisation Application

MAH
See Marketing Authorisation Holder

Marketing Authorisation
Authorisation to place a medicinal product on the market in a Member State issued by its Competent Authority or by EMA for the EU market.

Marketing Authorisation Application
(MAA) The application submitted to a Member State(s) for a Decentralised or Mutual Recognition Procedure or to EMA for the Centralised Procedure seeking permission to place a new product on the market.

Marketing Authorisation Holder
(MAH) The person who holds the marketing authorisation for placing a medicinal product on the market and is responsible for marketing the product. The MAH must be established in the EEA.

MDD
See *Medical Devices Directive*

MedDRA
Medical Dictionary for Regulatory Activities developed under the auspices of ICH. It is a medical terminology coding dictionary, important in the electronic transmission of adverse event reporting as well as in the coding of clinical trial data.

Medical Devices Directive
(MDD) The *Medical Devices Directive* (Directive 93/42/EEC) sets general requirements relating to the design and construction of medical devices and their accessories.

Member State
A member nation of the European Union. The EFTA States have adopted the complete *Acquis Communautaire* on medicinal products and are consequently parties to Community procedures; therefore, for the purposes of this book, the term Member State shall also include the EFTA countries.

MRA
See Mutual Recognition Agreement

MRL
Maximum residue limit

MUMS
Minor use, minor species

Mutual Recognition Agreement
(MRA) International agreement by which two or more countries agree to recognise one another's conformity assessments.

Mutual Recognition Procedure
Applicable to most conventional medicinal products, the Mutual Recognition Procedure is based upon the extension of an existing national marketing authorisation granted by one Member State (Reference Member State) to one or more additional Member States (Concerned Member States).

N

New Approach Directives
The European Council established a "New Approach" for technical harmonisation and standardisation to remove technical trade obstacles within the European Union in its Decision of 7 May 1985. The New Approach serves *inter alia* as the basis for the European Council Directives for medical devices that have been issued thus far with the object of removing existing trade obstacles and achieving high unified security standards.

Notice to Applicants
Procedures for marketing authorisation, regulatory guidelines and application dossier presentation and content for medicinal products for human use (Volume 2) and veterinary medicinal products (Volume 6). The *Notice to Applicants* has no legal force.

Notified Body
Certification organisation (e.g., independent testing house, laboratory or product certifier) authorised by the relevant Member State's Competent Authority to perform conformity assessment tasks specified in the medical device directives.

O

Official Journal
(OJ) *Official Journal of the European Union*. Contains details of all EU legislation, as well as draft legislation, information, notices and advertisements for public works and supplies contracts.

OJ
See *Official Journal*

OMCL
Official Medicines Control Laboratories (see EDQM)

Orphan Medicinal Products
A medicinal product that has a limited target population and treats a rare disease, thus limiting its commercial and financial potential. The *Orphan Medicinal Product Regulation* was adopted in December 1999, to stimulate the development in the EU of pharmaceuticals for the diagnosis, prevention and treatment of some 5,000 diseases that are classified as "rare" and affect not more than 5 in 10,000 persons in the EU.

OTC
Over-the-counter (products available without a prescription)

P

Paediatric Committee
(PDCO) Scientific committee within EMA that assesses the content of paediatric investigation plans and adopts opinions on them in accordance with Regulation (EC) No 1901/2006 as amended. This includes the assessment of applications for a full or partial waiver and assessment of applications for deferrals.

Paediatric Regulation
Regulation passed in 2006 to encourage the development and authorisation medicinal products to meet the special therapeutic needs of the paediatric population.

Patient Information Leaflet
(PIL) Provides a set of information, in a particular order, accompanying each medicine. It is usually the only source of information on how to use a medicine safely and effectively, when the patient actually takes the medicine.

PDCO
See Paediatric Committee

Periodic Safety Update Report
(PSUR) A periodic report, submitted at defined postauthorisation times, on the worldwide safety experience of a medicinal product.

PHARE
One of three pre-accession instruments funded by the EU to assist applicant countries in Central and Eastern Europe in preparing to join as Member States. Currently, it assists the Czech Republic, Estonia, Hungary, Latvia, Lithuania, Poland, Slovakia and Slovenia, as well as Bulgaria and Romania, which acceded in 2007. (Originally created in 1989 as Poland and Hungary: Assistance for Restructuring their Economies.)

Pharmacovigilance Working Party
(PhVWP) Reporting to the CHMP, the PhVWP facilitates coordination of MRP product pharmacovigilance across Member States and the development of consensus on conclusions and proposed actions when differences arise between Member States.

PhVWP
See Pharmacovigilance Working Party

PIC
Pharmaceutical Inspection Convention. The PIC and the Pharmaceutical Inspection Co-operation Scheme (PIC Scheme) operate together as PIC/S.

PIL
See Patient Information Leaflet

PMS
See Postmarket Surveillance

POM
Prescription-only Medicine

Postmarket Surveillance
(PMS) Systematic procedure by which a manufacturer records, evaluates and reports any incidents, proactively gathering product experience in the postmarketing phase. It is used as the basis for any necessary corrective actions.

PSUR
See Periodic Safety Update Report

Q

Qualified Person
A person at the Marketing Authorisation Holder's disposal who is responsible for ensuring that the quality of each batch of medicinal product is in accordance with the Marketing Authorisation's requirements.

R

Rapporteur and Co-rapporteur
Members of the CHMP, CVMP or COMP who assume responsibility for assessing Marketing Authorisation Applications, community referrals and requests for orphan drug designation.

Reference Member State
The Member State whose Assessment Report is the basis for the Mutual Recognition Procedure and Decentralised Procedure.

Regulation
A legal act that is entirely and directly binding on the Member States. Unlike a directive, it does not require transposition into national law and its provisions can come into force immediately.

RMS
See Reference Member State

S

SMEs
Small and medium-sized enterprises

SmPC
See Summary of Product Characteristics

SPC
See Supplementary Protection Certificate

Summary of Product Characteristics
(SmPC) The definitive statement between the Competent Authority and the Marketing Authorisation Holder regarding the medicinal or veterinary product. The summary of product characteristics contains a description of a medicinal product's properties and the conditions attached to its use. This includes: name, composition, pharmaceutical form and strength, therapeutic indication(s), adverse reactions, contraindications, shelf life, storage conditions and Marketing Authorisation Holder. It contains all information a prescriber/supplier needs for proper use of the medicinal or veterinary product. The content must be approved by the Competent Authority, and cannot be changed without the approval of the originating Competent Authority.

Supplementary Protection Certificate
(SPC) An SPC protects intellectual property rights following patent expiration and is available in the EU for medicinal products and plant protection products. An SPC can come into force only after the corresponding patent expires and for a maximum of five years, to grant a product not more than 15 years of market exclusivity. It is intended to compensate the holder for the extended period required for some products to be approved

T

Traditional Herbal Medicinal Products Directive
Requires traditional, over-the-counter herbal remedies to be manufactured to assured standards of safety and quality.

Treaty on European Union
The 1992 document that radically restructured the EC, formally established the European Union and committed the EC to Economic and Monetary Union (EMU) by 1999 at the latest. Also known as the *Maastricht Treaty*.

TSE
Transmissible spongiform encephalopathies

Type I Variation
Any of the "minor" variations listed in Annex I of Regulations (EEC) 1084/2003 (formerly 541/95) and (EEC) 1085/2003 (542/95) to documentation in an approved Marketing Authorisation. A Type IA or Type IB variation notification must be filed with EMA for any such change.

Type II Variation
Any change to the documentation in an approved Marketing Authorisation that is not a Type IA or Type IB Variation and is not regarded as an extension to the Marketing Authorisation.

U

Urgent Safety Restriction
An interim change to product information in the SmPC by the Marketing Authorisation Holder concerning indications, dosage, contraindications, warnings, target species and withdrawal periods resulting from new information about a medicinal product's safe use.

V

VICH
International Cooperation on Harmonisation of Technical Requirements for Registration of Veterinary Medicinal Products

Vigilance
The adverse incident reporting requirements and system for devices.

W

WHA
World Health Assembly

WHO
World Health Organisation

WSMI
World Self-Medication Industry

# Glossary

Index

A

ABPI Code (UK), 50
Abridged applications, 164–165
    and generic medicinal product market authorisation requirements, 209–210
Accessory
    as defined by MDD, 78, 88, 121–122
Active device, 90
Active implantable medical device
    compliance with conformity assessment procedures, 108–109
    regulatory scope, 129–130
Active Implantable Medical Devices Directive (90/385/EEC)
    authorised representative requirements, 116–117
    classification requirements, 88, 262
    clinical data and evaluation Annex 7 requirements, 100–102
    clinical investigation elements, 69, 103–105
    conformity assessment procedure requirements based on device risk classification, 108–109
    enforcement activities, 61–63
Active pharmaceutical ingredients
    and GMP requirements, 198–199
Active Substance Master File, 155
Adjuvants, 275–276
Advanced therapy medicinal products
    classification, 262
    clinical evaluation of, 100–102, 263
    definition of, 78, 130 (*See also* Vaccines, therapeutic)
    GMP requirements, 263
    hospital exemption, 264
    legal framework, 4–8, 12, 129–130, 256–257, 261–264
    market authorisation application submission requirements, 157
    postmarket surveillance/incident reporting provisions, 133–136, 141
    provisions for combined ATMPs, 264–265
    revision, 84–85
Advanced Therapy Medicinal Products Directive (Council Regulation (EC) No 1394/2007), 4, 6, 8
Adverse events and reactions (*See also* Pharmacovigilance)
    clinical trial reporting requirements for medicinal products/investigational medicinal products, 177–178
    device clinical investigation reporting requirements, 70
    medicinal product reporting requirements, 241–244
    medicinal/biological product enforcement requirements, 58–59
    vaccine product reporting requirements, 278–279
    veterinary medicinal product reporting requirements, 337–338
Advertising and promotion
    and definition of misleading, 51
    national legislation for medicinal products, 54–55
    nonprescription medicinal products requirements, 217–218
    prohibition of audiovisual commercial communications, 52
    regulatory scope and enforcement for medicinal products, 49–52, 60
AIMDD (*See* Active Implantable Medical Devices Directive (90/385/EEC))
Animal testing, 11, 304, 306
APIs (*See* Active Pharmaceutical Ingredients)
Association of the European Self-Medication Industry, 214

Index

ATMPs (*See* Advanced therapy medicinal products)
Australia
    MRA, 9
Austria
    national transposition of MDD labelling and language requirements, 144
Authorised representative
    compliance with IVDD requirements, 125
    definition and role, 73, 81
    role in conformity assessment, 116–117

B

Batch release
    OCABR testing requirements for human blood or plasma-derived medicinal products, 250, 252–253
Belgium
    national transposition of MDD labelling and language requirements, 144–145
Best Pharmaceuticals for Children Act (US), 46
Bibliographic applications, 165
    and Mutual Recognition Procedure submission process, 160
Biocidal products
    regulation, 8
Biocidal Products Directive (98/8/EC), 322
Bioequivalence, 207
Biological medicinal products
    and devices, 90
    clinical trial requirements, 273–274
    enforcement activities, 58–61
    regulation, 5–6
Biotechnology Working Party, 248, 250–251
    See also Human blood or plasma-derived medicinal products
Biotechnology-derived products
    and development pharmaceutics, 224
    Centralised Procedure authorisation requirements, 221–224
    demonstrating comparability, 227
    manufacturing requirements, 224–226
    preclinical and clinical testing requirements, 226–227
Blood derivatives (*See* Human blood and blood components)
Blood products (*See* Human blood or plasma-derived medicinal products)
Blood Products Working Group, 248
    See also Human blood or plasma-derived medicinal products
Blue Guide (EC Guide to New Approach directives), 69, 79
Bolar (Experimental and Testing) Provisions, 208–209

Borderline products (*See also* Combination products)
    and cosmetics requirements, 302–303
    and IVD products, 120
    and veterinary medicinal products, 322
    classification requirements and EC assessment process, 77, 82, 91
    foods and medicinal products issues, 315–316
Bovine spongiform encephalopathy, 2, 225
BP spill
    crisis management case study, 18, 20
BPWG (*See* Blood Products Working Group)
BSE (*See* Bovine spongiform encephalopathy)
Bulgaria
    national transposition of MDD labelling and language requirements, 145
BWP (*See* Biotechnology Working Party)

C

CABs (*See* Conformity assessment bodies)
Canada
    MRA, 9
CAPS (*See* Conformity Assessment Procedures)
Cascade Provision, 336
Case Report Forms, 103
CAT (*See* Committee for Advanced Therapies)
CE Mark
    and AIMD products, 131
    and compliance with Essential Requirements, 69, 79
    and IVD products, 119–120, 122, 124–125
    compliance with conformity assessment procedures, 7, 9
    enforcement, 63
CEN (*See* European Committee for Standardization)
CENELEC (*See* European Committee for Electrotechnical Standardization)
Centralised Procedure
    biotechnology-derived product authorisation requirements, 221–224
    medicinal product market authorisation application submission and review requirements, 5, 157–159, 185–189
    nonprescription medicinal product approval, 215
    orphan medicinal products application requirements, 288–289
    regulatory framework, 194
    renewal application submission requirements, 238–239
    variation application submission requirements, 235–237
    veterinary medicinal products application requirements, 325–331, 335
Certificate of European Pharmacopeia (CEP) (*See* Certificate of Suitability)

Certificate of Suitability, 198, 225
CHMP (*See* Committee for Medicinal Products for Human Use)
CIP (*See* Clinical Investigation Plan)
CJD
    See Transmissible spongiform encephalopathy
CJEU (*See* Court of Justice of the European Union)
Classification
    combination products, 294–298
    compliance with MDD, Annex IX requirements, 88–91
    device compliance with conformity assessment procedures and, 7, 9
Clinical evaluation
    and compliance with MDD/AIMDD requirements, 69–70, 100–102
Clinical Investigation Plan, 102–105
Clinical trials
    biotechnology-derived product requirements, 226–227
    device requirements, 102–105
    notification of adverse events, 177
    notification of amendments, 176–177
    overview and legal framework for medicinal product and investigational medicinal product requirements, 170–172
    vaccine product requirements, 273–274
Clinical Trials Directive (2001/20/EC)
    adverse events notification requirements, 177–178
    Competent Authority authorisation application provisions, 174–176
    establishment of EudraCT, 172–173
    GMP guidelines for investigational medicinal products, 170, 176
    lack of national harmonisation, 178
    notification of amendments provision, 176–177
    scope and definitions, 170–172
Clinical Trials Facilitation Group, 179
CMDh (*See* Coordination Group for Mutual Recognition and Decentralised Procedures-Human)
CMS (*See* Concerned Member State)
Coding
    for human tissue-engineered products, 265–266
Colours/Colorants, 305, 308
Combination products
    and classification disputes, 297–298
    case studies, 298–299
    national regulations, 295–296
    pharmaconsultation procedure, 297
    regulatory scope and classification of drug/device products, 90, 293–296
Combined ATMPs, 264–265
Commission Communication 2010/C82/01 (*See* Clinical Trials Directive (2001/20/EC))
Commission Regulation (EC) No 1084/2003 (*See* Variations)
Commission Regulation (EC) No 1085/2003 (*See* Variations)
Commission Regulation (EC) No 1234/2008 (*See* Variations)
Commission Regulation (EC) No 124/2009 (*See* Feed additives)
Commission Regulation (EC) No 429/2008 (*See* Feed additives)
Commission Regulation (EC) No 540/95 (*See* Adverse events and reactions)
Commission Regulation (EC) No 542/95 (*See* Variations)
Commission Regulation (EC) No 668/2009 (*See* Advanced Therapy Medicinal Products Directive (Council Regulation (EC) No 1394/2007))
Committee for Advanced Therapies
    and ATMP oversight, 70, 257, 261–262, 265
    role in medicinal product Centralised Procedure application review, 5–6
    role in reviewing combination product applications, 297
Committee for Medicinal Products for Human Use (*See also* European Medicines Agency)
    responsibilities and organizational structure, 184–185
    role in handling referrals, 166–167
    role in medicinal product Centralised Procedure application approval, 5, 157–159, 185–190, 194
    role in reviewing human tissue-engineered product applications, 257, 261
    role in reviewing plasma-derived medicinal product applications, 248, 250, 252
    role in reviewing variations applications, 237
    role on Paediatric Committee, 42–43
Committee for Orphan Medicinal Products
    position on prevalence and significant benefit, 289–290
    role in medicinal product Centralised Procedure application approval 5, 287-288
    role in providing protocol assistance, 290–291
    scope and responsibilities, 284–285, 287
Committee for Proprietary Medicinal Products (*See* Committee for Medicinal Products for Human Use)
Committee on Herbal Medicinal Products (*See also* Traditional Herbal Medicinal Products Directive)
    establishment of, 166, 218
    role in medicinal product Centralised Procedure application approval, 5, 7
Committee on Medicinal Products for Veterinary Use (*See also* Veterinary Medicinal Products Directive (2001/82/EC))
    role in medicinal product Centralised Procedure application approval, 5
    role in reviewing veterinary product applications 326-328, 335-336

Index

Common Technical Document (CTD)/electronic Common Technical Document (eCTD)
   medicinal product market authorisation application requirements, 154–156, 187–188
   renewal application requirements, 239
   veterinary medicinal product ASMF/DMF requirements, 332
Common Technical Specifications, 124
Community Code
   and impact of unclear provisions, 52–53
   and multimedia advertising provisions, 52
   articles 89 and 91, 52
   proposed EC legislative reforms, 53–54
   regulatory scope and requirements, 50–52
Community interest referral, 167
COMP (*See* Committee for Orphan Medicinal Products)
Comparability
   biotechnology-derived product guidelines, 227
Competent Authorities
   and Member State delegation, 70–72
   guidance development, 84
   national transposition of MDD notification requirements, 147–148
   role in ATMP authorisation, 264
   role in consensus building, 73
   role in device classification disputes, 82, 91
   role in device enforcement, 61–63
   role in enforcing advertising and promotion regulations, 50
   role in medicinal product clinical trial authorisation, 170, 174–176
   role in medicinal/biological product enforcement, 58–61
   role in nominating auditors for Joint Audit Programme, 201
   role in overseeing device clinical investigations, 103
   role in postmarketing surveillance/adverse incident reporting process, 134–141
   role in reviewing and issuing VAMF, 273
   role in reviewing combination product applications, 294–298
   role in reviewing nonprescription medicinal product classification
   role in veterinary medicinal product authorisation process, 325, 328
Compliance Group, 201–202
Concerned Member State
   role in Decentralised Procedure submission review process, 5, 162–164
   role in Mutual Recognition Procedure submission review process, 5, 159–161, 190–192
   role in reviewing generic medicinal product abridged applications, 209
   role in reviewing renewal applications, 237–238
   role in reviewing variation applications, 235–237
   role in reviewing veterinary medicinal product applications, 325–326
Concertation Procedure, 3, 186, 232
Conformity assessment bodies, 9
Conformity Assessment Procedures
   and applicability of standards, 94–96
   and handling classification disputes, 91
   and NB responsibilities, 71–72
   clinical data/clinical evaluation device requirements, 100–102
   Essential Requirements compliance and, 69, 93–94
   IVD requirements, 125
   module review, 112–115
   New Approach and Global Approach directives implementation, 7–9
   scope of MDD/AIMD/IVDD requirements based on device risk classification, 108–109, 111–112
Consensus, 94–94 (*See also* Standards)
Contergan, 2, 4
Coordination Group for Mutual Recognition and Decentralised Procedures-Human
   role in Decentralised Procedure application review process, 162, 326
   role in Mutual Recognition Procedure application review process, 161, 190–192, 326
Cosmetic products
   and CMRs use, 306
   animal testing requirements, 304, 306
   colorant requirements, 305, 308
   in combination with borderline products, 302–303
   labelling requirements, 303–304, 307–308
   legal framework, 11, 301–302
   marketing and premarket notification requirements, 303
   nanomaterial reporting requirements, 306
   Product Information File requirements, 306–307
   prohibited and restricted substances, 304–305
   US and EU regulations compared, 307–309
Cosmetic Products Notification Portal, 303
Cosmetics Directive (76/768/EEC)
   Annexes, 304–306
   evolution and scope, 11, 301–302
Cosmetics Product Regulation, 11
Council Regulation (EC) No 1394/2007/EC (*See* Advanced Therapy Medicinal Products Directive (Council Regulation (EC) No 1394/2007))
Council Regulation (EC) No 2377/90 (*See* Maximum residue limits)
Council Regulation (EEC) No 2309/93 (*See* Regulation (EC) No 726/2004)
Council Regulation (EEC) No 1768/92 (*See* Supplementary Protection Certificate)

Court of Justice of the European Union
    role in interpreting Community code, 50, 53, 55
    role in interpreting medical device law, 66, 77, 82
Creutzfeldt-Jakob disease (*See* Transmissible spongiform encephalopathy)
CRFs (*See* Case Report Forms)
Criminal sanctions, 61
Crisis management
    case studies, 19–20
    external crises, 18
    internal crises, 17–18
    leadership, 18–19
    overview, 17, 19
Cross Border Patients' Rights Directive (2011/24/EU), 32
CTD (*See* Common Technical Document (CTD)/electronic Common Technical Document (eCTD))
CTFG (*See* Clinical Trials Facilitation Group)
CTS (*See* Common Technical Specifications)
Custom-made devices, 79, 81, 88
CVMP (*See* Committee on Medicinal Products for Veterinary Use)
Czech Republic
    national transposition of MDD labelling and language requirements, 145

D

Data exclusivity, 207–208
Decentralised Procedure
    fees, 329
    medicinal product market authorisation application submission and review requirements, 5, 162–164, 185, 191–192
    referral process, 166
    regulatory framework, 194–195
    veterinary medicinal product application requirements, 325–326
Declaration of Conformity
    and compliance with IVDD Essential Requirements, 124–125
    and verification of medical device compliance, 69
Denmark
    national transposition of MDD labelling and language requirements, 145
Design dossier, 97, 124–125
Development Safety Update Report, 243
Device intended for clinical investigation, 81, 88
DG SANCO (*See* Directorate-General for Health and Consumer Protection)
Dietary supplements (*See* Foodstuffs)
Directive 1999/21/EC (*See* Foods for Special Medical Purposes)
Directive 2000/70/EC (*See* Human Blood and Human Plasma Derivatives Directive (2000/70/EC))
Directive 2001/18/EEC (*See* Genetically modified organisms)
Directive 2001/20/EC (*See* Clinical Trials Directive (2001/20/EC))
Directive 2001/82/EC (*See* Veterinary Medicinal Products Directive (2001/82/EC))
Directive 2001/83/EC (*See* Medicinal Products Directive (2001/83/EC))
Directive 2001/94/EC (*See* General Product Safety Directive (2001/94/EC))
Directive 2002/46/EC (*See* Food Supplements Directive)
Directive 2002/98/EC (*See* Human blood and blood components)
Directive 2003/63/EC (*See* Biological medicinal products; Medicinal Products Directive (2001/83/EC))
Directive 2003/94/EC (*See* Good Manufacturing Practice Directive (2003/94/EC))
Directive 2004/23/EC (*See* European Union Tissues and Cells Directive (2004/23/EC))
Directive 2004/24/EC (*See* Traditional Herbal Medicinal Products Directive (2004/24/EC))
Directive 2004/27/EC (*See* Decentralised Procedure; Good Manufacturing Practice; Medicinal Products Directive (2001/83/EC))
Directive 2004/28/EC (*See* Veterinary Medicinal Products Directive (2001/82/EC))
Directive 2004/33/EC (*See* Human blood and blood components)
Directive 2005/28/EC (*See* Clinical Trials Directive (2001/20/EC))
Directive 2005/61/EC (*See* Human blood and blood components)
Directive 2005/62/EC (*See* Human blood and blood components)
Directive 2006/114/EC (*See* Advertising and promotion)
Directive 2006/130/EC (*See* Veterinary Medicinal Products Directive (2001/82/EC))
Directive 2006/17/EC (*See* Active Implantable Medical Devices Directive (90/385/EEC); Human tissue-engineered products)
Directive 2006/86/EC (*See* Human tissue-engineered products)
Directive 2007/47/EC (*See* Medical Devices Directive (93/42/EEC))
Directive 2008/29/EC (*See* Medicinal Products Directive (2001/83/EC))
Directive 2009/120/EC (*See* Advanced Therapy Medicinal Products Directive (Council Regulation (EC) No 1394/2007))
Directive 2009/53/EC (*See* Medicinal Products Directive (2001/83/EC))

Index

Directive 2009/9/EC (*See* Veterinary Medicinal Products Directive (2001/82/EC))
Directive 2010/13/EU (*See* Advertising and Promotion)
Directive 2010/84/EU (*See* Medicinal Products Directive (2001/83/EC); Pharmacovigilance)
Directive 2011/24/EU (*See* Cross Border Patients' Rights Directive (2011/24/EU))
Directive 2011/62/EU (*See* Good Manufacturing Practice; Medicinal Products Directive (2001/83/EC))
Directive 65/65/EEC (*See* Medicinal Products Directive (2001/83/EC))
Directive 75/318/EEC
   See Medicinal Products Directive (2001/83/EC)
Directive 76/768/EEC (*See* Cosmetics Directive (76/768/EEC))
Directive 81/851/EEC (*See* Veterinary Medicinal Products Directive (2001/82/EC))
Directive 89/342/EEC (*See* Immunological Medicinal Products Directive (89/342/EEC))
Directive 89/381/EEC (*See* Human blood or plasma-derived medicinal products)
Directive 90/167/EC (*See* Medicated Feedstuffs)
Directive 90/219/EEC (*See* Genetically modified organisms)
Directive 90/220/EEC (*See* Genetically modified organisms)
Directive 90/385/EEC (*See* Active Implantable Medical Devices Directive (90/385/EEC))
Directive 91/356/EEC (*See* Good Manufacturing Practice)
Directive 91/412/EEC (*See* Veterinary Medicinal Products Directive (2001/82/EC))
Directive 92/26/EEC
   See Medicinal Products Directive (2001/83/EC)
Directive 92/27/EEC
   See Medicinal Products Directive (2001/83/EC)
Directive 92/28/EEC
   See Medicinal Products Directive (2001/83/EC)
Directive 93/42/EEC (*See* Medical Devices Directive (93/42/EEC))
Directive 98/79/EC (*See* In Vitro Diagnostic Devices Directive (98/79/EC))
Directive 98/8/EC (*See* Biocidal Products Directive (98/8/EC))
Directorate-General for Enterprise, 7, 248
Directorate-General for Health and Consumer Protection, 7, 184, 248, 266
Distribution
   and national transposition of MDD requirements, 148–150
Distributors
   as defined by New Approach directives, 73
   of cosmetics, 303
Divergent Decision Referral, 166

Donations
   human tissue-engineered product selection and testing requirements, 257–258
   plasma derived product testing requirements, 251–253
Drug/device combination product (*See also* Combination products)
   classification, 90
Drugs
   See Medicinal products
DSUR (*See* Development Safety Update Report)

E

EC Type-Examination, 113–118
eCTD (*See* Common Technical Document (CTD)/electronic Common Technical Document (eCTD))
EDQM (*See* European Directorate for the Quality of Medicines & Healthcare)
EFGCP (*See* European Forum for Good Clinical Practice)
EFPIA (*See* European Federation of Pharmaceutical Industries and Associations)
EFSA (*See* European Food Safety Authority)
EFTA (*See* European Free Trade Association)
EMA (*See* European Medicines Agency)
Embryonic stem cells (*See* Stem cells)
EN 13612:2002, 100
EN ISO 13485, 108, 115, 135, 140
EN ISO 14155:2010
   clinical investigation requirements, 100, 103
EN ISO 14971:2000, 140
Enforcement
   and GCP compliance, 60
   and GMP compliance, 59–60
   of advertising regulations, 60
   of medical devices, IVDs and AIMDs, 61–63
   of pharmacovigilance requirements, 60–61
   overview of legal provisions for pharmaceutical and biological products, 58–59
EPAR (*See* European Public Assessment Report)
EPO (*See* European Patent Organization)
ERP (*See* European Reference Medicinal Product)
Essential Requirements
   and custom-made device compliance requirements, 79, 81
   clinical data/clinical evaluation device compliance, 100–102
   IVDD compliance with, 122, 124
   manufacturer checklist requirement and, 93–94, 96–97
   medical device compliance with, 8–9, 69–70, 79, 81
   role and use of standards, 94–96

Ethics
    and Paediatric Regulation and guideline development, 41, 46
    impact on healthcare product regulatory developments, 2–3
Ethics Committee
    role in device clinical investigation, 103
    role in providing opinion on medicinal product clinical trial application submissions, 173–174, 177
ETSI (*See* European Telecommunications Standards Institute)
EU Clinical Trials Register, 173
EUCOMED, 75, 82
EUDAMED, 61, 141–142, 144
EudraCT
    and Paediatric Regulation provisions, 45, 172
    legal basis and scope, 172–173
EudraLex
    See Rules Governing Medicinal Products in the European Union
EudraVigilance, 244, 279
    Veterinary, 337
EUnetHTA (*See* European Network for Health Technology Assessment)
EUR-ASSESS Project, 34
EURODIS (*See* European Organisation for Rare Diseases)
EUROM, 75
European Agency for the Evaluation of Medicinal Products
    See European Medicines Agency
European Association of Notified Bodies for Medical Devices (Team-NB), 82
European Clinical Trial Database (*See* EudraCT)
European Commission
    decision-making role in granting Centralised Procedure, Mutual Recognition Procedure and Decentralised Procedure authorisations, 188–189, 191–192, 327–328
    issuance of New Approach directive guidance (Blue Guide), 69, 79
    launched High Level Pharmaceutical Forum (HLPF), 36–37
    New & Emerging Technology Working Group, 83–84
    overview of structure and responsibilities, 184
    proposed MDD modifications, 10
    referrals, 166
    role in clinical trial procedure developments, 178
    role in developing and enforcing MEDDEV guidelines, 82
    role in mandating standards development, 94–95
    Working Group on Classification and Borderline, 82, 91

European Committee for Electrotechnical Standardization, 73, 83, 94
European Committee for Standardization, 72–73, 83, 94, 266
European Conformity Mark or Conformité Européenne (CE) Mark (*See* CE Mark)
European Council Treaty
    as basis for New Approach Directives, 7
European Database for Medical Devices (*See* EUDAMED)
European Directorate for the Quality of Medicines & Healthcare
    role in overseeing API certification scheme, 198
    role in publishing Official Control Authority Batch Release procedures, 250–251, 253
European Federation of Pharmaceutical Industries and Associations
    European Code of Practice on the Promotion of Medicines, 51
    participated in clinical trial procedure development discussion with EC, 178
    participation in ICH, 202
European Food Safety Authority
    establishment, 11
    role in conducting scientific risk assessments, 312, 314–315
European Forum for Good Clinical Practice, 174
European Free Trade Association, 159
European Generic Medicines Association, 206
European Medicines Agency
    and paediatric research collaboration with FDA, 46
    collaboration with Member State HTA agencies, 31–33, 36–38
    establishment and role in administering Centralised Procedure, 5, 157–159, 185–189, 271
    GMP Inspection Services Group responsibilities, 201–202
    market application fees, 329–331
    organisational structure and responsibilities, 185
    presubmission meeting activity, 157–158, 187
    responsibility for the Committee for Advanced Therapies, 70
    role in implementing pharmacovigilance legislation, 242–244
    role in regulating paediatric use MAAs and establishing of Paediatric Committee, 42–46
    role in reviewing and approving veterinary medicinal products market applications, 325–328, 335
    role in reviewing orphan medicinal product applications for designation, 287–288
    role in reviewing variation applications, 234–237
    scientific review of Centralised Procedure applications, 158, 188

Index

unified application with US for orphan designation, 288
European Network for Health Technology Assessment and HTA Core Model, 33–35
    definition of HTA, 33
    history of, 32
European Organisation for Rare Diseases, 291
European Patent Organization, 208
European Pharmacopeia, 203, 250, 332
European Public Assessment Report, 159, 187, 189
European Reference Medicinal Product, 209–210
European Telecommunications Standards Institute, 73
European Union
    HTA agency structure and activities, 31–32
    Joint Audit Programme, 201
    overview of legislative process, 66, 153, 192, 194
    overview of structure, 184
European Union Tissues and Cells Directive (2004/23/EC)
    Member State transposition, 259–260
    scope and requirements, 256–259
    standards and coding provision, 265–266
EUTCD (*See* European Union Tissues and Cells Directive)
Evidence-generation plans, 27, 29
Exxon
    crisis management case study, 20

F

FDA (*See* US Food and Drug Administration)
Feed additives, 322–323
Field safety corrective action, 134, 136, 139
Financing mix, 23
Finland
    national transposition of MDD labelling and language requirements, 145
Fixed-combination applications, 166
Follow-up measures, 159, 232
Follow-up referral, 167
Food and Drug Administration (*See* US Food and Drug Administration)
Food supplements (*See* Foodstuffs)
Food Supplements Directive
    regulatory scope and definition, 11, 312–314
Foods for Special Medical Purposes, 316–317
Foodstuffs
    borderline issues, 315–16
    health claims, 315
    labelling, 313–314
    regulatory overview, 10–11, 312–313
    safety assessment of ingredients, 314–315

France
    medicinal product advertising and promotion regulations, 54
    national transposition of Competent Authority notification MDD requirements, 147
    national transposition of human tissue-engineered product requirements, 259
    pricing and reimbursement system, 24
FSCA (*See* Field safety corrective action)
FSD (*See* Food Supplements Directive)
FSMPs (*See* Foods for Special Medical Purposes)
FUMs (*See* Follow-up measures)

G

GCP (*See* Good Clinical Practice)
Gene therapy medicinal products
    regulation, 5–6
General Food Law Regulation (Regulation (EC) No 178/2002), 11, 313–314
General Product Safety Directive (2001/94/EC)
    relationship with medical device directives, 134
Generic applications, 164–165
Generic medicinal products
    market authorisation requirements, 209–210
    national initiatives and challenges, 210
    regulatory history and scope, 206–207
    veterinary, 329
Genetically modified organisms
    regulation, 5–6, 12, 276–277, 333
Germany
    and Competent Authority delegation, 70–71
    medicinal product advertising and promotion regulations, 52
    national transposition of device distribution requirements, 148–149
    national transposition of human tissue-engineered product requirements, 259–260
    pricing and reimbursement system, 25, 27–28
GHTF (*See* Global Harmonization Task Force)
Global Approach directives
    medical device regulation and, 7–9, 108
Global Harmonization Task Force (*See also* International Medical Device Regulators Forum)
    device harmonisation goals, 8
    role in establishing medical device vigilance system, 62, 136, 140, 142
    role of consensus standards in device regulation, 94
    Summary of Technical Documentation (STED) format, 125
Global Medical Device Nomenclature, 142
GMOs (*See* Genetically modified organisms)
GMP (*See* Good Manufacturing Practice)

Good Clinical Practice
    and Clinical Trials Directive provisions, 170
    and vaccine clinical trials, 273–274
    UK MHRA pharmaceutical/biological medicinal product enforcement, 60
Good Manufacturing Practice
    and vaccine manufacturing compliance, 272–273
    API requirements, 198–199
    ATMP requirements, 263
    compliance enforcement, 59–60
    cosmetic product requirements
    evaluation of medicinal product requirements and, 4–5, 198–203
    US FDA parallels with EU GMPs, 9
    veterinary medicinal product regulation and, 6, 338–339
Good Manufacturing Practice Directive (2003/94/EC), 5–6
Good Pharmacovigilance Practice, 244
GPSD (*See* General Product Safety Directive)
GVP (*See* Good Pharmacovigilance Practice)

H

Harmonisation
    and evolution of medicinal product regulations, 3–4
    clinical trial directive challenges with
    medical device regulatory development, 8, 69
    of medicinal product regulations, 153–154
    of pharmacopeias, 203
    of technical standards, 83
Hatch-Waxman Act (US), 208
Heads of Medicines Agencies, 178, 201
Health economics and outcomes research, 26–27, 29
Health insurance
    and pricing and reimbursement systems, 23–24
Health monitoring measures, 62
Health technology assessment
    and EUnetHTA Core Model development, methodology and concepts, 33–35
    and REA paradigm, 36–37
    compared to pricing and reimbursement 24-25
    definition of, 32–33
    history, 31–32
    reports, 35–36
Healthcare costs, 2–3
Healthcare establishments, 73
Healthcare products regulations
    evolution of, 1–4
    future developments, 12
Healthcare technology
    defined by INAHTA, 32
Helsinki Declaration, 2

Helsinki procedure, 82
HEOR (*See* Health economics and outcomes research)
Herbal medicinal products (*See* Traditional herbal medicinal products)
HMA (*See* Heads of Medicines Agencies)
HMPC (*See* Committee on Herbal Medicinal Products)
HTA (*See* Health technology assessment)
Human blood and blood components
    regulation, 4, 10–11, 250–251, 253
Human Blood and Human Plasma Derivatives Directive (2000/70/EC), 10
Human blood or plasma-derived medicinal products
    regulation, 5–6
Human subject protection
    impact on healthcare product regulatory developments, 2–3
Human tissue-engineered products
    and ATMP legislation, 261–264
    containing devices/combined ATMPs, 264–265
    legal framework, 5–6, 8, 256–257
Humanitarian medical devices, 291–292
Hybrid applications, 165

I

IB (*See* Investigators Brochure)
ICH (*See* International Conference on Harmonisation of Technical Requirements for Registration of Pharmaceuticals for Human Use)
ICREL (*See* Impact on Clinical Research of European Legislation)
IEC (*See* International Electrotechnical Commission)
IFPMA (*See* International Federation of Pharmaceutical Manufacturers & Associations)
IFU (*See* Instructions for Use)
IMDRF (*See* International Medical Device Regulators Forum)
Immunological medicinal products
    regulation, 5
Immunological Medicinal Products Directive (89/342/EEC), 5
Impact on Clinical Research of European Legislation project, 178
Implantable device (*See* Active implantable medical device)
Importers
    as defined by New Approach directives, 73
In vitro diagnostic devices
    and compliance with conformity assessment procedures, 108–109, 112
    and risk-based classification, 88, 122–124
    definition, 78, 120
    enforcement activities, 61–63
    labelling, e-labelling and language requirements, 125

Index

postmarket surveillance procedures, 133–136
registration requirements, 125
regulatory overview & scope, 119–122
In Vitro Diagnostic Devices Directive (98/79/EC)
 and authorised representative requirements, 117–118, 125
 and clinical evaluation requirements, 100–102
 and clinical investigation elements, 102–105
 conformity assessment procedure device classification requirements, 108–109, 112
 impact of New Approach/Global Approach directives, 8
 labelling, e-labelling and language requirements, 125
 postmarket surveillance/incident reporting provisions, 133–136, 141
 registration requirements, 125
 regulatory overview and scope, 119–122
 revisions, 126
INAHTA (*See* International Network of Agencies for Health Technology Assessment)
INCI (*See* International Nomenclature of Cosmetic Ingredients)
Incidents (*See also* Postmarket surveillance)
 reporting criteria & investigation requirements, 137–139
 types of, 136–137
Individual Case Safety Reports, 243–244
Informed consent
 applications, 166
 Paediatric Regulation provisions, 46
Inspections
Instructions for Use
 and National transposition of MDD requirements, 144–147
International Conference on Harmonisation of Technical Requirements for Registration of Pharmaceuticals for Human Use
 CTD/eCTD guidelines 154-156
 GMP guidelines, 202, 272
 overview, 202
 periodic safety reporting requirements, 243
International Cooperation on Harmonisation of Technical Requirements for Registration of Veterinary Medicinal Products, 323
International Electrotechnical Commission, 73, 83
International Federation of Pharmaceutical Manufacturers & Associations, 202
 Code of Pharmaceutical Marketing Practices, 50–51
International Generic Pharmaceutical Alliance, 206
International Medical Device Regulators Forum, 8, 140
International Network of Agencies for Health Technology Assessment
 defined health technology and HTA, 32–33

history of, 31–32
International Nomenclature of Cosmetic Ingredients, 304, 307–308
International Organization for Standardization, 83, 94–95, 202–203
Investigational medicinal products
 definition and clinical trial application requirements, 171, 174–176, 273–274
 GMP requirements
Investigators brochure
 and technical documentation requirements, 96
Ireland
 national transposition of device distribution requirements, 149–150
ISBT 28, 266
ISO (*See* International Organization for Standardization)
ISO 13485, 124
ISO 14971:2007, 124
ISO 15225, 142
Italy
 medicinal product advertising and promotion regulations, 52
 national transposition of Competent Authority notification MDD requirements, 147–148
 national transposition of human tissue-engineered product requirements, 260
 pricing and reimbursement system, 25–26
IVDD (*See* In Vitro Diagnostic Devices Directive)

J

James, Erika Hayes, 18
Japan
 crisis management case studies, 20
 MRA, 9
 participation in ICH, 202
Japanese Pharmacopeia, 203
Johnson & Johnson
 crisis management case study, 18–19
Joint Audit Programme (EU), 201

L

Labelling
 cosmetic products, 303–304
 foodstuffs, 11, 313–314
 IVDD requirements, 125
 national transposition of device language/IFU requirements, 144–147
 nonprescription medicinal product requirements, 215, 217
Language
 and IVDD requirements, 125

and National transposition of MDD requirements, 144–1147
Letter of Access, 156
Licence maintenance, 189, 191–192
Lot release
    testing requirements for biotechnology-derived products, 226
    vaccine requirements, 273, 277

M

Maastricht Treaty, 7
Mad cow disease (*See* Bovine spongiform encephalopathy)
MAH (*See* Marketing authorisation holder)
Manufacturers
    and clinical investigation device requirements, 100–105
    compliance with AIMDD submission requirements, 130–131
    compliance with IVDD submission requirements, 122–125
    definition of, 73, 81
    GMP and quality control requirements for vaccine products, 271–273
    incident reporting/postmarket surveillance responsibilities, 135–140
    responsibility for vaccine lot release requirements, 271–273, 277–278
    role in appealing combination product review, 297–298
Market exclusivity, 285–286
Market structure
    impact on healthcare product regulatory developments, 3, 66
Market Surveillance Operations Group, 141
Marketing authorisation
    advanced therapy product requirements, 6
    and accelerated assessment procedure request, 158
    and Centralised Procedure renewal requirements, 238–239
    and Mutual Recognition Procedure/Decentralised Procedure renewal requirements, 237–238
    conditional, 158–159
    cosmetic product requirements, 303
    Centralised Procedure submission process, 186–189
    Centralised, Decentralised and Mutual Recognition Procedure submission processes compared, 192
    CTD/eCTD application format requirements, 154–156
    Decentralised Procedure submission process, 191–192
    generic medicinal products requirements, 209–210
    human blood and plasma-derived medicinal product requirements, 252–253
    license maintenance requirements, 189, 191–192
    Mutual Recognition Procedure submission process, 159–161, 189–191
    overview of system for medicinal products, 3–5, 153–154, 185–186
    paediatric regulation requirements, 44–45
    referral process, 166–167
    renewals submission requirements, 237–239, 333
    specific obligations data requirements, 232
    submission process for various application types (generic, hybrid, bibliographic, etc), 164–166
    traditional herbal medicinal products registration procedures, 219
    variation submission requirements, 159, 232–237, 333
    veterinary medicinal products registration procedures, 324–328
Marketing authorisation holder
    compliance with pharmacovigilance requirements, 242–244, 278–279
    medicinal product application submission responsibilities, 154, 185, 187–188
    medicinal product postmarket responsibility to submit renewal applications, 237–239
    medicinal product postmarket responsibility to submit variation applications, 232—237
    PIP submission responsibilities, 42–45
    responsibility to provide pharmacovigilance data on veterinary medicinal products, 337
    vaccine/biological lot release testing responsibilities, 277–278
Maximum residue limits
    regulatory scope, 6, 333–335
    veterinary medicinal product marketing authorisation requirements, 333–337
MDD (*See* Medical Devices Directive (93/42/EEC))
MDEG (*See* Medical Device Expert Group)
MEDDEV
    development and enforcement of, 9
    Guideline 2.1/3 (Rev. 3), 77–78, 294, 296–297, 299
    Guideline 2.12 (Rev. 7), 135–136, 138–140
    Guideline 2.12/2 (Rev. 2), 69, 130, 135
    Guideline 2.4/1 (Rev. 9), 296
    Guideline 2.7.1 (Rev. 3), 101
    Guideline 2.7.3, 103
MedDRA (*See* Medical Dictionary for Regulatory Activities)
Medical Device Expert Group, 10, 296
Medical devices
    adverse incident reporting/postmarket surveillance requirements, 70
    and clinical evaluation requirements, 69–70, 100–102
    and clinical investigation plan, 102–105

Index

and compliance with conformity assessment
procedures, 108–109, 111–116
and NB responsibilities, 71–72
and role of standards, 94–96
classification of, 88–91
classification rules when used in combination
products, 294–296
combined with ATMPs, 264–265
definition, 75, 77–78, 294
EC proposed MDD modifications, 10
enforcement activities, 61–63
humanitarian, 291–292
impact of New Approach and Global Approach
regulations, 7–9, 66, 69–70
incorporating blood products, 253
intended to have a biological effect, 90
national transposition requirements for language
labelling/IFU & Competent Authority
notification/distribution, 143–150
overview of regulatory developments, 7–10, 12, 66,
69–71, 75, 77–79, 81–85
postmarket surveillance procedures, 133–136
requirements for devices intended for clinical
investigation, 81
Medical Devices Directive (93/42/EEC)
Annex IX classification provisions, 88–91
Competent Authority notification requirements,
147–148
clinical evaluation Annex X requirements, 69–70, 81,
100–102
clinical investigation elements, 102–105
combination product references, 294–295
conformity assessment procedure requirements based
on device risk classification, 108–109, 111–
116
custom-made device requirements, 79
enforcement provisions, 61–63
Essential Requirements checklist, 93–94, 96–97
evolution of, 7–9, 11
exclusions, 77–78
human blood or blood products derivatives
amendment, 253
impact combined ATMPs regulation, 264–265
interpretations and revisions, 82–85
Member State enforcement provisions, 70–71, 83
national transposition requirements for language
labelling/IFU & Competent Authority
notification/distribution, 143–150
NB requirements, 71
postmarket surveillance/incident reporting
requirements, 134–136, 141
scope and definitions, 75, 77–79, 81, 294
Medical Devices Vigilance System, 134, 136 (*See also*
Postmarket surveillance; Vigilance)

Medical Dictionary for Regulatory Activities, 244
Medicated feedstuffs, 322–323, 339
Medicinal products
advertising and promotion requirements, 49–55
clinical trial requirements, 170–172
Centralised Procedure marketing authorisation
submission process, 157–159, 186–189
defined, 294
Decentralised Procedure marketing authorisation
submission process, 162–164, 191–192
enforcement activities, 58–61
evolution of regulatory framework, 1–6
GMP requirements
Mutual Recognition Procedure marketing
authorisation submission process, 159–161,
189–191
overview of market authorisation system & submission
requirements, 153–156, 185–186
overview of postmarketing and pharmacovigilance
activities, 231–232
regulated in combination products, 294–296
Medicinal Products Directive (2001/83/EC)
advanced therapy medicinal products amendments,
4–6
advertising and promotion provisions, 49–50
and handling borderline food product issues, 315–316
data exclusivity provisions, 207, 209
evolution of, 4–5, 153, 198
GMP requirements, 4–5, 198–203
herbal medicinal product requirements amendment,
4, 7
human blood or plasma-derived medicinal products
amendments, 5–6
medicinal product defined, 294
nonprescription medicinal product requirements,
214–215, 217–218
pharmacovigilance requirements, 4, 241
Medicines and Healthcare Products Regulatory Authority
(*See also* UK)
advertising and promotion medicinal product
regulation, 50, 52, 54
clinical investigation guidance for devices, 101–102
GCP and GMP medicinal/biological product
enforcement activities, 59–60
Member States (*See also* Specific countries)
and HTA agency structure and activities, 31–33,
36–38
and NB oversight, 71–72
Competent Authority role in reviewing veterinary
medicinal product applications, 328
national transposition of EUTCD, 259–260
national transposition requirements for device
language labelling/IFU & Competent
Authority notification/distribution, 143–150

regulation of combination products, 296–297
reimbursement and pricing for vaccine products, 279–280
responsibility for human tissue-engineered product donation and procurement, 263–264
responsibility for transposition of IVDD requirements, 119
responsibility for transposition of MDD requirements, 70–71, 83
responsibility/competence for pricing and reimbursement policy, 24
role in medical device regulatory enforcement, 70–71
role in overseeing lot release testing, 273
MHRA (*See* Medicines and Healthcare Products Regulatory Authority)
Minor use, minor species, 335
Mixed marketing applications, 166
MRAs (*See* Mutual Recognition Agreements)
MRLs (*See* Maximum residue limits)
Multistate Procedure, 186, 232
MUMS (*See* Minor use, minor species)
Mutual Recognition Agreements, 9–10
Mutual Recognition Facilitation Group (*See* Coordination Group for Mutual Recognition and Decentralised Procedures-Human)
Mutual Recognition Procedure
    fees, 329
    generic medicinal product abridged application requirements, 209
    medicinal product marketing authorisation application submission and review requirements, 5, 159–161, 185, 189–191
    referral process, 166
    regulatory framework, 194
    veterinary medicinal product application requirements, 324–326

N

National Procedure, 5, 164
    veterinary medicinal product application requirements, 324–325, 329
National transpositions (*See also* specific Member States) and MDD compliance, 143–144, 150
NB-MED
    role and responsibilities, 71–72
    technical documentation guidelines, 97–98
NBOG (*See* Notified Body Operations Group)
Netherlands
    national transposition of Competent Authority notification MDD requirements, 148
    national transposition of MDD labelling and language requirements, 145–146
New Approach directives
    and conformity assessment procedures, 108
    definition of importers and distributors, 73
    historical overview, 66, 69, 129
    key principles, 69–70
    medical device regulation and, 7–9
    revisions, 70
    role of standards, 94
New Zealand
    MRA, 9
No observable adverse effect level, 334–335
Noninvestigational medicinal products, 171
Nonprescription medicinal products
    advertising requirements, 217–218
    instructions for use, labelling and packaging requirements, 215, 217
    legislative scope, 214–215
Norway
    national transposition of MDD labelling and language requirements, 146
Notified Bodies
    accreditation requirements, 70, 84
    role in AIMD submission review, 131
    role in combined ATMP review, 265
    role in conformity assessment procedures, 9, 93, 97–98, 109, 111–116
    role in device classification disputes, 91
    role in device clinical evaluation process, 69
    role in device enforcement, 62–63
    role in guidance development, 82
    role in IVD submission review, 124–125
    role in reviewing combination product applications, 294–297
Notified Body Operations Group, 111
Novel Food Regulation, 314–315
Nutrition and Health Claims Regulation (Regulation (EC) No 1924/2006, 315

O

Odwalla Foods
    crisis management case study, 20
Office of Technology Assessment (US)
    establishment, 31
Official Control Authority Batch Release, 250, 252–253, 278
Official medicines control laboratories, 250, 253, 273, 277–278
Orphan Medicinal Product Regulation (Regulation (EC) No 141/2000)
    annual report provision, 291
    orphan designation criteria and opinion, 286–288
    research and development incentives, 285–286, 290
    scope, 5, 284–286
    transfer of sponsorship provision, 291

Index

Orphan medicinal products
    designation procedure and requirements, 287–288
    EU vs. US legislation, 286
    market authorisation application requirements, 288–289
    market exclusivity extension under Paediatric Regulation, 44
    regulatory overview, 5, 284–286, 289–290
Over-the-Counter products (See Nonprescription medicinal products)

P

Packaging
    nonprescription medicinal product requirements, 217
Paediatric Committee
    role in medicinal product Centralised Procedure application approval, 5, 42–43, 45
Paediatric Investigation Plan
    application procedure, 43–44
    scope and requirements, 42
    waivers and deferrals, 43
Paediatric Regulation (Regulation (EC) No 1901/2006)
    compared with US pediatrics regulations, 46
    extended intellectual property protection, 44
    legal basis for EudraCT, 5, 172
    marketing authorisation requirements, 44–45
    orphan medicinal product market exclusivity provision, 44
    regulatory scope and requirements, 4–5, 41–42
Paediatric Use Marketing Authorisation, 45
Patents, 208
PDCO (See Paediatric Committee)
Pediatric Research Equity Act (US), 46
Periodic Safety Update Reports, 242–243, 338
Pharmaceutical Inspection Cooperation Scheme
    overview, 198–199
    Pharmaceutical Inspectorate scope and responsibilities, 199–200
Pharmaceutical products (See Medicinal products)
Pharmacovigilance (See also Adverse events and reactions)
    and Paediatric Regulation provisions, 45
    enforcement requirements, 60–61
    human blood and plasma-derived medicinal product requirements, 253
    legal framework, 241–242
    medicinal product/investigational medicinal product reporting requirements, 4–5
    renewals application requirements, 237–239
    vaccine product requirements, 278–279
    variations application requirements, 232–237
    veterinary medicinal product requirements, 337–338
Pharmacovigilance Regulation, 278–279
Pharmacovigilance Risk Assessment Committee, 242

PhEur (See European Pharmacopeia)
PIC/S (See Pharmaceutical Inspection Cooperation Scheme)
PIP (See Paediatric Investigation Plan)
Plasma Master File, 252
Plasma-derived medicinal products
    market authorisation application requirements, 251–253
    postmarket requirements, 253
    scope and legal framework, 248, 250–251
    sourcing and manufacturing control requirements, 251–252
PMCF (See Postmarket Clinical Follow-Up)
PMCPA (See Prescription Medicines Code of Practice Authority)
PMOA (See Principal mode of action)
Portugal
    national transposition of Competent Authority notification MDD requirements, 148
Postmarket clinical follow-up, 70, 135
Postmarket surveillance (See also Medical Devices Vigilance System; Vigilance)
    Competent Authority enforcement, 136–139
    device adverse incident reporting and vigilance system requirements, 70
    overview of device regulatory procedures, 133–135
    veterinary medicinal product requirements, 338
PRAC (See Pharmacovigilance Risk Assessment Committee)
Preclinical testing
    biotechnology-derived product requirements, 226
Predicate device, 98
Premix (See Medicated feedstuffs)
Prescription Medicines Code of Practice Authority, 50
Prevalence, 288–289
Pricing
    and reimbursement policy responsibility, 24
    defined and compared to reimbursement and HTA, 24–25
    ex-factory and reimbursed, 24–26
    for vaccine products, 279–280
    models compared, 25, 29
Principal mode of action
    as basis for regulating combination products, 294, 296
    definition
    role in combined ATMP product classification, 265
    role in device classification, 7, 77, 88
Principal payer, 23–24
Protocol assistance, 290–291
PSURs (See Periodic Safety Update Reports)
Public safety
    impact on healthcare product regulatory developments, 2–3
PUMA (See Paediatric Use Marketing Authorisation)

Q

QP (*See* Qualified Person)
QRD (*See* Quality Review of Documents)
Qualified Person
    medicinal product marketing authorisation responsibilities, 158
    role in certifying clinical batch material releases, 176, 273
Quality assurance
    and vaccine manufacturing requirements, 271–273
    device production, 114–115
Quality Review of Documents, 155
Quality systems
    and compliance with IVDD requirements, 124
    and device compliance conformity assessment procedures, 108, 115
    regulatory guidelines for medicinal products, 198–199, 202

R

REA (*See* Relative Effectiveness Assessment)
Reference Member State
    role in Decentralised Procedure submission review process, 5, 162–164, 192
    role in Mutual Recognition Procedure submission review process, 5, 159–161, 189–191
    role in reviewing generic medicinal product abridged applications, 209
    role in reviewing renewal applications, 237–238
    role in reviewing variation applications, 235–237
    role in reviewing veterinary medicinal product applications, 325–326
Referrals
    and medicinal product market authorisation process, 166–167
Regulation (EC) No 1223/2009 (*See* Cosmetics Product Regulation)
Regulation (EC) No 1234/2008 (*See* Variations; Variations Regulation)
Regulation (EC) No 1235/2010 (*See* Pharmacovigilance)
Regulation (EC) No 178/2002
Regulation (EC) No 1830/2003 (*See* Genetically modified organisms)
Regulation (EC) No 1831/2003 (*See* Feed additives)
Regulation (EC) No 1924/2006 (*See* Nutrition and Health Claims Regulation (Regulation (EC) No 1924/2006)
Regulation (EC) No 1925/2007 (*See* Foodstuffs, safety assessment of ingredients)
Regulation (EC) No 1950/2006 (*See* Veterinary Medicinal Products Directive (2001/82/EC))
Regulation (EC) No 258/97 (*See* Novel Food Regulation)
Regulation (EC) No 470/2009 (*See* Maximum residue limits)
Regulation (EC) No 726/2004
    biotechnology-derived product market authorisation requirements via Centralised Procedure, 221–22
    data exclusivity requirements, 208
    expanded applicability to orphan medicinal products, 5
    generic product provisions, 206–208
    implementation of, 4–5
    market authorisation requirements and established EMA, 194
    pharmacovigilance requirements, 198, 241
Regulation (EC) No 1394/2007 (*See* Advanced Therapy Medicinal Products Directive (Council Regulation (EC) No 1394/2007))
Regulation (EC) No 141/2000 (*See* Orphan medicinal products; Regulation (EC) No 726/2004)
Regulation (EC) No 178/2002 (*See* General Food Law Regulation)
Regulation (EC) No 1901/2006 (*See* Paediatric Regulation (Regulation (EC) No 1901/2006))
Regulation (EC) No 1829/2003 (*See* Genetically modified organisms)
Regulation (EC) No 1830/2003 (*See* Genetically modified organisms)
Reimbursement
    and pricing policy responsibility, 24
    defined and compared to pricing and HTA, 24–25
    for vaccine products, 279–280
    models compared, 25–26, 29
    overview of, 23–24
Relative Effectiveness Assessment, 36–37
Release testing (*See* Lot release)
Renewals
    legal framework under Centralised Procedure, 238–239
    legal framework under Mutual Recognition Procedure and Decentralised Procedure, 237–238
Residual solvents, 332–333
Responsible Person, 303
Reusable surgical instrument, 89–90
Risk management
    plans for vaccine product pharmacovigilance, 278–279
    role in device regulation, 135
RMS (*See* Reference Member State)
Romania
    pricing and reimbursement system, 25
Rules Governing Medicinal Products in the European Union
    clinical trial requirements, 274
    evolution of, 3–4

Index

GMP and quality system requirements, 198–199, 202, 273, 338
human blood and plasma-derived medicinal product requirements, 250, 252
Notice to Applicants (NTA) overview, 153
pharmacovigilance requirements, 60, 241, 278
veterinary medicinal product requirements, 323, 325

S

Safeguard Clause, 62, 141
Self-medication
　scope and political support for, 214
Significant benefit, 290
Snow Brand Milk Products Co.
　crisis management case study, 20
Software device classification, 8, 77, 90
Somatic cell therapy medicinal products
　regulation, 4–5, 262
Spain
　national transposition of Competent Authority notification MDD requirements, 148
　national transposition of device distribution requirements, 150
　national transposition of human tissue-engineered product requirements, 260
　pricing and reimbursement system, 28–29
Specimen receptacles, 78, 121
Sponsor
　role in clinical trial authorisation process, 171–178
　role in orphan medicinal product authorisation process, 287
　role in proving prevalence in orphan medicinal product designation process, 288–289
Standalone applications
　and Mutual Recognition Procedure submission process, 160
Standards
　application in device conformity assessment procedures and consensus development process, 94–97
　harmonisation of technical, 83, 94–95
　human tissue-engineered products, 265–266
　overview of organisations, 72–73
Stem cells
　legal framework, 260–261
Supplementary Protection Certificates, 207–208
　and paediatric research IP extensions, 44
Surgically invasive device, 89
Suspected adverse drug reactions, 337–338
Sweden
　medicinal product advertising and promotion regulations, 52
　national transposition of human tissue-engineered product requirements, 260
Swedish Council on Technology Assessment in Health Care, 31
Switching
　prescription to nonprescription status, 215
Switzerland
　MRA, 9
　national transposition of MDD labelling and language requirements, 146

T

Technical file
　and device regulatory requirements, 97
　and IVDD regulatory requirement, 124–125
Thalidomide, 2 (*See also* Contergan)
Third-party conformity assessment (*See* Notified Bodies)
Tissue and Cells Regulatory Committee Expert Working Group, 266
Tissue establishments, 257, 263
Traceability
　human tissue-engineered product requirements, 258, 263, 266
Traditional herbal medicinal products
　regulation of, 5, 7, 218–219
Traditional Herbal Medicinal Products Directive (2004/24/EC), 4, 166, 218–219, 316 (*See also* Committee on Herbal Medicinal Products)
Transmissible spongiform encephalopathy, 2, 225, 252, 332
Transparency Directive, 24, 36, 280
Treaty on the Functioning of the European Union, 24, 32, 66
Treaty of Lisbon, 66
Trend reporting, 139–140
TSE (*See* Transmissible spongiform encephalopathy)
Tylenol
　crisis management case study, 18–19

U

UK (*See also* Medicines and Healthcare Products Regulatory Authority)
　advertising and promotion medicinal product regulation, 50, 52, 54
　defined rulings on borderline/combination products, 296–297
　GMP compliance enforcement through MHRA, 59–60
　national transposition of human tissue-engineered product requirements, 260, 263–264, 266
　national transposition of MDD labelling and language requirements, 147

pricing and reimbursement system, 24–27
US Food and Drug Administration
    and paediatric research collaboration with EMA, 46
    compared with EU paediatric regulations, 46
    GMP parallels with EU GMPs, 9
    participation in ICH, 202
    standards development, 95
    unified application with EU for orphan designation, 289
US Pharmacopeia, 203
US/EU Mutual Recognition Agreement, 9

V

Vaccine antigen master file, 6, 273–274
Vaccine Working Party, 271
Vaccines
    clinical trials, 273–274
    DNA, 276–277
    influenza, 279
    manufacturing and quality control/GMP requirements, 271–273
    market authorisation requirements, 274–275
    nonclinical development aspects, 274
    pharmacovigilance and risk management plan requirements, 278–279
    policy-making activities, 280
    reimbursement and pricing, 279–280
    scope and development, 271
    Therapeutic, 277
VAMF (*See* Vaccine antigen master file)
Variations
    biotechnology-derived product requirements
    generic product requirements, 210
    medicinal product marketing authorisation application requirements, 159, 232–237
    veterinary medicinal product marketing authorisation requirements, 333

Variations Regulation, 232–33
Veterinary medicinal products
    Active Substance Master File/Drug Master File, 332
    classified as borderline products, 322
    clinical requirements, 336
    compliance with GMP requirements, 338–339
    dossier compared with human medicinal products dossier, 331–332
    generic, 329
    market authorisation renewals and variations, 333
    pharmacovigilance requirements, 337–338
    regulatory scope, 6–7, 320, 322
Veterinary Medicinal Products Directive (2001/82/EC) (*See also* Committee on Medicinal Products for Veterinary Use)
    market authorisation requirements, 328–329
    regulatory scope, 6–7, 320–321, 324
    revisions, 324
VHP (*See* Voluntary Harmonisation Procedure)
VICH (*See* International Cooperation on Harmonisation of Technical Requirements for Registration of Veterinary Medicinal Products)
Vigilance, 62, 136–138, 140 (*See also* Medical Devices Vigilance System; Postmarket surveillance)
    and compliance with IVDD requirements, 124, 136
Viral safety
    clearance of biotechnology-derived products, 225–226
    clearance of plasma-derived products, 250, 252
Voluntary Harmonisation Procedure, 179
VWP (*See* Vaccine Working Party)

W

Well-established use, 165
World Health Organization
    definition of self-medication, 214
    Ethical Criteria for Medicinal Drug Promotion, 50
World Self-Medication Industry, 214

Index